Langenbecks Archiv für Chirurgie

vereinigt mit Bruns' Beiträge für Klinische Chirurgie

Forumband 1993

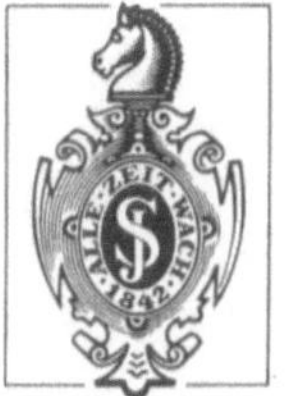

Chirurgisches Forum '93

für experimentelle und klinische Forschung

110. Kongreß der Deutschen Gesellschaft für Chirurgie
München, 13.–17. April 1993

Wissenschaftlicher Beirat

H. G. Beger, Ulm
(Vorsitzender)
U. Brückner, Ulm
M. Heberer, Basel
B. Kremer, Kiel
Ch. Ohmann, Düsseldorf
B. v. Specht, Freiburg
L. Sunder-Plassmann, Ulm
W. Wayand, Linz

Schriftleitung

H. G. Beger unter Mitarbeit von
M. Büchler, M. H. Schoenberg und M. Storck

Herausgeber

H. M. Becker
Präsident des 110. Kongresses
der Deutschen Gesellschaft für Chirurgie

H. G. Beger
Vorsitzender der Sektion Experimentelle Chirurgie

W. Hartel
Generalsekretär der Deutschen Gesellschaft für Chirurgie

Springer-Verlag
Berlin Heidelberg New York London Paris
Tokyo Hong Kong Barcelona Budapest

Schriftleitung:

Professor Dr. Hans G. Beger
Chirurgische Klinik I, Klinikum der Universität Ulm,
Steinhövelstraße 9, W-7900 Ulm

Mitarbeiter der Schriftleitung:

Priv.-Doz. Dr. Markus Büchler
Priv.-Doz. Dr. Michael H. Schoenberg

Chirurgische Klinik I, Klinikum der Universität Ulm,
Steinhövelstraße 9, W-7900 Ulm

Dr. M. Storck
Chirurgische Klinik II, Klinikum der Universität Ulm,
Steinhövelstraße 9, W-7900 Ulm

Herausgeber:

Professor Dr. H. M. Becker
Gefäßchirurgische Abteilung, Städtisches Krankenhaus München-Neuperlach,
Oskar-Maria-Graf-Ring 51, W-8000 München 83

Professor Dr. Hans G. Beger
Chirurgische Klinik I, Klinikum der Universität Ulm,
Steinhövelstraße 9, W-7900 Ulm

Professor Dr. W. Hartel
Steinhölzle 16, W-7901 Westerstetten-Vorderdenkental

Mit 103 Abbildungen

ISBN-13: 978-3-540-56533-8 e-ISBN-13: 978-3-642-78122-3
DOI: 10.1007/978-3-642-78122-3

24/3130-5 4 3 2 1 0 – Gedruckt auf säurefreiem Papier

Vorwort

Chirurgische Forschung – bestehend aus den Komponenten Grundlagenforschung, klinische Forschung und Entscheidungsfindung (theoretische Chirurgie) – ist der Motor des Fortschrittes in der klinischen Chirurgie. Die Leistungsfähigkeit der Chirurgie, die ja ein auf die Praxis orientiertes, von handwerklicher Leistung abhängiges, technisches Fach der Medizin im Sinne einer Therapiewissenschaft ist, beruht ganz überwiegend auf ihrer naturwissenschaftlichen Methode der Erkenntnisgewinnung und der Umsetzung von neuen Erkenntnissen in bessere klinische Therapieergebnisse.

Das Chirurgische Forum hat in der deutschen Chirurgie und zum Deutschen Chirurgenkongreß in diesem Sinne eine herausragende und zunehmende Bedeutung als Präsentations- und Diskussionsforum für neueste Ergebnisse. Der Forumband ist dementsprechend der alljährliche Spiegel der wissenschaftlichen Aktivitäten und Forschungsergebnisse aus dem Bereich der chirurgischen Fächer – Allgemein-/Viszeralchirurgie, Gefäßchirurgie, Unfallchirurgie, Herz- und Thoraxchirurgie und der chirurgischen Intensivmedizin.

Der Forumband 1993 ist John H. Gibbon, Jr., gewidmet, dem Erfinder des Prinzips der extrakorporalen Zirkulation mittels Herz-Lungen-Maschine. John Gibbon hat die klinische Medizin durch neue Erkenntnisse über Physiologie und Pathophysiologie von Herz-Kreislauf-Funktionen wesentlich erweitert und durch die Erfindung der Herz-Lungen-Maschine die Herzchirurgie, so wie sie sich heute zu einem chirurgischen Schwerpunktfach entwickelt hat, begründet. Professor Harris B. Shumacker, Jr., Delray Beach, FL 33483, USA, danken wir für die lebendige Laudatio.

Für das Forum '93 wurden 348 Beiträge angemeldet, gegenüber 1992 entspricht das einer Steigerung um 12,6%. Die Abstracts verteilten sich auf die Bereiche Endokrinologie 2%, Herz-Lunge-Gefäße 5%, Leber-Galle-Pankreas 9%, Magen-Darm 12%, Onkologie 16%, perioperative Pathophysiologie 18%, Transplantation 20%, Traumatologie 14% und laparoskopische Chirurgie 4%. Die Arbeiten zur laparoskopischen Chirurgie, dem neuen großen Thema in der klinischen Chirurgie, spiegeln den überwiegend klinischen Entwicklungstand und das Fehlen von Arbeiten zur experimentellen Grundlegung wider.

Das zunehmende Interesse ausländischer Chirurgen am Deutschen Chirurgenkongreß und hier insbesondere der Forumsdiskussion spiegelt sich wider in der sprunghaft angestiegenen Zahl von 25 Beiträgen aus dem Ausland, davon 13 aus dem nicht deutschsprachigen Ausland. 29,3% der Abstracts, entsprechend 102 Vorträgen, wurden vom Beirat und den Gutachtern in das endgültige Programm des Deutschen Chirurgenkongresses einbezogen. Jede Anmeldung wurde durch mindestens 4 Gutachter anonym beurteilt. Der Forumssausschuß dankt den folgenden auswärtigen Gutachtern für die rasche und sachgerechte Begutachtung:

W. Eigler, Essen
A. Encke, Frankfurt
G. Feifel, Homburg
R. Hetzer, Berlin

G. Muhr, Bochum	H.D. Röher, Düsseldorf
Th. Junginger, Mainz	M. Rothmund, Marburg
E. Kraas, Berlin	R. Siewert, München
F. Köckerling, Erlangen	H. Troidl, Köln
H. Pichlmaier, Köln	H. Tscherne, Hannover

Der Redaktionsstab der Schriftleitung zusammen mit Frau M. Zuleger und Frau M. Wild hat zuverlässig und schnell zur zeitgerechten Fertigstellung des Forumbandes beigetragen. Mein besonderer Dank geht an Herrn Schwaninger und den Springer Verlag für den reibungslosen Druck des Forumbandes.

H. G. Beger, Ulm

John Heysham Gibbon, Jr. *(1903–1973)*

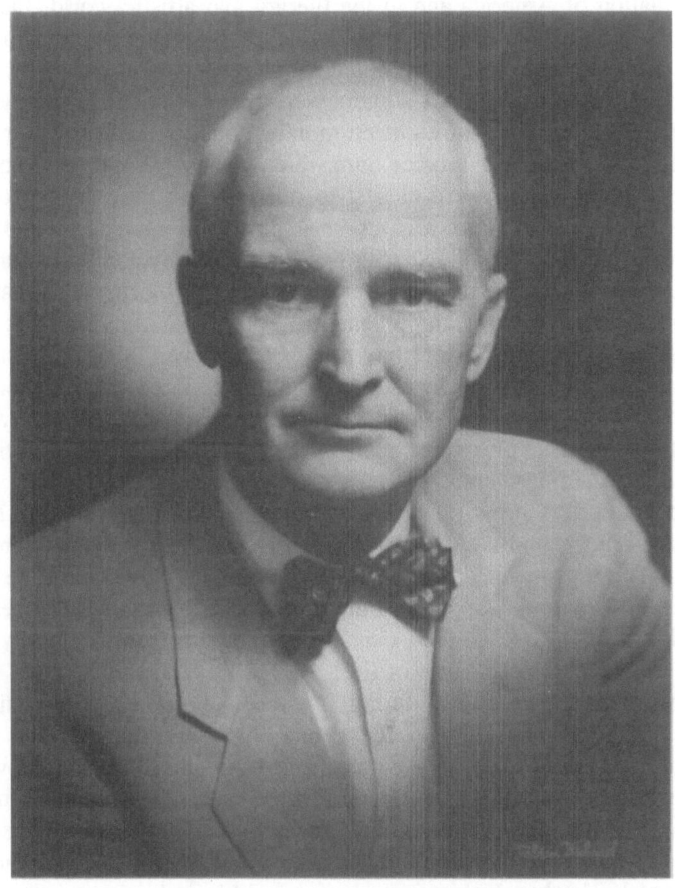

When John Heysham Gibbon, Jr. was born in Philadelphia, Pennsylvania, on September 29, 1903, his parents could hardly have anticipated that their first son would make a contribution which would form the basis for current cardiac surgery. They had every reason to believe, however, that he would have a bright future, even a distinguished one; the family background of both parents, Marjorie Gibbon and John Heysham Gibbon, indicated that this might prove true.

Marjorie Gibbon was one of five beautiful and attractive daughters of Margaret McFadden Young of a leading Pittsburgh family and Lt. General Samuel B. M. Young, one of the most prominent figures in the Spanish-American War, the Indian Conflicts, the Phillipine Insurrection, and the War Between the States. The Gibbon family, which had emigrated to Philadelphia from England in 1684 had numbered among its members outstanding doctors and military officers, a mineralogist, an explorer. By direct descent and marriage they were related to men who had played an important role in the formation of America and in the literary and artistic world. Jack's father was a nationally recognized surgeon, a distinguished professor and chairman of the department of surgery at the Jefferson Medical College.

Jack's boyhood was a happy one. Winters were spent in the city, summers on the farm in suburban Media. Jack was eighteen months younger than his sister Marjorie, eighteen months older than his brother Sam, three years senior to his brother Bob. In his childhood he and Sam were closest to one another; later Jack became very close to Marjorie. Lynfield Farm was an ideal place for youngsters and gave the Gibbon children a place for roaming about freely and for developing enduring tastes and capabilities. There were ponies, horses, hunters, cattle, sheep, fields, gardens, the barn, and Crum Creek later to become beautiful Spington Reservoir. Jack was wiry and daring and most competitive. He had to be best at everything and usually was, tops in climbing the ridgepole of the barn, in walking across the tree fallen over the creek, in riding, indeed, in all physical activities, and in chess as well. As a little fellow he had a violent, explosive temper, an attribute later replaced entirely by a calm, peaceful, even temperment.

The Gibbon youngsters grew up in an affectionate, warm, stimulating household surrounded by adoring parents and admiring family and friends. They were not, however, spoiled. In contrast, they were made to understand clearly that the standards set by their parents' examples applied to them as well-old fashioned virtues, playing the game fairly, being a good soldier, chivalry, patriotism. It was a family of doers, not idle recipients of the good things of life.

Jack's interests changed abruptly during summer camp when he was fifteen and ready for entry into Princeton, largely due to one of the camp counselors' influence. Previously concerned almost entirely with physical pursuits, Jack was now burning with intellectual interests, philosophy, literature, and poetry. It was as if a new world had been opened before him. His letters, and especially those to Marjorie, were aplomb with stanzas from poems he had discovered, and even more with philosophical topics. In the summer of 1921 when Jack was seventeen and Marjorie nineteen the two had a wonderful summer wandering about Europe, walking through Normandy, discussing weighty matters, French history in which Marjorie was intensely interested, and philosophy which occupied Jack's free moments. He was reading William James' *Varieties of Religious Experience* at the time and he and Marjorie were making plans for him to attend medical school in Edinburgh and she to keep house for the two of them.

It was with such a background that he entered Jefferson Medical College after graduating from Princeton. He slipped into medicine more or less effortless, as a matter of course. John Lardner, Jack's great-great-grandfather through his father's grandmother was a London doctor. His great-great-grandfather on this father's side, born in Pennsylvania and educated in medicine in Edinburgh was the first American doctor in a direct line of five down to Jack. His father and his only paternal uncle were practicing physicians, his father a leading American surgeon, president of the American Surgical Association and other professional organizations. It was a natural move for Jack to make.

His aim in life, nevertheless, was not firmly determined and towards the end of his first year in medical school he gave serious consideration to quitting and pursuing some other course, such as writing. Fortunately, however, he paid heed to his father's advice to continue his medical education, that he wouldn't have to practice medicine if he didn't want to do so but would "write no worse" for having a medical degree – fatherly admonition which steered him in the right direction. He continued in school, graduated in medicine in 1927, and obtained an internship at the Pennsylvania Hospital, the first hospital established in the United States. He was on the right course.

Jack had given no serious thought to research but, fortunately, this interest was aroused during his internship year by the clinical studies of Dr. Joseph Hayman who was investigating the relative effects of potassium chloride and sodium chloride in the diet of a severely hypertensive patient. Jack's role in this simple study was limited to taking the patient's blood pressure at intervals. While doing this, however, he came quite unexpectedly to the exciting awareness that controlled experimentation, careful observation, and valid conclusions could lead to new knowledge. Just as philosophy and poetry had set him afire in earlier years, this realization lighted a new zeal which would remain with him through life. When he consulted John B. Flick, surgeon to the Pennsylvania Hospital and his father's partner, with the question whether it might be possible to combine research and surgical practice as a career objective, he was given assurance that this was entirely feasible. John Flick went further and made the valuable suggestion that he apply to Dr. Edward B. Churchill for a research fellowship with him at the Harvard Medical School. This appealed to Jack who recognized that such a move would provide an opportunity to learn the answers to two important questions, whether he would like surgical research, and whether he had any talent for it. Churchill granted the appointment and Jack was finally on track.

In February 1930, Jack began his research career in a small laboratory in the Gate House of the Boston City Hospital. His first project, suggested by Churchill, was an inquiry into the relationship between pulmonary artery pressure and blood flow in the presence of experimentally produced arteriovenous fistulas, a proposal which would lead to other studies of pulmonary circulation and cardiac function. When Churchill became director of one of the two surgical services at the Massachusetts General Hospital a few months after Jack's arrival in Boston, he was moved to a laboratory on the top floor of the Bullfinch Building there. It was at this institution, in February 1931, that Jack conceived the idea of developing a machine capable of oxygenating the blood of man extracorporeally so it could be returned to the body and take over temporarily the function of the heart and lungs.

A patient who had developed a massive pulmonary embolus after a cholecystectomy was taken to the operating room for observation and Jack was assigned the duty of following her vital signs and notifying his chief when he felt her condition had worsened to the point when a pulmonary embolectomy seemed indicated. The procedure was carried out skillfully by Churchill the following morning but ended fatally. Gibbon described well how the concept originated. "During that long night, helplessly watching the patient struggle for life as her blood became darker and her veins more distended, the idea naturally occurred to me that if it were possible to remove continuously some of the blue blood from the patient's swollen veins, put oxygen into that blood and allow carbon dioxide to escape from it, and to inject continuously the now-red blood back into the patient's arteries, we might have saved her life. We would have bypassed the obstructing embolus and performed part of the work of the patient's heart and lungs outside the body."

The idea of partially bypassing the heart and lungs expanded almost immediately to that of taking over their entire function, an idea which continued to be a driving force in Gibbon's life until it was brought to fruition twenty-two years afterward.

Another event of great consequence not only in Jack Gibbon's personal life but in his entire research effort took place during the year in Boston, his marriage to Mary Hopkinson, Churchill's technician, daughter of Charles Hopkinson, renowned American portrait painter. Maly, as she was known to their friends, continued to work by Jack's side in all his laboratory investigations, a true research partner.

Upon their return to Philadelphia in the spring to 1931, arrangements were made for Jack to work in the laboratories of the University of Pennsylvania School of Medicine. This he did in the afternoons, devoting the mornings to the practice of surgery, and thus confirming John Flick's affirmation of the feasibility of combining research with clinical surgery. To his regret, he did not have the facilities and support necessary to pursue the heart-lung project but he kept active and carried out other interesting investigations, some in conjunction with Eugene M. Landis who later became professor of physiology at Harvard.

When he could tolerate no longer his inability to tackle the heart-lung research which remaind foremost in his mind, he asked Churchill for another year with him. His request was granted, although Churchill was quite unenthusiastic, to say the least, about his proposed study. Indeed, heardly anyone he consulted felt that his project was one he should undertake. His friend Eugene Landis was the exception.

While Jack and Maly were assembling apparatus and beginning the construction of the first heart-lung machine, Jack completed his review of the pertinent literature. He knew, of course, that much had been done with respect to the extracorporeal oxygenation of blood and with perfusion of organs and parts of the body. The list of investigators was impressive, LeGallois, Brown-Sequard, Brodie, Ludwig, Schmidt, von Frey, Gruber, Jacobi, Hamel, Embly, Martin, Richards, Drinker, Bayliss, Daly, Thorpe, and others, and their contributions were significant. Their work, because of the limited capacity of the oxygenators which they had devised, was, however, of limited practical help to Gibbon in his effort to make an apparatus suitable for use in man. The Russian investigator, Brukhonenko, had, indeed, in 1929 asked whether it would not be possible to develop the means and techniques for working upon the human heart, but he used only biological oxygenators for his own experiments, and the aviator, Charles Lindberg, has posed the same question at the same time but his research was limited to small organ perfusion. From a practical point of view, Jack had to begin almost anew.

The initial efforts to acquire equipment and work alone in a one-room laboratory were told graphically both by Jack and by Maly. He recalled them in this way:

"Imagine for a moment the way research was carried out ... in the 1930s. The Federal Government was not then pouring out hundreds of millions ... to perform research ... I bought an air pump in a second hand shop down in East Boston for a few dollars, and used it to activate finger cot blood pumps. Valves were made from solid rubber corks with the small end cut transversely three quarters through to form a flap about 2 mm thick. With the flap held up, a cork borer was passed through the center of the stopper, thus creating a channel for the stream of blood. These simple valves worked well. Plastic materials were not available, so our circuit was largely rubber and glass. Heparin had just become available, but its antagonist, protamine, was not ... "

Maly wrote: "To do these experiments we had to be at the laboratory bright and early, as they continued all that day and sometimes well into the evening. We could only manage about three ... a week. First we had to smoke a kymograph record and get it in place on the operating table. Then, we had to bring a cat down to the laboratory from its upstairs laboratory and anesthetize it ... perform a tracheotomy and connect the animal to an artificial respirator while a 'Drinker Heart-Lung Preparation' was done ... These preparations usually took four or five hours ... ."

They began with a rotating drum oxygenator, and with studies upon cats since their original apparatus was not adequate for larger animals. Funds were so short they often roamed the streets at night with bait and nets looking for stray cats for their studies! After a productive year in Boston it was necessary to return to Philadelphia but this time the work could be continued in the Harrison Research Laboratories at Pennsylvania. Later in 1970 Gibbon wrote:

"In reviewing the 13 articles that we wrote upon the subject of the heart-lung machine, ... I was struck by the fact that in the first year we worked on the problem, 1934–35, we encountered, discussed and partially solved most of the continuing difficulties that plagued us over the next 19 years ..."

Over time, helpful changes were made in all aspects of the apparatus, the oxygenator, pumps, control mechanisms, and by 1939 he was able to report to the meeting of the American Association for Thoracic Surgery that he had reached a real milestone and that cats had survived indefinitely after a period of total bypass of heart and lungs during which their function had been taken over completely by the extracorporeal machine. He was in a position to think ahead to a device which would permit open heart operations im man. In discussing his presentation, Leo Eloesser, a former president of the organization, said it reminded him of Jules Verne's dreamy visions which seem impossible to accoplish when they were presented and which became real achievements later.

Just as the work reached this promising stage, the United States entered World War II. Jack had accepted a commission in the 52nd Evacuation Hospital which had been organized by the Pennsylvania Hospital. Many wondered why a man engaged in important research, married and father of four children, and not well off financially, should have chosen to volunteer for duty. He had been brought up in a family in which partriotism was held high, one with a proud military heritage. His father had had a distinguished military career. His maternal grandfather, General Young, had earned such appointments as President of the War College Board, member and sometimes presiding officer of Joint Army and Navy Board, and Chief of Staff of the Army. His father's uncle, John Gibbon, who also was engaged in the Spanish-American War, the Indian Wars and the War Between the States, commanded the famous Iron Brigade and had his finest moment when he stopped Pickett's charge at Gettysburg. It is doubtful, nevertheless, that these considerations entered into Jack's decision at a conscious level. Joining the army was simply the right thing for him to do. Activated on January 5, 1942, on the seas by January 23, his unit served in the South Pacific Theater during the entire War. Jack was invalided home with an excruciatingly painful herniated disk after approximately thirty months overseas, and finished his military service in the States as chief of surgery at the Mayo General Hospital.

The work on the heart-lung machine was resumed immediately upon his return to Philadelphia. Jack was an assistant professor of surgery at Pennsylvania but early in 1946 he was made professor and director of surgical research at Jefferson. Ten years later he became the Samuel D. Gross Professor of Surgery and chairman of the department. The development of the heart-lung machine progressed, in no small part from the cooperation Gibbon secured with the International Business Machines Corporation and its board chairman, Mr. Thomas J. Watson. Expert engineering and badly needed financial help were at last available. Still, each step forward only was the result of numerous tests and changes in design. The discovery by two of Jack's young assistants that better oxygenation could be achieved when blood was filmed on screens rather than on a smooth surface led to their use in 1950, first as a vertical cylinder and then as vertical plates suspended in parallel inside a clear plastic chamber. The Gibbon laboratories had become a Mecca for those interested in the new project and Jack was pleased to share with them the advances which were being made, the troubles which were encountered, and his ideas for future study.

The work progressed, dogs could be used instead of cats, survivals were occuring after longer periods of total cardiopulmonary bypass, and in May 1952 Jack felt that he could say at the meeting of the Thoracic Association that he was approaching the time when the heart-lung machine could be employed safely in treating human patients. Finally, on May 6, 1953, 19 years after the work was first begun he operated successfully upon Cecelia Bavolek whose large atrial septal defect had necessitated hospitalization six times within the previous six months. During a period of 27 minutes of total cardiorespiratory bypass the defect was closed and she recovered uneventfully. It had been established once and for all that the heart-lung machine could be used successfully for open heart surgery in man. The basis for current cardiac surgery had been laid.

Many might have wished to publicize this important event. Jack did not. He summarized his work and his experiences with four clinical efforts at a symposium on recent advances in cardiovascular physiology and surgery in Minneapolis in September 1953, and his remarks were published, not in a widely read national and international journal, but in *Minnesota Medicine*. That was all. Jack had at last reached his goal, and he could turn over the future of open heart surgery to "younger hands".

What did Gibbon's contribution mean to surgery? It opened the gates to an entirely new field, that of careful, deliberate, unhurried operations within the cardiac chambers, on the neural pathways which regulate the heart's orderly activity, and to the vessels supplying it with the substances it requires. To be sure, great progress had been made. Most of the extracardiac congenital anomalities had been brought within the realm of surgical palliation or cure, some stenotic valvular lesions could be treated by blind intracardiac manipulations, and, especially with the aid of hypothermia, some brief and relatively simple procedures could be accomplished within the open heart. Heart surgery as we know it today, however, had to wait for the heart-lung machine and it is this apparatus which has formed the basis for this wide and ever-expanding field.

In addition, it has increased the extent, safety, and effectiveness of certain operations in general, neurological, and non-cardiac vascular surgery.

There are other areas, too, in which Gibbon's contribution has had a significant impact. Nothing has made us more aware of the importance of the physiopathologic alterations associated with the disorders we treat and with the operative procedures we employ in treating them – the bleeding and coagulation factors, body water and electrolyte disturbances, difficulties in renal function, respiratory and metabolic problems, tissue and organ perfusion, the circulation and its distribution to various body segments and its changes with various stimuli, to name some. Few if any areas of medicine have fostered more the introduction and progressive improvement of intensive care units and the pre- und postoperative care of the patient. The cardiac surgery it made possible had been unsurpassed in bringing together as working teammates, physicians, pediatricians, radiologists, chemists, physicists, engineers, industrialists. Furthermore, the heart-lung machine and the area it has opened has done much to promote good feeling, compassionate relationships between doctors and their patients. Man had always revered the heart as a very special organ.

The heart-lung machine has other messages. It emphasizes the importance of research, the necessity for animal research, the need for laboratories and their support. It stresses the value of accurate diagnosis and a planned operative procedure. It focuses attention upon the best possible patient management before, during, and after the operation. It makes evident that medical progress does not arise out of thin air, but through ideas and their determined and thoughtful pursuit.

In 1967 Gibbon retired from the Chair of Surgery and spent the rest of his life on Lynfield Farm. There he was surrounded by family and friends. He could play tennis, swim, work in the garden, read to his heart's content, entertain the frequent guests who came to see him and Maly, and undertake more seriously than before painting for which he had developed a passion. He spent more and more time in his studio and with progressive success. He was especially interested in portrait painting and received a number of commissions. His committment to the surgical societies and to community and government affairs continued. He travelled extensively. They were happy days.

What sort of man was this John H. Gibbon, Jr. who entered medicine with such hesitancy and rose to the top of it, who would untertake a research project when nearly everyone discouraged him from doing so, who could pursue an idea so steadfastly over such a long period and yet could abandon it when he felt his country called him to serve, just as the project seemed near successful completion, not knowing whether he would live to finish it? He was not well understood except by his intimates. His tall, erect statue, patrician face, clear blue eyes, and his quiet, gentlemanly conduct led some to feel that he was too reserved, unapproachable. Those who saw him unwind while entertaining his friends about the swimming pool or on the tennis court found him a relaxed, warm, feeling person. Those who had his most private thoughts knew him as a man with very deep feelings and deep love. He liked people who were doing things. He liked ideas, research, valid conclusions. He liked books, literature, poetry, paintings. He liked sports. He had strong convictions. He thought a professorship of surgery was an obligation as well as an opportunity and he had no use for those who did not fulfill the obligations their positions demanded. He was interested in bright young people and in fostering their careers. He sought no reward for what he did. He knew that the accomplishment was itself reward enough. Awards did come to him, to be sure, many of them, high ones, cherished ones. He accepted them with no undue pride but rather with a somewhat surprised satisfaction.

Those who had the privilege of knowing this man remember him well and not just as a person who made one of the epoch-making contributions of out time. We remember him as a dedicated investigator, teacher, and clinical surgeron. We remember him as a professor who used his highly respected name and position for making his department the best possible teaching, training, and research unit, not for personal enrichment. We think of him as a patriot who served his country in time of war. We remember him as a liberal, feeling person, deeply concerned with matters he considered just. We recall him as a loving, sympathetic father and adoring husband. We retain vivid memories of him as a genial host, at cocktails and dinner, on strolls through the garden and about the farm, in games of tennis, by the pool, at sheep-dippinh time, in long, intimate, warm, stimulating conversations. We think of him as a man who always seemed, despite the seriousness of work or play, to bubble over with the excitement and enthusiasm of youth. We think of him as a man who could wear the mantle of greatness with easy grace.

The German Society of Surgery and the German Society of Surgical Research happily pay hommage to John H. Gibbon, Jr., developer of the heart-lung machine, father of current cardiac surgery.

Harris B. Shumaker, Jr., M.D.
Delray Beach, USA

VII. Leber – Galle – Pankreas

VIII. Transplantation II

Table of Contents

VI. Transplantation I

Adjuvante Strahlentherapie nach Resektion eines Plattenepithelkarzinoms der Speiseröhre. Eine prospektiv randomisierte Studie

Adjuvant Postoperative Radiation Therapy Following Resection of Squamous Cell Carcinoma of the Esophagus. A Prospective Randomized Trial

H.-U. Zieren[1], J.M. Müller[1], H. Pichlmaier[1] und R.-P. Müller[2]

[1]Allgemeine, Abdominal-, Gefäß- und Thoraxchirurgie, Universität Köln (Direktor: Prof. Dr. Dr. H. Pichlmaier)
[2]Klinik und Poliklinik für Strahlentherapie, Universität Köln (Direktor: Prof. Dr. R.-P. Müller)

Zielsetzung

Trotz vieler Fortschritte in der chirurgischen Therapie des Speiseröhrenkarzinoms sind die Langzeitergebnisse mit einer durchschnittlichen 5-Jahres-Überlebensrate von etwa 20% seit Jahrzehnten unverändert unbefriedigend [2]. Nachdem verschiedene nicht-kontrollierte Studien auf eine Verbesserung der Spätprognose durch eine adjuvante postoperative Strahlentherapie hinwiesen [5], wurde der Effekt der adjuvanten Strahlentherapie in einer kontrollierten Studie untersucht.

Methodik

Studienanlage: Die Studie wurde als prospektiv randomisierte Phase-III-Studie angelegt. Bei einem angestrebten Signifikanzniveau von alpha = 0,05 und einer Power des Testes von 80% (1-beta) war zum Nachweis einer Verdopplung der 5-Jahres-Überlebensrate von 20% auf 40% eine Fallzahl von 80 Patienten pro Behandlungsgruppe nötig. Zwischenauswertungen sollten alle 12 Monate erfolgen. Die Studie sollte abgebrochen werden, wenn die Überlebenswahrscheinlichkeit in einem Therapiearm auf einem Signifikanzniveau von $p<0,01$ größer war oder die Ergebnisse anderer Studien vorlagen, die die Weiterführung der eigenen Studie verboten.

In die Studie wurden, beginnend mit dem 1.6.1988, alle Patienten aufgenommen, bei denen ein Plattenepithelkarzinom der thorakalen Speiseröhre in einem Tumorstadium II bis IV nach UICC in kurativer Absicht reseziert wurde. Patienten mit Tu-

Chirurgisches Forum 1993
f. experim. u. klinische Forschung
Becker/Beger/Hartel (Hrsg.)

moren des Stadiums I wurden von der Studie ausgeschlossen, da Stadium-I-Tumoren im eigenen Krankengut selten sind und der statistisch signifikante Nachweis bzw. Ausschluß einer Verbesserung der ohnehin relativ guten Langzeitprognose nur durch eine Rekrutierungsphase von über 10 Jahren möglich gewesen wäre. Ein weiteres Ausschlußkriterium bestand im präoperativen Nachweis von Fernmetastasen.

Als Zielkriterien wurden die Überlebensraten und die Lebensqualität der Patienten gewählt. Die Lebensqualität der Patienten wurde parallel durch Selbst- und Fremdbewertung erfaßt. Die Selbsteinschätzung der Patienten erfolgte mit der deutschsprachigen Fassung des EORTC "Quality-of-Life Questionnaire" [1]. Die Fremdeinschätzung der Lebensqualität wurde nach dem Quality-of-Life Index von Spitzer [3] vorgenommen. Die Lebensqualität wurde präoperativ, zum Zeitpunkt der Entlassung aus der stationären Behandlung und weiter in dreimonatigen Abständen erfaßt.

Studienablauf: Die Indikation zur Ösophagektomie, die Wahl der Resektions- und des Rekonstruktionsverfahrens erfolgte unabhängig von der Studie aufgrund erhobener Befunde. Nachdem das abschließende pathologische Tumorstaging vorlag, wurden die Patienten nach dem Resektionsverfahren (stumpfe Dissektion vs. abdomino-thorakale Resektion) und dem Tumorstadium (Stad. II–IV) in Untergruppen mit vergleichbarer Prognose stratefiziert und schließlich durch Randomisierung ermittelt, ob bei dem einzelnen Patienten eine postoperative Bestrahlung durchgeführt werden sollte oder nicht.

Adjuvante Strahlentherapie: Die postoperative Strahlentherapie begann zwischen 3 und 6 Wochen nach der Resektion. Das Bestrahlungsfeld umfaßte zunächst das gesamte ehemalige Ösophagusbett einschließlich der lokalen Lymphabflußgebiete (Tumoren oberhalb der Trachealbifurkation: incl. beider Supraclaviculargruben, Tumoren unterhalb der Trachealbifurkation: incl. Truncus-coeliacus-Region). Dieses Feld wurde zunächst mit 30,6 Gy bestrahlt. Nach Feldverkleinerung auf das ehemalige Tumorbett mit einem cranio-caudalen Sicherheitsabstand von 5 cm erfolgte die Dosiserhöhung auf 55,8 Gy. Die tägliche Einzeldosis betrug 1,8 Gy in 31 Sitzungen.

Nachsorge: Postoperativ wurden die Patienten in dreimonatigen Abständen einem kompletten Tumorstaging unterzogen (Labor incl. Tumormarker, Röntgen-Thorax, Sono-Abdomen, Ösophago-Gastroskopie, CT-Thorax).

Statistische Auswertung: Die Wahrscheinlichkeit für das gesamte und das rezidivfreie Überleben wurde nach Kaplan-Meier berechnet und mittels Log-Rank-Test verglichen. Die Ergebnisse der Lebensqualitätserfassung wurden mit dem Kruskall-Wallis-Test verglichen. Das Signifikanzniveau wurde auf 5%, d.h. $p<0,05$, festgelegt.

Ergebnisse

Patientengut: In die Studie wurden 68 Patienten aufgenommen. 33 Patienten wurden adjuvant bestrahlt (RAD) und 35 als Kontrollgruppe (KON) nicht adjuvant behandelt. Beide Therapiegruppen waren hinsichtlich Geschlecht und Alter der Patienten,

Operationsverfahren, postoperative Komplikationen sowie Lokalisation, Stadium und Differenzierung der Tumoren vergleichbar. Bei 52 Patienten (RAD: 25 Pat., KON: 27 Pat.) wurde eine stumpfe Dissektion und bei 16 Patienten (RAD: 8 Pat., KON: 8 Pat.) eine abdomino-thorakale Ösophagektomie durchgeführt. Bei 32 Patienten (RAD: 16, KON: 16) bestand ein Tumorstadium II, bei 24 Patienten (RAD: 11, KON: 13) ein Stadium III und bei 12 Patienten (RAD: 6, KON: 6) ein Stadium IV.

Follow-up: Zum Zeitpunkt der vorliegenden Auswertung betrug der zeitliche Abstand zur Operation mindestens 1 Jahr. 25 Patienten der Bestrahlungsgruppe und 28 Patienten der Kontrollgruppe waren nach $11,0 \pm 6,2$ Monaten bzw. $10,5 \pm 6,8$ Monaten verstorben. 8 Patienten der Bestrahlungsgruppe und 7 Patienten der Kontrollgruppe lebten nach $23,6 \pm 12,1$ bzw. $25,4 \pm 12,0$ Monaten postoperativ.

Langzeitergebnisse: Die 1-, 2- und 3-Jahres-Überlebensraten waren in der Bestrahlungsgruppe (57%, 29%, 22%) und in der Kontrollgruppe (53%, 31%, 20%) nahezu identisch. Sowohl in der Bestrahlungs- als auch in der Kontrollgruppe waren die 1-, 2- und 3-Jahres-Überlebensraten von Patienten mit einem Tumorstadium II (RAD: 80%, 48%, 35%, KON: 87%, 53%, 38%) signifikant besser als von Patienten mit einem Tumorstadium III (RAD: 41%, 23%, 18%, KON: 47%, 27%, 19%) und einem Tumorstadium IV (RAD: 25%, 17%, 0%, KON: 28%, 0%, 0%). Auch bei der Analyse des rezidivfreien Überlebens fanden sich zwischen beiden Therapiearmen weder in den Haupt- noch in den Untergruppen signifikante Unterschiede. Die 1-, 2- und 3-Jahres-Raten für das rezidivfreie Überleben betrugen in der Bestrahlungsgruppe 39%, 22% und 19% und in der Kontrollgruppe 33%, 23% und 20%.

Lebensqualität: Die Erfassung der Lebensqualität zeigte für die Bestrahlungs- und die Kontrollgruppe über den gesamten Beobachtungszeitraum insgesamt vergleichbare Tendenzen. 3 Monate postoperativ bewerteten jedoch die Patienten der Bestrahlungsgruppe ihre globale Lebensqualität auf der 7-stufigen Skala (1 = sehr schlecht, bis 7 = ausgezeichnet) signifikant schlechter als die Patienten der Kontrollgruppe (RAD: Mittelwert $3,8 \pm 1,5$, Median: 3; KON: Mittelwert $4,6 \pm 1,2$, Median: 4). Darüber hinaus klagten Patienten der Bestrahlungsgruppe nach 3 und 6 Monaten signifikant häufiger über Schluckstörungen. Entsprechend traten bougierungspflichtige narbige Stenosen der ösophago-gastralen Anastomose in der Bestrahlungsgruppe signifikant häufiger auf als in der Kontrollgruppe (RAD: 18 Pat., 55%, KON: 10 Pat., 29%).

Diskussion

In der vorliegenden Untersuchung fanden sich keine signifikanten Unterschiede in der gesamten und der rezidivfreien Überlebensrate zwischen Patienten, die adjuvant bestrahlt wurden und Patienten, die keine adjuvante Therapie erhielten. Diese Ergebnisse wurden durch eine mittlerweile publizierte französische Multicenterstudie an einem größeren Krankengut bestätigt [4]. Da die postoperative Strahlentherapie zu einem – wenn auch nur kurzfristigen – Verlust an Lebensqualität führte und narbige Anastomosenstenosen nach der Strahlentherapie signifikant häufiger auftraten, wurde die eigene Studie nach Vorliegen der Ergebnisse der Multicenterstudie vor Erreichen der vom Statistiker geforderten Fallzahl abgebrochen.

Zusammenfassung

In einer prospektiv randomisierten Studie wurden die Auswirkungen einer adjuvanten Strahlentherapie nach potentiell kurativer Resektion eines Plattenepithelkarzinoms der thorakalen Speiseröhre untersucht. Nach Bildung von Untergruppen mit vergleichbarer Prognose wurden 33 Patienten postoperativ bestrahlt und mit einer Kontrollgruppe von 35 nicht adjuvant behandelten Patienten verglichen. Weder in den gesamten noch in den rezidivfreien Überlebensraten fanden sich zwischen Bestrahlungs- und Kontrollgruppe signifikante Unterschiede. Da bougierungspflichtige narbige Anastomosenstenosen in der Bestrahlungsgruppe signifikant häufiger auftraten als in der Kontrollgruppe (55% vs. 29%) und bestrahlte Patienten ihre eigene Lebensqualität 3 Monate postoperativ signifikant schlechter beurteilten als Patienten der Kontrollgruppe, kann eine routinemäßige postoperative Strahlentherapie nach kurativer Resektion eines Speiseröhrenkarzinoms nicht empfohlen werden.

Summary

Postoperative radiation therapy following curative resection of squamous cell carcinoma of the esophagus was investigated in a prospective randomized study. 33 patients received postoperative radiation therapy and were compared to a control group of 35 patients who received no adjuvant treatment following surgery. No statistically significant differences were noted concerning overall and disease-free survival rates between both treatment groups. The incidence of fibrotic strictures of the esophagogastric anastomosis was significantly higher in the radiation group (55% vs. 29%). Patients in the radiation group assessed their own quality of life 3 months after surgery significantly lower than patients in the control group. Due to these results postoperative radiation therapy cannot be advocated as an adjuvant therapy following curative resection for squamous cell carcinoma of the esophagus.

Literatur

1. Aaronson NK, Bakker W, Stewart AL, van Dam FSAM, van Zandwijk N, Yarnold JR, Kirkpatrick A (1987) Multidimensional approach to the measurement of quality of life in lung cancer. Clinical trials. In: Aaronson NK, Beckmann J (eds) The quality of life of cancer patients. Raven Press, New York, p 63–82
2. Müller JM, Erasmi H, Stelzner M, Zieren U, Pichlmaier H (1990) Surgical therapy of esophageal carcinoma. Br J Surg 77:845–857
3. Spitzer WO, Dobson AJ, Hall J, Chestermann E, Levi J, Shepherd R, Battista RN, Catchlove BR (1981) Measuring the quality of life of cancer patients. A concise QL-index for use by physicians. J Chron Dis 34:585–597

4. Téniére P, Hay J-M, Fingerhut A, Fagniez P-L (1991) Postoperative radiation therapy does not increase survival after curative resection for squamous cell carcinoma of the middle and lower esophagus as shown by a multicenter controlled trial. Surg Gynecol Obstet 173:123–130
5. Zieren H-U, Müller JM, Pichlmaier H, Müller R-P, Staar S (1991) Welchen Wert haben adjuvante Behandlungen im chirurgischen Therapiekonzept des Speiseröhrenkarzinoms? Med Welt 42:761–767

Dr. med. H.-U. Zieren, Chirurgische Universitätsklinik Köln,
Joseph-Stelzmann-Straße 9, W-5000 Köln 41

Die multimodale Behandlung beim lokal fortgeschrittenen Ösophaguscarcinom – Ergebnisse einer Pilotstudie

Multimodal Treatment of Locally Advanced Esophageal Carcinoma – Results of a Pilot Study

M.K. Walz[1], H. Wilke[2], M. Stahl[2], W. Niebel[1], U. Schmidt[3] und F.-W. Eigler[1]

[1]Abteilung für Allgemeine Chirurgie, Universitätsklinik Essen
[2]Innere Klinik und Poliklinik (Tumorforschung), Universitätsklinik Essen
[3]Institut für Pathologie, Universitätsklinik Essen

Einleitung

Die Gesamtprognose des Ösophaguscarcinoms ist nach wie vor ungünstig. Selbst bei den hoch-ausgewählten, resezierend behandelten Patienten liegt die 5-Jahres-Überlebenswahrscheinlichkeit nur bei 20% [1].

Da das Ösophaguscarcinom überwiegend in einem fortgeschrittenen Tumorstadium mit bereits stattgehabter Metastasierung diagnostiziert wird [1, 2], erscheint das Konzept einer kombinierten präoperativen Chemo-Radiotherapie – wie erstmals 1981 von Steiger und Mitarb. (zit. nach [3]) beschrieben – vielversprechend. Wir haben seit März 1991 ein multimodales Therapiekonzept beim lokal fortgeschrittenen, nicht-fernmetastasierten Ösophaguscarcinom angewandt, über dessen Frühergebnisse hier berichtet wird.

Patienten und Methodik

Von März 1991 bis Juni 1992 wurden 28 Patienten (25 Männer, 3 Frauen; Alter 59,6 ± 7,6 [44–71] Jahre) mit einem lokal fortgeschrittenen Ösophaguscarcinom in die Studie zur neoajduvanten Chemo-Radiotherapie aufgenommen. Die Carcinome waren 2mal im cervicalen Ösophagus, 5mal im oberen thorakalen, 11mal im mittleren thorakalen und 6mal im unteren thorakalen Ösophagus lokalisiert. Die Malignome wurden in der prätherapeutischen Probeexzision überwiegend als mittelgrading differenziert beurteilt (G1: 0, G2: 15, G3: 6, keine Aussage: 7).

Die Aufnahmekriterien in die Studie waren:

1. Tumorstadium T3/T4NXM0 oder T2NXM0 mit einer Längenausdehnung $\geq$ 5 cm,
2. Alter $\leq$ 70 Jahre,
3. grundsätzliche medizinische Operabilität,
4. hinreichende Knochenmarkreserve (Leukozyten $\geq$ 4.000/mm^3, Thrombozyten $\geq$ 100.000/mm^3),
5. Einverständnis des Patienten.

Chirurgisches Forum 1993
f. experim. u. klinische Forschung
Becker/Beger/Hartel (Hrsg.)

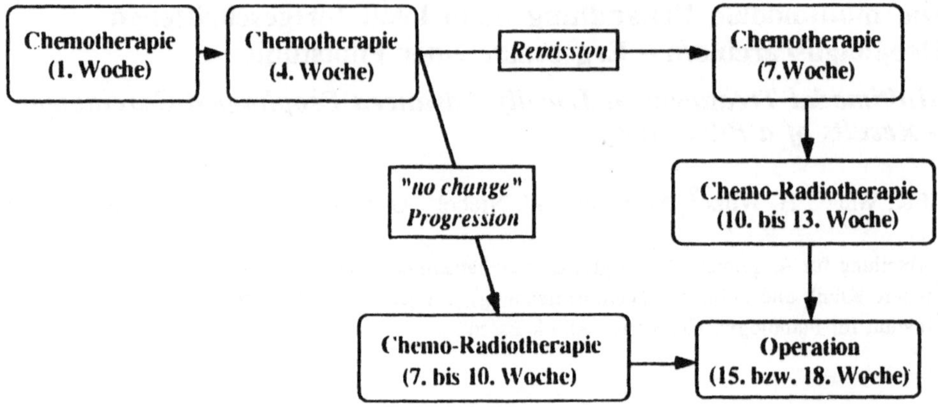

Abb. 1. Multimodales Therapiekonzept beim lokal fortgeschrittenen Ösophaguscarcinom

Das Behandlungsschema ist Abb. 1 zu entnehmen: zunächst wurden 2 bzw. 3 Kurse Chemotherapie (Leukovorin 300 mg/m^2, Etoposid [VP-16] 100 mg/m^2, 5-Fluorouracil 500 mg/m^2, Cisplatin 30 mg/m^2 jeweils für 3 Tage in der 1., 4. und ggf. 7. Woche) gegeben. Bei klinischer Progression oder fehlender Tumorrückbildung ("no change") nach 2 Chemotherapiekursen wurde eine kombinierte Chemo-Radiotherapie ab der 7. Woche, bei Ansprechen des Tumors ab der 10. Woche (nach 3 Kursen Chemotherapie) durchgeführt (Etoposid [VP-16] 100 mg/m^2 [Tag 4–6], Cisplatin 50 mg/m^2 [Tag 2 u. 8]; parallel beginnend lokoregionäre Radiatio mit Photonen [20 Einzeldosen à 2 Gv in 4 Wochen). Bei Patienten, die wegen Operationsablehnung oder Inoperabilität nicht operiert wurden (Abb. 2), wurde eine erhöhte Strahlendosis von 60–67 Gy appliziert. Der operative Eingriff wurde in der 15. bzw. 18. Woche nach Therapiebeginn vorgenommen. Die Ösophagusresektion erfolgte standardisiert als En-bloc-Resektion mit Lymphadenektomie über einen rechts-thorakalen Zugang. Nach Umlagerung wurde über eine mediane Laparotomie die Resektion der kleinen Magenkurvatur einschließlich einer Lymphadenektomie des Lig. gastro-duodenale und des Truncus coeliacus vorgenommen. Die Nahrungspassage wurde mittels eines Schlauchmagenhochzugs im hinteren Mediastinum mit cervicaler Ösophago-Fundostomie (zweischichtige Handnaht) wiederhergestellt, alternativ eine Colon-Interposition mit Ösophago-Colostomie und Colo-Enterostomie vorgenommen.

Die Resektionspräparate wurden auf einem Präpariertisch intraoperativ längs eröffnet und in aufgespanntem Zustand formalin-fixiert. Die histologische Begutachtung erfolgte in jedem Falle anhand zahlreicher (>30) Präparate aus Ösophagus- und Magenwand unter Einschluß der mitresezierten lokoregionären Lymphknoten.

Nach Entlassung aus der stationären Behandlung wurden alle Patienten in 3monatigem Abstand klinisch, radiologisch und endoskopisch nachuntersucht.

Die statistischen Berechnungen wurden mit dem IBM-Großrechner des Westdeutschen Tumorzentrums unter Anwendung der SAS-Software (SAS Inc.; Cary, South Carolina, USA) vorgenommen.

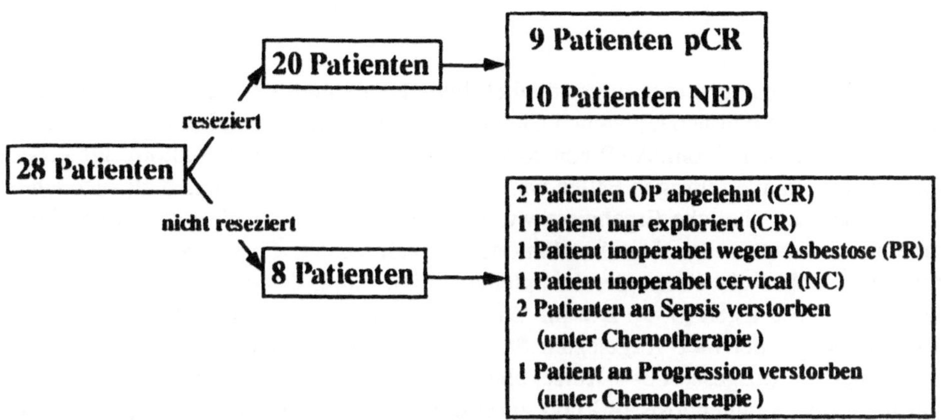

Abb. 2. Verlauf nach Aufnahme in die Studie zur neoadjuvanten Chemo-Radiotherapie; *(p)CR:* (pathol.) komplette Remission; *NED* ("no evidence of disease"): tumorfrei nach Operation bei mikros. oder makros. Tumorrest; *PR:* partielle Remission; *NC* ("no change"): fehlende Tumorrückbildung

Ergebnisse

Von 28 in die Studie aufgenommenen Patienten wurden 20 Patienten ösophagusreseziert (19mal R0, einmal R2); 8 Patienten wurden aus verschiedenen Gründen nicht reseziert (Abb. 2). Die neoadjuvante Chemoradiotherapie konnte bei insgesamt 25 Patienten vollständig durchgeführt werden (15 Pat.: 3 Chemotherapiekurse, 10 Pat.: 2 Chemotherapiekurse vor kombinierter Chemo-Radiotherapie).

Zwei Patienten verstarben am 19. bzw. 21 postoperativen Tag an einer Pneumonie bzw. einer Mediastinitis infolge einer partiellen Interponatsnekrose. Insgesamt wurden bei 10 Patienten postoperative Komplikationen beobachtet (4 Recurrensparesen, 3 Anastomoseninsuffizienzen, 3 Pneumonien, 1 Chylothorax).

Die histologische Aufarbeitung ergab in 9 Fällen eine komplette Remission (Abb. 2). Bei 11 Patienten fanden sich noch makroskopische (2 Pat.) oder mikroskopische Tumorreste (9 Pat.), bei einem dieser Patienten lediglich in einem Lymphknoten bei carcinom-negativem Befund im Bereich der Ösophaguswand. In Lymphknoten war bei 6 Patienten Tumorgewebe nachweisbar, bei 14 Patienten bestanden keine Lymphknotenmetastasen.

Nach einer medianen Nachbeobachtungszeit von 10 Monaten nach Therapiebeginn sind 7 von 28 Patienten verstorben (3 präoperativ, 2 perioperativ, 2 bei Tumorprogression nach 2 bzw. 16 Monaten). Die beiden Patienten, die den operativen Eingriff bei klinisch kompletter Remission abgelehnt hatten, leben 12 bzw. 17 Monate nach Therapiebeginn ohne Tumornachweis.

Derzeit (31.12.92) leben insgesamt 21 Patienten, 17 sind tumorfrei; bei 4 Patienten bestehen Rezidive bzw. Tumorreste. Die kumulative Überlebenswahrscheinlichkeit beträgt nach 12 Monaten 78%, nach 22 Monaten 68%.

Diskussion

Die Ergebnisse belegen eine ungewöhnlich hohe lokale und lokoregionäre Wirksamkeit der angewandten neoadjuvanten Chemo-Strahlentherapie beim lokal fortgeschrittenen Ösophaguscarcinom. An 9 von 20 Resektaten (45%) war kein Tumorrestgewebe nachweisbar, in allen übrigen Fällen waren deutliche Tumorregressionen zu verzeichnen. Tendenziell ähnliche Ergebnisse wurden in jüngerer Zeit auch von anderen Autoren nach Anwendung einer kombinierten neoadjuvanten Chemo-Strahlentherapie mitgeteilt, wobei die Raten der kompletten, mikroskopisch verifizierten Remissionen um 21–36% lagen [3–5]. Die im Vergleich zu diesen Studien verbesserte lokale Ansprechrate in der hier vorgelegten Studie dürfte am ehesten auf die intensivierte Chemotherapie (insgesamt 3–4 Kurse, alle 3 Wochen) in Kombination mit der relativ hohen lokalen Strahlendosis (40 Gy) zurückzuführen sein. Wegen der Aggressivität sollte diese Vorbehandlung vorerst nur innerhalb von klinischen Studien angewandt werden.

Nach kombinierter neoadjuvanter Therapie wurden bisher 2-Jahres-Überlebenswahrscheinlichkeiten um 47–66% mitgeteilt, nach 3 Jahren lebten noch 33–46% der Patienten [3–5]. Diese Ergebnisse liegen deutlich über denen der meisten Untersuchungen ohne Vorbehandlung (Übersicht bei [2]). Eine ähnliche Tendenz zeichnet sich auch in der hier vorliegenden Studie ab, obwohl – im Gegensatz zu den früheren Arbeiten [3–5] – ausschließlich lokal fortgeschrittene Tumoren behandelt wurden. Ob letztlich eine Verbesserung der Langzeitergebnisse im Vergleich zu nicht-vorbehandelten Patienten erreicht werden kann, bleibt noch abzuwarten. Darüberhinaus stellt sich die Frage, ob zukünftig bei der hohen Rate pathologisch kompletter Remissionen ein operativ-resezierendes Vorgehen generell notwendig ist. Die dargestellten Ergebnisse wie auch die Mitteilungen der Literatur legen eine randomisierte Prüfung dieses Therapiekonzepts gegen eine alleinige Chemostrahlentherapie nahe.

Zusammenfassung

Bei 28 Patienten mit lokal fortgeschrittenem Ösophaguscarcinom wurde eine neoadjuvante Chemo-Radiotherapie durchgeführt. Drei Patienten verstarben präoperativ an Sepsis bzw. Tumorprogression. Bei fünf weiteren Patienten wurde keine Resektion vorgenommen (Operationsablehnung, Inoperabilität), so daß 20 Patienten für eine Ösophagusresektion verblieben. Zwei Patienten verstarben an postoperativen Komplikationen. An 9 von 20 Resektaten fand sich eine komplette Remission, 10mal konnten Tumorreste vollständig reseziert werden. Die kumulative 2-Jahresüberlebenswahrscheinlichkeit liegt um 68%. Die Ergebnisse belegen die hohe lokale und lokoregionäre Wirksamkeit dieser neoadjuvanten Therapiemodalität, die allerdings prä- und perioperativ mit einer erhöhten Komplikationsrate einhergeht; günstige Auswirkungen auf die Langzeitprognose zeichnen sich ab.

Summary

Twenty-eight patients with locally advanced carcinoma of the esophagus were treated preoperatively with combined chemoradiotherapy. Three patients died preoperatively of sepsis or tumor progression. Five other carcinomas were not resected for different reasons (refusal of operation, inoperability). Of 20 patients resected, nine showed a complete remission, as demonstrated by histological examination. Two patients died postoperatively of pneumonia or mediastinitis. The cumulative 2-year survival rate is about 68%. The results demonstrate a high efficacy of this multimodal treatment for locally advanced esophageal cancer accompanied by an increased level of pre- and perioperative complications. An improvement for long-term survival seems to be possible.

Literatur

1. Pichlmaier H, Müller JM, Zieren U (1992) Plattenepithelcarcinom des Oesophagus. Behandlungskonzept der Chirurgischen Klinik der Universität zu Köln. Chirurg 63:701–708
2. Schumpelick V, Faß J, Truong S, Dreuw B, Treutner KH (1992) Behandlungsergebnisse des Ösophaguscarcinoms. Chirurg 63:715–721
3. Orringer MB, Forastiere AA, Perez-Tamayo C, Urba S, Takasugi BJ, Bromberg J (1990) Chemotherapy and radiation therapy before transhiatal esophagectomy for esophageal carcinoma. Ann Thorac Surg 49:348–55
4. McFarlane SD, Jill LD, Jolly PC, Kozarek RA, Anderson RP (1988) Improved results of surgical treatment for esophageal and gastroesophageal junction carcinomas after preoperative combined chemotherapy and radiation. J Thorac Cardiovasc Surg 95:415–22
5. Neunheim KS, Petruska PJ, Roy TS, Andrus CH, Johnson FE, Schlueter JM, Baue AR (1992) Preoperative chemotherapy and radiotherapy for esophageal carcinoma. J Thorac Cardiovasc Surg 103:887–895

Dr. med. M.K. Walz, Abteilung für Allgemeine Chirurgie, Universitätsklinikum Essen, Hufelandstraße 55, W-4300 Essen

Expression von Lewis-y-Antigen: Ein neuer prognostischer Parameter beim nicht-kleinzelligen Bronchialkarzinom?

Expression of Lewis-y Antigen: A New Prognostic Parameter in Non-Small-Cell Lung Cancer?

B. Passlick[1], K. Pantel[2], J.R. Izbicki[1], F. Liewald[3], O. Karg[4] und G. Riethmüller[2]

[1] Chirurgische Klinik, Klinikum Innenstadt, Ludwig-Maximilians-Universität München (Direktor: Prof. Dr. L. Schweiberer)
[2] Institut für Immunologie, Ludwig-Maximilians-Universität München (Direktor: Prof. Dr. G. Riethmüller)
[3] Abt. für Gefäß-, Thorax- und Herzchirurgie, Universität Ulm (Direktor: Prof. Dr. L. Sunder-Plassmann)
[4] Zentralkrankenhaus Gauting, Gauting (Leiter der Thoraxchirurgischen Abteilung: Prof. Dr. O. Thetter)

Einleitung

Die Expression von Blutgruppen-Determinanten A und B, sowie deren Vorläuferantigene (Lewis-y und x, sowie andere H-Antigene) hat bei einigen epithelialen Tumoren prognostische Bedeutung [1]. Neuere experimentelle Untersuchungen zeigen, daß Blutgruppen-Kohlehydrate die Invasions- und Metastasierungsfähigkeit von Tumorzellen erhöhen können, indem sie als Liganden für Adhäsionsmoleküle fungieren [2]. In der vorliegenden Arbeit untersuchten wir deshalb, ob Tumoren von Patienten mit operablem nicht-kleinzelligen Bronchialkarzinom ein mit der Blutgruppe H assoziiertes Antigen (Lewis-y-Antigen) exprimieren und ob diese Expression von prognostischer Bedeutung ist.

Material und Methoden

Unmittelbar nach der makroskopischen Beurteilung des Operationspräparates wurden von 80 Patienten mit nicht-kleinzelligem Bronchialkarzinom (42 Adenokarzinome, 31 Plattenepithelkarzinome, 5 Adenosquamöse Karzinome, 2 Großzellige Karzinome) eine repräsentative Probe des Tumors entnommen, mit flüssigem Stickstoff schockgefroren und bei −80°C gelagert. 4–6 μm dicke Gefrierschnitte wurden mit dem monoklonalen Antikörper (mAb) ABL-364 (IgG3, freundlicherweise von Dr. Loibner, Sandoz, Wien, zur Verfügung gestellt [3]) und der immunhistochemischen Alkalische Phosphatase-Anti-Alkalische Phosphatase (APAAP) Technik gefärbt. Unspezifische Färbungen wurden durch die Verwendung von Isotypkontrollen ausgeschlossen. Ein Tumor wurde als positiv gewertet, wenn mehr als 5% der Tumorzellen gefärbt waren.

Chirurgisches Forum 1993
f. experim. u. klinische Forschung
Becker/Beger/Hartel (Hrsg.)

Von 48 Tumoren wurde der DNS-Ploidiestatus bestimmt. Die Untersuchung erfolgte in gleicher Weise wie kürzlich beschrieben [4]. Die Tumornachsorge der Patienten wurde nach den Richtlinien des Tumorzentrums München durchgeführt, entweder in unserer Abteilung oder bei den niedergelassenen Kollegen.

Ergebnisse

Von 80 untersuchten Tumoren exprimierten 39 (48,2%) das durch den mAb ABL-364 definierte Antigen. Die Expression des Lewis-y-Antigens war dabei unabhängig von der Tumorhistologie (Adenokarzinom vs. Plattenepithelkarzinom), dem Differenzierungsgrad des Tumors, sowie dem T- und N-Stadium des Patienten. Eine deutliche Korrelation zeigte sich zum DNS-Ploidiestatus des Tumors (Tabelle 1). Von 24 untersuchten ABL-364 positiven Tumoren waren 14 (58,3%) aneuploid, jedoch nur 5 von 24 (20,8%) der negativen Tumoren ($p < 0{,}001$, χ^2-Test).

Tabelle 1. DNS-Ploidiestatus von ABL-364 positiven und ABL-364 negativen Bronchialkarzinomen

DNS Ploidiestatus	ABL-364 positiv[a] (n=24)	ABL-364 negativ (n=24)
aneuploid	14 (58,3%)[b]	5 (20,8%)
euploid	10 (41,7%)	19 (79,2%)

[a] Gefrierschnitte von nicht-kleinzelligen Bronchialkarzinomen wurden mit dem mAb ABL-364 und der APAAP-Methode gefärbt und mit dem Lichtmikroskop ausgewertet. Wenn mehr als 5% der Tumorzellen gefärbt waren, wurde der Tumor als positiv gewertet.

[b] $p < 0{,}001$ im Vergleich zu ABL-364 negativen Tumoren (χ^2-Test).

Von den 80 Patienten konnten postoperativ 69 (34 ABL-364 positiv, 35 ABL-364 negativ) bis zu 27 Monate (Median: 14) klinisch nachuntersucht werden. Dabei zeigte sich, daß die Expression des Lewis-y-Antigens mit einer schlechteren Prognose assoziiert ist (Abb. 1). Bei 55,8% der ABL-364 positiven Patienten trat ein Tumorrezidiv auf, dagegen nur bei 25,7% der Patienten mit einem ABL-364 negativen Tumor ($p = 0{,}02$, log-rank-Test). Ebenso verstarben innerhalb des Beobachtungszeitraums 44,1% der positiven Patienten an ihrem Tumorleiden, jedoch nur 20,0% der Patienten mit ABL-364 negativen Tumoren ($p = 0{,}05$, log-rank-Test).

Zusammenfassung

Da die Expression von Blutgruppen-Determinanten bei einigen epithelialen Tumoren prognostische Bedeutung hat, untersuchten wir die Expression eines Lewis-y-assoziierten Antigens auf nicht-kleinzelligen Bronchialkarzinomen mit Hilfe des monoklonalen Antikörpers ABL-364 und der immunhistologischen APAAP-Methode.

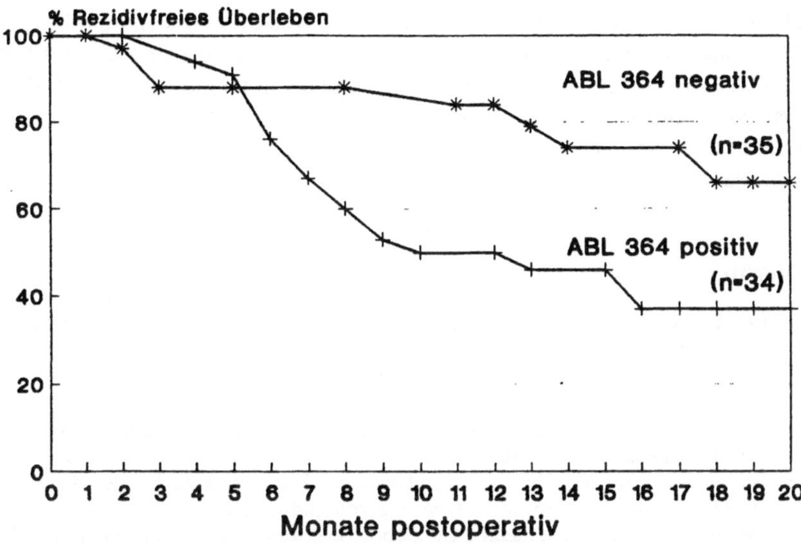

Abb. 1. Dargestellt ist der Anteil rezidivfreier Patienten mit ABL-364 negativen und ABL-364 positiven Tumoren. Mediane Beobachtungszeit: 14 Monate. Der Unterschied zwischen positiven und negativen Patienten ist signifikant mit p = 0,02 (Log-rank-Test)

Das Antigen wurde von 39 (48,2%) von 80 untersuchten Tumoren exprimiert, wobei dessen Expression nicht mit konventionellen Risikofaktoren wie der Histologie und dem Differenzierungsgrad des Tumors oder dem T- und N-Stadium des Patienten korrelierte. Eine deutliche Korrelation zeigte sich dagegen zum DNS-Ploidiestatus des Tumors ($p < 0{,}001$). Vorläufige Nachuntersuchungen zeigen, daß die Expression des Lewis-y-Antigens mit einer schlechteren Prognose assoziiert ist. Patienten mit Lewis-y-Antigen positiven Tumoren erleiden früher ein Tumorrezidiv (p = 0,02) und versterben eher an ihrem Tumorleiden als Patienten mit Lewis-y-Antigen negativen Tumoren (p = 0,05). Zusammenfassend scheint die Expression des, durch den mAb ABL-364 definierten, Lewis-y-assoziierten Antigens ein mit einer genetischen Instabilität assoziiertes Ereignis zu sein, welches mit einer schlechteren Prognose des nicht-kleinzelligen Bronchialkarzinoms einhergeht.

Summary

The expression of blood group antigens has prognostic significance in some epithelial tumors, including non-small-cell lung cancer (NSCLC). Therefore, we evaluated the expression of a blood group H associated antigen (Lewis-y) on primary tumors from patients with NSCLC. By using immunohistochemistry (alkaline phosphatase – antialkaline phosphatase, APAAP technique) together with the monoclonal antibody ABL-364, we found positive staining on 39 out of 80 (48.2%) tumors. The expression of the Lewis-y-related antigen correlated neither with the histology and differentiation grades of the tumor nor with the T and N stage of the patient, while a strong correlation to the DNA ploidy status of the tumor was observed ($P < 0.001$). Preliminary follow-up studies demonstrated that the expression of the Lewis-y antigen correlated with an increased relapse rate ($P = 0.02$) and a shorter survival ($P = 0.05$). In conclusion, the expression of the Lewis-y antigen by NSCLC cells seems to be associated with an increased genetic instability and correlates with a poorer prognosis in patients with NSCLC.

Literatur

1. Lee JS, Ro JY, Sahin AA, Hong WK, Brown BW, Mountain CF, Hittelman WN (1991) Expression of blood group antigen A – A favourable prognostic factor in non-small cell lung cancer. N Engl J Med 324:1084–1090
2. Miyake M, Hakomori SI (1991) A specific cell surface glycoconjugate controlling cell motility: evidence by functonal monoclonal antibodies that inhibit cell motility and tumor cell metastasis. Biochemistry 30:3328–3334
3. Blaszcyk-Thurin M, Thurin J, Hindsgaul O, Karlsson KA, Steplewski Z, Koprowski H (1987) Y and blood group B type 2 glycolipid antigens accumulate in a human gastric carcinoma cell line as detected by monoclonal antibody. J Biol Chem 262:372–379
4. Liewald F, Sunder-Plassmann L, Valet G, Wulf G, Weiss M, Schildberg FW (1992) Durchflußcytometrische Analyse beim nicht-kleinzelligen Bronchialkarzinom und deren prognostische Bedeutung. Chirurg 63:205–210

Dr. B. Passlick, Chirurgische Klinik und Poliklinik, Klinikum Innenstadt, Nußbaumstraße 20, W-8000 München 2

Überexpression des Epidermal Growth Factor Rezeptors und seiner Liganden beim humanen Pankreaskarzinom

Overexpression of the Epidermal Growth Factor Receptor and Its Ligands in Human Pancreatic Cancer

H. Friess[1], M. Büchler[2], Y. Yamanaka[1], M. Ebert[2], H.G. Beger[2] und M. Korc[1]

[1]Department of Medicine, University of California Irvine, Irvine, USA
[2]Abteilung für Allgemeine Chirurgie, Universität Ulm

Das duktale Pankreaskarzinom, mittlerweile die vierthäufigste Todesursache bei Tumorerkrankungen, ist durch seine zunehmende Inzidenz und überaus schlechte Prognose charakterisiert [1]. Die Ursachen für die Aggressivität, schnelle Tumorzellproliferation, das hohe Metastasierungspotential und Resistenz gegenüber konservativen onkologischen Therapiemaßnahmen sind nicht bekannt. Wachstumsfaktoren und deren Rezeptoren spielen bei der malignen Zelltransformation und Tumorzellproliferation eine Schlüsselrolle. Der Epidermal Growth Factor Rezeptor (EGFR) ist ein transmembranes Protein mit Tyrosin-Kinase Aktivität, und seine Überexpression ist mit malignem Zellwachstum und gesteigertem Metastasierungspotential verbunden [2]. Epidermal Growth Factor (EGF) und Transforming Growth Factor alpha (TGF-α) stimulieren den EGFR und ihre Überexpression befähigt Zellen ebenfalls zu malignem Wachstum [2]. Die Bedeutung dieser Wachstumsfaktoren in der Pathogenese des humanen Pankreaskarzinoms ist nicht bekannt. Ziel unserer Untersuchung war es daher, die Expression und Verteilung des EGF Rezeptors und seiner beiden Liganden EGF und TGF-α beim humanen Pankreaskarzinom zu analysieren.

Patienten und Methoden

Pankreaskarzinomgewebe von 22 Patienten (12 Frauen, 10 Männer) mit einem mittleren Alter von 59 Jahren (range: 23–69 Jahre) wurde in unsere Untersuchung einbezogen. Normales Pankreasgewebe von 12 Organspendern (4 Frauen, 8 Männer, mittleres Alter: 34 Jahre (range: 18–50 Jahre)) diente als Kontrolle.

Die Studie wurde von den Ethikkommissionen der Universität Ulm und der University of California Irvine, USA, begutachtet.

Immunhistochemie: Nach Fixation von frisch entnommenem Pankreasgewebe in Bouin'scher Lösung und Paraffineinbettung wurden 5 μm Paraffinschnitte mit spezifischen monoklonalen Antikörpern gegen EGFR (Sigma, Chemical Co., St. Louis, Verdünnung 1:400), EGF (Amgen Inc., Thousand Oaks, Verdünnung 1:200) und TGF-α (Oncogene Science Inc., Uniondale, Verdünnung 1:50) inkubiert und die resultierende Immunreaktion durch eine Streptavidin-Biotin-Peroxidasereaktion visuali-

Chirurgisches Forum 1993
f. experim. u. klinische Forschung
Becker/Beger/Hartel (Hrsg.)

siert. Zur besseren Beurteilung der Gewebestrukturen erfolgte eine Gegenfärbung mit Hämatoxylin.

In situ Hybridisierung: Deparaffinierte 5 μm Gewebeschnitte wurden 10 min mit 1 μg/ml Proteinase K (Boehringer Mannheim) und nachfolgend für 10 min mit 0,5 × SSC (1 × SSC = 150 mM NaCl, 15 mM Na-Citrat, pH 7,0) vorbehandelt. Nach Vorhybridisierung über 3 h bei 42°C wurden die Präparate 18 h bei 50°C unter Zusatz der radioaktiv markierten (^{32}PCTP) cRNA-Sonden für EGFR, EGF oder TGF-α (120.000 cpm) und 50 μg tRNA hybridisiert. Nach 2maligem Waschen der Gewebeschnitte für 30 min, RNAse-Behandlung (20 μg/ml), und weiteren Waschschritten in 0,1 × SSC, 10 mM β-Mercaptoethanol und 1 mM EDTA, erfolgte die Beschichtung der Präparate mit Autoradiographieflüssigkeit und die Exposition für 5–10 Tage. Die Gewebeschnitte wurden danach ebenfalls mit Hämatoxylin gegengefärbt und die mRNA-Expression mittels Videoimage Analyse quantifiziert [2].

Northern blot Analyse: Nach elektrophoretischer Auftrennung von 20 μg Gesamt-RNA in einem 1,2% Agarose/1,8 M Formaldehyd Gel, Elektrotransfer auf Nylon Membranen (GeneScreen, Du Pont) und UV cross-linking, wurden die Filter vorhybridisiert, mit spezifischen radioaktiv markierten cRNA- (^{32}PCTP, 1 × 10^6 cpm/ml) oder cDNA- (32PdCTP, 1 × 10^6 cpm/ml) Sonden 18 h hybridisiert und gewaschen. Die autoradiographischen Banden wurden mittels Laser-Densitometrie quantifiziert [2].

Zur Synthese der Antisense cRNA-Sonden diente ein 0,86 kb BamHI/EcoRI Fragment von humaner EGFR cDNA, ein 0,56 kb EcoRI Fragment von humaner EGF cDNA und ein 1,3 kb Fragment von humaner TGF-α cDNA. Maus 7S cytoplasmale cDNA (0,19 kb BamHI Fragment), welche mit humaner ribosomaler RNA kreuzhybridisiert, wurde zur Beurteilung von Unterschieden in den elektrophoretisch aufgetrennten RNA Mengen herangezogen.

Ergebnisse

Immunhistochemie: EGFR Immunoreaktivität fand sich im normalen Pankreas in nahezu allen Gangepithelien (apikal). Acinuszellen zeigten Immunostaining für EGFR im Bereich der Zellmembran und partiell im Cytoplasma (Abb. 1A). EGF und TGF-α Immunoreaktivität wurde an der Zellmembran und im Cytoplasma von allen Gangzellen und in den meisten Acinuszellen gefunden. Im Tumorgewebe wiesen alle karzinomatösen Gangepithelien an der apikalen Zelloberfläche eine verstärkte Immunoreaktivität für EGFR auf (Abb. 1B).

In situ Hybridisierung: In Gang- und Acinuszellen des normalen Pankreas fanden sich niedrige Spiegel von EGFR und EGF mRNA, wohingegen TGF-α mRNA in beiden Zelltypen in höheren Spiegeln aufgefunden wurde. In Acinuszellen waren alle drei mRNAs überwiegend basalwärts lokalisiert, während in Gangepithelien vor allem eine apikale Lokalisation wiedergefunden wurde. Pankreaskarzinomzellen wiesen eine signifikante Erhöhung ($p < 0{,}001$) der mRNAs für EGFR, EGF und TGF-α auf.

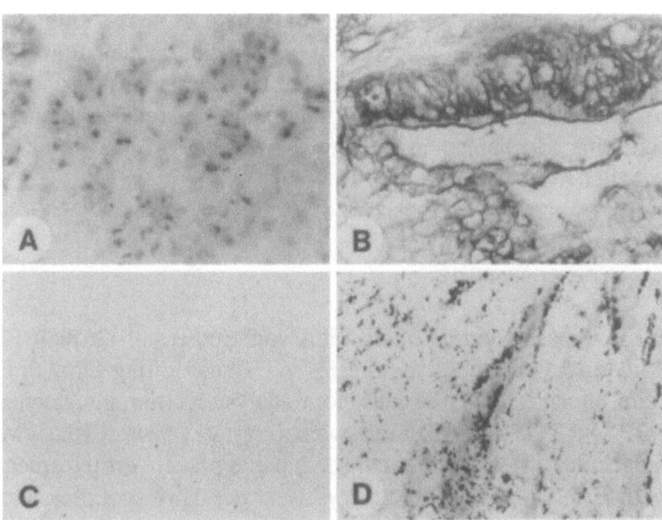

Abb. 1. A, B: Immunhistochemie. Epidermal Growth Factor Rezeptor (EGFR) im normalen Pankreas (**A**) und im Pankreaskarzinomgewebe (**B**). Das Tumorgewebe (**B**) weist eine deutlich verstärkte Immunoreaktivität für EGFR auf. Vergrößerung × 100. **C, D**: In situ Hybridisierung. Epidermal Growth Factor Rezeptor (EGFR) mRNA im normalen Pankreas (**C**) und beim Pankreaskarzinom (**D**). Während sich im normalen Pankreas (**C**) nur geringe Spiegel von EGFR mRNA finden, ist im Tumorgewebe eine deutliche Überexpression erkennbar. Vergrößerung × 100

Mittels Videoimage Analyse war für EGFR eine 17fache, für EGF eine 25fache und für TGF-α eine 4fache Zunahme der mRNA Spiegel verifizierbar.

Northern blot Analyse: Im normalen Pankreas waren niedrige mRNA Spiegel für EGFR und EGF und vergleichsweise hohe Spiegel für TGF-α nachweisbar. Verglichen mit diesem gesunden Kontrollgewebe fanden sich im Pankreaskarzinomgewebe eine 3-, 10- und 15fache mRNA-Erhöhung ($p < 0{,}001$) für EGFR, TGF-α und EGF.

Diskussion

Das Pankreaskarzinom gehört zu den aggressivsten Malignomerkrankungen und mehr als 80% der Patienten sind 3–6 Monate nach der Diagnosestellung bereits verstorben. Die Ursachen für die hohe Malignität sind nicht bekannt. Studien an isolierten Rattenacini deuten darauf hin, daß der EGFR und EGF bei der physiologischen Pankreasregulation eine Rolle spielen [3]. Des weiteren tragen diese Wachstumsfaktoren zur Zelldifferenzierung und Wachstuumsregulation bei. In humanen Pankreaskarzinomzellinien ist der EGFR überexprimiert und die Synthese von TGF-α gesteigert [4]. Diese Überexpression von Wachstumsfaktoren und Wachstumsrezeptoren befähigt Zellen zu malignem Zellwachstum. Beim Mammakarzinom ist die vermehrte Expression von EGFR mit einem gesteigerten Metastasierungspotential verbunden, und beim Blasenkarzinom zeigen EGFR überexprimierende Tumoren eine erhöhte Invasivität [2]. Unsere Untersuchungen zeigen zum ersten Mal, daß der EGFR und seine stimulierenden Liganden EGF und TGF-α beim humanen Pankreaskarzinom simultan überexprimiert sind. Dies legt die Vermutung nahe, daß Pankreaskarzinomzellen über autokrine und parakrine Mechanismen ihr aggressives Wachstumsverhalten selbst steuern und unterhalten können.

Zusammenfassung

Die Expression und Lokalisation von Epidermal Growth Factor Rezeptor (EGFR), Epidermal Growth Factor (EGF) und Transforming Growth Factor-α (TGF-α) wurde beim humanen Pankreaskarzinom analysiert. Immunhistochemisch waren der EGFR, EGF und TGF-α im Tumorgewebe verstärkt nachweisbar. Mittels in situ Hybridisierung konnte gezeigt werden, daß die erhöhten Proteinspiegel für EGFR, EGF und TGF-α mit der vermehrten Synthese der korrespondierenden mRNAs einhergehen. Beim Pankreaskarzinom waren im Vergleich zum normalen Pankreas die durch Northern blot Analyse ermittelten mRNA Spiegel für EGFR 3fach, für EGF 15fach und für TGF-α 10fach erhöht. Unsere Untersuchungsergebnisse deuten darauf hin, daß der EGFR, EGF und TGF-α in der Pathogenese des humanen Pankreaskarzinoms eine Rolle spielen und zum aggressiven Verlauf dieser Erkrankung beitragen.

Summary

The expression and distribution of epidermal growth factor receptor (EGFR), epidermal growth factor (EGF), and transforming growth factor α (TGF-α) were analyzed in human pancreatic cancer. Immunohistochemistry showed that EGFR, EGF, and TGF-α were expressed in higher levels in pancreatic cancer than in the normal pancreas. In situ hybridization revealed that the increased protein levels for EGFR, EGF, and TGF-α were accompanied by increased levels of the corresponding mRNAs. Northern blot analysis showed that there was a 3-, 15-, and 10-fold increase, respectively, in mRNA levels encoding EGFR, EGF, and TGF-α in pancreatic cancer compared with normal controls. Our results suggest that EGFR, EGF, and TGF-α play a role in the pathogenesis of human pancreatic cancer and may contribute to the aggressiveness of this disease.

Literatur

1. Gudjonsson B (1987) Cancer of the pancreas. 50 years of surgery. Cancer 60:2284–2303
2. Korc M, Chandrasekar B, Yamanaka Y, Friess H, Büchler M, Beger HG (1992) Overexpression of the epidermal growth factor receptor in human pancreatic cancer is associated with concomitant increases in the levels of epidermal growth factor and transforming growth factor alpha. J Clin Invest 90:1352–1360
3. Korc M, Matrisian LM, Planck SR, Magun BM (1983) Binding of epidermal growth factor in rat pancreatic acini. Biochem Biophys Res Commun 111:1066–1073

4. Sainsbury JRC, Sherbet GV, Farndon JR, Harris AL (1985) Epidermal-growth-factor receptors in human brain tumors. Lancet i:364–366

Dr. med. H. Friess, University of California Irvine, Department of Medicine, Division of Endocrinology and Metabolism, Med. Sci. I, C 240, Irvine, CA 92717, USA

4. Sainsbury JRC, Sherbet GV, Farndon JR, Harris AL (1985) Epidermal-growth-factor receptors in human [illegible] tumours. [illegible] [illegible]

Dr. med. H. Fries, University of California Irvine, Department of Medicine, Division of Endocrinology and Metabolism, Med. Sci. I C 240, Irvine, CA 92717, USA

Positronen-Emissionstomographie – ein neues Verfahren in der Diagnostik des Pankreaskarzinoms

Positron Emission Tomography – A New Procedure in the Diagnosis of Pancreatic Cancer

R. Isenmann[1], M. Büchler[1], H. Frieß[1], M. Ebert[1], J. Langhans[2] und H.G. Beger[1]

[1]Abteilung für Allgemeinchirurgie, Chirurgische Klinik I
(Ärztl. Direktor: Prof. Dr. H.G. Beger), Universität Ulm
[2]Abteilung für Nuklearmedizin (Leiter: Prof. Dr. S.N. Reske), Universität Ulm

Einleitung

Die Prognose des Pankreaskarzinoms ist schlecht, die 5-Jahresüberlebensrate ist die niedrigste aller gastrointestinalen Malignome. Die Suche nach neuen diagnostischen Methoden, die neben den gängigen Kriterien wie Kontrastmittel-CT und ERCP eine zuverlässige und frühzeitige Diagnosestellung erlauben, erscheint deshalb gerechtfertigt.

Die Positronen-Emissionstomographie (PET) ist ein bildgebendes Verfahren, bei welchem die beim radioaktiven Zerfall von Positronen-Strahlern freiwerdende Energie registriert und mittels eines Rechners graphisch dargestellt wird. Die in dieser Arbeit verwendete, mit Fluor-18 markierte 2-Deoxyglucose, reichert sich selektiv in Malignomen an. Ziel der Untersuchung war es, mit diesem Verfahren Pankreaskarzinome darzustellen und die Wertigkeit der diagnostischen Methode, insbesondere in der Differenzierung zur chronischen Pankreatitis, zu evaluieren.

Patienten und Methoden

Insgesamt wurden von Februar bis Dezember 1992 42 Patienten (33 Männer, 9 Frauen, mittleres Alter 56 Jahre) präoperativ einer PET-Untersuchung unterzogen. Intraoperativ wurde ein Pankreaskarzinom bei 25 Patienten histologisch gesichert, 17 litten an einer chronischen Pankreatitis (Tabelle 1).

Tabelle 1. Tumorstadien (UICC-Klassifizierung) der 25 Patienten mit Pankreaskarzinom

Patienten	
Stadium I	0
Stadium II	3
Stadium III	12
Stadium IV	10

Chirurgisches Forum 1993
f. experim. u. klinische Forschung
Becker/Beger/Hartel (Hrsg.)

10 der Karzinompatienten hatten zum Zeitpunkt der Operation bereits Fernmetastasen (8 Leberfiliae, 2 Peritonealkarzinose).

Alle erhielten bei der präoperativen PET-Untersuchung 200–400 mBq F-18 2-Deoxylglucose (FDG) intravenös verabreicht. 60 min später wurde die Aktivitätsverteilung des Radiotracers im Oberbauch mittels PET-Scanner (Siemens ECAT 931/15) registriert und bildlich aufgezeichnet. Eine Aktivitätsanreicherung in der Pankreasloge wurde als Kriterium für das Vorliegen eines Pankreaskarzinoms erachtet. Gleichzeitig wurde auf das Vorhandensein weiterer Herde im Sinne von Fernmetastasen geachtet.

Die intraoperativ gewonnenen histologischen Befunde wurden mit den präoperativen PET-Befunden verglichen und ausgewertet.

Ergebnisse

Tabelle 2. Ergebnisse bei 25 Patienten mit Pankreaskarzinom und 17 mit chronischer Pankreatitis

		PET	
		positiv	negativ
Chron. Pankreatitis	n=17	4	13
Pankreaskarzinom	n=25	23	2
Sensitivität		92,0%	
Spezifität		76,5%	
Positiver Vorhersagewert		85,2%	
Negativer Vorhersagewert		86,7%	

13/17 Patienten mit chronischer Pankreatitis (76,4%) zeigten, wie erwartet, keine Aktivitätsanreicherung in der Pankreasloge, der PET war richtig negativ. Bei 4/17 Patienten dieser Gruppe (23,6%) war die Untersuchung falsch positiv (Tabelle 2).

Bei 23/25 Patienten mit Pankreaskarzinom (92,0%) ergab sich ein richtig positives Untersuchungsergebnis, lediglich bei 2 Patienten (8,0%) war der PET-Befund falsch negativ.

Die Sensitivität der Untersuchungsmethode beträgt somit für das Pankreaskarzinom 92%, die Spezifität liegt bei 76,5%. Der positive Vorhersagewert beträgt 85,2%; d.h. bei positivem Untersuchungsergebnis liegt die Wahrscheinlichkeit, daß wirklich ein Pankreaskarzinom vorliegt, bei 85%.

Bei 6 der 8 Patienten mit Leberfiliae wurden diese auch im PET gesehen. Bei beiden Patienten mit Peritonealkarzinose war bereits im PET der Verdacht geäußert worden.

Diskussion

Inzidenz und Prognose des Pankreaskarzinoms rechtfertigen die Suche nach neuen Diagnosemethoden, mit denen die Erkrankung frühzeitig und zuverlässig diagnostiziert werden kann. Die Positronen-Emissionstomographie ermöglicht mittels radioaktiver Tracer-Substanzen die bildgebende Darstellung von Stoffwechselprozessen. Seit den Untersuchungen von Warburg [1] ist bekannt, daß maligne Tumoren eine erhöhte Glukoseaufnahme und Metabolisierung aufweisen. Es konnte bereits vor längerer Zeit gezeigt werden, daß 2-Deoxyglucose (DG) sich in simultaner Weise verhält [2]. Mit Positronen-Strahlern markierte DG wurde deshalb in Verbindung mit einem PET-Scanner zur Diagnostik von kolorektalen Tumoren und deren Metastasen erfolgreich verwendet [3].

Untersuchungen mit PET bei Pankreaserkrankungen wurden erstmals von Syrota und Mitarb. vorgenommen, die als Radiotracer C-11 markiertes L-Methionin verwendeten [4]. Mit dieser Substanz, die in den Proteinstoffwechsel des Pankreas eingeschleust wird, war eine Unterscheidung zwischen den verschiedenen Pankreasmorphologien nicht möglich. Untersuchungen dieser Problemstellung mit FDG unter standardisierten Bedingungen stammen von der Aachener Arbeitsgruppe und ergaben an einer kleinen Patientengruppe ermutigende Ergebnisse bezüglich der Unterscheidung zwischen chronischer Pankreatitis und Pankreaskarzinom [5].

In der vorliegenden Arbeit konnten wir an einem großen Patientenkollektiv zeigen, daß PET mit FDG als Routineverfahren zur Diagnostik des Pankreaskarzinoms geeignet ist und daß mit dieser Untersuchungsmethode eine Differenzierung zur chronischen Pankreatitis möglich ist. Die Methode erlaubt ebenfalls die Darstellung von Fernmetastasen.

Eine Erklärung für die falsch positiven bzw. falsch negativen Ergebnisse in unserer Studie konnte bisher noch nicht gefunden werden.

Welche Rolle die neue Untersuchungsmethode im Prozeß der diagnostischen Entscheidungsfindung in Zukunft spielen wird, ist anhand der vorliegenden Ergebnisse noch nicht sicher abzuschätzen. Hier sind weitergehende Studien und insbesondere der Vergleich mit den etablierten Diagnosemethoden Kontrastmittel-CT und ERCP notwendig. Außerdem sollte die Wertigkeit der neuen Untersuchungsmethode, insbesondere bei frühem Karzinomstadium, genauer evaluiert werden.

Zusammenfassung

Insgesamt 42 Patienten mit Pankreaserkrankungen (25 mit Pankreaskarzinom, 17 mit chronischer Pankreatitis) unterzogen sich präoperativ einer Positronen-Emissionstomographie (PET) mit Fluor-18 markierter 2-Deoxyglukose (FDG). Eine Aktivitätsanreicherung im Bereich der Pankreasloge galt als Kriterium für das Vorliegen eines Pankreaskarzinoms; fehlte diese, so deutete dies auf eine chronische Pankreatitis hin. Postoperativ wurden die PET Ergebnisse mit der intraoperativ gewonnenen Histologie verglichen und ausgewertet. Bei 23 der Patienten mit Pankreaskarzinom war die präoperativ im PET gestellte Diagnose richtig. Für die chronische Pankreatitis galt dies bei 13 von 17 Patienten. Daraus errechnet sich eine Sensitivität von 92%, der positive Vorhersagewert für das Pankreaskarzinom liegt bei 85,2%.

PET mit 18-FDG ist somit als nicht-invasive Methode zur Differenzierung zwischen Pankreaskarzinom und chronischer Pankreatitis geeignet.

Summary

In 42 patients with either cancer of the pancreas ($n = 25$) or chronic pancreatitis ($n = 17$), positron emission tomography (PET) with ^{18}F-labeled 2-deoxyglucose (18-FDG) was performed preoperatively. Activity enhancement in the pancreatic region was regarded as a criterion for pancreatic cancer, and no enhancement was expected in patients with chronic pancreatitis. PET results and the diagnosis established by histological examination of surgical specimens were compared after operation. In 23 of the patients with pancreatic cancer, the PET diagnosis was correct. This was also the case in 13 of the 17 patients with chronic pancreatitis.

The sensitivity of PET for pancreatic cancer was 92%, and the positive predictive value was 85.2%.

PET with 18-FDG seems to be a suitable noninvasive diagnostic procedure to differentiate between chronic pancreatitis and cancer of the pancreas.

Literatur

1. Warburg O (1931) The metabolism of tumors. Richard R. Smith Inc., New York, pp 129–169
2. Som P, Atkins HL, Bandoypadhyay D et al. (1980) A fluorinated glucose analog, 2-fluoro-2-deoxy-D-glucose (F-18): Nontoxic tracer for rapid tumor detection. J Nucl Med 21:670–675
3. Yonekura Y, Benua RS, Brill AB et al. (1982) Increased accumulation of 2-deoxy-2-(18F)fluoro-D-glucose in liver metastasis from colon carcinoma. J Nucl Med 23:1133–1137
4. Syrota A, Duquesnoy RT, Paraf A, Kellershohn C (1982) The role of positron emission tomography in the detection of pancreatic disease. Radiology 143:249–253
5. Klever R, Bares R, Faß J, Büll U, Schumpelick V (1992) Zur Wertigkeit der Positronen-Emissions-Tomographie (PET) mit 18-Fluordesoxyglucose (18-FDG) zur Differentialdiagnose von Pankreaskarzinom/Pankreatitis: Erste klinische Erfahrungen. Langenbecks Arch Chir [Suppl] 1992:11–14

Dr. R. Isenmann, Abteilung für Allgemeinchirurgie, Chirurgische Klinik I, Universität Ulm, Steinhövelstraße 9, W-7900 Ulm

"In-vivo" Untersuchungen zur Anabolie des Proteinstoffwechsels maligner Kolontumoren beim Menschen: Beziehungen zur Pathohistologie

In Vivo Investigations of Anabolic Protein Metabolism in Malignant Human Colon Tumors: Relations to Histopathology

E. Hagmüller[1], H.J. Günther[1], D. Ockert[1], H. Kollmar[1], Y. Ghoos[2] und H.D. Saeger[1]

[1]Chirurgische Universitätsklinik, Klinikum Mannheim, Universität Heidelberg
[2]Universitaire Ziekenhuizen, Leuven, Belgium

Zielsetzung

Die möglichen Ursachen der allseits bekannten "Tumorkachexie" sind bis heute nicht eindeutig geklärt und beruhen zum Teil auf Vermutungen bezüglich der metabolischen Interaktion zwischen Malignom und Tumorträger. So waren Tumoren in der Vergangenheit wiederholt als "Stickstoffallen" bezeichnet worden, obwohl ein überzeugender quantitativer Nachweis hierzu nicht erbracht werden konnte – weder experimentell noch "in-vivo". Die wenigen Untersuchungen zum Proteinstoffwechsel von Tumoren beschränkten sich bisher auf die Errechnung sogenannter "fraktioneller Syntheseraten" [4, 5] und beschrieben deshalb die Proteinkinetik nur qualitativ und inkomplett, da der gleichzeitig ablaufende tumorale Proteinabbau nicht erfaßt und somit das Maß der tumoralen "Anabolie" nicht angegeben werden konnte. Weiterhin liegen bezüglich der Aufnahme und Abgabe von Aminosäuren durch Tumoren des Menschen nur wenige Mitteilungen vor. In eigenen Untersuchungen zeigte sich, daß Kolontumoren des Menschen verzweigtkettige Aminosäuren in signifikant höherem Maße aufnahmen als gesundes Kolongewebe bzw. periphere Gewebe [2, 3]. Um den Stoffwechsel dieser Aminosäuren im Tumor, die Proteinkinetik und insbesondere das Ausmaß der tumoralen Anabolie erstmals quantitativ zu erfassen, wurde ein Tracer-Modell mit ^{13}C-Leuzin für Untersuchungen an Kolontumoren des Menschen modifiziert und angewandt.

Methodik

Die Daten der Studie stammen von 15 Patienten mit resektablen Kolontumoren (Coecum 6, Colon ascendens 4, Colon sigmoideum 5). Untersucht wurden 8 Männer und 7 Frauen mit einem Durchschnittsalter von 66 bzw. 61 Jahren nach 24stündiger Nahrungsrestriktion; kein Patient war unterernährt. Alle intraoperativen Untersuchungen umfaßten die Ermittlung der tumoralen und peripheren Austauschraten der Aminosäuren sowie die Analysen zur Proteinkinetik.

Chirurgisches Forum 1993
f. experim. u. klinische Forschung
Becker/Beger/Hartel (Hrsg.)

Ermittlung der Austauschraten: Während der Operation erfolgte die Analyse der transtumoralen Aminosäurenbilanzen durch direkte Messung der Tumordurchblutung ("venous-outflow"-Technik) und zur Aminosäurenbestimmung (Biotronic LC 600) durch Entnahme arteriellen sowie tumorvenösen Blutes aus der kanülierten "tumordrainierenden Vene". Dazu wurden die tumordrainierenden Gefäße (Arterie und Vene) im Mesokolon schonend freigelegt und die seitlich einstrahlenden, normales Kolon drainierenden Gefäße ligiert. Postoperativ ermittelten wir das Gewicht der Tumoren nach deren sorgfältiger Präparation. Das Produkt aus der Tumordurchblutung und den jeweiligen arteriovenösen Konzentrationsdifferenzen ergab die quantitativen Austauschraten. Zum Vergleich wurden die Austauschraten der peripheren Gewebe am Arm ebenfalls intraoperativ ermittelt (Blutabnahme aus "deep vein", Durchblutungsmessung mittels Venenverschlußplethysmographie).

Proteinkinetik: Zur Analyse der Proteinkinetik des Tumors (und der peripheren Gewebe am Arm) wurde ^{13}C-Leuzin als Tracer verwendet. Das an der Carboxylgruppe mit dem stabilen Isotop ^{13}C markierte Leuzin wird beim Abbau zunächst zu α^{13}C-Ketoisokapronat (^{13}C-KIC) deaminiert und dann oxidiert unter irreversibler Abspaltung von $^{13}CO_2$, welches ins Blut abgegeben wird. Die intravenöse Gabe von ^{13}C-Leuzin (Bolus: 1 mg/kg KG, Infusion: 0,64 mg/kg KG $\times$ h) wurde 90 min vor Operationsbeginn gestartet. Intraoperative Blutentnahmen aus der Tumorvene, einer tiefen Armvene, arteriell und zentralvenös, erlaubten über die Bestimmungen der jeweiligen Anreicherungen (^{13}C-Leu, ^{13}C-KIC, $^{13}CO_2$) und Konzentrationen (Leu, KIC, CO_2) die Berechnungen zur Proteinkinetik für die Tumoren, die peripheren Gewebe am Arm und für den Gesamtkörper. Die Analyse der Anreicherungen (^{13}C-Leu, ^{13}C-KIC im Serum, $^{13}CO_2$ im Serum und Ausatemluft) erfolgten mit Hilfe eines Gaschromatografie/Massenspektrometers.

Das Narkoseverfahren war "total intravenös" mit Propofol/Fentanyl; Inhalationsanästhetika wurden nicht verwendet. In das Beatmungssystem wurde ein Gerät zur indirekten Kalorimetrie eingebracht zwecks kontinuierlicher Bestimmung der CO_2-Konzentrationen in der Atemluft und des Atemminutenvolumens.

Alle Berechnungen zur Proteinkinetik der Tumoren und der peripheren Gewebe am Arm erfolgten nach einem dazu eigens entwickelten Tracermodell, welches inzwischen auch von Bennet [1] beschrieben wurde. Die entsprechenden Berechnungen für den Gesamtkörper basierten auf dem "reciprocal-pool model" des Leuzinstoffwechsels [3]. Voraussetzung für die Analysen zur Proteinkinetik war das Vorliegen eines metabolischen Fließgleichgewichtes; dieses war in allen Fällen spätestens 90 min nach Start der Isotopeninfusion gegeben, gekennzeichnet durch das Erreichen eines konstanten Plateaus der Anreicherungen von ^{13}C-Leuzin, ^{13}C-Ketoisokapronat zentralvenös sowie $^{13}CO_2$ in der Ausatemluft.

Ergebnisse

Die Durchblutung der untersuchten Kolonkarzinome lag im arithmetischen Mittel bei $56,8 \pm 26,4$ (SD) ml/100g $\times$ min und war damit um etwa den Faktor 16 größer als die durchschnittliche Durchblutung der peripheren Gewebe mit $3,53 \pm 0,87$ (SD). Das

Gewicht der Tumoren betrug im Schnitt $80,2 \pm 33,8$ (SD) g; der kleinste wog 30 g, der größte 150 g. Größere Karzinome waren verhältnismäßig schlechter durchblutet als kleinere – entsprechend einer negativen Korrelation zwischen der Tumordurchblutung und der Tumormasse ($r = -0,724$; $p = 0,0023$).

Betreffend der quantitativen Austauschraten von Aminosäuren zeigten sich deutliche Unterschiede zwischen Tumor und Peripherie. Vorwiegend essentielle Aminosäuren – und hier vor allem die verzweigtkettigen – sowie Glutamin wurden von den Tumoren aufgenommen, während diese Aminosäuren von den peripheren Geweben abgegeben wurden. Tumoral in hohem Maße freigesetzt wurde die Aminosäure Alanin (Tabelle 1).

Tabelle 1. Tumoraler und peripherer Austausch von Aminosäuren. Mittelwerte ± SEM (nmol/100g × min), p = Irrtumswahrsch. nach dem Wilcoxon-Test

	Karzinome	Peripherie	p
Alle Aminosäuren	374 ± 1999	−425 ± 127	0,46 n.s.
Essentielle AS	1681 ± 586	−107 ± 58	0,0085
Nicht essentielle AS	−1086 ± 1321	−304 ± 71	0,81 n.s.
Verzweigtkettige AS	1523 ± 233	−49 ± 37	0,0001
Leuzin	662 ± 127	−5 ± 24	0,0001
Glutamin	1232 ± 259	−90 ± 25	0,0001
Alanin	−1303 ± 384	−110 ± 14	0,0002

Bei isolierter Betrachtung der tumoralen Bilanzen für Aminosäuren konnte festgestellt werden, daß niedrig differenzierte, vorwiegend muzinöse Kolonkarzinome Aminosäuren in signifikant höherem Maße dem Blut entzogen als dies für mittelgradig bzw. hochdifferenzierte Kolonmalignome der Fall war (Tabelle 2). Dies betraf gleichsinnig sowohl die Gruppe der essentiellen als auch die Gruppe der nicht essentiellen Aminosäuren. Grundsätzlich wurden jedoch essentielle Aminosäuren von den Kolontumoren in der Regel aufgenommen, während nicht essentielle Aminosäuren vorwiegend von hochdifferenzierten Karzinomen ins Blut freigesetzt wurden.

Tabelle 2. Aminosäurenaustausch und Nettobilanz differenziert in 2 pathohistologische Gruppen. Gruppe I: n=8, gute Prognose, $T_2N_0M_0$-$T_3N_0M_0$, G_1-G_2, nicht mucinös, keine Lymphang. carc.; Gruppe II: n=7, schlechtere Prognose, $T_2N_1M_0$-$T_4N_3M_0$, G_3, 6× muzinös, 3× Lymphang. carc.; Mittelwerte ± SEM (nmol/100g × min), p = Irrtumswahrsch. bei U-Test nach Mann/Whitney

	Gruppe I	Gruppe II	p
Alle Aminosäuren	−3933 ± 2489	5376 ± 1671	0,012
Essentielle AS	111 ± 579	3250 ± 575	0,005
Nicht essentielle AS	−3700 ± 1735	1917 ± 1159	0,012
Verzweigtkettige AS	926 ± 131	2205 ± 320	0,003
Leuzin	358 ± 51	1009 ± 198	0,013
Glutamin	724 ± 143	1812 ± 452	0,018
Nettobilanz (Anabolie)	122 ± 163	1442 ± 374	0,007

Mittels des angewendeten ^{13}C-Leuzin-Tracermodells konnten die einzelnen Größen der Proteinkinetik von Tumoren des Menschen quantifiziert werden (Tabelle 3). Der tumorale Proteinumsatz war extrem gesteigert – so lag die tumorale Proteinsyntheserate gegenüber den Werten für die peripheren Gewebe um den Faktor 14 höher, für die tumorale Proteinabbaurate (Breakdown) um den Faktor 10. Das Ausmaß der ermittelten tumoralen Nettobilanz (Differenz aus Proteinsynthese- und Proteinabbaurate = Anabolie oder Katabolie) zeigte eine erhebliche Anabolie der Kolontumoren auf, wobei dieser Wert für niedrig differenzierte und verschleimende Adenokarzinome noch deutlich höher ausfiel. Katabole Verhältnisse fanden sich dagegen bezüglich der peripheren Gewebe am Arm und bezüglich des Gesamtkörpers. Relativ gering im Verhältnis zur tumoralen Syntheserate zeigte sich die Leuzinoxidationsrate, die nur 7,5% der Syntheserate ausmachte; das tumoral aufgenommene Leuzin trug somit nur in geringem Maße zur energetischen Versorgung der Malignome bei.

Tabelle 3. Proteinkinetik für Tumoren, periphere Gewebe und Gesamtkörper. Mittelwerte ± SEM (nmol/100g × min), $p < 0,001$ Tumoren vs Peripherie, Wilcoxon-Test

	Karzinome	Peripherie	Gesamtkörper
Breakdown	1801 ± 516	177 ± 56	152 ± 10
Synthese	2170 ± 498	154 ± 65	137 ± 10
Oxidation	162 ± 22	15 ± 2	15 ± 2
Nettobilanz	369 ± 129	−23 ± 22	−15 ± 2

Die erstmals quantitativ ermittelten, hohen Syntheseraten bestätigen die wenigen bisher vorliegenden Daten über gesteigerte fraktionelle Syntheseraten bei Tumoren [4, 5]. Neben der Forcierung der tumoralen Syntheseraten stellten wir durch unsere Untersuchungen jedoch zusätzlich fest, daß das Ausmaß der tumoralen Proteinabbaurate ebenfalls sehr hoch ist – wenn auch geringer als die Syntheserate. Es konnte somit erstmals die Höhe der Anabolie des Proteinstoffwechsels (Nettobilanz) von Malignomen beim Menschen "in-vivo" bestimmt werden. Die Ergebnisse zeigen dabei auf, daß Kolontumoren zum Teil erhebliche Mengen an Aminosäuren aufnehmen und davon einen großen Teil, netto betrachtet, in Tumorprotein einbauen – in wesentlicher Abhängigkeit von der Pathohistologie. Diese Resultate sind von Bedeutung für die Ernährung des Tumorkranken sowie zur Weiterentwicklung von diagnostischen Methoden (z.B. PET, NMR-Spektroskopie).

Zusammenfassung

Bei 15 Patienten mit Kolontumoren wurde die tumorale Proteinkinetik mittels des Tracers ^{13}C-Leuzin quantitativ erfaßt. Die tumorale Proteinsyntheserate war im Vergleich zur Syntheserate der peripheren Gewebe bzw. des Gesamtkörpers excessiv erhöht, dasselbe betraf die tumorale Proteinabbaurate. Es zeigte sich ein erhebliches Maß (Nettobilanz) an Anabolie für die Kolonkarzinome. Tumoral aufgenommen wurden essentielle, vor allem verzweigtkettige Aminosäuren. Schlecht differenzierte, prognostisch ungünstige Kolontumoren nahmen größere Mengen von Aminosäuren auf als hoch differenzierte Malignome; entsprechend höher lag für die prognostisch ungünstigen Karzinome das Maß der tumoralen Anabolie.

Summary

In 15 patients with colon carcinomas, tumoral protein kinetics have been measured quantitatively using ^{13}C-leucine. We were able to demonstrate extremely high values of tumoral protein synthesis in comparison to the synthesis rates of the peripheral tissues and the whole body. The same was true for the tumoral breakdown rate and for the net balance as a parameter of tumoral anabolism. Essential amino acids and, in particular, branched chain amino acids were taken up by the colon carcinomas. In poorly differentiated tumors we noted higher uptake rates of amino acids than in well-differentiated carcinomas. Corresponding to these uptake rates higher values of tumoral anabolism were determined in tumors with low differentiation.

Literatur

1. Bennet WM, Connacher AA, Scrimgeour CM, Rennie MJ (1990) The effect of amino acid infusion on leg protein turnover assessed by L-(^{15}N)phenylalanine and L-(1-^{13}C)leucine exchange. Eur J Clin Invest 20:41–50
2. Hagmüller E, Saeger H-D, Barth H-O, Seßler M, Holm E (1989) Neue Aspekte des Tumorstoffwechsels: Substrataustausch maligner Colontumoren beim Menschen. Langenbecks Arch Chir [Suppl] Chir Forum '89:525–529
3. Hagmüller E (1992) Der Stoffwechsel von malignen Kolontumoren beim Menschen – "In-vivo" Untersuchungen zum quantitativen Substrataustausch sowie zum Aminosäurenstoffwechsel mit Hilfe einer modifizierten ^{13}C-Leuzin-Tracertechnik. Medizinische Habilitationsschrift, Universität Heidelberg
4. Heys SD, Park KGM, McNurlan MA, Milne E, Eremin O, Wernerman J, Keenan RA, Garlick PJ (1991) Stimulation of protein synthesis in human tumors by parenteral nutrition: evidence for modulation of tumor growth. Br J Surg 78:483–487
5. Shaw JHF, Humberstone DA, Douglas RG, Koea J (1991) Leucine kinetics in patients with benign disease, non-weight-losing cancer, and cancer cachexia: studies at the whole-body and tissue level and the response to nutritional support. Surgery 109:37–50

Dr. med. habil. E. Hagmüller, Oberarzt, Chirurgische Universitätsklinik, Klinikum Mannheim, Fakultät für Klinische Medizin, Universität Heidelberg, Theodor-Kutzer-Ufer, W-6800 Mannheim

VLA-Adhäsionsrezeptoren beim kolorektalen Karzinom

VLA Adhesion Receptors in Colorectal Cancer

R.J. Weinel[1], A. Rosendahl[1], K. Neumann[2] und M. Rothmund[1]

[1]Klinik für Allgemeinchirurgie, Philipps-Universität Marburg
[2]Abteilung für Pathologie, Philipps-Universität Marburg

Einleitung

Eine, im Vergleich zum Normalgewebe veränderte Interaktion von Tumorzellen mit den adhäsiven Proteinen der extrazellulären Matrix ist mitverantwortlich für die Fähigkeit von Tumorzellen zu invasivem Wachstum und zur Metastasierung. Dieser Kontakt zwischen Zellen und extrazellulärer Matrix wird durch Rezeptoren für adhäsive Proteine auf der Zelloberfläche vermittelt.

Für die Interaktion zwischen Zellen und den Matrixbestandteilen Laminin, Collagen und Fibronektin sind vornehmlich Adhäsionsrezeptoren aus der VLA-Gruppe der Integrine verantwortlich [1]. Wir untersuchten immunhistologisch Rezeptoren für Collagen (VLA $\alpha 2$), Fibronektin (VLA $\alpha 5$) und Laminin (VLA $\alpha 6$) in normaler Kolonmukosa, Kolonadenomen und Kolonkarzinomen. Dabei gingen wir der Frage nach, welche Unterschiede es in Expression und Verteilung dieser Rezeptoren in normaler Kolonmukosa und neoplastisch verändertem Kolonepithel gibt.

Methode

Proben für die Immunhistologie wurden von frischen Resektionspräparaten von 15 Patienten mit kolorektalen Karzinomen entnommen. Die Proben wurden in flüssigem Stickstoff eingefroren und bei $-70°$ gelagert.

Die immunhistologischen Untersuchungen wurden mittels der Avidin-Biotin-Komplextechnik unter Zuhilfenahme spezifischer monoklonaler Antikörper durchgeführt. Als Chromogen diente DAB.

Die Stärke der Antigen-Expression auf den Zellen wurde semiquantitativ mittels einer 4-Punkte-Skala erfaßt (–, +, + +, + + +). Der Anteil der positiven Zellen wurde ebenfalls semiquantitativ mittels einer 4-Punkte-Skala erfaßt (1 = 0–15%, 2 = 15–50%, 3 = 50–85%, 4 = 85–100% der Zellen gefärbt). Die Lokalisation der Antigen-Expression auf den Zellen wurde beschrieben als basalmembranseitig (BM), lateral (L), apikal (A) oder diffus (D).

Chirurgisches Forum 1993
f. experim. u. klinische Forschung
Becker/Beger/Hartel (Hrsg.)

Ergebnisse (Tabelle 1)

Der Collagen-Rezeptor VLA $\alpha 2$ war in normaler Kolonmukosa auf weniger als 50% der Zellen schwach, überwiegend basalmembranseitig orientiert nachweisbar. Bei Adenomen zeigten nur einzelne Zellen eine schwache Färbung für VLA $\alpha 2$. Die Expression von VLA $\alpha 2$ beim Kolonkarzinom war heterogen. Während einzelne Zellen eine mäßigstarke, diffuse Expression von VLA $\alpha 2$ zeigten, war das Antigen in etwa 50% der Zellen nicht nachweisbar.

Tabelle 1. Ergebnisse. Expression und Verteilung von VLA-$\alpha 2$ und -$\alpha 6$ in normaler Kolonmukosa, Kolonadenomen und Kolonkarzinomen. Zusammengefaßte Ergebnisse der immunhistologischen Untersuchung

	Antigene (Antikörper)		
Gewebe	VLA-$\alpha 2$ (10-G-11)	VLA-$\alpha 5$ (SAM I)	VLA-$\alpha 6$ (GoH_3)
normale Mukosa n = 15	+ / 2 BM, (D, A)	+ / 3 BM	+ + / 3 BM (D)
Kolonadenom n = 5	+ / 1 BM	– / 4	+ / 3 Dm (BM)
Kolonkarzinom n = 15	+ + / 1 + / 1 – / 2 D	– / 4	+ + / 2 + / 2 D

Die meisten Zellen der normalen Kolonmukosa zeigten eine schwache, basalmembranseitig orientierte Expression des Fibronektinrezeptors VLA $\alpha 5$. In Adenomen und Kolonkarzinomen war VLA 5 nicht nachweisbar.

Der Lamininrezeptor VLA $\alpha 6$ war in normaler Kolonmukosa auf den meisten Zellen mäßig stark und überwiegend basalmembranseitig exprimiert. Die Intensität der Expression von VLA $\alpha 6$ bei Adenomen war schwach mit einer überwiegend diffusen Verteilung des Antigens auf der Zelloberfläche. Kolonkarzinome wiesen eine heterogene, schwache bis mäßig starke Expression von VLA $\alpha 6$ mit diffuser Verteilung des Antigens auf der Zelloberfläche auf.

Diskussion

Die im Vergleich zum Normalgewebe heterogene Expression und diffuse Verteilung von VLA $\alpha 2$ und $\alpha 6$ beim Kolonkarzinom stehen im Einklang mit einer bei malignen Tumoren veränderten Zell-Matrix-Interaktion, welche für die Fähigkeit der Tumorzellen zu invasivem Wachstum von Bedeutung ist. In experimentellen Systemen konnte gezeigt werden [2], daß eine verstärkte Expression von VLA $\alpha 2$ einhergeht mit einem zunehmenden Metastasierungspotential von Tumorzellen. Bei Plattenepithelkarzinomen und Lungentumoren wurde im Vergleich zum Normalgewebe eine verstärkte Expression des Laminin-Rezeptors VLA $\alpha 6$ beschrieben [3]. Experimentelle Befunde beschreiben eine Rolle für VLA $\alpha 6$ bei der Migration von Tumorzellen in der interstitiellen Matrix [4]. Wir fanden eine, im Vergleich zu normaler Kolonmukosa heterogene Expression von VLA $\alpha 2$ und VLA $\alpha 6$ beim Kolonkarzinom. Dabei zeigten Subpopulationen von Tumorzellen eine im Vergleich zur normalen Mukosa verstärkte Expression der Antigene. Womöglich handelt es sich hierbei um Subpopulationen von Tumorzellen mit einem besonders ausgeprägten Potential zur Metastasierung oder zu invasivem Wachstum.

Der Verlust des Fibronektin-Rezeptors VLA $\alpha 5$ ist in anderen Zellsystemen als ein mit der neoplastischen Transformation der Zellen einhergehendes Ereignis beschrieben [5]. Da im Kolon VLA $\alpha 5$ bereits bei Adenomen nicht mehr nachweisbar ist, erscheint der Fibronektin-Rezeptorverlust ein frühes Ereignis in der neoplastischen Transformation von Kolonepithelien zu sein.

Zusammenfassung

Wir untersuchten die Expression von Rezeptoren für Kollagen (VLA $\alpha 2$), Fibronektin (VLA $\alpha 5$) und Laminin (VLA $\alpha 6$) in normaler Kolonmukosa, bei Kolonadenomen sowie bei Kolonkarzinomen. Wir fanden eine im Vergleich zum Normalgewebe heterogene Expression und diffuse Verteilung von VLA $\alpha 2$ und VLA $\alpha 6$ beim Kolonkarzinom. Dies steht im Einklang mit einer bei malignen Tumoren veränderten Zell-Matrix-Interaktion. In experimentellen Zellsystemen wurde über einen Verlust von VLA $\alpha 5$ bei der neoplastischen Transformation von Zellen berichtet. Der Verlust dieses Rezeptors bereits bei Kolonadenomen weist darauf hin, daß es sich hierbei um ein frühes Ereignis in der neoplastischen Transformation von Kolonepithelien handelt.

Summary

The expression of receptors for collagen (VLA$\alpha 2$), fibronectin (VLA$\alpha 5$), and laminin (VLA$\alpha 6$) was investigated immunohistochemically in normal mucosa, adenomas, and carcinomas of the colon. Compared with normal mucosa, VLA$\alpha 2$ and VLA$\alpha 6$ showed heterogenous expression and diffuse distribution in colon carcinoma. This is in accordance with changes in cell matrix interaction of cancer cells. Neoplastic transformation in experimental cell systems has been reported to be accompanied by a loss of VLA$\alpha 5$. As VLA$\alpha 5$ is already lost in colonic adenomas, this seems to be an early event in the neoplastic transformation of colon epithelial cells.

Literatur

1. Weinel RJ, Rosendahl A, Neumann K, Chaloupka B, Erb D, Rothmund M, Santoso S (1992) Expression and function of VLA-α2, -α3, -α5 and -α6-integrin receptors in pancreatic carcinoma. Int J Cancer 52:827–833
2. Chan BMC, Matsuura N, Takada Y, Zetter BR, Hemler ME (1991) In vitro and in vivo consequences of VLA-2 expression on rhabdomyosarcoma cells. Science 251:1600–1602
3. Feldman LF, Shin KC, Natale RB, Todd RF (1991) β1 integrin expression on human small cell lung cancer cells. Cancer Res 51:1065–1070
4. van Waes C, Kozarsky KF, Warren AB et al. (1991) The A9 antigen associated with aggressive human squamous carcinoma is structurally and functionally similar to the newly defined integrin $\alpha 6\beta 4$. Cancer Res 51:2395–2402
5. Schreiner C, Fisher M, Hussein S, Juliano RL (1991) Increased tumorgenicity of fibronectin receptor deficient chinese hamster ovary cell variants. Cancer Res 51:1738–1740

Diese Arbeit wurde gefördert durch die Deutsche Krebshilfe Dr. Mildred-Scheel-Stiftung (W52/89/Ro1).

Dr. med. R.J. Weinel, Klinik für Allgemeinchirurgie, Philipps-Universität Marburg, Baldingerstraße, W-3550 Marburg

Expression des endothelialen Wachstumsfaktors VEGF in Coloncarcinomen

Expression of the Vascular Endothelial Growth Factor in Colonic Carcinoma

M.W. Strik[1], S. Eggstein[1], A. Imdahl[1], H. Weich[2] und B.U. v.Specht[1]

[1]Chirurgische Klinik mit Poliklinik, Universität Freiburg (Direktor: Prof. Dr. E.H. Farthmann)
[2]Institut für Molekulare Zellbiologie, Freiburg

Einleitung

Bösartige Tumoren sind Gewebeneubildungen, die nicht in die Architektur des Gewebes, bzw. des Organs, integriert sind, dem sie ursprünglich entstammen. Da die Versorgung mit Nährstoffen per diffusionem nur maximal auf 0,5 bis 1 mm möglich ist, muß eine Neueinsprossung von Gefäßen erfolgen. Angiogenese ist eine Abfolge von Ereignissen, wie die enzymatische Degradation der Basalmembran von Blutgefäßen, Chemotaxis und die Proliferation endothelialer Zellen [1]. Initiiert wird dieser Ablauf von Wachstumsfaktoren, die einen direkten Effekt auf endotheliale Zellen ausüben. Hierzu zählen acidic und basic FGF, TGF-α, TGF-β und PD-ECGF, die jedoch nur nach dem Zugrundegehen der produzierenden Zelle auf die Endothelzellen wirksam werden können.

Der vor nicht allzu langer Zeit entdeckte "vascular endothelial growth factor" (VEGF), auch Vasculotropin genannt, ist bisher der einzige bekannte endotheliale Wachstumsfaktor, der von intakten Zellen sezerniert werden kann [2]. Seine Zielzellen-Spezifität beschränkt sich auf Gefäßendothelzellen.

Inzwischen kennt man vier verschiedene Formen dieses Wachstumsfaktors, die durch alternatives splicing desselben Gens gebildet werden. Die häufigste Form ist ein Protein aus 165 Aminosäuren (AS), seltener sind ein 121 AS-Protein mit einer Deletion von 44 AS und eine längere Form von 189 AS mit einem 24 AS Insert. Vor wenigen Monaten wurde ein weiterer Clon mit einem 41 AS Insert gegenüber der 165 AS Form identifiziert [3]. Neben der Induktion des endothelialen Zellwachstums und Gefäßproliferation steigert die VEGF Familie auch die Gefäßpermeabilität, wobei die zwei kürzeren Formen einen stärkeren Effekt auf das endotheliale Zellwachstum haben, die längeren Formen vor allem die Gefäßpermeabilität steigern.

Die Expression dieses Wachstumsfaktors könnte ein Prognosefaktor für die Malignität und Metastasierungspotenz eines Tumors darstellen. Ziel der vorliegenden Studie war es, in Coloncarcinom-Zellinien und in Tumorproben von Coloncarcinomen die Expression der mRNA des VEGF nachzuweisen und mit dem jeweiligen Tumorstadium zu korrelieren.

Chirurgisches Forum 1993
f. experim. u. klinische Forschung
Becker/Beger/Hartel (Hrsg.)

Material und Methoden

Aus 6 humanen Kolonkarzinom-Zellinien und insgesamt 22 Kolonkarzinom Proben (OP-Präparate) wurde die Gesamt-RNA extrahiert. Bei den bearbeiteten Tumorproben handelte es sich um Adenokarzinome unterschiedlichen Differenzierungsgrades und Tumorstadiums, vom hochdifferenzierten, lokalisierten bis zum entdifferenzierten, diffus metastasierten Karzinom. Diese wurden durch Random-Primer initiierte Reverse Transcription in cDNA umgeschrieben und anschließend in die Polymerase Kettenreaktion (PCR) eingesetzt. Für diese wurden zwei hochspezifische 20mer Oligonucleotidprimer ausgewählt (5'-TCGGGCCTCCGAAACCATGA-3'; 5'-CCTGGTGAGAGATCTGGTTC-3'). Das erhaltene Amplifikationsgemisch wurde elektrophoretisch aufgetrennt. Zum Nachweis der Spezifität der auf diese Weise erhaltenen DNA-Fragmente wurden diese einer Restriktionsanalyse mit den Restriktionsenzymen BSM I und FOK I unterzogen. Außerdem erfolgte eine Southern-Blot Hybridisierung mit einem spezifischen, internen 20mer Oligonucleotid. Als Positivkontrolle diente RNA der Lymphom-Zellinie U 937, bei der die Expression der VEGF RNA bereits nachgewiesen wurde [4].

Ergebnisse

Die Positivkontrolle (U 937) zeigte nach PCR-Amplifikation Banden von 650 und 520 bp Länge. Diese hatten die geforderten Restriktionsstellen und sowohl die Originalfragmente, als auch die Restriktionsfragmente hybridisierten in der erwarteten Weise mit dem internen Oligonucleotid. Von den untersuchten 6 Zellinien zeigten 5 Zellinien die mRNA des VEGF. Bei 22 untersuchten Tumorproben ließ sie sich in insgesamt 17 Tumoren nachweisen. Auch die Zellinien und die Tumorproben wiesen diese Restriktionen und Hybridisierungen auf. Ein Bezug zwischen der Expression des VEGF und dem Differenzierungsgrad der Tumorproben ließ sich nicht herstellen.

Diskussion

Angiogenese ist ein unabdingbarer Teil der Tumorentwicklung. Durch andere Studien wurde bereits der Zusammenhang der Expression von VEGF und Angiogenese nachgewiesen. Auch fand sich die VEGF mRNA bereits in verschiedenen Sarkomen. Die vorliegenden Daten zeigen, daß VEGF mRNA auch von humanen Kolonkarzinomen exprimiert werden. Dies legt den Schluß nahe, daß dieser Wachstumsfaktor eine wesentliche Rolle in der Entwicklung von Kolonkarzinomen innehat. Vorausgesetzt, daß VEGF erforderlich ist für die Entwicklung eines malignen Tumors, bleibt unklar, warum dieser Wachstumsfaktor nicht in allen Tumorproben und Zellinien gefunden werden konnte. Eine Möglichkeit ist, daß die Tumorzellen den Wachstumsfaktor nur zu bestimmten Zeiten, wenn Angiogenese erforderlich ist, produzieren. So konnten Ferrara et al. zeigen, daß die Formen des VEGF in verschiedenen Zellinien unterschiedlich stark exprimiert werden [2]. Trotzdem sich anhand der verwandten Methoden kein Bezug zwischen der Expression und dem Differenzierungsgrad der Tumoren herstellen ließ, bleibt die Frage, ob ein quantitativer Unterschied in der Expression durch diese Tumoren vorliegt, noch zu beantworten. Dies muß anhand entsprechender Methoden untersucht werden.

Zusammenfassung

Tumorangiogenese ist eine entscheidende Voraussetzung für die Tumorentwicklung ab einem bestimmten Stadium. Der endotheliale Wachstumsfaktor VEGF (Vascular Endothelial Growth Factor) stellt eine Faktorenfamilie dar, die durch alternatives splicing vier Proteine verschiedener Größe bildet. Diese induzieren einerseits das endotheliale Zellwachstum, andererseits steigern sie die Gefäßpermeabilität. Es konnte mittels molekularbiologischer Methoden nachgewiesen werden, daß dieser Wachstumsfaktor auch von Kolonkarzinomzellinien und von soliden Kolonkarzinomen exprimiert wird. Dies legt den Schluß nahe, daß diesem Wachstumsfaktor eine wichtige Bedeutung in der Entwicklung dieses Tumors zukommt.

Summary

Angiogenesis is an important step in the development of a malignant tumor at a certain stage. The vascular endothelial growth factor (VEGF) is a family of growth factors that consists of four different proteins encoded by alternative splicing. These proteins induce endothelial cell growth and increase vascular permeability. Using the polymerase chain reaction we detected VEGF in colonic carcinoma cell lines and in solid colonic carcinomas. We conclude that this growth factor is of importance in the development of colonic carcinomas.

Literatur

1. Ausprunk DH, Folkman J (1977) Migration and proliferation of endothelial cells in preformed and newly formed blood vessels during angiogenesis. Microvasc Res 14:52–65
2. Ferrara N, Henzel HW (1989) Pituitary follicular cells secrete a novel heparin-binding growth factor specific for vascular endothelial cells. Biophys Res Commun 161:851–858
3. Houck KA, Ferrara N, Winer J, Cachianes G, Li B, Leung DW (1991) The vascular endothelial growth factor family: Identification of a fourth molecular species and characterization of alternative splicing of RNA. Mol Endo 5-12:1806–1814
4. Weindel K, Marme D, Weich HA (1992) AIDS-associated Kaposi's sarcoma cells in culture express vascular endothelial growth factor. Biochem Biophys Res Commun 183(3):1167–1174

Dr. M.W. Strik, Klinik für Allgemeine Chirurgie mit Poliklinik, Universität Freiburg, Hugstetterstraße 55, W-7800 Freiburg

Endosonographische Differenzierung eines Rektumadenoms von einem -karzinom mittels computerunterstützter Ultraschallbildanalyse

Endosonographic Differentiation of Rectal Adenoma and Carcinoma with Computer-Assisted Tissue Characterization

Chr. Kuntz[1], F. Glaser[1], M. Fein[2], I. Zuna[2] und Ch. Herfarth[1]

[1]Chirurgische Universitätsklinik Heidelberg (Ärztl. Dir.: Prof. Dr. Ch. Herfarth)
[2]Schwerpunkt 5, DKFZ, Heidelberg (Sprecher: Prof. Dr. W.J. Lorenz)

Zielsetzung

Die endosonographische Differentialdiagnose Rektumadenom und -karzinom ist – im Gegensatz zur Infiltrationstiefenbestimmung von Rektumkarzinomen – umstritten [1, 4]. Histologisch unterscheiden sich kleine Rektumkarzinome von -adenomen durch Infiltration in die Lamina muscularis mucosae. Sonographisch ist diese Infiltration wegen der geringen Dicke der Lamina muscularis mucosae nicht darstellbar. Als Unterscheidungskriterium muß die Echostruktur des Tumors (Homogenität, Echogenität) verwandt werden: Adenome (uT0) erscheinen endosonographisch homogen und echoreich, kleine Karzinome auf dem Boden villöser Adenome (uT1, uT2) dagegen inhomogen echoreich mit echoarmen Arealen [2, 3]. Aufgrund dieser Unterscheidung beträgt die Treffsicherheit des endorektalen Ultraschalls (EUS) zum Nachweis eines Malignomes auf dem Boden eines breitbasigen Adenomes im Krankengut der Chir. Universitätsklinik Heidelberg zwar 91%, ein Zusammenhang zwischen Echostruktur und Histologie wird jedoch von mehreren Autoren bestritten [1, 4].

Ziel dieser Arbeit war es, die Parameter Homogenität und Echogenität durch *c*omputer*u*nterstützte *U*ltraschallbild*a*nalyse (CUUA) zu objektivieren und für die endosonographische Unterscheidbarkeit zwischen Rektumadenomen und -karzinomen zu evaluieren.

Patienten und Methode

Bei 39 Patienten mit einem Durchschnittsalter von 66 Jahren wurden eine endorektale Sonographie in Steinschnittlage mit einem 7,0 MHz Schallkopf (Type 1846, Bruel & Kjaer) durchgeführt. Die präoperative Diagnostik hatte bei 17 Patienten ein Adenom und bei 22 Patienten ein Karzinom ergeben. Alle endosonographischen Untersuchungen erfolgten unter Standardbedingungen: Amplitudenauflösung 8 bit entsprechend 256 Grauwertstufen, Focuslänge 2–5 cm, konstante "time gain compensation (tgc)". Das charakteristischste Ultraschallbild jedes Tumors wurde digital erfaßt und mittels

Chirurgisches Forum 1993
f. experim. u. klinische Forschung
Becker/Beger/Hartel (Hrsg.)

eines "frame grabbers" auf einer Diskette gespeichert. Die Analyse dieser B-scan Bilder erfolgte auf einer Hewlett-Packard-"workstation". Auf ihr konnte jedes Bild erneut aufgerufen und eine "region of interest (ROI)" in den sonographisch typischsten Tumorbezirk gelegt werden. In dieser ROI wurden 72 statistische Parameter, die alle auf den Grauwert, die Makro- und Mikrostruktur eines Ultraschallbildes Bezug nehmen, berechnet. Deren Signifikanz, ein Adenom von einem Karzinom zu trennen, wurde mit dem t-Test und die besten Parameter mit einer anschließenden Diskriminanzanalyse errechnet (Abb. 1). Danach erfolgte mit diesen Parametern die Reklassifizierung aller Tumoren sowie der Vergleich mit dem postoperativen histologischen Ergebnis.

Ergebnisse

Die postoperative histologische Diagnose der 39 untersuchten Tumoren ergab 8 Adenome und 31 Karzinome. Bei 9 Patienten mit der präoperativ bioptisch gesicherten Diagnose eines Adenoms lagen in 4 Fällen ein pT1 und 5mal ein pT2 Karzinom vor. Nach der Diskriminanzanalyse ließ sich die Anzahl der 72 Parameter bezüglich Grauwert, Mikro- und Makrostruktur auf 2 hochsignifikant trennende reduzieren (mittlerer Grauwert, Verlaufslängenzuteilung). Die Reklassifizierung der Tumoren mit diesen 2

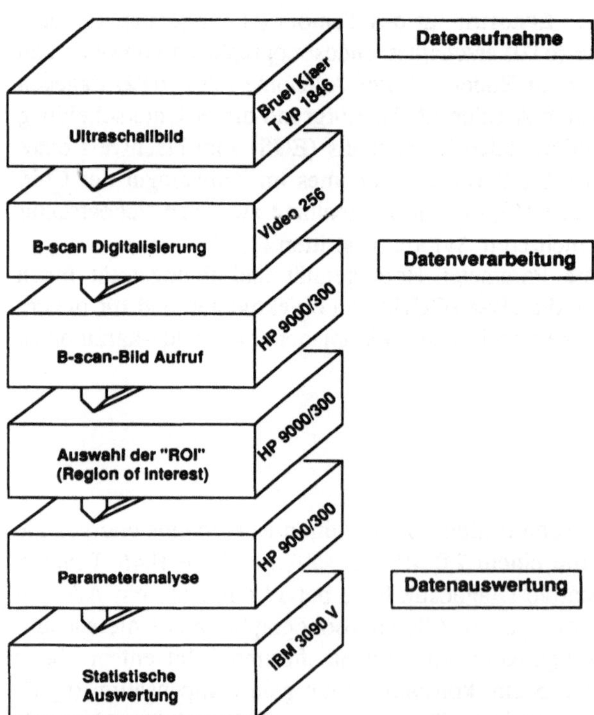

Abb. 1. Schematische Darstellung der computerunterstützten Ultraschallbildanalyse

Parametern erkannte 7 der 8 Adenome und 28 von 31 Karzinomen richtig (Tabelle 1). Alle 9 Tumoren, die präoperativ bioptisch als Adenom und postoperativ als Karzinom eingestuft waren, wurden mittels CUUA als Karzinom richtig erkannt. Die Sensitivität der CUUA zur Erkennung eines Karzinoms anhand der Echostruktur beträgt 90%, die Spezifität 89%, der positive Vorhersagewert 97% und der negative 70%.

Tabelle 1. Vergleich der präoperativen Ergebnisse mittels CUUA (computerunterstützte Ultraschallbildanalyse) mit dem postoperativ histologischen Resultat (pT0, pT1/2)

	n	Adenom (CUUA)	Karzinom (CUUA)
pT 0	8	7	1
pT 1/2	31	3	28

Zusammenfassung

Die computerunterstützte Ultraschallbildanalyse von Rektumtumoren kann auf dem Boden der unterschiedlichen Echostruktur ein Adenom von einem Karzinom mit einer Treffgenauigkeit von 90% unterscheiden. Mit ihrer Hilfe ist außerdem möglich, ein Malignom auf dem Boden eines breitbasigen Adenoms mit einer Genauigkeit von 94% zu bestimmen. Die vorgestellten Ergebnisse bestätigen somit 1. die These der sonographischen Unterscheidbarkeit und 2. die untersucherabhängigen klinischen Ergebnisse des endorektalen Ultraschalls in der Unterscheidung eines Rektumadenoms von einem Rektumkarzinom.

Summary

Endosonographic computer-assisted tissue characterization (CATC) of rectal tumors is able to differentiate between rectal adenoma and carcinoma because of the echostructure alone. The accuracy rate is 90%. With CATC it is also possible to recognize a malignant tumor in a sessile adenoma with an accuracy rate of 94%. The presented data confirm the thesis of endosonographic differentiation and the clinical results depending on who performs the examination obtained by endorectal ultrasound in differentiating between a rectal adenoma and carcinoma.

Literatur

1. Buess G, Heintz A, Frank K, Strunk H, Kuntz Chr, Junginger Th (1989) Neue endosonographische Untersuchungstechnik zur Verbesserung der Beurteilung kleiner Rektumtumoren. Chirurg 60:851–855
2. Glaser F, Kleikamp G, Schlag P, Möller P, Herfarth Ch (1989) Die Endosonographie in der präoperativen Beurteilung rektaler Tumoren. Chirurg 60:856–861
3. Strunk H, Heintz A, Frank K, Kuntz Chr, Buess G, Braunstein S (1990) Endosonographisches Staging von Rektumtumoren. Fortsch Röntg 153:373–378

4. Tio T, Weijers O, Hulsmann F, Jonkers L, Collins E, Sie LH, Tytgat GNJ (1992) Endosonography of colorectal disease. Endoscopy 24:309–314

Dr. Chr. Kuntz, Chirurgische Universitätsklinik, Im Neuenheimer Feld 110, W-6900 Heidelberg

Allgemeine Stressreaktion bei konventioneller und bei laparoskopischer Cholezystektomie

General Stress Response to Conventional and Laparoscopic Cholecystectomy

F. Glaser[1], Ch. Kuntz[1], F. Klee[2], H.J. Buhr[1], G. Sannwald[1] und Ch. Herfarth[1]

[1]Chirurgische Universitätsklinik (Direktor: Prof. Dr. Ch. Herfarth), Heidelberg
[2]Krankenhaus Salem (Chefarzt: Prof. Dr. S. Wysocki), Heidelberg

Zielsetzung

Seit Einführung der laparoskopischen Cholezystektomie (LCE) 1987 sind nur drei prospektive, *randomisierte* Studien [1, 2, 3] publiziert worden, mit dem Ziel, klinische Ergebnisse der konventionellen Cholezystektomie (KCE) mit der LCE zu vergleichen. Weitere randomisierte Vergleiche zwischen LCE und KCE scheitern an den bekannten Vorteilen der LCE und dem hierdurch ausgelösten gezielten Operationswunsch der Patienten [4]. Ziel dieser prospektiven, nicht randomisierten, aber kontrollierten Studie war es, über einen Vergleich der humoralen Stressreaktion eine objektive Bewertung der LCE zu erreichen.

Patienten und Methodik

Es wurden, vom 1. Mai bis 1. September 1992, in einem Krankenhaus der Regelversorgung, alle Patienten erfaßt, die wegen symptomatischer Cholezystolithiasis zur elektiven Cholezystektomie anstanden. In die Studie aufgenommen wurden Patienten im Alter von 30 bis 70 Jahren. Ausgeschlossen wurden Patienten mit akuter Cholezystitis, Pankreatitis, Choledocholithiasis oder malignen Erkrankungen. Die Auswahlkriterien zur KCE und die Therapie der Patienten wurden durch das Studienprotokoll nicht verändert, sondern durch Ärzte vorgenommen, die nicht mit der Studie befaßt waren. Indikationen zur KCE waren 1.) Voroperationen im Oberbauch, 2.) Verdacht auf Choledocholithiasis, 3.) verdickte Gallenblasenwand und 4.) Zystikussteine.

Zu folgenden Zeitpunkten wurde Blut abgenommen: am Tag vor der Operation, zwischen 18 und 19 Uhr und eine Stunde präoperativ (Ausgangswerte), während der

Chirurgisches Forum 1993
f. experim. u. klinische Forschung
Becker/Beger/Hartel (Hrsg.)

Präparation des Ductus cysticus, sechs Stunden nach Operationsende und am ersten und zweiten postoperativen Tag, zwischen 7.00 Uhr und 7.30 Uhr.

Die Konzentrationen von freiem Adrenalin und freiem Noradrenalin wurden chromatographisch (HPLC), adrenokortikotropes Hormon (ACTH) und gesamtes Cortisol durch Radioimmunoassay, Glukose enzymatisch und die Interleukine im Serum enzymimmunometrisch bestimmt. Die Reaktion jedes einzelnen Patienten wurde aus den intra- und postoperativen Konzentrationsänderungen der Variablen, im Vergleich zu den präoperativen Ausgangswerten, berechnet. Auf diese Weise wurde der Effekt von unterschiedlichen Ausgangswerten in den Gruppen reduziert.

Die KCE erfolgte über einen Rippenbogenrandschnitt; intraoperativ wurde routinemäßig cholangiographiert. Die LCE entsprach weitgehend der von Dubois beschriebenen Technik.

Der Stichprobenumfang wurde prospektiv so berechnet, daß (bei einem α-Fehler von 5%) eine Teststärke von 80% vorlag. Die Mittelwerte der Variablen wurden zu den vier oben genannten Zeitpunkten nach Beginn der Operation miteinander verglichen. Die Berechnung von Signifikanzen erfolgte mit dem U-Test nach Wilcoxon und dem Fisher-Exact-Test. Darüberhinaus wurde, wegen multiplen Testen zu jedem Vergleichszeitpunkt, das Signifikanzniveau nach Bonferroni-Holm korrigiert. Werte sind als Mittelwerte (S.E.M.) angegeben.

Ergebnisse

60 Patienten wurden gemäß den prospektiven Kriterien in die Studie aufgenommen. 40 Patienten wurden laparoskopisch operiert, 18 konventionell, 2 mußten nachträglich wegen intraoperativer Choledochusrevision ausgeschlossen werden. Präoperativ ergaben sich keine signifikanten Unterschiede zwischen den Gruppen bezüglich Geschlechterverteilung, Alter, Körpergewicht, Körpergröße, Dauer der biliären Symptome, Diagnosen, Medikation, allgemeinen Labordaten sowie den Ausgangswerten der überwachten Stressparameter. Die perioperative Behandlung war für beide Gruppen statistisch nicht unterschiedlich in Bezug auf Prämedikation, perioperative Medikamenten- und Antibiotikagabe, Dauer des Eingriffs und Operationszeitpunkt. Signifikant reduziert waren in der LCE Gruppe die intraoperative Thiopentaldosis pro Patient (315(10)mg versus 357(17)mg; $p = 0,04$), die Droperidoldosis pro Patient (9,1(0,5)mg versus 11,2(0,7)mg; $p = 0,01$) und die Pancuroniumdosis pro Patient (5,2(0,2)mg versus 6,2(0,3)mg; $p = 0,01$). Postoperativ war die Anzahl der Morphinäquivalente je Patient nach LCE signifikant niedriger als bei der KCE (4,1(1,2) versus 15,3(2,4); $p < 0,001$). Die signifikant kleineren intra- und postoperativen Konzentrationsänderungen der humoralen Stressparameter nach LCE sind in Tabelle 1 aufgeführt. Intraoperativ und sechs Stunden postoperativ zeigten sich nach LCE niedrigere Konzentrationsänderungen von Interleukin-1 beta (IL-1β) und Interleukin-6 (IL-6), was ebenso wie die geringeren IL-6 Anstiege am ersten und zweiten postoperativen Tag nach LCE für ein geringeres Gewebetrauma durch die LCE spricht. Am ersten postoperativen Tag besteht zudem ein signifikant reduzierter Katecholamin- und Glukoseanstieg nach LCE. Dieses Verhalten der Katecholamine paßt gut zu den, im zeitlichen Verlauf nachlassenden, Auswirkungen der signifikant höheren Anästhetikadosis,

die die Patienten in der KCE Gruppe erhielten. Der höhere Glukoseanstieg nach KCE im Vergleich zur LCE kann als Folge des gleichsinnigen Katecholaminverhaltens interpretiert werden. Am zweiten postoperativen Tag sind die Noradrenalinveränderungen in der KCE Gruppe noch immer ausgeprägter als nach LCE. Bei den intra- und postoperativen ACTH-, Cortisol- und IL-8-Konzentrationen zeigten sich ebenfalls reduzierte Anstiege in der Gruppe der LCE, die Unterschiede zwischen den Gruppen waren jedoch nicht signifikant.

Tabelle 1. Signifikant unterschiedliche intra- und postoperative Konzentrationsänderungen humoraler Stressparameter nach laparoskopischer (LCE) und konventioneller Cholezystektomie (KCE). Angegeben sind die Mittelwerte (S.E.M.). * Die p-Werte wurden mit dem U-Test nach Wilcoxon ermittelt

	Intraoperativ		
Variable	LCE (n=40)	KCE (n=18)	p-Wert*
Interleukin-1β (ng/l)	−0,10 (0,05)	1,21 (0,81)	< 0,001
	6 h nach Operationsende		
Variable	LCE (n=40)	KCE (n=18)	p-Wert*
Interleukin-1β (ng/l)	0,02 (0,07)	0,63 (0,20)	< 0,01
Interleukin-6 (ng/l)	16,8 (7,7)	29,0 (8,3)	< 0,01
	Erster postoperativer Tag		
Variable	LCE (n=40)	KCE (n=18)	p-Wert*
Adrenalin (nmol/l)	0,05 (0,03)	0,26 (0,07)	< 0,01
Noradrenalin (nmol/l)	0,57 (0,21)	1,40 (0,39)	< 0,01
Glukose (mg/dl)	14 (3)	40 (8)	< 0,01
Interleukin-6 (ng/l)	17,8 (3,8)	52,8 (13,3)	< 0,01
	Zweiter postoperativer Tag		
Variable	LCE (n=40)	KCE (n=18)	p-Wert*
Noradrenalin (nmol/l)	0,55 (0,17)	1,59 (0,27)	< 0,001
Interleukin-6 (ng/l)	6,4 (1,8)	28,4 (6,4)	< 0,001

Zusammenfassung

In einer prospektiven, kontrollierten Studie wurden zur Objektivierung des perioperativen Stresses nach LCE und KCE biochemische Stressparameter im Blut von Patienten bestimmt, die wegen symptomatischer Cholezystolithiasis operiert wurden. Ausschlußkriterien waren die akute Cholezystitis, Choledocholithiasis, Pankreatitis und Malignome. Verglichen wurden die Parameter von 40 laparoskopisch und 18 konventionell operierten Patienten. Beide Gruppen waren bezüglich Patientencharakteristika und perioperativen Therapiedaten vergleichbar. Sowohl intra- als auch postoperativ konnte eine reduzierte Stressantwort in der LCE Gruppe, signifikant für IL-1β, IL-6, Adrenalin, Noradrenalin und Glukose, nachgewiesen werden.

Summary

To objectify perioperative stress response to laparoscopic (LCE) and conventional cholecystectomy (CCE), a prospective, controlled trial was planned and biochemical stress parameters were measured in the blood of patients who had undergone elective surgery for symptomatic cholecystolithiasis. Patients with acute cholecystitis, pancreatitis, choledocholithiasis, or malignant disease were excluded from the study. Values from 40 patients after LCE and from 18 patients after CCE were compared. Both groups had statistically similar patient characteristics and perioperative care. The LCE group showed a significantly lower stress response with respect to interleukin-1β, interleukin-6, epinephrine, norepinephrine, and glucose.

Literatur

1. Pennincks F, Aerts R, Kerremans R, Konincks PR (1991) Laparoscopic cholecystektomy: some advantages or just an artifice of new technology? HPB-Surg 3:291–295
2. Frazee RC, Roberts JW, Okeson GC, Symmonds REm Snyder SK, Hendricks JC, Smith RW (1991) Open versus laparoscopic cholecystectomy. A comparison of postoperative pulmonary function. Ann Surg 213:651–654
3. Kunz R, Orth K, Vogel J, Steinacker JM, Meitinger A, Brückner U, Beger HG (1992) Laparoskopische Cholezystektomie versus Mini-Lap-Cholezystektomie. Ergebnisse einer prospektiven, randomisierten Studie. Chirurg 63:291–295
4. Neugebauer E, Troidl H, Spangenberger W, Dietrich A, Lefering R, and the Cholecystectomy Study Group (1991) Conventional versus laparoscopic cholecystectomy and the randomized controlled trial. Br J Surg 78:150–154

Dr. F. Glaser, Chirurgische Universitätsklinik Heidelberg, Im Neuenheimer Feld 110, W-6900 Heidelberg 1

Beurteilung eines Gewebetraumas mit Hilfe von Aktivierungsstrukturen auf der Zellmembran von Leukozyten. Ein Vergleich: Laparoskopische Chirurgie versus konventionelle Chirurgie

Evaluation of Tissue Trauma with the Help of Activation Markers on the Cell Membrane of Leukocytes. A Comparison: Laparoscopic Versus Conventional Cholecystectomy

D. Decker[1], M. Schöndorf[2], P. Decker[1], F. Bidlingmaier[2], A. Hirner[1] und A. von Rücker[2]

[1]Chirurgische Klinik der Universität Bonn (Direktor: Prof. Dr. A. Hirner)
[2]Institut für Klinische Biochemie der Universität Bonn (Direktor: Prof. Dr. F. Bidlingmaier)

Einleitung

Die Schwere eines Gewebetraumas oder elektiven chirurgischen Eingriffs wird auch heute im wesentlichen durch den klinischen Verlauf beurteilt. Zusätzlich bedient man sich bei der klinischen Evaluierung eines Traumas unterschiedlicher *Score*-Schemen [1]. Bei der biochemischen Quantifizierung eines Traumas gibt es bisher nur sehr unspezifische Meßgrößen (z.B. CRP, Coeruloplasmin oder Neopterin). Die Cytokine (z.B. TNF, IL-1, IL-6, IL-8), von denen man sich anfangs eine bessere Quantifizierung traumatischer Vorgänge erhofft hat, zeigen ebenfalls keine befriedigende Korrelation [2, 3].

Auf der Suche nach besser quantifizierbaren Meßgrößen wurden im folgenden biochemisch-immunologische Aktivierungsprozesse untersucht, die sich auf der Membranoberfläche von Leukozyten abspielen. Bei einem Gewebetrauma werden durch humorale (Immun-)Mediatoren diverse Proteinstrukturen auf der Zellmembran verändert exprimiert. Sie können als Maß für die primäre Entzündungsphase verwendet werden und scheinen mit der Schwere der Gewebeschädigung zu korrelieren.

Operationsverfahren – Patientenauswahl

Bei den folgenden Untersuchungen wurden prospektiv 12 laparoskopisch und 10 konventionell durchgeführte Cholezystektomien untersucht. Diese Operationsverfahren unterscheiden sich deutlich in ihrer Klinik und schienen deshalb besonders gut geeignet, biochemische Trauma-Meßgrößen zu überprüfen. In die Studie aufgenommen wurden Patienten im Alter zwischen 35 und 55 Jahren mit einer Cholelithiasis der Klassifikation 0–II nach McSherry. Die Einteilung der Patienten in die einzelnen Gruppen erfolgte nach eingehender Aufklärung.

Chirurgisches Forum 1993
f. experim. u. klinische Forschung
Becker/Beger/Hartel (Hrsg.)

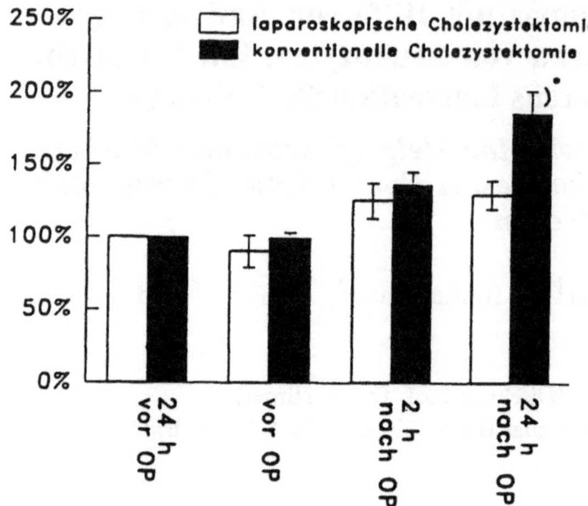

Abb. 1. Veränderungen der Leukozytenzahl in Abhängigkeit vom Zeitpunkt der Blutentnahme bei Cholezystektomien. Zur besseren Vergleichbarkeit wurden die Werte, die 24 h vor der Operation gewonnen wurden, gleich 100% gesetzt. Die Balken geben den Mittelwert ± SEM an.)*: $p < 0{,}05$ beim Vergleich der unterschiedlichen Operationsverfahren

Methodik

Die Blutentnahmen für die durchflußzytometrische Bestimmung ausgewählter Aktivierungsmarker auf Leukozyten erfolgten 24 h vor Operation, unmittelbar vor Hautschnitt, 2 h nach Hautschnitt und 24 h nach der Operation. Die zellulären Aktivierungsmerkmale wurden mit Hilfe fluoreszierender monoklonaler Antikörper im Durchflußzytometer (Becton Dickinson, FACScan) bestimmt [4].

Ergebnisse

Ausgehend von der Gesamtleukozytenzahl wurden mit Hilfe der Streulichtanalyse des Durchflußzytometers zunächst die drei Zellpopulationen Lymphozyten, Monozyten und Granulozyten dargestellt. Abbildung 1 zeigt, daß bei den konventionell operierten Patienten erst 24 h nach dem chirurgischen Eingriff eine signifikante Erhöhung der Leukozytenzahl von ca. 45% gegenüber laparoskopisch operierten Patienten auftritt. Lymphozyten, Monozyten und Granulozyten verhielten sich untereinander ähnlich wie die Leukozyten. Im Rahmen eines Screenings wurde zunächst auf zellulären Subsets die Aktivierungsmerkmale bestimmt.

Bei den Lymphozyten erfolgte eine Subtypisierung, die auch sonst routinemäßig für die Immunstatusbestimmung eines Patienten durchgeführt wird. Sie beinhaltet die Bestimmung der NK-Zellen ($CD3^-/CD16^+$ + $CD56^+$), der B-Lymphozyten ($CD3^-/CD19^+$), der T-Lymphozyten ($CD3^+$) sowie deren Subpopulationen, die T-Helfer Zellen ($CD3^+/CD4^+$) und T-Suppressor Zellen ($CD3^+/CD8^+$). Auf den NK-Zellen wurden die Zelloberflächenmerkmale CD11b (der Komplement-Rezeptor CR-

3), CD25 (der Interleukin-2-Rezeptor), CD54 (das Adhäsionsmolekül ICAM-1) und CD71 (der Transferrin-Rezeptor) untersucht. Auf B- und T-Lymphozyten wurden neben CD25, CD54 und CD71 auch CD30 (das Aktivierungsantigen Ki-1), HLA-DR (der Haupthistokompatibilitätskomplex II) und CD56 (das Adhäsionsmolekül NCAM) untersucht. *Bei den Monozyten* wurden neben den schon erwähnten Membraneigenschaften CD11b, CD25, CD71 und HLA-DR auch CD14 (der LPS-Rezeptor) und CD16 (der Antikörper-Fc-Rezeptor) untersucht. Das Aktivierungsantigen CD67 wurde *auf Granulozyten* bestimmt.

Mittels der Multivarianz-Regressionsanalyse wurden aus den vorliegenden Daten die drei Aktivierungsmerkmale bestimmt, die am besten den Unterschied zwischen laparoskopischer und konventioneller Cholezystektomie widerspiegelten. Dies waren der Interleukin-2-Rezeptor CD25, das Aktivierungsantigen KI-1 CD30 und der Transferrin-Rezeptor CD71. Die Zell-Subpopulation, auf der sich diese Zellmerkmale am prägnantesten veränderten, waren T-Lymphozyten ($CD3^+$).

2 h nach dem Hautschnitt war der IL-2 Rezeptor CD25 bei konventioneller Operationstechnik 1,6fach höher als bei laparoskopischen Operationen. Das Aktivierungsantigen CD30 zeigte einen vierfach höheren Anstieg bei konventionellen Cholezystektomien. Beim Transferrin-Rezeptor CD71 wurde ein 2fach höherer Anstieg beobachtet.

Zur besseren Anschaulichkeit wurde ein Aktivierungsindex eingeführt, der die Daten eines Patienten zu einem Zeitpunkt miteinander multipliziert [Aktivierungsindex = f(CD25) × f(CD30) × f(CD71)]. Abbildung 2 zeigt, daß mit diesem Index sehr leicht zwischen den verschiedenen Operationsverfahren unterschieden werden kann. Auftretende methodische Schwankungen können besser ausgeglichen werden. 24 h nach der Operation haben sich die Aktivierungsvorgänge weitgehend normalisiert, wobei nach konventionellen Operationen eine noch höhere Restaktivität zu beobachten ist. Dies ist vermutlich Ausdruck des geringeren Traumas bei laparoskopischen Operationen.

Diskussion

Die laparoskopische Cholezystektomie ist in den letzten Jahren zum Standardoperationsverfahren geworden. In der Literatur gibt es mehrere Erfahrungsberichte, die zeigen, daß laparoskopische Operationstechniken mit geringeren Schmerzen, geringeren subjektiven Beschwerden des Patienten, meist besserem kosmetischen Ergebnis, verkürztem stationären Aufenthalt, früherer Rückkehr des Patienten zur normalen körperlichen Aktivität und geringem Trauma verbunden sind. Zur Beurteilung des Traumas wurde das klinische Bild bzw. der klinische Verlauf herangezogen (vgl. Überblick in [1]).

Untersuchungen mehrerer Arbeitsgruppen haben in den vergangenen Jahren gezeigt, daß sich während eines Gewebetraumas die Dichte von Cytokin-Rezeptoren (TNF, IL-1, IL-2), Komplement-Rezeptoren (CR3: CD11b), Antikörper-Rezeptoren (Fc-Anteil: CD64), Adhäsionsmoleküle (ICAM1: CD54), Transferrin-Rezeptoren (CD71) und andere Moleküle (CD64, CD66) rasch auf Leukozyten verändern können [3, 5–7]. Ähnlich konnte gezeigt werden, daß durch ein Gewebetrauma sich z.B. der quantitative Anteil an Cd4-Helfer-T-Lymphozyten, CD8-Suppressor-T-Lymphozyten, CD19-B-Lymphozyten und HLA-DR-Monozyten verändern [6, 7]. Wir konnten bei unseren

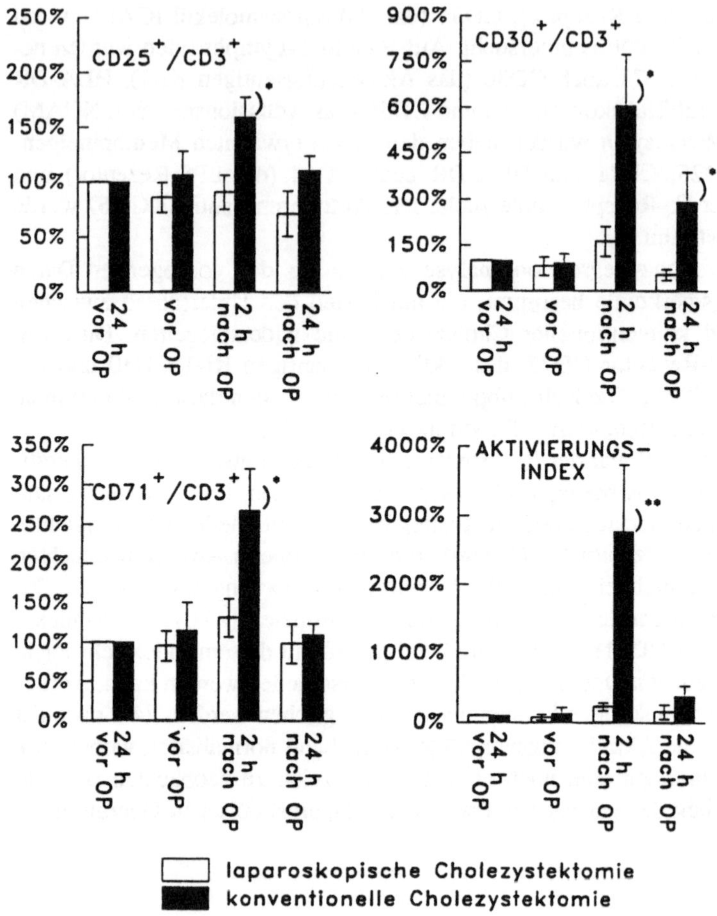

Abb. 2. Veränderungen bei T-Lymphozyten-($CD3^+$)-Subsets mit den Oberflächenmerkmalen CD25, CD30 und CD71 in Abhängigkeit vom Zeitpunkt der Blutentnahme bei Cholezystektomien. Der Aktivierungsindex faßt die Veränderungen der gezeigten Oberflächenmerkmale eines Patienten durch Multiplikation zusammen (vgl. Text). Die Zellzahlen, die 24 h vor der Operation gewonnen wurden, wurden gleich 100% gesetzt. Die Balken geben den Mittelwert ± SEM an.)*: $p < 0{,}05$;)**: $p < 0{,}01$ beim Vergleich der unterschiedlichen Operationsverfahren

Untersuchungen zeigen, daß sich die Expression mehrerer Aktivierungsmerkmale auf Lymphozyten, Monozyten und Granulozyten nach der Cholezystektomie verändern. Mit Hilfe eines Aktivierungsindexes konnte zwischen dem laparoskopischen und traditionellen Operationsverfahren während der frühen Entzündungsphase hoch signifikant ($p < 0{,}01$) unterschieden werden. Obwohl unsere Ergebnisse an einer kleinen Patientenzahl ermittelt wurden und als vorläufig zu betrachten sind, lassen sie erkennen, daß Zellaktivierungsprozesse als Maß für die primäre Entzündungsphase verwendet und zur Beurteilung der Schwere einer Gewebeschädigung nach operativem Eingriff genutzt werden können.

Zusammenfassung

Ziel der vorliegenden Untersuchung war festzustellen, ob die laparoskopische Cholezystektomie biochemisch gegenüber der konventionellen Cholezystektomie als die schonendere Operationsmethode identifiziert werden kann. Hierzu wurden Aktivierungsmarker auf der Membranoberfläche von Leukozyten mit Hilfe fluoreszierender monoklonaler Antikörper und der Durchflußzytometrie prä-, intra- und postoperativ untersucht. Erste Ergebnisse bei 12 laparoskopischen und 10 konventionellen Cholezystektomien zeigen, daß drei Aktivierungsmarker auf Leukozyten (der IL-2 Rezeptor CD25, das Aktivierungs-Antigen CD30 und der Transferrin-Rezeptor CD71) nach konventionellem Eingriff signifikant erhöht sind. Oberflächenantigene auf Leukozyten scheinen nach diesen ersten Ergebnissen geeignet, verschiedene Operationsverfahren biochemisch zu quantifizieren.

Summary

The purpose of this study was to determine whether laparoscopic cholecystectomy, in comparison to conventional surgery, is the optimal treatment from a biochemical standpoint. Therefore, activation markers on the surface of leukocytes were measured before, during, and after surgery with the help of fluorescent monoclonal antibodies and flow cytometry. Preliminary results with 12 laparoscopic and ten conventional cholecystectomies show that three activation markers (CD25, the IL-2 receptor; CD30, the activation antigen Ki-1; and CD71, the transferrin receptor) are significantly increased after conventional surgery. Surface antigens on leukocytes may be capable of quantifying various surgical procedures according to these preliminary results.

Literatur

1. Barkun JS, Barkun AN, Sampalis JS, Fried G, Taylor B, Wexler MJ, Goresky CA, Meakins JL (1992) Randomised controlled trial of laparoscopic versus mini cholecystectomy. Lancet 340:1116–1119
2. Faist E, Ninnemann J, Green D (eds) Immune consequences of trauma, shock and sepsis. Springer, Berlin (1989)
3. Rubin LA, Nelson DL (1990) The soluble interleukin-2 receptor: Biology, function, and clinical application. Ann. Intern. Med. 113:619–627
4. Keren DF (1989) Flow cytometry in clinical diagnosis. ASCP Press, Chicago
5. Fasano MB, Cousart S, Neal S, McCall CE (1991) Increased expression of the interleukin 1 receptor on blood neutrophils of humans with the sepsis syndrome. J Clin Invest 88:1452–1459
6. Werfel T, Witter W, Götze O (1991) CD11b and CD11c antigens are rapidly increased on human natural killer cells upon activation. J Immunol 146:2423–2427
7. Wilmore DW (1991) Homeostasis: Bodily changes in trauma and surgery. In: Sabiston DC Jr (ed) Textbook of Surgery. Saunders, Philadelphia, pp 19–33

Dr. D. Decker, Chirurgische Universitätsklinik Bonn, Sigmund-Freud-Straße 25, W-5300 Bonn

Peri- und postoperative Mediatorenfreisetzung: laparoskopische versus laparotomische Cholecystektomie

Peri- and Postoperative Mediator Release: Laparoscopic Versus Laparotomic Cholecystectomy

F. Schütze, C. Osswald, D. Berger, R. Kunz und H.G. Beger

Abteilung für Allgemeinchirurgie, Universität Ulm

Einleitung

Nach laparoskopischen Operationen zeigen Patienten deutlich verbesserte Rekonvaleszenzen im Vergleich zu konventionellen Verfahren. An 42 cholecystektomierten Patienten wurde in einer randomisierten Studie untersucht, ob der unterschiedliche klinische Verlauf sich anhand von peri- und postoperativen Akutphase- und anderen Laborparametern objektivieren läßt.

Funktion der Akutphasenproteine ist die Elimination infektiöser Partikel bzw. der Abbau zerstörter Gewebsanteile durch Induktion des Immun-, Komplement-, Gerinnungs-, Fibrinolyse- und Hormonsystems. Die Interleukine, insbesondere das Interleukin-6 (IL-6) sowie der Tumornekrosefaktor (TNF), werden bei jedem Gewebstrauma, entsprechend des Umfanges, freigesetzt und bieten damit die Möglichkeit der Graduierung eines Traumas [1, 2]. Endotoxin im Gastrointestinaltrakt als größtem Reservoir ist ein wichtiger Trigger der gesamten Mediatoren und könnte so als Auslöser der Akut-Phase-Reaktion eine Rolle spielen [3].

Patienten und Methoden

Von 42 Patienten (w 29, m 13, Durchschnittsalter 44,9 Jahre) wurden 22 laparoskopisch (LCCE) und 20 konventionell mit Minilaparotomie (MCCE) cholecystektomiert. Beide Gruppen unterscheiden sich nicht signifikant in Alter, Geschlecht, Größe, Gewicht und Risikofaktoren (Tabelle 1). Bestimmt wurden IL-6 und TNF (Quantikine-IL-6- bzw. TNF-Immuno-Assay der Fa. R & D Systems, Minneapolis) via Enzymimmunoassay sowie das Endotoxin mittels chromogen modifiziertem Limulus-Amöbozyten-Lysat-Test [4], außerdem folgende Laborparameter durch Standardmethoden: Das C-reaktive Protein, Leukozyten und Thrombozyten, Leberwerte (GOT, GPT, AP und gGT) und der Sauerstoffpartialdruck.

Venöse Blutentnahmen erfolgten direkt nach Narkoseeinleitung, perioperativ 20 minütig bis zur Hautnaht, postoperativ stündlich über 3 h, die arterielle Blutgasanalyse erfolgte 1 Tag präoperativ und am 1. postoperativen Tag.

Chirurgisches Forum 1993
f. experim. u. klinische Forschung
Becker/Beger/Hartel (Hrsg.)

Tabelle 1. Patientendaten

OP-Typ	Pat. Zahl	Männl.	Weibl.	Alter		Größe		Gewicht	
				(∅)	Median	(∅)	Median	(∅)	Median
LCCE	22	7	15	45,1	47,5	169,5	169	76,36	75,5
MCCE	20	6	14	44,8	45	166	164,5	72,2	70,5

Ergebnisse

Ein signifikanter Anstieg des Endotoxins war im LCCE-Kollektiv nicht nachweisbar, während sich in der MCCE-Gruppe bei allen intra- und postoperativ ermittelten Endotoxinplasmaspiegeln signifikante Anstiege im Vergleich zum präoperativen Ausgangswert (p zwischen 0,0003 und 0,016) fanden. Parallel hierzu kommt es zu einem signifikanten perioperativen Anstieg (p 0,00068 bis 0,026) des IL-6 in der Laparotomiegruppe.

Tabelle 2. Plasmakonzentrationen der ermittelten Akutphaseparameter

Parameter	LCCE	p	MCCE	p
Endotoxin (EU/ml):				
präoperativ	0,01	0	0,01	0
1. intra-OP 20'	0,01	n.s.	0,045	0,016
2. intra-OP 40'	0,01	n.s.	0,07	0,00051
3. intra-OP 60'	0,01	n.s.	0,045	0,0093
intra-OP-Max	0,02	n.s.	0,085	0,0003
post-OP-Max	0,01	n.s.	0,07	0,00051
IL-6 (pg/ml)::				
präoperativ	9	0	9	0
1. intra-OP 20'	9	n.s.	9,5	0,026
2. intra-OP 40'	9	n.s.	15	0,0076
3. intra-OP 60'	9	n.s.	9	n.s.
intra-OP-Max	9,5	n.s.	15	0,0055
post-OP-Max	7,5	0,0013	20	0,00068
TNF (pg/ml)::				
präoperativ	5	0	4	0
1. intra-OP 20'	5	n.s.	4	n.s.
2. intra-OP 40'	5	n.s.	4	n.s.
3. intra-OP 60'	5	n.s.	4	n.s.
intra-OP-Max	8	0,004	5	0,0055
post-OP-Max	5	n.s.	6	0,01

Statistische Überprüfung nach Wilcoxon-Ranks-Test im Sinne einer longitudinalen Unterscheidung (n.s. = nicht signifikant im Vergleich zum präoperativen Ausgangswert). Präoperativer Wert nach Narkoseeinleitung entnommen

Bei den laparoskopisch Cholecystektomierten läßt sich eine Erhöhung der IL-6 Plasmakonzentration erst postoperativ nachweisen, während sich intraoperativ keine signifikante Veränderung zum Vorbefund ergibt. Keine signifikanten Veränderungen zeigte der perioperative TNF-Spiegel in beiden Kollektiven, wobei in beiden der intra-OP Maximalwert signifikant erhöht war (Tabelle 2).

Das CRP zeigte erwartungsgemäß in den ersten 6 h keinen Anstieg in beiden Kollektiven, Ausgangs- und Kontrollwerte lagen im Normbereich ohne signifikante Veränderungen.

Bei den Routineparametern fanden sich keine signifikanten Veränderungen für die gGT, GPT und die Thrombozytenzahl. Signifikante Anstiege der Leukozytenzahl waren in beiden Kollektiven nachweisbar, die laparotomierten stiegen signifikant mehr als die laparoskopierten Patienten ($p = 0{,}04$). Ein ähnliches Verhalten ließ sich für GOT und Ap nachweisen (Tabelle 3). Der pO_2 zeigte in beiden Kollektiven einen Abfall ohne signifikante Differenz.

Tabelle 3

Parameter	LCCE	MCCE
Leukozyten		
präoperativ	6800	6800
postoperativ	9750	10400
GOT (U/ml)		
präoperativ	9	9
postoperativ	16	22
AP (U/ml)		
präoperativ	111	95,5
postoperativ	105	100

Die hier am Beispiel der Cholecystektomie erbrachten Ergebnisse beweisen die geringere Gewebstraumatisierung durch laparoskopische Verfahren. Die intra- bzw. postoperative Endotoxinämie im Sinne einer frühzeitigen Translokation aus dem Gastrointestinaltrakt läßt sich im Gegensatz zur MCCE nicht nachweisen. Die zeitlich verzögerte IL-6-Freisetzung fällt ebenfalls deutlich geringer aus. Die reduzierte Mediatorfreisetzung verringert den peri- und postoperativen Streß im Gesamtorganismus.

Zusammenfassung

Laparoskopische Operationsverfahren, hier am Beispiel der Cholecystektomie im Vergleich zur Mini-Lap-Cholecystektomie, führen zu einer deutlich geringeren Akutphasereaktion und damit zur Verringerung des operativen Traumas. Am Beispiel des Interleukin-6, des Endotoxins und des TNF konnte die deutlich reduzierte Mediatorfreisezung bei endoskopischen Operationsverfahren demonstriert werden.

Summary

Reduced acute-phase reaction in laparoscopic operations compared with routine procedures, in this case cholecystectomy, was demonstrated by measuring interleukin-6, tumor necrosis factor (TNF) and endotoxin in patients undergoing gallbladder surgery.

Literatur

1. Ninnemann JL (1987) Trauma, sepsis and the immune response. J Burn Care Rehabil 8:462–468
2. Ramadori G, Meyer zum Büschenfelde KH (1990) Die Akut-Phase-Reaktion und ihre Mediatoren, Teil II: Tumor-Nekrose-Faktor alpha und Interleukin-6. Z Gastroenterol 28:14–21
3. Berger D, Beger HG (1991) Neue Aspekte zur Pathogenese und Behandlung der Sepsis und des septischen Schocks. Chirurg 62:783–788
4. Berger D, Schleich S, Seidelmann M, Beger HG (1991) Demonstration of an interaction between transferrin and lipopolysaccharide - An in vivo study. Eur Surg Res 23:309–316

F. Schütze, Abteilung Allgemeinchirurgie, Universität Ulm, Steinhövelstraße 9, W-7900 Ulm

Experimentelle laparoskopische Rektumresektion
Experimental Laparoscopic Resection of the Rectum

P. Metzger[1], E.M. Gamal[1], J. Kiss[1], R. Imre[1], I. Furka[2] und I. Mikó[2]

[1]Chirurgische Klinik der Ärztlichen Fortbildungsuniversität, Budapest, Ungarn (Direktor: Prof. Dr. J. Kiss)
[2]Institut für Experimentelle Chirurgie, Medizinische Universität, Debrecen, Ungarn (Direktor: Prof. Dr. I. Furka)

Mit der weltweiten Verbreitung der laparoskopischen Technik durch die laparoskopische Appendektomie [1] und Cholezystektomie [2] wurde die Idee geboren, auch weitere Eingriffe laparoskopisch durchzuführen. Die wichtigste Voraussetzung, dies zu erfüllen, wäre die Klärung der technischen Details dieser Operationen. Die herkömmlichen Operationen am Magen, Oesophagus, Dickdarm und Rektum sind weitgehend standardisiert und werden mit guten Früh- und Spätergebnissen durchgeführt. Um dasselbe zu erreichen, muß die laparoskopische Technik noch verfeinert und gesichert werden. Die experimentelle Arbeit bei Tierversuchen bietet sich als ideale Möglichkeit an, um die laparoskopische Handhabung zu erlernen und die neuen laparoskopischen Instrumente in die alltägliche Arbeit einzuführen. Durch die Entwicklung laparoskopisch einsetzbarer Klammernahtgeräte sind nun auch resezierende und rekonstruktive Eingriffe an intestinalen Hohlorganen der laparoskopischen Methode zugänglich gemacht worden. Nach der Einführung der laparoskopischen Technik in der Magenchirurgie [3, 4, 5] sind auch die ersten Ergebnisse von laparoskopischen Eingriffen am Dickdarm erschienen [6, 7, 8, 9]. Ohne ausführliche Erprobung einer neuen Operationsmethode am Tiermodell wird keine solche Operationstechnik beim Menschen angewendet.

Operationstechnik

Die Tiere (Hunde) wurden in Vollnarkose und Rückenlagerung unter sterilen Bedingungen laparoskopiert. Es wurden 5 Zugänge gesetzt: ein 10-mm-Trokar im Nabelbereich für die Optik, zwei 12-mm-Trokare im rechten und linken Mittelbauch für die Anwendung der Klammernahtgeräte und Arbeitsinstrumente, wie Schere, Nadelhalter, Faßzangen usw., sowie zwei 5-mm-Trokare beidseits im Unterbauch für die Assistenzinstrumente. Der Operationstisch wurde in 30gradige Trendelenburg'sche Position gebracht.

Zunächst wurden das Sigma und Rektum mit zwei Babcock'schen Klemmen positioniert und die Mesosigmae an der Kante der Aorta durchtrennt. Die Arteria mesenterica inferior wurde stammnahe zwischen den Clips durchtrennt. Das Rektum wurde bis zur geplanten Resektionslinie freigelegt. Zur Präparation der Mesosigmae wur-

Chirurgisches Forum 1993
f. experim. u. klinische Forschung
Becker/Beger/Hartel (Hrsg.)

den Schere und Elektrokoagulationshaken angewendet. Das Klammernahtgerät (Endo GIA-3, Fa. USSC.) wurde über einen 12-mm-Trokar im rechten Mittelbauch eingeführt und das Rektum zwischen die beiden Branchen des Klammergeräts plaziert. Nach dem Schließen setzt das Gerät je drei Klammernahtreihen zu beiden Seiten der Resektionslinie; es besitzt jedoch nur eine Länge von 3 cm, weshalb zwei Applikationen erforderlich waren, um das Rektum vollständig zu durchtrennen. Das freigelegte Rektum wurde durch eine linksseitige Mini-Laparotomie aus der Bauchhöhle entfernt und reseziert. Nach der Resektion wurde der Kopf eines EEA Staplers extrakorporal in den Dickdarm plaziert und mit einer Tabaksbeutelnaht befestigt. Nachdem der Dickdarm mit dem Kopf des Klammergeräts in die Bauchhöhle zurückgelegt worden war, wurde die Bauchdecke zugenäht und das Pneumoperitoneum wiederhergestellt. Das EEA Klammernahtgerät wurde unter Bildkontrolle durch das Rektum eingeführt und mit dem Spieß durch die Klammernahtreihen plaziert. Nach der Entfernung des Spiesses wurden die zwei Teile des Geräts mit Hilfe einer Babcock-Klemme zusammengeführt und so eine End-zu-End Kolorektostomie intrakorporal hergestellt. Nach der abschließenden Spülung des Abdomens wurden keine Drainagen gelegt.

Der weitere Verlauf gestaltete sich in drei Fällen bei primärer Wundheilung problemlos, die Tiere tolerierten den Kostaufbau gut, mit normaler Darmpassage. Bei einem Hund hat ein im Rektum liegendes Knochenteil die Anastomose perforiert und so eine Anastomoseninsuffizienz verursacht.

Diskussion

Die hohe Akzeptanz der minimal-invasiven Chirurgie, sowohl bei Patienten als auch bei Chirurgen, hat sich in den vergangenen Jahren am Beispiel der laparoskopischen Appendektomie und Cholezystektomie gezeigt. Die allgemein anerkannten Vorteile (kürzerer Krankenhausaufenthalt, geringere Schmerzhaftigkeit, weniger Wundkomplikationen, raschere Rekonvaleszenz) könnten auch bei erweiterten laparoskopischen Eingriffen zum Vorteil der Patienten sein. Trotzdem hat sich diese Technik in der Rektum-Chirurgie noch nicht einwandfrei durchgesetzt [8].

Die laparoskopische Technik ist weitgehend noch nicht standardisiert. Es wird heftig diskutiert, ob die intrakorporale Anastomosentechnik sicher genug sei oder nicht [8]. Es ist auch fraglich, ob die via Laparoskop durchgeführte Lymphdissektion der bei offenem Bauch durchgeführten gleichwertig ist.

Die laparoskopischen Instrumente müssen noch weiterentwickelt werden. Die zur Zeit noch relativ teueren Instrumente begrenzen auch die experimentellen Möglichkeiten.

Die laparoskopische Anwendung der sogenannten Tristapler Technik hat sich in unseren Tierexperimenten als technisch möglich erwiesen, obwohl eine Endo-GIA mit 6 cm langen Klammernahtreihen mehr Sicherheit bei der Anwendung geben würde.

Die technische Durchführbarkeit und der funktionelle Heilerfolg der laparoskopischen Rektumresektion wurden anhand der tierexperimentellen Ergebnisse bewiesen. Die Entwicklung der Operationstechnik steht noch am Beginn: sie bedarf noch der Erprobung und Verbesserung. Um die Komplikationsrate so niedrig wie möglich zu halten und gute klinische Ergebnisse zu erreichen, sollte die Weiterentwicklung dieser

Technik in spezialisierten Zentren erfolgen. Erst die so standardisierte Technik sollte sich unter den praktizierenden Chirurgen verbreiten.

Zusammenfassung

Dank der Entwicklung laparoskopisch einsetzbarer Klammernahtgeräte und der zunehmenden Erfahrung mit der neuen Operationstechnik wurden Eingriffe am Rektum auch möglich. Es wird über vier, an Hunden durchgeführte, laparoskopische Rektumresektionen berichtet. Die Operationstechnik wird beschrieben. Sie erfolgt nach den aus der offenen Abdominalchirurgie bekannten Regeln. Diese Technik erfordert neben einem aufwendigen Instrumentarium auch einen in der laparoskopischen Technik erfahrenen Chirurgen. Obwohl diese Methode in erfahrenen Händen sicher durchzuführen ist, ist der Schwierigkeitsgrad jedoch nicht zu unterschätzen. Wo ausreichende klinische Erfahrungen noch nicht vorliegen, kann diese Technik nicht zur allgemeinen Anwendung empfohlen werden.

Summary

Due to the development of laparoscopic suture techniques and an increasing experience in operation procedures, laparoscopic operation of rectal tumors has become possible. This study reports four laparoscopic resections of the rectum in dogs. The operation technique is described, whereby the technique used was similar to those techniques used in open abdominal surgery. The described technique is only possible with sophisticated instruments and a surgeon experienced in laparoscopic techniques. Although under these circumstances the operation can be performed safely, the difficulties should not be underestimated. So far, since clinical experience is still lacking for this technique, it should not be used generally for rectum operations.

Literatur

1. Götz F, Pier A, Bacher C (1991) Die laparoskopische Appendektomie: Indikationen, Technik und Ergebnisse bei 653 Patienten. Chirurg 62:253–256
2. Périssat J, Collet D, Belliard R, Dost C, Bikandou G: Die laparoskopische Cholecystektomie: Operationstechnik und Ergebnisse der ersten 100 Operationen. Chirurg 61:723–728
3. Shapiro S, Gordon L, Dayhovsky L, Grundfest W, Chandra M (1991) Development of laparoscopic anterior seromyotomy and right posterior truncal vagotomy for ulcer prophylaxis. J Laparoendosc Surg 1:277
4. Schönleben K, Brune I, Günther M (1991) Rekonstruktive laparoskopische Eingriffe an Dünndarm und Magen. Chir Praxis 44:303–310
5. Brune IB, Schönleben K (1992) Laparoskopische Seit-zu-Seit Gastrojejunostomie. Chirurg 63:577–580
6. Beart RW (1992) Laparoscopic-assisted colon resection. In: Cormann LM (ed) Colon and rectal surgery. Lippincott, Philadelphia, 1993, pp 552–564
7. Coopermann A, Katz V, Zimmon D, Botero G (1991) Laparoscopic colon resection: a case report. J Laparoendoscopic Surg 1:221

8. Jacobs, Verdeja JC, Goldstein HS (1991) Minimally invasive colon resection (laparoscopic colectomy). Surg Laparosc Endosc 1:144
9. Cooperman AM, Zucker KA (1991) Laparoscopic guided intestinal surgery. In: Zucker KA (ed) Surgical Laparoscopy, pp 304–310

P. Metzger, Chirurgische Klinik, Ärztliche Fortbildungsuniversität, Budapest, Ungarn

Verbesserter in vivo Nachweis neuroendokriner Dünndarmtumoren und ihrer Metastasen mit einem 111-Indium markierten Somatostatin Analogon

Improved In Vivo Localization of Neuroendocrine Tumors of the Midgut and Their Metastases with ^{111}In Labeled Analog of Somatostatin

G. Schürmann[1], U. Raeth[1], M. Böhme[1], U. Dörr[2], H. Bihl[2] und H. Buhr[1]

[1]Chirurgische und Medizinische Universitätsklinik, Universität Heidelberg
[2]Klinik für Nuklearmedizin, Katharinenhospital, Stuttgart

Einleitung

Artdiagnostik und Lokalisation neuroendokriner (NE) Tumoren des Gastrointestinaltraktes sind insbesondere im Fall fehlender Hormonaktivität schwierig. NE-Tumoren verfügen über Bindungsstellen mit hoher Affinität für Somatostatin (SMS) [1], und durch exogen zugeführtes SMS kann die Hormonproduktion und das Wachstum dieser Tumoren supprimiert werden. Der SMS-Rezeptorreichtum von NE-Tumoren kann unter Verwendung von synthetischem SMS als Radioligand für die in vivo Tumorlokalisationsdiagnostik genutzt werden. Dies gelang zunächst mit dem 123-Jod markierten SMS-Analogon Tyr-3-Octreotide (Code-Nr. 204-090, Firma Sandoz, Basel) [2, 3]. Der klinische Einsatz von 123-Jod Octreotide war durch hohe Kosten, kurze Halbwertszeit und technische Probleme beschränkt. Die Weiterentwicklung dieser Methode führte zur Synthese eines neuen SMS-Analogons [DTPA-D-Phe1]-Octreotide ("Pentatreotide") [4], das eine vereinfachte Markierung mit 111-Indium erlaubt. Im folgenden berichten wir über unsere Ergebnisse beim klinischen Einsatz der SMS-Rezeptorszintigraphie mit dem neuen Analogon.

Methoden

Patienten: Wir untersuchten 15 Patienten mit nachgewiesenen neuroendokrinen Dünndarm-Tumoren folgender ursprünglicher Lokalisation des Primärtumors: Ileum n = 11, Appendix n = 1, Colon ascendens n = 3. Bei 6 von 15 Patienten war der Primärtumor zum Zeitpunkt der Szintigraphie in situ (im folgenden als "Kollektiv

Chirurgisches Forum 1993
f. experim. u. klinische Forschung
Becker/Beger/Hartel (Hrsg.)

PT" (Primärtumor) bezeichnet). Bei 3 Patienten dieses Kollektivs lagen zusätzlich Lebermetastasen vor. Bei 9 anderen Patienten war der Primärtumor ursprünglich R0-reseziert worden (im folgenden als "Kollektiv oPT" (ohne Primärtumor) bezeichnet). Intraabdominelle Metastasen wurden jedoch im weiteren Verlauf dieser Patienten durch Ultraschall, CT oder Relaparotomie in 6 Fällen diagnostiziert; diese Tumormanifestationen bestanden auch zum Zeitpunkt der Szintigraphie. 9 Patienten hatten ein Karzinoidsyndrom. Eine bei diesen Patienten durchgeführte SMS-Therapie wurde 12 bis 36 h vor der Szintigraphie abgesetzt.

Rezeptorszintigraphie: Als Radioligand wurde das mit 111-Indium markierte [DTPA-D-Phe1]-Octreotide ("Pentatreotide"; SDZ 215-811, OctreoscanR111, Firma Mallinckrodt, Holland) verwendet. Es wurden im Durchschnitt 125 MBq 111-Indium Pentatreotide als i.v.-Bolus injiziert. Plantare Teil- und Ganzkörperaufnahmen erfolgten 30 min, 4 h und 24 h post injectionem.

Ergebnisse

Kollektiv PT. Die szintigraphische Darstellung des Primärtumors gelang bei 5 von 6 Patienten. Abhängig von der Tumorgröße zeigte sich eine homogene bis mäßig inhomogene Tracerakkumulation. Der Primärtumor, der szintigraphisch nicht zur Darstellung kam, war histologisch-bioptisch ein hochproliferativer entdifferenzierter Tumor mit mesenterialer Infiltration. Lebermetastasen, die bei 3 Patienten bestanden, waren in allen 3 Fällen szintigraphisch positiv. Außerdem kamen im Kollektiv PT bei 2 Patienten Mediastinalmetastasen und bei 3 weiteren Patienten Wirbelsäulenmetastasen zur Darstellung, ohne daß diese Befunde vorher bekannt waren. 2 Fälle von BWS/LWS Metastasen sind derzeit noch ungesichert, in allen anderen Fällen konnten die Befunde bestätigt werden.

Kollektiv oPT. Lebermetastasen, die bei 6 von 9 Patienten, deren Primärtumor zum Zeitpunkt der Untersuchung reseziert war, bekannt waren, kamen in allen 6 Fällen zur Darstellung. Intestinal fanden wir erwartungsgemäß keine suspekten Anreicherungen, jedoch bestand in 2 Fällen der Verdacht auf abdominelle Lymphknotenmetastasen (nicht gesichert).

Diskussion

Mit der Anwendung von 111-Indium Pentatreotide (OctroscanR111) konnten wesentliche Nachteile des früheren Radioliganden 123-Jod Tyr-3 Octreotide überwunden werden. Neben einer längeren Halbwertszeit des neuen Nuklids (2,8 d versus 13 h) gilt dies insbesondere für eine günstigere Biodistribution. Unter Octreotide mit vorwiegend biliärer Ausscheidung kam es zu einem deutlichen hepatobiliären Aktivitätsanstieg, der Lebermetastasen kaschieren konnte. Von Pentatreotide werden innerhalb von 24 h 80–90% der applizierten Dosis renal eliminiert [5], wodurch auch der in Spätaufnahmen erkennbare Aktivitätsanstieg im Colonrahmen (infolge biliärer Elimination) deutlich reduziert wurde. Für die jetzt noch bestehende Hintergrundaktivität in der Milz sind möglicherweise lienale SMS-Rezeptoren verantwortlich. Kürzlich radioimmunographisch nachgewiesene SMS-Rezeptoren in anderen Organen (gastrointestinale Mucosa, gastrointestinale Lymphfollikel) scheinen hingegen als Hintergrund in der SMS-Ganzkörperrezeptorszintigraphie keine Rolle zu spielen. Verlängerte Halbwertszeit und günstigere Biodistribution gegenüber dem früher verwendeten 123-Jod-Tyr-3-Octreotide ermöglichen eine Darstellung SMS-rezeptorpositiver Tumoren noch nach 24 h, wenn die Hintergrundaktivität durch renale Ausscheidung von Pentatreotide minimal ist.

Auch die klinischen Ergebnisse haben sich im Vergleich der eigenen Serien durch die Anwendung von Pentatreotide verbessert. In der jetzigen Serie hatte die Rezeptorszintigraphie eine Sensitivität von 85%. Alle Lebermetastasen waren szintigraphisch positiv. Nicht zur Darstellung kamen lediglich ein entdifferenzierter Primärtumor und eine miliare Peritonealkarzinose. Demgegenüber waren in der früheren 123-Jod Octreotide Serie Lebermetastasen nur bei 10 von 14 Patienten szintigraphisch positiv und auch Knochenmarksmetastasen kamen in 2 Fällen nicht zur Darstellung [4]. Joseph und Mitarb. [6] ermittelten bei 38 Patienten mit teilweise metastasierenden gastroenteropankreatischen NE-Tumoren SMS-rezeptorszintigraphisch (Pentatreotide) eine Nachweisrate von 91% bei Gastrinomen (n = 11), 73% bei "Karzinoiden" (n = 11), 81% bei hormoninaktiven Tumoren (n = 14) und 50% bei Insulinomen (n = 2). Anderen Autoren gelang die rezeptorszintigraphische Darstellung von Gastrinomen nur in vereinzelten Fällen (P. Hammond, Royal Postgraduate Medical School, Hammersmith Hospital, London; persönliche Mitteilung).

Es wurde mit der SMS-Rezeptorszintigraphie auch die Hoffnung verbunden, daß ein Szintigraphieergebnis den Erfolg einer SMS-Therapie voraussagt, da beide Methoden u.a. von Status und Dichte der SMS-Rezeptoren eines NE-Tumors abhängen. Hierfür bestand in unserer früheren Serie keine eindeutige Evidenz. Fünf Patienten mit positiver Rezeptorszintigraphie sprachen auf die SMS-Therapie an, 4 weitere Patienten zeigten ein diskrepantes Verhalten zwischen SMS-Szintigraphie und SMS-Therapie [4]. Trautmann berichtete über 12 Patienten mit positiver SMS-Szintigraphie und fehlendem Ansprechen auf eine SMS-Therapie und über 2 weitere Patienten mit umgekehrtem Verhalten. Eine mögliche Erklärung hierfür wäre, daß durch beide Verfahren unterschiedliche SMS-Rezeptoren besetzt werden. Bisher wurden 3 SMS-Rezeptorsubtypen beschrieben, und es sind wahrscheinlich mindestens 2 weitere Subtypen vorhanden. Die klinische Konsequenz sollte derzeit lauten, die Indikation zur SMS-Therapie nicht von der szintigraphischen Darstellbarkeit der Tumoren abhängig zu machen.

Die 111-Indium Pentatreotide-Rezeptorszintigraphie ist somit auf Grund hoher Sensitivität und verbesserter Durchführbarkeit eine sinnvolle Methode zur in vivo Lokalisation neuroendokriner Tumoren. Ihr klinischer Einsatz ist insbesondere bei Verdacht auf das Vorliegen von neuroendokrinen Tumoren und im Follow-up dieser Patienten indiziert.

Zusammenfassung

Neuroendokrine Tumoren können in vitro und in vivo lokalisiert werden, indem man ihre Bindungsstellen für Somatostatin radiographisch markiert. In der vorliegenden Studie wurden 15 Patienten mit neuroendokrinen Midgut-Tumoren szintigraphisch untersucht unter Verwendung des 111-Indium markierten Somatostatin Analogons [DTPA-D-Phe1]-Octreotide (OctreoscanR111, Mallinckrodt, Holland). Bei 5 von 6 Patienten mit Primärtumoren in situ gelang die rezeptorszintigraphische Darstellung. Alle 9 Fälle von Lebermetastasen waren szintigraphisch positiv. Sieben weitere Tumormanifestationen wurden durch die Szintigraphie erstmals entdeckt (Mediastinum n = 2, Wirbelsäule n = 3, Abdomen n = 2) mit nachfolgender Bestätigung in bisher 4 Fällen. Verlängerte Halbwertszeit (2,8 d) und günstigere Biodistribution gegenüber dem früher verwendeten 123-Jod-Tyr-3-Octreotide ermöglichen eine Darstellung SMS-rezeptorpositiver Tumoren noch nach 24 h, wenn die Hintergrundaktivität durch renale Ausscheidung von [111-Indium-DTPA-D-Phe1]-Octreotide minimal ist.

Summary

Neuroendocrine tumors may be localized in vivo by labeling their binding sites for somatostatin with radioligands. Fifteen patients with neuroendocrine tumors of the midgut were investigated scintigraphically by means of a ^{111}In-radiolabeled synthetic analog of somatostatin [DPTA-D-Phe1]-octreotide (OctreoscanR111, Mallinckrodt, Holland). In five of six patients with primary tumors in situ and in all nine patients with liver metastases, the tumors were localized correctly. Seven other tumor localizations, so far unknown, were discovered by receptor scintigraphy (mediastinum, n = 2; vertebral column, n = 3; abdomen, n = 2). Because of its longer half-life (2.8 days) and an altered biodistribution compared with the older ^{123}I-octreotide, [^{111}In-DTPA-D-Phe1]octreotide allows somatostatin receptor-bearing tumors to be visualized after 24 h, when interfering background radioactivity is minimized by renal clearance.

Literatur

1. Reubi JC, Kvols L, Krenning E, Lamberts SW (1990) Distribution of somatostatin receptors in normal and tumor tissue. Metabolism [Suppl 2] 39:78–81
2. Lamberts SW, Bakker WH, Reubi JC, Krenning EP (1990) Somatostatin-receptor imaging in the localization of endocrine tumors. N Engl J med 323:1246–49
3. Schürmann G, Raeth U, Böhme W, Wiedenmann B, Bihl H, Buhr H (1992) In vivo Nachweis neuroendokriner Tumoren und ihrer Metastasen mit einem 123-Jod markierten Somatostatin Analogon. Langenbecks Arch Chir [Suppl] Chir Forum '92:1–4
4. Bakker WH, Krenning EP, Reubi JC, Breeman WA, Setyono-Han BB, de Jong M, Kooij PP, van Hagen PM, Marbach P, Visser TJ, Pless J, Lamberts SW (1991) In vivo application of [111-Indium-DTPA-D-PHE1]-octreotide for detection of somatostatin receptor-positive tumors in rats. Life Sciences 19:1593–1601
5. Krennung EP, Bakker WH, Kooij PP, Breeman WA, Oei HY, de Jong M, Reubi JC, Visser TJ, Bruns C, Kwekkeboom DJ, Reijs AE, van Hagen PM, Koper JW, Lamberts SW (1992) Somatostatin receptor scintigraphy with indium-111-DTPA-D-Phe-1-Octreotide in

man: metabolism, dosimetry and comparison with iodine-123-Tyr-3-Octreotide. J Nucl Med 33:652–658

6. Joseph K, Stapp J, Reinecke J, Hoffken H, Benning R, Neuhaus C, Trautmann ME, Schwerk WB, Arnold R (1992) Rezeptorszintigraphie bei endokrinen gastroenteropankreatischen Tumoren. Dtsch Med Wochenschr 117:1025–1028

Dr. G. Schürmann, Chirurgische Universitätsklinik, Kirschnerstraße 1,
W-6900 Heidelberg

Zur Bedeutung von C-neu und p53 bei endokrinen Tumoren

The Significance of C-neu and p53 in Endocrine Tumors

D. Simon, P.E. Goretzki und H.D. Röher

Klinik für Allgenmein- und Unfallchirurgie, Heinrich-Heine-Universität Düsseldorf

Einleitung

Die Dignitätsbeurteilung und prognostische Einschätzung von endokrinen Tumoren ist schwierig. Gefäß- und Kapselinvasion oder Kernpolymorphie sind bei endokrinen Tumoren keine sicheren Malignitätskriterien. Neben patientenbezogenen Daten (Alter, Geschlecht, etc.) ist daher die Beurteilung der Tumorbiologie von großer Bedeutung. Hier bieten Onkogene und Tumorsuppressorgene einen möglichen Ansatz zur Lösung des Problems. Sie kodieren Proteine, die das Wachstum der Zelle regulieren. Mutationelle Aktivierung von G-Proteinen (ras und GSP) spielen in der Entwicklung von endokrinen Tumoren eine wesentliche Rolle [1, 2].

Neben TSH ist z.B. der epidermale Wachstumsfaktor (EGF) von Bedeutung für die Proliferationsaktivität von Thyreozyten; EGF-Rezeptoren (EGF-R) sind an endokrinen Tumoren nachgewiesen. Das menschliche *neu*-Onkogen (HER2 und erB-2) weist eine starke Homologie zum EGF-R auf, allerdings ist der Ligand des Membranrezeptors (p185) nicht bekannt. Bei Mammakarzinomen korreliert die Expression von *neu*-Onkogenen mit einer schlechten Prognose und *neu* gilt als prädiktiver Faktor für das Auftreten einer hämatogenen Metastasierung. Die Expression von *neu* und EGF-R ist heterogen verteilt und unabhängig voneinander [3].

P53 ist die häufigste genetische Veränderung in menschlichen Tumoren. Bei endokrinen Tumoren ist seine Bedeutung noch nicht hinreichend geklärt. Problematisch ist hierbei die Tatsache, daß es im Gegensatz zu anderen Onkogenen eine Vielzahl von Mutationen (n = 93) gibt; je nach Mutante entsteht ein inaktiviertes oder aber aktiviertes (gain of function) Protein. Bei Colonkarzinomen ist eine Kooperation von p53 mit ras-Mutationen bekannt [4]. Der p53-Mutation kommt möglicherweise eine Bedeutung in der Entdifferenzierung von malignen Tumoren zu [5].

Ziel dieser Untersuchung war es daher, die Bedeutung von p53 und *neu* für die Entwicklung endokriner Tumoren zu ermitteln.

Material und Methode

Unmittelbar postoperativ in flüssigem Stickstoff schockgefrorenes Tumorgewebe von 133 Tumoren wurden untersucht. Es handelte sich hierbei um 52 differenzierte Schilddrüsenkarzinome (DTC), 5 Strumen, 24 Nebennierenrindentumoren (NNR), 7 NNR-Karzinome, 19 Phäochromozytome, 7 gesunde Nebennieren, 5 Karzinoide,

Chirurgisches Forum 1993
f. experim. u. klinische Forschung
Becker/Beger/Hartel (Hrsg.)

3 Insulinome, 4 Epithelkörperchenadenome und 7 nicht endokrine Tumoren (Leber/Ösophagus zur Kontrolle). 5 μm dicke Kryostatschnitte wurden immunhistochemisch mit der Avidin-Biotin-Komplex (ABC) Methode aufgearbeitet. Für *neu* wurde ein monoklonaler Antikörper eingesetzt, für p53 wurde ein Panel von verschiedenen Antikörpern (pAb 240,421,1801,DO7,CM1) verwendet. Die Inkubation mit dem Primärantikörper dauerte 18 h bei 4°C, als Chromogen wurde Diaminobenzpyridin (DAB) genommen. Als Kontrollgewebe dienten Fibroblasten (negativ) und Leber-, Ösophagus- und Mammakarzinome (positiv).

Ergebnisse

Von den 133 Geweben waren insgesamt 10 endokrine Tumoren (7,5%) (6 DTC, 1 NNR-Ca, 2 Karzinoide, 1 Phäochromozytom) positiv für p53. 9 der 10 Tumoren waren maligne (9/64; 14%). Eine positive Reaktion war bei Antikörper pAb 1801 und CM1 nachweisbar. Die Färbung war nukleär und heterogen im Tumor verteilt.

C-*neu* fand sich in 22 Tumorgeweben (22/133; 16,5%), davon waren 16 DTCs, 3 Phäochromozytome, 2 NNR-Karzinome und 1 NNR-Adenom. Alle benignen Tumoren bis auf 1 großes (10 × 6 × 3 cm) hormoninaktives NNR-Adenom und 2 Phäochromozytome waren negativ für *neu*, positiv hingegen waren 19 maligne endokrine Tumoren (19/64; 29,7%). Die Färbung war membranbetont und ebenfalls heterogen verteilt.

Diskussion

An Schilddrüsenkarzinomzellinien (FTC-133) konnte der EGF-Rezeptor (EGF-R) und die proliferative Aktivität von EGF nachgewiesen werden. Das *neu*-Onkogen besitzt eine 50%ige Homologie zum EGF-R und eine über 80%ige in der Tyrosinkinase-Domäne. Dies weist darauf hin, daß *neu* (erbB-2) einen Rezeptor für einen noch nicht bekannten Wachstumsfaktor kodiert. In 22 endokrinen Tumoren konnte eine Überexpression von *neu* festgestellt werden, davon 19mal in malignen Tumoren. Bei den 3 benignen Tumoren handelte es sich um 2 Phäochromozytome und 1 hormoninaktiven NNR-Tumor. Alle 3 Tumoren waren relativ groß (< 5 cm), so daß eine Malignität, die mit herkömmlichen Kriterien nicht immer eindeutig festzulegen ist, nicht ausgeschlossen ist. Die beiden positiven NNR-Karzinome waren fortgeschrittene Tumoren mit bereits bestehender Metastasierung. Bei den Schilddrüsenkarzinomen handelte es sich dagegen um 5 papilläre, 5 follikuläre und 6 medulläre Karzinome mit teilweise guter Differenzierung und unterschiedlichen Tumorstadien. Die Überexpression von *neu* alleine ergab an den hier untersuchten endokrinen Tumoren im Gegensatz zu Untersuchungen am Mammakarzinom keine Korrelation zur Prognose. Es konnte lediglich eine heterogene Verteilung im Tumorgewebe nachgewiesen werden, was auf eine mögliche Heterogenität des Tumors hinweist.

G-Proteinmutationen spielen eine zentrale Rolle in der Entstehung und Propagation von Tumoren. In Schilddrüsentumoren sind $G_s$alpha (GSP) und ras (p21), welches im weiteren Sinne zur G-Protein Superfamilie zu zählen ist, von besonderer Bedeutung.

Die mutationelle Aktivierung von GSP und ras führt zur konstitutionellen Aktivierung des Rezeptors und damit zur Proliferation. Von Colonkarzinomen ist eine Kooperation von ras mit mutiertem p53 bekannt. Auf Grund der verlängerten Halbwertszeit von mutiertem p53 eignet es sich besonders zum immunhistochemischen Nachweis. Immunhistochemisch waren 10 von insgesamt 119 endokrinen Tumoren (8,4%) positiv für p53. Bei einem Tumor handelte es sich um ein Phäochromozytom. So lag bei 9/64 (14%) der malignen endokrinen Tumoren eine Überexpression von p53 vor. 6 dieser 9 Tumoren zeigten ein fortgeschrittenes Tumorstadium mit Fernmetastasen, 3 Tumoren waren wenig differenziert (G3). P53 Mutationen sind somit in endokrinen Tumoren selten, scheinen jedoch ein Indikator für eine schlechte Prognose bei endokrinen Tumoren darzustellen.

Der Vergleich von p53 positiven und *neu* positiven Tumoren zeigt eine Überexpression *beider* Proteine in 3 Tumoren (3/64 mal.Tu; 4,7%); alle 3 Tumoren sind Schilddrüsenkarzinome mit einem geringen Differenzierungsgrad (G3).

Zusammenfassung

In einem Drittel der endokrinen Tumoren findet sich eine Überexpression von *neu*-Onkogen, was seine Rolle bei der Entstehung endokriner Tumoren unterstreicht. P53 dagegen ist eine eher selten auftretende Mutation in endokrinen Tumoren (7,5%) und korreliert mit einer schlechten Prognose der Tumoren. Neun von 10 positiven Tumoren waren maligne, 6 hiervon wiesen Fernmetastasen und 3 eine Entdifferenzierung auf. Die Überexpression von p53 und *neu* fanden wir bei nur drei wenig differenzierten (G3) Schilddrüsenkarzinomen. Die Überexpression von p53 und c-*neu* verbietet unseres Erachtens eine eingeschränkte Radikalität bei bisher als "low risk" eingestuften Patienten.

Summary

In one third of all endocrine tumors overexpression of *neu* oncogene was demonstrated, which underlines its role in tumor development. In contrast to this, p53 is a rather rare mutational event in these patients. Nine out of ten positive tumors were malignant, six of them had distant metastases, and three showed low tumor grading (G3). Overexpression of both p53 and *neu* was shown in three poorly differentiated (G3) thyroid carcinomas. This indicates a dedifferentiation and forbids a limited radicality in patients formerly designated as being "low risk".

Literatur

1. Lyons J, Landis CA, Harsh G, Vallar L, Grünewald K, Feichtinger H, Duh QY, Clark OH, Kawasaki E, Bourne HR, McCormick F (1990) Two G protein mutations in human endocrine tumors. Science 249:655–9

2. Goretzki PE, Lyons J, Stacy-Philips S, Rosenau W, Demeure M, Clark OH, McCormick F, Röher HD, Bourne HR (1992) Mutational activation of ras and GSP oncogenes in differentiated thyroid cancer and their biological implications. World J Surg 16:576-82
3. de Potter CR, Beghin C, Makar AP, Vandekerckhove D, Roels HJ (1990) The neu-oncogene protein as a predictive factor for haematogenous metastases in breast cancer patients. Int J Cancer 45:55–8
4. Hinds PW, Finlay CA, Quartin RS, Baker SJ, Fearon ER, Vogelstein B, Levine AJ (1990) Mutant p53 DNA clones from human colon carcinomas cooperate with ras in transforming primary rat cells: A comparison of the "hot spot" mutant phenotypes. Cell Growth Differ 1(12):571–80
5. Sidransky D, Mikkelsen T, Schwechheimer K, Rosenblum ML, Cavanee W, Vogelstein B (1992) Clonal expansion of p53 mutant cells is associated with brain tumor progression. Nature 335:46–47

Dr. med. D. Simon, Abteilung für Allgemein- und Unfallchirurgie, Heinrich-Heine-Universität Düsseldorf, Moorenstraße 5, W-4000 Düsseldorf

Der Pulsatile-Fluß-Index (PFI) zur Objektivierung des Effekts der präoperativen Plummerung bei Morbus Basedow

The Use of Pulsatile Flow Index to Evaluate the Effect of Preoperative Iodine Intake in Graves' Disease

U. Krause[1], K.W. Sievers[2], T. Plajer[2] und Th. Olbricht[3]

[1]Abteilung für Allgemeine Chirurgie (Direktor: Prof. Dr. F.W. Eigler), Universitätsklinikum – GHS, Essen
[2]Röntgendiagnostisches Zentralinstitut (Direktor: Prof. Dr. E. Löhr), Universitätsklinikum – GHS, Essen
[3]Abteilung für Endokrinologie (Direktor: Prof. Dr. D. Reinwein), Universitätsklinikum – GHS, Essen

Einleitung

Plummer führte 1923 die orale Jodidgabe ein als Operationsvorbereitung bei M. Basedow. Die "Plummerung" ist heute nicht mehr weit verbreitet, da bei euthyreoter Stoffwechsellage ein zusätzlicher durchblutungsmindernder Effekt bezweifelt wird [3, 4]. Seit Einführung der Duplex-Doppler-Sonographie in die Schilddrüsendiagnostik läßt sich die Durchblutung recht genau nicht-invasiv messen und damit ein Effekt des Jodid überprüfen [2].

Methodik

Bei 22 schilddrüsengesunden Probanden wurde mittels Duplex-Doppler-Sonographie der Blutfluß in der A. thyreoidea superior beidseits bestimmt, danach bei 24 Kranken mit Morbus Basedow nach thyreostatischer Vorbehandlung (Euthyreose) und bei gestellter Operationsindikation. Die Messungen erfolgten vor und nach 10-tägiger hochdosierter oraler Jodidgabe (600–750 mg gesamt). Die Untersuchungen erfolgten an einem Sonoline 2 Duplex Doppler (Siemens, Erlangen) mit einem 7,5 MHz Sektorschallkopf. Die Auswertung erfolgte über die Bestimmung des Integrals der Pulskurve, die, dividiert durch die maximale Amplitude und die Frequenz, den Pulsations-Fluß-Index ergeben, nach der Formel:

$$PFI = \frac{A}{Y\ max + T}\ .$$

Weitere Berechnungen der Einzel- und Mittelwerte erfolgten mittels eines IBM-kompatiblen Statistikprogramms computergestützt. Signifikanztests erfolgten nach dem Students' T-Verfahren.

Chirurgisches Forum 1993
f. experim. u. klinische Forschung
Becker/Beger/Hartel (Hrsg.)

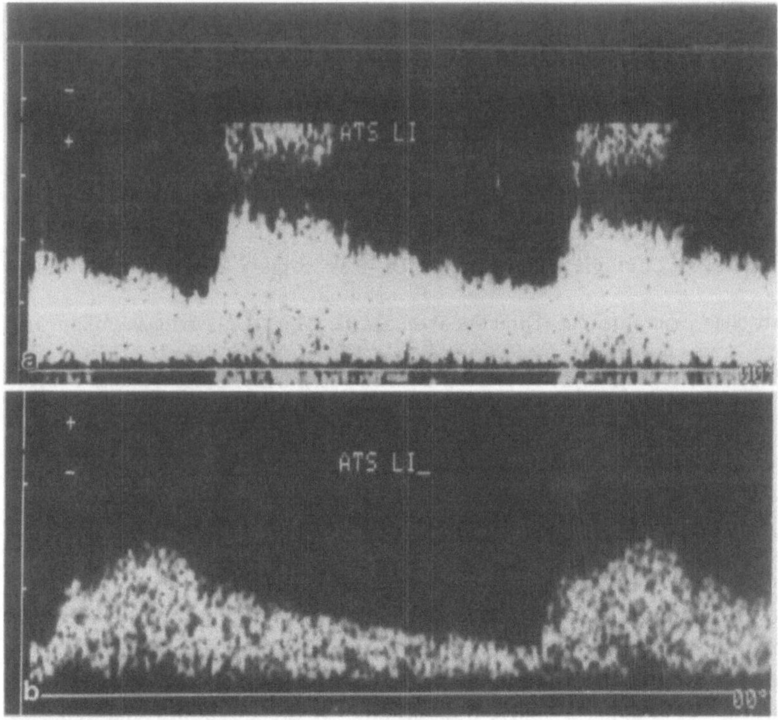

Abb. 1. a Pulskurve eines Patienten mit M. Basedow vor Jodtherapie: deutliche Abflachung ohne Abgrenzung der diastolischen Frequenz. PFI = 0,7. **b** Pulskurve nach Jodtherapie: Nachweis einer postsystolischen Kerbe. Der Frequenzanstieg ist schneller. PFI = 0,53

Ergebnisse

Bei allen untersuchten Patienten (bzw. Probanden) konnte ein verwertbares Signal im Bereich der A. thyreoidea superior ermittelt werden. In der Kontrollgruppe war ein abgerundeter systolischer Kurvenverlauf mit deutlicher Abgrenzung der Diastole typisch. Bei den Basedow-Patienten war diese Differenzierung nicht mehr möglich (Abb. 1a), nach Plummerung aber reversibel (Abb. 1b).

Die Auswertung des PFI ergab folgende Mittelwerte: Die gesunden Probanden (n = 22) hatten einen Index-Mittelwert von 0,46 mit einer Standard-Abweichung von 0,11. Der mittlere PFI bei den Basedow-Patienten betrug vor Plummerung 0,65 mit einer Standardabweichung von 0,08, d.h. 41% höher als in der Kontrollgruppe. Der Unterschied ist signifikant ($p < 0,001$). Nach Plummerung betrug der mittlere Index im gleichen Kollektiv 0,56 (± 0,1 SD), entsprechend einem Abfall um 14%. Der Unterschied ist signifikant ($p < 0,05$). Bei drei der untersuchten 24 Patienten war ein leichter Anstieg feststellbar (s. Abb. 2), zweimal ein- und einmal doppelseitig.

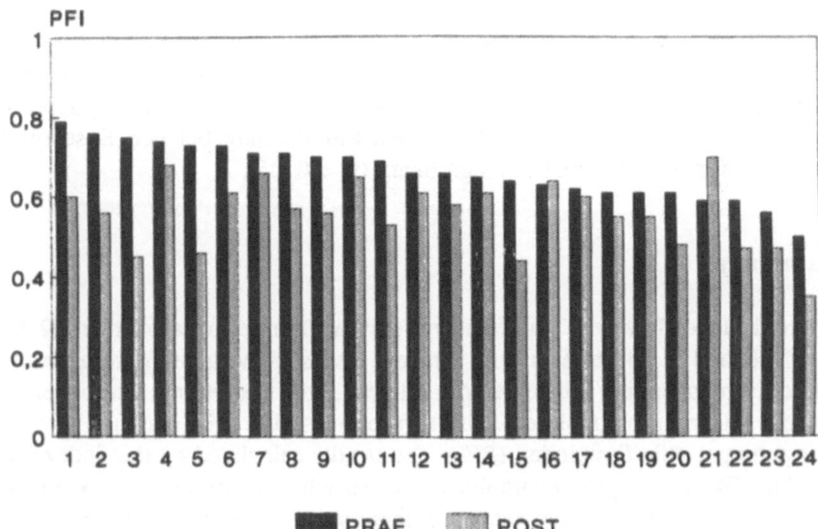

Abb. 2. Darstellung der prä- und posttherapeutischen PFI-Werte bei 24 Patienten mit M. Basedow, jeweils doppelseitig gemessen

Diskussion

Die Operationsvorbereitung mit Jodid bei Morbus Basedow gilt heute als entbehrlich, da sich ein durchblutungsmindernder Effekt über die Normalisierung des Stoffwechsels hinaus schwer nachweisen ließ [3, 4]. Seit Einführung der Duplex-Doppler-Sonographie hat sich diese Situation geändert [2]. Die Verwendung eines Index zur Quantifizierung des Blutflusses bei dieser Methode ist essentiell, um anatomiebedingte Fehler (z.B. Gefäßdurchmesser, Untersuchungswinkel) auszuschließen. Der PFI hat sich in unserer Arbeitsgruppe bereits als brauchbarer Index in der Nierendiagnostik bewährt [5]. Die hier mitgeteilten Ergebnisse zeigen, daß der PFI auch für die Beurteilung der Schilddrüsendurchblutung ein brauchbarer Parameter ist, sowohl bei eu- wie bei hyperthyreoter Stoffwechsellage. Darüber hinaus konnten wir nachweisen, daß die hochdosierte Jodidgabe bei Morbus Basedow auch nach zuvor erreichter Euthyreose die Schilddrüsendurchblutung vermindert. Zu ganz ähnlichen Ergebnissen kamen Arntzenius u. Mitarb., allerdings bei euthyreoten Patienten [1].

Ob sich die qualifizierbare Durchblutungsminderung in einen operationstechnischen Vorteil, d.h. einen verminderten Blutverlust umsetzen läßt, wird z.Zt. in einer prospektiv-randomisierten klinischen Studie untersucht.

Zusammenfassung

Bei 22 gesunden Probanden und danach bei 24 Morbus Basedow-Kranken wurde die Schilddrüsendurchblutung nicht-invasiv mittels Duplex-Doppler-Sonographie gemessen, bei letzteren vor und nach Plummerung zur Operationsvorbereitung. Alle Patienten waren euthyreot nach Thyreostatika-Vorbehandlung. Die Meßwerte wurden mittels eines Index semiquantitativ verglichen (PFI = pulsatiler Fluß-Index). Letzterer erwies sich als gut reproduzierbar. Die Morbus Basedow-Patienten hatten eine um 41% stärkere Schilddrüsendurchblutung als die gesunde Kontrollgruppe, berechnet aufgrund des Index. Der PFI-Abfall nach Plummerung bei den Basedow-Patienten betrug 14% und war statistisch signifikant ($p < 0,05$).

Summary

Thyroid blood flow was studied using duplex Doppler ultrasound in 22 healthy individuals and in 24 patients with Graves' disease. The latter were examined before and after preoperative intake of oral iodine (Lugol's solution). The patients were euthyroid following pretreatment with thyreostatics. The data obtained were calculated using the pulsatile flow index (PFI). The results calculated by this index were reproducible. The patient group with Graves' disease had a 41% higher blood flow than the control group. After iodine treatment, there was a 14% decrease compared with the initial mean values from the same patients. The difference was statistically significant ($P < 0.05$).

Literatur

1. Arntzenius AB, Smit LJ, Schipper J, von der Heide D, Meinders AE (1991) Inverse relation between iodine intake and thyroid blood flow: color doppler flow imaging in euthyroid humans. J Clin Endocrinol Metab 73:1951–1055
2. Hodgson KJ, Lazarus JH, Wheeler MH, Woodcock JP, Owen GM, McGregor AM, Hall R (1988) Duplex scan-derived thyroid blood flow in euthyroid and hyperthyroid patients. World J Surg 12:470–475
3. Marigold JH, Morgan AK, Earle DJ, Young AE, Croft DN (1985) Lugol's iodine: its effect on thyroid blood flow in patients with thyrotoxicosis. Br J Surg 72:45–47
4. Marmon L, Au FC (1989) The preoperative use of iodine solution in thyrotoxic patients prepared with propanolol. Is it necessary? Am J Surg 55:629–631
5. Sievers KW, Cazenave CR, Kaude JV, Crokar BP (1987) Pulsatile flow index (PFI): its importance in the evaluation of renal transplant dysfunction with duplex ultra sound. J Med Imaging I:294–298

Priv.-Doz. Dr. U. Krause, Abteilung für Allgemeine Chirurgie,
OPZ II Universitätsklinikum Essen, Hufelandstraße 55, W-4300 Essen 1

Einfluß der Leu-M1-Immunreaktivität auf die Prognose des C-Zell-Karzinoms der Schilddrüse

Influence of Leu-M1 Immunoreactivity on the Prognosis of C-Cell Carcinoma of the Thyroid

A. Frilling[1], V. Bay[2], H.-D. Röher[3] und S. Schröder[4]

[1]Abteilung für Allgemeinchirurgie, Universität Hamburg
[2]I. Chirurgische Abteilung, Allgemeines Krankenhaus, Hamburg-Harburg
[3]Abteilung für Allgemein- und Unfallchirurgie, Universität Düsseldorf
[4]Institut für Pathologie, Universität Hamburg

Unter den Schilddrüsenkarzinomen beansprucht das C-Zell-Karzinom (Synonym: medulläres Karzinom) wegen seiner biologischen Besonderheiten eine Sonderstellung. Da der Tumor kein Radiojod speichert und nur eine sehr geringe Ansprechrate auf perkutane Radiatio oder Chemotherapie aufweist, nimmt der chirurgische Eingriff einen besonderen therapeutischen Stellenwert ein. Wegen der sehr unterschiedlichen Krankheitsverläufe mit rezidivfreien Zeitspannen von wenigen Monaten bis zu mehreren Jahrzehnten ist gerade bei dieser Geschwulst intensiv nach Faktoren gesucht worden, die eine bessere Prädiktion des biologischen Verhaltens gestatten. Neben allgemeinen Tumorprognoseparametern wie Alter, Geschlecht und Tumorstadium und für das C-Zell-Karzinom spezifischen Parametern wie Tumorform (sporadisch vs. familiär) und Calcitoninspiegel im Serum wird eine erhebliche prognostische Relevanz auch den immunzytochemisch erfaßbaren Tumoreigenschaften beigemessen [5]. Nachdem bereits beim papillären Schilddrüsenkarzinom der prognosebestimmende Effekt des myelomonozytären Leu-M1-Antigens nachgewiesen werden konnte [4], haben wir die Bedeutung der Leu-M1-Positivität im Tumorgewebe auch bei Patienten mit einem C-Zell-Karzinom überprüft.

Methodik

Die Untersuchung erfolgte am paraffineingebetteten Primärtumorgewebe von zwei verschiedenen Patientenkollektiven. Das erste bestand aus 39 Patienten, deren Tumorgewebe im Institut für Pathologie der Universität Hamburg untersucht wurden. Das zweite Kollektiv umfaßte 21 Patienten, die wegen eines C-Zell-Karzinoms in der Abteilung für Allgemein- und Unfallchirurgie der Universität Düsseldorf ope-

Chirurgisches Forum 1993
f. experim. u. klinische Forschung
Becker/Beger/Hartel (Hrsg.)

riert wurden. Der immunzytochemische Leu-M1-Nachweis wurde im ersten Kollektiv mittels eines monoklonalen Antikörpers (Fa. Becton-Dickinson, Heidelberg, Deutschland, Verdünnung 1:30) nach der Avidin-Biotin-Peroxidasekomplex-Methode geführt. Im zweiten Kollektiv wurde ein monoklonaler Antikörper (Fa. Dako, Kopenhagen, Dänemark, Verdünnung 1:100) in der direkten Peroxidase-Antiperoxidase-Methode angewandt. Die Auszählung Leu-M1-positiver Zellen pro 100 Tumorzellen fand bei 100facher Vergrößerung mit einem Okularmikrometer statt. Die statistische Analyse erfolgte im ersten Kollektiv mit dem Cox-Regressionsmodell und der Kaplan-Meier-Methode und im zweiten Kollektiv mit dem Mann-Whitney-U-Test. Als signifikant galten Ergebnisse mit $p < 0,05$.

Ergebnisse

Kollektiv 1 (n=39 Patienten): Epithelanfärbung für das Leu-M1-Antigen war deutlich nachweisbar (> als 15% der Zellen) im Tumorgewebe von 16 Patienten (41%). Bei 5 Fällen (13%) zeigte sich nur eine mäßige Anfärbung (weniger als 15% der Tumorzellen) und in 18 (46%) bestand keine positive Reaktion. Eine Leu-M1-Expression fand sich häufiger bei Männern als bei Frauen und bei jüngeren (< 45 Jahren) im Vergleich zu älteren Patienten. Bei den postoperativ tumorfreien Patienten betrug die Leu-M1-Immunreaktivität 12%. Eine signifikant höhere Leu-M1-Positivität lag bei Patienten vor, die ein Tumorrezidiv entwickelten (18%, $p < 0,05$) oder die am Tumor verstarben (33%, $p < 0,025$).

Kollektiv 2 (n=21 Patienten): Bei 13 Patienten (62%) konnte eine unterschiedlich stark ausgeprägte Leu-M1-Reaktivität gezeigt werden; 8 Patienten (38%) hatten Leu-M1-negative Tumoren. Beim Vergleich der sporadischen und der familiären Tumorform zeigte sich eine intensivere Immunreaktivität bei den Patienten mit einem sporadischen Karzinom. Die Leu-M1-Immunreaktivität betrug bei den an dem Tumorleiden verstorbenen Patienten 31% ($p < 0,04$), bei den Patienten mit einem Karzinomrezidiv 16% ($p < 0,05$) und bei den tumorfreien Patienten 9%.

Diskussion

Das Leu-M1-Antigen wurde zunächst in myelomonozytären Zellen [1] und später auch in den Reed-Sternberg-Zellen des Morbus Hodgkin entdeckt. Neuere Studien erbrachten den Nachweis von Leu-M1-Antigen in den epithelialen Zellen der Haut, im Gastronintestinal- und Urogenitaltrakt, im Gehirn und in verschiedenen endokrinen Organen [2]. Der monoklonale Leu-M1-Antikörper identifiziert den protein- oder lipidgebundenen Zuckerrest Karbohydrat-Lakto-N-Fukopentaose III. Fukosehaltigen Glykokonjugaten wird eine wichtige Rolle bei der malignen Zelltransformation zugesprochen. Über die prognostische Bedeutung des Leu-M1-Antigens liegen kontroverse Berichte vor. Während eine starke Leu-M1-Immunreaktivität beim Morbus Hodgkin mit einer guten Prognose einhergeht, wurde beim papillären Schilddrüsenkarzinom bei positivem Antigennachweis eine höhere Tumorrezidivrate festgestellt [4]. Eine negative Korrelation der Leu-M1-Immunreaktivität mit der Tumorprognose konnte auch in unseren beiden Kollektiven von Patienten mit C-Zell-Karzinom gezeigt werden. Die Leu-M1-Reaktivität war bei Patienten mit einem Tumorrezidiv mit 18% bzw. 16% signifikant höher als bei tumorfreien Patienten, bei denen sie 12% bzw. 9% betrug. Mit 33% bzw. 31% war der Unterschied noch deutlicher bei den verstorbenen Patienten. Auch Neuhold et al. [2] stellten in ihrem Kollektiv von 47 Patienten mit einem sporadischen C-Zell-Karzinom eine prognoserelevante Bedeutung des Leu-M1-Antigens fest. Eine signifikant höhere Leu-M1-Positivität lag bei den Patienten mit Tumoren größer als 4 cm und bei Vorliegen von Lymphknotenmetastasen vor. Während bei allen 5 am Tumorrezidiv bereits verstorbenen Patienten eine starke Leu-M1-Reaktivität nachweisbar war, lebten alle Patienten mit Rezidivtumoren, bei denen nur eine schwache oder fehlende Antigenpositivität festzustellen war. Da die Ausdehnung des chirurgischen Eingriffes beim Primärtumor entsprechend der C-Zell-Karzinomform und des Tumorstadiums festgelegt ist, ergeben sich therapeutische Konsequenzen aus der Ausprägung der Leu-M1-Expression in erster Linie bei Vorliegen eines Tumorrezidivs. Bei positiver Leu-M1-Immunreaktivität wäre bei diesen Patienten ein besonders aggressives therapeutisches Vorgehen im Sinne einer ausgedehnten Mikrodissektion des lymphatischen Gewebes zu befürworten.

Zusammenfassung

An zwei Kollektiven von Patienten mit einem C-Zell-Karzinom wurde die prognostische Bedeutung des Leu-M1-Antigens nachgewiesen. Bei tumorfreien Patienten lag die Leu-M1-Immunreaktivität bei 12% (Kollektiv 1) bzw. 16% (Kollektiv 2). Eine signifikant höhere Leu-M1-Reaktivität zeigte sich bei den Patienten, die an dem Tumor verstorben sind (33% bzw. 31%) oder ein Tumorrezidiv entwickelt haben (18% bzw. 16%). Eine hohe Leu-M1-Expression deutet auf ein aggressives Tumorverhalten hin und erfordert ein besonders radikales chirurgisches Vorgehen.

Summary

The prognostic significance of Leu-M1 antigen was demonstrated in two groups of patients suffering from medullary thyroid carcinoma. Markedly increased Leu-M1 immunoreactivity occurred in the tumor tissue of patients who died from the cancer (33% and 31%, respectively) or who developed tumor recurrencies (18% and 16%, respectively), as compared with symptom-free surviving patients (12% and 9%, respectively). Significant Leu-M1 reactivity indicates high tumor malignancy and justifies radical surgical procedures.

Literatur

1. Hanjan SNS, Kearney JF, Cooper MD (1982) A monoclonal antibody (MMA) that identifies a differentiation antigen on human myelomonocytic cells. Clin Immunol Immunopathol 23:172–188

2. Neuhold N, Längle F, Gnant M, Hollenstein U, Niederle B (1992) Relationship of CD15 immunoreactivity and prognosis in sporadic medullary thyroid carcinoma. J Cancer Res Clin Oncol 118:629–634
3. Schröder S, Schwarz W, Rehpenning W, Dralle H, Bay V, Böcker W (1988) Leu-M1 immunoreactivity and prognosis in medullary carcinomas of the thyroid gland. J Cancer Res Clin Oncol 114:291–296
4. Schröder S, Schwarz W, Rehpenning W, Löning T, Böcker W (1987) Prognostic significance of Leu-M1 immunostaining in papillary carcinomas of the thyroid gland. Virchows Arch (Pathol Anat) 411:435–439
5. Takami H, Bessho T, Kameya T, Mimura T, Ito K, Abe O, Hosoda H, Shikata J (1988) Immunohistochemical study of medullary thyroid carcinoma: relationship of clinical features to prognostic factors in 36 patients. World J Surg 12:572–579

PD Dr. A. Frilling, Abteilung für Allgemeine Chirurgie, Universitäts-Krankenhaus, Martinistraße 52, W-2000 Hamburg 20

Einfluß verschiedener Zytostatika und elektromagnetischer Felder auf die Proliferation humaner Mammakarzinomzellen

Influence of Different Antiblastic Drugs and of Electromagnetic Fields on Proliferation of Human Breast Cancer Cells

S. Johann, S. Mikorey-Lechner, W. Kraus und G. Blümel

Institut für Experimentelle Chirurgie, Technische Universität, München

Einleitung

Der positive Einfluß elektromagnetischer Felder (EMF) auf die Heilung von Pseudarthrosen, Prothesenlockerungen und Hüftnekrosen ist mittlerweile unbestritten. Nicht geklärt sind jedoch die Auswirkungen von EMF auf Tumorwachstum und Zellproliferation. Um diesem Problem näherzukommen, wurden in vitro zwei Tumorzellinien, die humanen Mammakarzinomzellinien MCF7 und MDA, auf Änderungen nach intermittierendem EMF (6 h an/6 h aus) untersucht. Hierzu wurden die mitochondriale Aktivität als Parameter für die Proliferation einer Zelle herangezogen. Gleichzeitig wurde der Einfluß verschiedener Zytostatika in Verbindung mit EMF auf die mitochondriale Aktivität untersucht.

Material und Methoden

Die beiden humanen Mammakarzinomzellinien MCF7 (ATCC HTB 22) und MDA (ATCC MDA-MB-231, HTB 26) wurden in RPMI 1640 mit 10% FKS bei 37°C und 5% CO_2 vermehrt. Die Zellen wurden zweimal wöchentlich passagiert und die Vitalität mit Hilfe der Trypanblau-Färbung bestimmt. Zu Testbeginn wurden die Mammakarzinomzellen in 96-Lochplatten in verschiedenen Konzentrationen eingesät und bis zu 14 Tagen unter Standardbedingungen bebrütet.

Zur Erzeugung eines EMF wurden zwei solenoide Magnetspulen (Magnetodyn Funktionsgenerator M70S; 20 Hz, 50 Gauss) in einen Brutschrank so eingebracht, daß keine Änderung der Kulturbedingungen (38°C, 5% CO_2) resultierte [1]. Zur Konstanthaltung der Temperatur wurde ein Haake Wasser-Kühlsystem verwendet. Temperaturunterschiede zwischen Kontroll- und Testzellen waren geringer als $0,15$°C. Kontrollzellen wurden unter identischen Bedingungen bei fehlendem EMF gehalten.

Die mitochondriale Aktivität der Mammakarzinomzellen wurde mittels MTT-Test [2] bestimmt. Hierzu wurden zu jeder Probe 10 μl Methylthiazolyl-Tetrazoliumbromid (MTT; 5 mg/ml PBS) pipettiert, nach 4 h die von lebenden Zellen gebildeten Formazankristalle in 200 μl 0,04 M HCl gelöst und die Proben mittels Plattenphotometer bei 550 nm gemessen.

Chirurgisches Forum 1993
f. experim. u. klinische Forschung
Becker/Beger/Hartel (Hrsg.)

Um die Wirkung von Zytostatika auf Zellkulturen zu bestimmen, wurden zu 50 μl Zellsuspension 50 μl Zytostatikumlösung pipettiert. Folgende Zytostatika wurden verwendet: Carboplatin, 5-Fluorouracil und Cyclophosphamid zu 250 μg/ml, Mitoxantronhydrochlorid, Adriblastin, Mitomycin, Methotrexat-Dinatrium und Epirubicinhydrochlorid zu 25 μg/ml.

Ergebnisse

Mammakarzinomzellen wurden zu 100, 200, 500 und 1000 Zellen/ml in 6fach Ansätzen in 96-Lochplatten pipettiert und sowohl mit, als auch ohne den Einfluß eines EMF für 14 Tage inkubiert. Nach dieser Zeit zeigten MCF7-Zellen, die unter dem Einfluß eines EMF standen, eine signifikante Steigerung der mitochondrialen Aktivität um das 1,3 bis 2,0fache gegenüber den Kontrollzellen (Abb. 1). Gleiche Ergebnisse wurden bei den MDA-Zellen erzielt.

MCF7-Zellen, die alternativ 3 Tage unter Einfluß des EMF standen und anschließend 3 Tage ohne den Einfluß eines EMF wuchsen, zeigten eine niedrigere mitochondriale Aktivität als 6 Tage EMF inkubierte Zellen, aber eine höhere Aktivität als die Kontrollzellen.

MCF7-Zellen (1000 Zellen/Loch) sowie MDA-Zellen (800 Zellen/Loch) wurden 7 Tage mit und ohne EMF inkubiert. Der gleichzeitige Zusatz von Zytostatika führte zu einer Reduktion der mitochondrialen Aktivität um 50–93%, wobei EMF-inkubierte

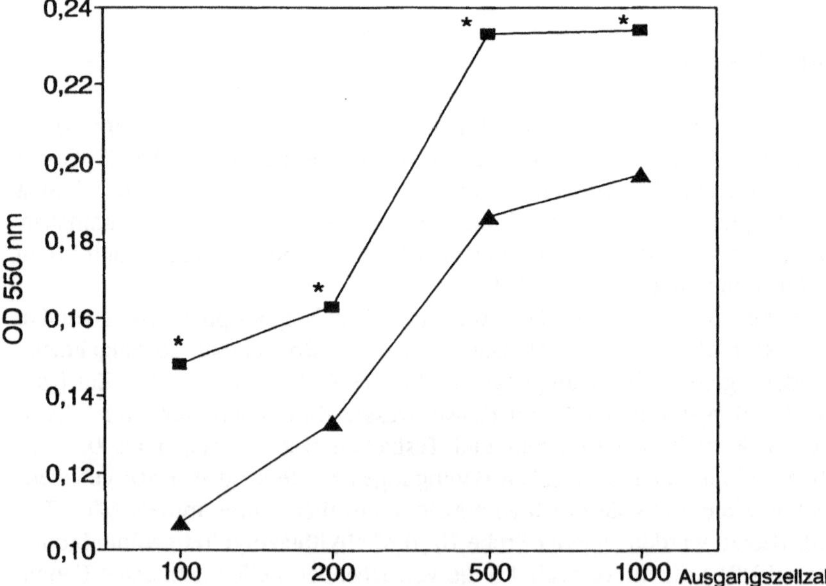

Abb. 1. Mitochondriale Aktivität der MCF7-Zellen nach 14 Tagen Inkubation ohne EMF (-▲-) und unter dem Einfluß (-■-) eines EMF in Abhängigkeit von der Zellzahl (Ausgangszellzahl/ml). $\alpha = 0,05$

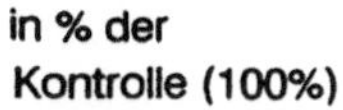

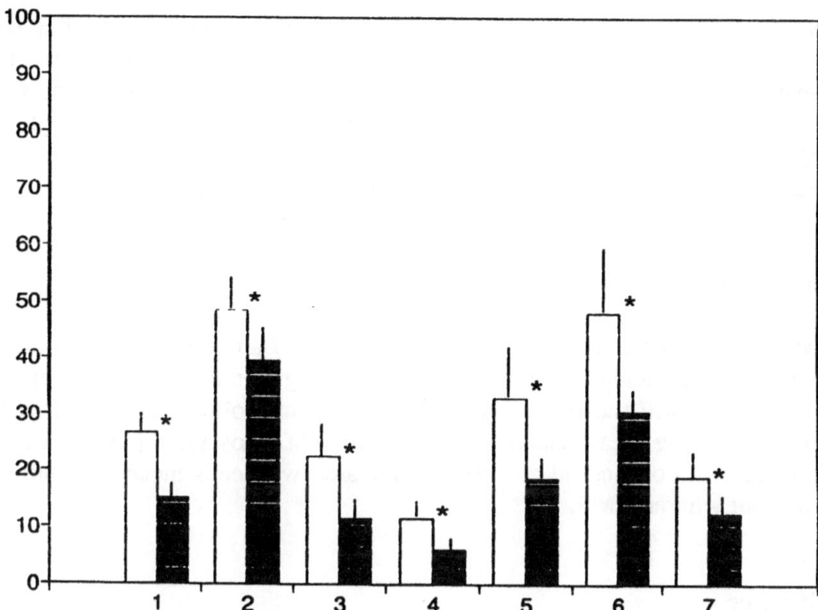

Abb. 2. Mitochondriale Aktivität der MCF7-Zellen (1000 Zellen/Loch) ohne (□) den Einfluß eines EMF und unter (■) dem Einfluß eines EMF bei gleichzeitiger Zugabe verschiedener Zytostatika. *1* Doxorubicin; *2* Methotrexat; *3* Mitomycin; *4* Mitoxantron; *5* Cyclophosphamid; *6* Carboplatin; *7* 5-Fluorouracil; $\alpha = 0,05$

Zellen eine signifikant niedrigere mitochondriale Aktivität aufwiesen (bis zu 60%) als Kontrollzellen (Abb. 2).

Diskussion

Unsere Ergebnisse zeigen, daß EMF in der Lage sind, zu einem gesteigerten MTT-Umsatz zu führen. Der MTT-Umsatz ist ein Maß für die mitochondriale Aktivität, die wiederum proportional zur Zellzahl und somit zur Proliferation ist [2]. Eine Erhöhung der Proliferation unter EMF kann schon nach 2 Tagen beobachtet werden (Ergebnisse nicht gezeigt). Kontroverse Ergebnisse, abhängig von dem Gebrauch verschiedener Zellinien und unterschiedlichem EMF, werden in der Literatur beschrieben. So stimuliert als auch hemmt ein pulsierendes EMF die zelluläre DNS-Synthese in chinesischen Hamsterzellen abhängig von der magnetischen Feldstärke [3].

Bei gleichzeitigem Einfluß von Zytostatika und EMF zeigen die Mammakarzinomzellen eine verringerte Proliferation als Zellen, die nur mit Zytostatika alleine inkubiert wurden. Ähnliche Ergebnisse stellen Petrini et al. [4] vor, die eine verringerte ^{3}H-Thymidin Inkorporation in MCF7 Zellen nach EMF- und Doxorubicin-Applikation beschreiben.

Zusammenfassung

2 Mammakarzinomzellinien (MCF7 und MDA) wurden ohne den Einfluß eines elektromagnetischen Feldes (EMF) und unter dem Einfluß eines EMF über 14 Tage inkubiert. Zellen, die unter dem Einfluß eines EMF standen, zeigten eine signifikante Erhöhung der Proliferation im Vergleich zu den Kontrollzellen. Bei gleichzeitiger Gabe von verschiedenen Zytostatika resultierte eine niedrigere Proliferation der EMF Zellen im Gegensatz zu den nicht EMF inkubierten Zellen.

Summary

Two different human breast cancer cell lines (MCF7 and MDA) were incubated for 14 days with and without the influence of electromagnetic fields (EMF). Cells under the influence of EMF showed a significant increase in proliferation compared to control cells. Incubating breast cancer cells with different cytostatic drugs and EMF led to a decrease in mitochondrial activity as compared with cells incubated with antiblastic drugs but without EMF.

Literatur

1. Kraus W (1984) Magnetfeldtherapie und magnetisch induzierte Elektrostimulation in der Orthopädie. Orthopäde 13:78–92
2. Mosmann T (1983) Rapid colorimetric assay for cellular growth and survival: application to proliferation and cytotoxicity assays. J Immunol Meth 65:55–63
3. Takahashi K, Kaneko I, Date M, Fukuda E (1986) Effect of pulsing electromagnetic fields on DNA synthesis in mammalian cells in culture. Experientia 42:185–186
4. Petrini M, Mattii L, Sabbatini A, Carulli G, Grassi B, Cadossi R, Ronca G, Conte A (1990) Multidrug resistance and electromagnetic fields. J Bioelectricity 9:209–212

Dr. S. Johann, Institut für Experimentelle Chirurgie, Technische Universität München, Ismaninger Straße 22, W-8000 München 80

Tumorzell-Proliferation und Prognose beim Mammakarzinom

Tumor Cell Proliferation and Prognosis in Mammary Carcinoma

H. Schimmelpenning[1], E. Eriksson[2] und G. Auer[2]

[1]Klinik für Allgemeinchirurgie, Johann-Wolfgang Goethe Universität, Frankfurt
[2]Abteilung für Tumorpathologie, Karolinska Institutet, Stockholm

Einleitung

Das klinische Verhalten von Mammakarzinomen ist oft schwierig vorherzusagen. Daher wurden und werden viele Versuche unternommen, um in Ergänzung zu den herkömmlichen histopathologischen Kriterien weitere zuverlässige und reproduzierbare Prognoseparameter zu finden. In diesem Zusammenhang zeigte sich, daß sowohl der cytometrisch gemessene Kern-DNS Gehalt, als auch zellkinetische Daten nützliche Informationen beinhalten können [1].

In verschiedenen Untersuchungen hat man gefunden, daß der Kern-DNS Gehalt eng mit dem klinischen Verlauf von Mammakarzinomen korreliert. Patientinnen mit DNS-diploiden Tumoren haben in der Regel einen günstigen Verlauf. Im Gegensatz dazu ist die Tumorprogression bei Patientinnen mit DNS-aneuploiden Tumoren deutlich aggressiver.

Die Proliferationsrate maligner Tumoren kann auf verschiedene Weise ermittelt werden. Es stehen jetzt unter anderem monoklonale Antikörper gegen das 36 kd, S-Phasen-assoziierte Kernprotein PCNA (proliferating cell nuclear antigen) zur Verfügung. Das Protein ist ein Hilfsprotein der DNS-Polymerase delta und notwendig für die zelluläre DNS-Synthese.

Vor diesem Hintergrund wurde in der vorliegenden, retrospektiven Studie die immunhistochemische Expression des S-Phase-assoziierten PCNA und der Kern-DNS Gehalt in Tumorzellen von Patientinnen mit langfristigen klinischen Verlaufsangaben ermittelt.

Methodik

Die Untersuchung umfaßte eine Serie von 209 Patientinnen mit invasiven Mammakarzinomen und klinischen Verlaufsangaben zwischen 13 und 19 Jahren. Die chirurgische Behandlung war bei allen Fällen eine radikale Mastektomie mit axillärer Lymphknotendissektion.

Die immunhistochemische PCNA-Färbung wurde mit dem monoklonalen Antikörper PC10 in der Avidin-Biotin-Peroxidase Komplex Technik und Diaminobenzidin als Chromogen durchgeführt (Novacastra Laboratories, Newcastle upon Tyne, UK). In verschiedenen Studien wurde die Anwendbarkeit dieses Antikörpers in kon-

Chirurgisches Forum 1993
f. experim. u. klinische Forschung
Becker/Beger/Hartel (Hrsg.)

ventionell fixiertem Paraffinmaterial nachgewiesen [2]. In jedem der 209 Präparate wurden mit dem Mikroskop 10 Gesichtsfelder (Vergrößerung ×400) innerhalb des Tumors ausgewählt und der Anteil an PCNA-immunreaktiven Zellen in 5% Intervallen ermittelt.

Der Kern-DNS Gehalt wurde in nach Feulgen gefärbten Feinnadelpunktaten der Karzinome bildanalytisch gemessen und nach Auer in vier Histogrammtypen klassifiziert [3]. Typ I Histogramme hatten einen umschriebenen diploiden Peak. Typ II Histogramme hatten einen Peak in der G_2/M Region, oder je einen Peak in der G_0/G_1 und in der G_2/M Region. Histogramme von Typ III hatten einen Peak in der G_0/G_1 Region und eine deutliche Verteilung von Zellen in der S-Phase Region dieses diploiden Peaks. Typ IV Histogramme zeigten deutlich aneuploide DNS-Verteilungsmuster auch über die G_2/M Region hinaus.

Die statistische Analyse von immunhistochemischen Ergebnissen und deren Relation zu anderen Tumoreigenschaften wurde mit Hilfe des Chi-Square Testes durchgeführt. Für die Berechnung der prognostischen Signifikanzen wurden Kaplan-Meier Kurven, bzw. Cox's Regressionsanalysen verwendet.

Tabelle 1. Beziehung zwischen dem Anteil PCNA-immunreaktiver Tumorzellen und histopathologischen Tumoreigenschaften in 209 Fällen mit invasiven Mammakarzinomen

	Anteil der PCNA-immunreaktiven Tumorzellen				
	< 5%	< 10%	< 15%	> 20%	
Tumorgröße					
< 2 cm	40	37	12	20	P = 0,02
2–5 cm	16	10	10	21	
> 5 cm	6	2	5	5	
mehrere[a]	4	3	0	1	
unbekannt[a]	6	5	2	4	
Lymphknotenstatus					
pN0	38	37	17	23	n.s.
pN +	33	19	12	28	
Differenzierungsgrad					
Ductal Grad I	7	5	3	0	P < 0,01
Grad II	30	20	11	17	
Grad III	25	27	10	25	
Andere Karzinome[a]	10	15	5	8	
DNS-Histogramm[b]					
I	23	19	9	5	P = 0,009
II[a]	13	9	5	8	
III[a]	7	5	4	6	
IV	29	24	11	32	

[a] Nicht in der statistischen Analyse enthalten
[b] nach Auer [3]
n.s. = nicht signifikant

Ergebnisse

Der Anteil der PCNA immunreaktiven Zellen innerhalb der 209 primären Mammakarzinome variierte von weniger als 5% bis zu 60% der Tumorzellen.

Die Beziehung zwischen PCNA-Immunreaktivität und verschiedenen histopathologischen Characteristika ist in Tabelle 1 zusammengefaßt. Es fand sich ein signifikanter Zusammenhang zwischen PCNA-Expression, Tumorgröße, Differenzierungsgrad und DNS-Histogramm Typ. Schlecht differenzierte Karzinome wiesen eine höhere PCNA-Immunreaktivität auf als hoch differenzierte Tumoren. Bei 25 von 79 niedrig differenzierten Karzinomen waren mehr als 20% der Tumorzellen PCNA-immunreaktiv. In der Gruppe der hoch differenzierten Tumoren waren dagegen maximal 15% der Tumorzellen PCNA gefärbt und es gab keinen Fall mit 20% immunreaktiver Tumorzellen. Bei nur 5 von 56 DNS-diploiden Tumoren (Auer Typ I) waren mehr als 20% der Tumorzellen PCNA-immunreaktiv, während dies bei 32 von 98 DNS-aneuploiden Karzinomen (Auer Typ IV) der Fall war. Kein Zusammenhang bestand zwischen PCNA-Expression und Lymphknotenstatus.

Für eine Gruppe von Patientinnen lieferte die PCNA-Immunreaktivität zusammen mit dem Kern-DNS-Gehalt prognostische Zusatzinformationen. Von 22 Patientinnen mit DNS-nahe-diploiden Karzinomen hoher Zuwachsrate (Auer Typ III) waren in sechs Fällen mehr als 20% der Tumorzellen PCNA-immunreaktiv. Bei fünf dieser Patientinnen entwickelten sich innerhalb von zwei Jahren Fernmetastasen und sie verstarben innerhalb von drei Jahren. Im Gegensatz dazu entwickelten sich bei keiner der 16 Patientinnen mit weniger als 20% PCNA-Expression innerhalb der ersten zwei Jahre Fernmetastasen, sondern erst signifikant später ($p = 0{,}0001$). In einer Multivariatanalyse waren Lymphknotenstatus ($p < 0{,}01$), Tumorgröße ($p < 0{,}01$) und DNS-Histogramm Typ ($p = 0{,}001$) von prognostischer Bedeutung.

Interpretation und Schlußfolgerung

In der vorliegenden Studie fanden sich interessante Zusammenhänge zwischen PCNA-Immunreaktivität und Tumoreigenschaften, die üblicherweise als schlechte prognostische Zeichen gelten. Es liegt daher die Vermutung nahe, daß auch die PCNA-Expression prognosebestimmend sein könnte. Eine generelle Zunahme der proliferativen Aktivität muß aber nicht notwendigerweise zu einer generellen Zunahme des Tumorwachstums führen. Es erscheint möglich, daß die hohe PCNA-Expression in niedrig differenzierten Tumoren nicht lediglich Ausdruck von gesteigerter proliferativer Aktivität ist. Vielmehr ist sie Ausdruck für die Aktivierung von DNS-Reparationsmechanismen in diesen genetisch instabilen Tumoren, die häufig durch aneuploide DNS-Verteilungsmuster gekennzeichnet sind.

In einer Gruppe von Patientinnen liefert die PCNA-Expression jedoch zusammen mit dem DNS-Verteilungsmuster zusätzliche prognostische Information. In nahediploiden, genetisch stabilen Tumoren reflektiert die PCNA-Expression daher offensichtlich rasche Tumorproliferation, während sie in aneuploiden, genetisch instabilen Tumoren den Ablauf von DNS-Reparationsmechanismen anzeigt.

Zusammenfassung

In dieser retrospektiven Studie an 209 Patientinnen mit invasiven Mammakarzinomen und langfristigen klinischen Verlaufsangaben fand sich eine signifikante Beziehung von PCNA-Immunreaktivität zu Tumorgröße, Differenzierungsgrad und DNS-Verteilungsmuster. In einer Gruppe von Patientinnen mit nahe-diploiden Tumoren vom DNS-Histogramm Typ III lieferte hohe PCNA-Expression darüberhinaus prognostische Zusatzinformatin (p = 0,0001).

Summary

In the present retrospective study on 209 patients with invasive mammary carcinomas and long-term clinical follow-up data, we found a significant interrelationship between proliferating cell cuclear antigen (PCNA) immunoreactivity and tumor size, tumor grade, and DNA distribution pattern. In a subgroup of patients with near-diploid tumors of histogram type III, high PCNA expression also provided additional prognostic information ($P = 0.0001$).

Literatur

1. Fallenius AG, Auer GU, Carstensen JM (1988) Prognostic significance of DNA measurements in 409 consecutive breast cancer patients. Cancer 62:331–341
2. Hall PA, Levison DA, Woods AL, Yu CCW, Kellock DB, Watkins JA, Barnes DM, Gillett CE, Camplejohn R, Dover R, Waseem NH, Lane DP (1990) Proliferating cell nuclear antigen (PCNA). Immunolocalization in paraffin sections: an index of cell proliferation with evidence of deregulated expression in some neoplasms. J Pathol 162:285–294
3. Auer G, Eriksson E, Azavedo E, Caspersson T, Wallgren A (1984) Prognostic significance of nuclear DNA content in mammary adenocarcinomas in humans. Cancer Res 44:394–396

H. Schimmelpenning, Klinik für Allgemeinchirurgie, Johann-Wolfgang Goethe Universität, Theodor-Stern-Kai 7, W-6000 Frankfurt a.M. 70

Untersuchungen zur Wahl des Zytostatikums für die isolierte hypertherme Extremitätenperfusion – Chemosensitivitätstests an 5 humanen Melanom-Zellinien

Investigations Regarding the Choice of the Cytostatic Agent in Hyperthermic Isolated Limb Perfusion. Chemosensitivity Testing on Five Human Melanoma Cell Lines

Th. Meyer[1], J. Göhl[1], W. Hohenberger[1], C. Christl[2], G. Bernhardt[2], Th. Spruß[2] und H. Schönenberger[2]

[1]Klinik und Poliklinik für Chirurgie, Universität Regensburg
[2]Institut für Pharmazie, Universität Regensburg

Einleitung

Die isolierte hypertherme Zytostatikaperfusion gilt als geeignete Therapieform lokoregionärer Rezidive von Extremitätenmelanomen. Auswahl und Dosierung bisher verwendeter Substanzen basierte dabei u.a. auf Ergebnissen bei der systemischen Therapie metastasierter Melanome und orientierte sich vor allem am beobachteten klinischen Effekt bei vertretbarer lokaler Toxizität. Als Standardtherapeutikum gilt derzeit Melphalan [5]. Nachdem das Zytostatikum von entscheidender Bedeutung für den Erfolg der multifaktoriell beeinflußten Extremitätenperfusion ist, haben wir ein Konzept entwickelt, das auf experimenteller Grundlage eine Auswahl des Zytostatikums nach objektiven Kriterien ermöglichen soll. An einem repräsentativen Panel humaner Melanom-Zellinien werden diverse zytostatisch wirksame Substanzen getestet. Die effektiven Agenzien werden dann intraperitoneal und/oder peritumoral Melanom-tragenden Nacktmäusen verabreicht. Die hier wirkungsstärksten Substanzen werden mittels isolierter Extremitätenperfusionen an Melanom-tragenden Nacktratten mit Verlaufskontrolle des Tumorwachstums und pharmakokinetischen Untersuchungen inklusive Perfusat- und Gewebespiegelmessungen weiter untersucht. Über die Ergebnisse der Chemosensitivitätstests an fünf humanen Melanom-Zellinien soll im Folgenden berichtet werden.

Material und Methode

Fünf humane Melanom-Zellinien, SK-MEL-2, -3, -5, -24, -28 (American Type Culture Collection, Rockville, Md., USA), wurden auf ihre Sensitivität gegenüber Cisplatin (cDDP), Carboplatin (CBDCA), Dacarbazin (DIC), Dactinomycin (DACT), Doxorubicin (ADM), Melphalan (L-PAM), Methotrexat (MTX), Mitoxantron (DHAQ) und Vinblastin (VBL) getestet. Es wurde ein standardisierter kinetischer Mikroassay basierend

Chirurgisches Forum 1993
f. experim. u. klinische Forschung
Becker/Beger/Hartel (Hrsg.)

auf einer Kristallviolett-Färbung verwendet. Die Zellen wurden in 96-Loch Mikrotiter-Platten in definierter Dichte ausgesät. Nach 48–72 h wurde das Kulturmedium abgesaugt und durch Medium, das die Testsubstanz oder das jeweilige Lösungsmittel enthielt, ersetzt. Die Substanzen wurden als 1000fach konzentrierte Stammlösung zugegeben. Auf jeder Platte dienten die Reihen 5 und 6 (n = 16) als Kontrollen, jeweils zwei vertikale Reihen (n = 16) wurden einer Konzentration exponiert. Die Exposition erstreckte sich sowohl über 250–350 h (sog. *Langzeitexposition*, LZE) ohne einen weiteren Medienwechsel, als auch in 10 000fach höherer Konzentration über 1 h (sog. *Kurzzeitexposition*, KZE) mit nachfolgendem Medienwechsel. Nach verschiedenen Inkubationszeiten wurden die Zellen mit 1% Glutardialdehyd fixiert und bei 4°C aufbewahrt. Am Ende des Experimentes wurden alle Platten gleichzeitig mit 0,02% Kristallviolett gefärbt, dann wurde die Extinktion bei 578 nm gemessen. Die Ergebnisse, d.h. die Substanzwirkung, werden als Auftragung der korrigierten T/C-Werte gegen die Zeit nach folgender Formel dargestellt:

$$(T/C)_{\mathrm{corr}}(\%) = \left[(A_{\mathrm{T}} - A_{\mathrm{c,0}})/(A_{\mathrm{c}} - A_{\mathrm{c,0}})\right] \cdot 100$$

(A_T = mittlere Extinktion der behandelten Zellen, A_c = mittlere Extinktion der Kontrollen, $A_{c,0}$ = mittlere Extinktion zum Zeitpunkt der Substanzzugabe).

Ergebnisse

Der Kristallviolett-Assay erlaubt eine Unterscheidung von zytostatischen und zytoziden Effekten. Es wurden nur *zytozide* Substanzwirkungen als therapeutisch relevant und erfolgversprechend gewertet. Die jeweils im zeitlichen Verlauf erhaltenen minimalen korrigierten T/C-Werte finden sich in Tabelle 1. Beim Vergleich von LZE und KZE, einhergehend mit einer Steigerung der Konzentration in der Regel um eine 10er-Potenz bei einstündiger Expositionsdauer, behält nur ADM seine zytozide Wirkung bei allen Zellinien, lediglich VBL und DHAQ erzielen ähnlich gute Ergebnisse (5/5 vs. 4/5 und 4/5 vs. 4/5 Zellinien). Überraschend ist der starke Wirkungsverlust von CBDCA mit zytozidem Effekt bei 5/5 Linien in der LZE (60 μM) auf lediglich 1/5 Linien in der KZE, selbst bei 100fach höherer Konzentration (0,5 mM). cDDP bleibt in der Effektivität relativ konstant (3/5 vs. 2/5) bei allerdings 10fach niedrigerer äquiaktiver Konzentration im Vergleich zu CBDCA. Die gute Ansprechbarkeit der Zellinien auf DACT bei der LZE (0,5 nM) kann bei der KZE (50 nM) erst bei 100facher Konzentration annähernd reproduziert werden (5/5 vs. 3/5), die Dosierungen liegen aber noch im klinisch relevanten Bereich. L-PAM bestätigt seine Eignung für die isolierte Perfusion und zeigt eine Steigerung von 1/5 Zellinien bei der LZE auf 3/5 Zellinien bei der KZE (5 μM vs. 50 μM). MTX wirkt sowohl bei der LZE als auch bei der KZE in relativ hoher Konzentration bei jeweils 2 Zellinien zytozid. DIC war bei der LZE in Konzentrationen von 0,5–5 μM bei keiner Linie wirksam. Auf die KZE wurde deshalb verzichtet.

Bei Betrachtung der einzelnen Zellinien erweist sich SK-MEL-3 (4/9 und 1/8 Substanzen mit zytozider Wirkung) sowohl bei der LZE als auch bei der KZE als am resistentesten. Die Zellinie wurde aus einer Lymphknoten-Metastase einer 42jährigen

Tabelle 1. Im zeitlichen Verlauf erzielte minimale korrigierte T/C-Werte bei Langzeitexposition (*oben*) und bei Kurzzeitexposition (*unten*)

	SK-MEL-2	SK-MEL-3	SK-MEL-5	SK-MEL-24	SK-MEL-28	Zytozider Effekt / Zellinien gesamt
0.1 µM VBL	- 50	- 5	- 57	- 42	- 6	5 / 5
1 µM ADM	- 60	- 26	- 80	- 65	- 73	5 / 5
0.5 nM DACT	- 20	- 76	- 48	- 17	- 20	5 / 5
60 µM CBDCA	- 67	- 42	- 48	- 26	- 9	5 / 5
0.5 µM DHAQ	- 43	+ 10	- 3	- 20	- 59	4 / 5
5 µM CDDP	- 30	+ 2	- 33	- 46	+ 4	3 / 5
10 µM MTX	- 10	+ 64	- 57	+ 30	+ 23	2 / 5
5 µM L-PAM	+ 1	+ 30	+ 38	- 23	+ 31	1 / 5
5 µM DIC	+ 55	+ 75	+ 84	+ 88	+ 97	0 / 5
Zytozide Substanzwirkung / Substanzen gesamt	7 / 9	4 / 9	7 / 9	7 / 9	5 / 9	

	SK-MEL-2	SK-MEL-3	SK-MEL-5	SK-MEL-24	SK-MEL-28	Zytozider Effekt / Zellinien gesamt
1 µM VBL	- 66	+ 7	- 72	- 31	- 41	4 / 5
10 µM ADM	- 72	- 27	- 70	- 39	- 45	5 / 5
50 nM DACT	- 28	+ 2	- 46	- 4	+ 5	3 / 5
0.5 mM CBDCA	- 12	+ 17	+ 27	+ 2	+ 25	1 / 5
5 µM DHAQ	- 58	+ 3	- 25	- 42	- 4	4 / 5
50 µM cDDP	+ 9	+ 11	- 28	- 32	+ 7	2 / 5
0.1 mM MTX	- 47	+ 49	- 49	+ 12	+ 24	2 / 5
50 µM L-PAM	- 59	+ 16	+ 5	- 51	- 17	3 / 5
DIC	n i c h t g e t e s t e t					
Zytozide Substanzwirkung / Substanzen gesamt	7 / 8	1 / 8	6 / 8	6 / 8	4 / 8	

Frau isoliert, die bereits mit Methyl-CCNU vorbehandelt worden war. An zweiter Stelle bezüglich der Resistenz folgt SK-MEL-28 (5/9 und 4/8), die übrigen Zellinien sind untereinander ähnlich chemosensibel und insgesamt relativ empfindlich. Vergleicht man die einzelnen Zellinien hinsichtlich der Anzahl der wirksamen Substanzen, so stellt man fest, daß sie sich für die jeweilige Zellinie bei der LZE und

KZE kaum verändert. Mit Ausnahme von CBDCA und L-PAM bleibt das Wirkprofil des jeweiligen Zytostatikums bei den einzelnen Zellinien in etwa erhalten.

Diskussion

Melphalan gilt heute als Standardtherapeutikum für die Extremitätenperfusion beim malignen Melanom. Die klinischen Ergebnisse verschiedener Autoren sind jedoch aufgrund zahlreicher Variablen nur bedingt vergleichbar. Gibt es eine Alternative zum Melphalen?

Umfangreiche, mit diversen klonogenen und nicht-klonogenen Assays vorgenommene Untersuchungen ergeben lediglich eine 61–67%ige Korrelation der in vitro-Ergebnisse mit einer klinisch zu beobachtenden Tumor*remission*. Der Vorhersagewert für eine Tumor*resistenz* liegt aber bei 91–97% [4]. Ein Ansprechen *in vivo* sollte bei einem, im Zellkulturexperiment erzielbaren *zytoziden* Effekt, eher wahrscheinlich sein, als wenn sich nur eine Proliferationshemmung einstellt. Unter diesem Aspekt empfehlen sich aufgrund der vorliegenden Chemosensitivitätstests vor allem VBL, DHAQ, ADM und auch DACT und cDDP für weiterführende Untersuchungen. Diese Substanzen führten bei den meisten Zellinien zu einer Zytolyse, wobei der Effekt auch in der Kurzzeitexposition im wesentlichen erhalten blieb.

Vinca-Alkaloide und *Dactinomycin* wurden bisher in der Regel nur in Kombination bei der isolierten Extremitätenperfusion eingesetzt [5]. Damit kann der Anteil dieser Substanzen am Therapieerfolg nicht abgeschätzt werden.

Mitoxantron, ein neueres Zytostatikum, wurde vor kurzem in einer pharmakokinetischen Studie an 5 Patienten mit einem solitären malignen Melanom am Bein bei adjuvanten Perfusionen nach Tumorexzision und Lymphknotendissektion getestet [3]. Mitoxantron eignet sich wegen der in vitro nachgewiesenen Zytotoxizität an Melanomzellen, der Steigerung der Wirksamkeit unter hyperthermen Bedingungen, der hohen Aufnahme in das perfundierte Gewebe und der niedrigen systemischen Plasmaspiegel als Folge der geringen Leckrate gut für die isolierte, hypertherme Perfusion. Umfangreichere Erfahrungen mit längerem Nachbeobachtungszeitraum liegen jedoch bisher nicht vor.

Doxorubicin, wie Mitoxantron ein Anthracyclin-Derivat, wird bei der regionalen Chemotherapie der Weichteilsarkome in Form der intraarteriellen Infusion oder der isolierten Perfusion verwendet. Es wurde allerdings von einer teilweisen Präzipitation mit Heparin berichtet, die die Anwendung bei der Perfusion limitiert [2]. Bei Betrachtung der in vitro-Ergebnisse von ADM und DHAQ tritt ein zytozider Effekt von DHAQ bereits bei der halben äquiaktiven Konzentration im Vergleich zu ADM ein. Die Bedeutung dieser Beobachtung, z.B. verminderte lokale Toxizität bei gleicher Wirksamkeit, muß erst im Tierexperiment untersucht werden.

Vor kurzem wurde die Wirksamkeit und Toxizität von *Cisplatin* mit Melphalan und anderen Substanzen verglichen [5]. Nach 5 von 6 therapeutischen Perfusionen kam es zu einem Lokalrezidiv (bzw. einer ausbleibenden Tumorremission), ebenso wie nach 2 von 4 prophylaktischen Perfusionen. Bei 4 Patienten entwickelte sich eine höhergradige toxische Gewebereaktion. Die Gründe hierfür könnten in einer inadäquaten Cisplatin-Dosierung oder in suboptimalen Gewebetemperaturen zu suchen sein, insgesamt ist aber Cisplatin sicherlich nicht das Mittel der Wahl für die hypertherme Perfusion beim malignen Melanom.

Dacarbazin, eines der Standard-Chemotherapeutika bei der systemischen Therapie des metastasierten Melanoms, wirkt nach bisherigem Kenntnisstand hauptsächlich über eine Methylierung der Nucleinsäuren nach Metabolisierung der Ausgangssubstanz in der Leber. Alternativ kann durch Photoaktivierung ein in vitro zytotoxisches Derivat entstehen, auch wurde in vitro bei Anwesenheit aktiver DNA-Polymerase α eine direkte DNA-Schädigung nachgewiesen. Eine Lichtexposition erfolgte bei unseren Experimenten nur kurzzeitig bei dem Herstellen der Lösung, der Substanzzugabe und der obligaten mikroskopischen Wachstumskontrolle. Dabei trat praktisch keine zytostatische Wirkung ein. Es gibt noch keinen schlüssigen Beweis, daß der photolytische Zerfall oder die direkte DNA-Schädigung für die Tumorwirkung in vivo eine Rolle spielen. Nach neueren Berichten [1] zeigte DIC eine dem Melphalan deutlich unterlegene bzw. der alleinigen lokalen Exzision gleiche Wirkung. Möglicherweise waren die Ergebnisse früherer Autoren Folge der Hyperthermie oder eines systemischen Lecks mit konsekutiver metabolischer Aktivierung von DIC in der Leber [5].

Zusammenfassung

Die Sensitivität fünf humaner Melanom-Zellinien gegenüber Melphalen (L-PAM), Dacarbazin (DIC), Methotrexat (MTX), Vinblastin (VBL), Dactinomycin (DACT), Doxorubicin (ADM), Mitoxantron (DHAQ), Cisplatin (cDDP) und Carboplatin (CB-DCA) wurde mittels eines standardisierten kinetischen Microassays untersucht. Unter Berücksichtigung der bei isolierter hyperthermer Extremitätenperfusion erreichbaren Plasmaspiegel erscheinen VBL, DHAQ, ADM, DACT und cDDP für weiterführende, pharmakokinetisch kontrollierte in vivo-Studien erfolgversprechend.

Summary

Sensitivity of five human melanoma cell lines towards melphalan (L-PAM), dacarbazine (DIC), methotrexate (MTX), vinblastine (VBL), dactinomycin (DACT), doxorubicin (ADM), mitoxantrone (DHAQ), cisplatin (cDDP) and carboplatin (CDBCA) was tested by means of a standardized kinetic microassay. With respect to achievable plasma concentrations in hyperthermic isolated limb perfusion VBL, DHAQ, ADM, DACT and cDDP seem promising for further pharmacokinetically controlled in vivo-studies.

Literatur

1. Edwards MJ, Boddie AW Jr, Ames FC, McBride CM (1990) Isolated limb perfusion for stage 1 melanoma of the extremity: a comparison of melphalan and dacarbazine (DTIC). South Med J 82:985–987

2. Krementz ET, Ryan RF, Muchmore JH et al. (1992) Hyperthermic regional perfusion for melanoma of the limbs. In: Balch CM, Houghton AN, Milton GW et al. (eds) Cutaneous melanoma, 2nd edition. Lippincott, Philadelphia, Pennsylvania, pp 403–426
3. Nagel JD, Krüger I, Ghussen F, Bode U (1991) Clinical pharmakokinetics of mitoxantrone in hyperthermic, isolated perfusion of the leg. Cancer Chemother Pharmacol 29:155–158
4. Phillips RM, Bibby MC, Double JA (1990) A critical appraisal of the predictive value of in vitro chemosensitivity assays. J Natl Cancer Inst 82:1455–1468
5. Thompson JF, Gianoutsos MP (1992) Isolated limb perfusion for melanoma: effectiveness and toxicity of cisplatin compared with that of melphalan and other drugs. World J Surg 16:227–233

Th. Meyer, Klinik und Poliklinik für Chirurgie, Universität Regensburg,
Franz-Josef-Strauß-Allee, W-8400 Regensburg

Kombination von Zytokinen mit aktiv-spezifischer Immuntherapie – Prävention von zerebralen Melanommetastasen im Mausmodell

Combination of Cytokines with Active-Specific Immunotherapy. Prevention of Cerebral Murine Melanoma

L. Staib[1], W. Harel[2] und M.S. Mitchell[2]

[1]Chirurgische Klinik 1, Universitätsklinik Ulm (Ärztl. Direktor: Prof. Dr. H.G. Beger)
[2]Comprehensive Cancer Center, University of Southern California, Los Angeles, USA

Die Entwicklung von Hirnmetastasen bei Patienten mit metastasiertem malignen Melanom, die unter aktiv-spezifischer Immuntherapie eine Tumorremission zeigten, bereitet ein besonderes therapeutisches Problem [1]. Es ist bisher nicht bekannt, ob die Immunisierung gegen Tumoren das Zentralnervensystem, z.B. aufgrund der Blut-Hirn-Schranke, nicht erreicht, oder ob lokale Faktoren (Suppressorfaktoren, Mangel an Zytokinen, verminderte Antigenpräsentation) die Immunantwort aktivierter T-Lymphozyten und Makrophagen verhindert. In dem von uns entwickelten Mausmodell zur aktiv-spezifischen Immuntherapie des Melanoms konnten wir in den Randbereichen der zerebralen Melanommetastasen CD4- und CD8-positive T-Lymphozyten sowie melaningefüllte Makrophagen nachweisen. Außerdem zeigte sich ein protektiver Effekt des Melanomvakzins gegenüber Hirnmetastasen [2]. Es stellte sich daher die Frage, ob der Effekt des Vakzins durch Kombination mit zerebral aktiven Zytokinen [3], wie Interleukin-1 (IL-1), Interferon-gamma (IFNg) und Tumor-Nekrose-Faktor-alpha (TNFa) verstärkt werden kann.

Methode

Immunisierung. C57/BL6-Mäuse (H-2^b) (VAC-Gruppe, n = 75) wurden wie beschrieben [2] intraperitoneal mit einem syn- und allogenen Mausmelanomzell-Vakzin immunisiert. Dazu wurden in einer Dosis von $2,5 \times 10^6$ Zellen/Injektion mit 4000 rad bestrahlte syngene G3.12-BM2-Zellen (H-2^b) sowie allogene Cloudman-Zellen (H-2^q) mit dem unspezifischen Immunstimulans Detox (Fa. Ribi, Montana, USA) gemischt und den Mäusen subkutan injiziert.

Der Erfolg der Immunisierung wurde durch die seitengetrennte subkutane Injektion von je 10.000 vitalen G3.12- und Cloudman-Zellen festgestellt: Als immun gegen Melanome galt ein Tier, wenn innerhalb von 60 Tagen kein Tumor wuchs. Wachstum eines G3.12-Tumors bedeutete: keine spezifische Immunisierung; Wachstum eines Cloudman-Tumors: mangelhafte Antigen-Expression des allogenen Tumors, Ergebnis nicht verwertbar. Kontrolltieren (PBS-Gruppe, n = 29) wurde statt Vakzin intraperitoneal PBS injiziert. Zehn Tiere dieser Gruppe wurden als Stichprobe nachfolgend subkutan seitengetrennt mit je 10.000 vitalen G3-12- und Cloudman-Zellen inokuliert.

Chirurgisches Forum 1993
f. experim. u. klinische Forschung
Becker/Beger/Hartel (Hrsg.)

Intrazerebrale Tumorinokulation. Mäusen der VAC- und der PBS-Gruppe wurden unter Inhalationsanästhesie in einer Hamiltonspritze 200 vitale G3.12-Zellen in 20 μl Volumen intracerebral injiziert, um experimentelle Melanom-Hirnmetastasen zu erzeugen. Die Tiere wurden postmortal (oder 60 Tage nach Tumorzellinokulation) seziert und auf Melanom-Hirnmetastasen sowie extrazerebrale Metastasen hin untersucht. Die erstellten Überlebenskurven wurden mit einem Log-Rank-Test auf statistische Signifikanz getestet.

Zytokintherapie. Einen Tag nach intrazerebraler Tumorinokulation wurden die Tiere der PBS- und der VAC-Gruppe randomisiert einer der folgenden Therapiegruppen zugeteilt: *PBS-Gruppe*: PBS (n = 10), IL-1/IFNg/TNFa (n = 9). *VAC-Gruppe*: PBS (n = 10), IL-1/IFNg/TNFa (n = 10), IL-1/IFNg (n = 9), IL-1/TNFa (n = 10), IFNg/TNFa (n = 9), IL-1 (n = 9), IFNg (n = 9), TNFa (n = 9).

Rekombinantes humanes *Interleukin-1β* (spezif. Aktivität 10^8 U/mg; Immunex Corp., Seattle, Washington, USA) wurde in einer Dosis von 360 ng/die über 8 Tage subkutan injiziert. Rekombinantes murines *Interferon-gamma* (spezif. Aktivität $13,1 \times 10^6$ U/mg; Genentech Inc., South San Francisco, California, USA) wurde in einer Dosis von 40.000 IU/die über 5 Tage intraperitoneal appliziert. Rekombinanter humaner *Tumor-Nekrose-Faktor alpha* (spezif. Aktivität 10^8 U/mg; Biosource International, Camarillo, California, USA) wurde in einer Dosis von 20.000 IU/die über 5 Tage intraperitoneal appliziert.

Ergebnisse

Immunisierung. Kein Tier aus der VAC-Gruppe entwickelte innerhalb von 60 Tagen subkutane G3.12- oder Cloudman-Melanome. Alle als Stichprobe aus der PBS-Gruppe ausgewählten und subkutan inokulierten Tiere (n = 5) verstarben innerhalb von 40 Tagen an subkutanen G3.12-Melanomen.

Intrazerebrale Tumorinokulation. Die intrazerebrale Injektion von vitalen G3-12-Zellen in immunisierte und Kontrollmäuse hatte keine methodisch bedingte Letalität zur Folge (Blutung, Infektion).

Zytokintherapie. Die Häufigkeit von intrazerebralen syngenen Melanomen ist in Abb. 1 dargestellt. Die PBS-Behandlung führte bei 10/10 Tieren der PBS-Gruppe zu letalen Hirnmetastasen, jedoch nur bei 2/10 Tieren der VAC-Gruppe ($p < 0,05$). Die Applikation der drei Zytokine IL-1, IFNg und TNFa in Kombination verhinderte in der PBS-Gruppe Hirnmetastasen in 4/9 Tieren und in der VAC-Gruppe bei allen 10 Tieren signifikant gegenüber der PBS-Behandlung ($p < 0,05$). Bei metastasenfreien Tieren waren 60 Tage nach Tumorinokulation makroskopisch keine zerebralen oder extrazerebralen Melanommetastasen nachweisbar, während befallene Tiere neurologisch symptomatisch wurden und nach zwei bis drei Tagen verstarben. Intrazerebrale Melanommetasasen wurden in allen Hirnregionen beobachtet. Extrazerebrale Metastasen wurden nicht beobachtet. Die Zytokintherapie hatte keine erkennbaren Nebenwirkungen oder eine therapiebedingte Letalität zur Folge. In Abb. 2 ist die relative Häufung

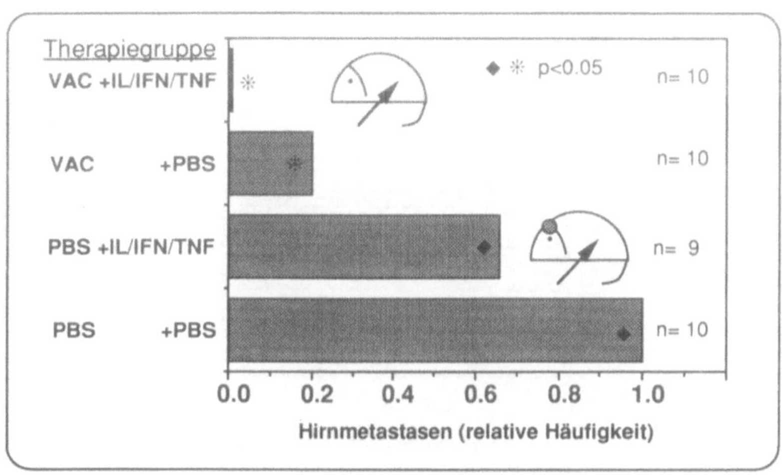

Abb. 1. Häufigkeit zerebraler Melanom-Metastasen nach Inokulation mit 200 syngenen Melanomzellen (G3.12). C57BL/6-Mäuse wurden mit bestrahlten syn- und allogenen Melanomzellen und Detox über 5 Wochen immunisiert (VAC-Gruppe) oder mit PBS ip. injiziert (PBS-Gruppe). Nach der Tumorzellinokulation erhielten die Tiere systemisch PBS oder Interleukin-1, Interferon-Gamma oder Tumor-Nekrose-Faktor-alpha. Hirnmetastasen traten in der Vakzin-Gruppe seltener auf als in der PBS-Gruppe. Die Kombination von IL-1, TNFa und IFNg verringerte das Auftreten von zerebralen Metastasen in beiden Gruppen signifikant (*,◆ $p < 0{,}05$, log-rank-Test der Überlebenszeiten)

von G3.12-Hirnmetastasen bei Tieren der VAC-Gruppe dargestellt, die Zytokine in unterschiedlichen Kombinationen erhielten. Die Gabe eines einzelnen Zytokins oder der Kombination von IL/TNF bzw. IL/IFN ist der PBS-Behandlung bei zuvor immunisierten Tieren gleichwertig ($p > 0{,}05$). Die Kombination von Vakzin mit TNF/IFN oder IL/TNF/IFN führte zu einer signifikanten ($p < 0{,}05$) Reduktion von Hirnmetastasen, da alle Tiere ($n = 9$ bzw. $n = 10$) tumorfrei blieben.

Diskussion

Der tumorprotektive Effekt der aktiv-spezifischen Immuntherapie (ASI) gegenüber syngenen zerebralen Melanommetastasen ließ sich im Mausmodell durch Kombination mit Interferon-gamma und Tumor-Nekrose-Faktor-alpha (sowie Interleukin-1) steigern. Wir konnten in früheren Untersuchungen zeigen, daß die ASI mit Melanomvakzin im Mausmodell [2] und beim Menschen [4] CD4- und CD8-positive T-Lymphozyten erzeugt, die gemeinsam mit Makrophagen die Blut-Hirn-Schranke überwinden können. Es ist denkbar, daß durch die systemische Gabe zweier oder mehrerer Zytokine im zuvor spezifisch immunisierten Organismus eine verstärkte Aktivierung der tumorlysierenden T-Lymphozyten und Makrophagen hervorgerufen wird. Die zerebralen Wirkungen von TNFa, IL-1 und IFNg liegen u.a. in der Aktivierung, Antigenexpressionserhöhung (MHC I und II) und Zytokinsekretionsförderung von Astrozyten, Microglia und Oligodendrogliazellen (Übersicht bei [3]). Ein mehr-

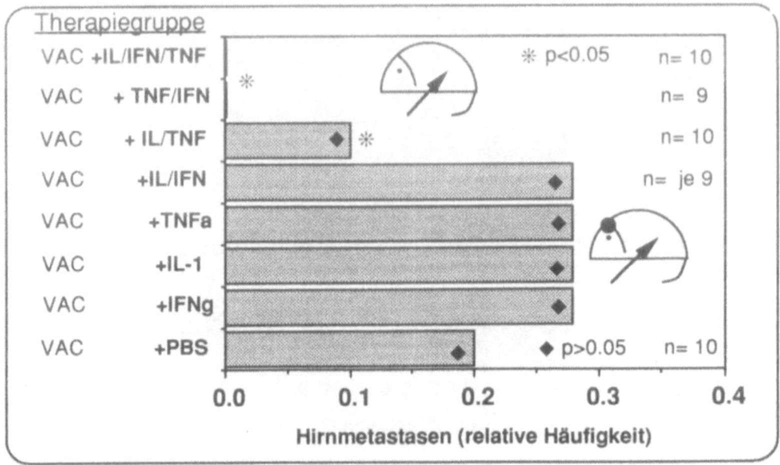

Abb. 2. Häufigkeit zerebraler Melanom-Metastasen nach Inokulation mit 200 syngenen Melanomzellen (G3.12). C57BL/6-Mäuse wurden mit bestrahlten syn- und allogenen Melanomzellen und Detox über 5 Wochen immunisiert (VAC-Gruppe). Nach der Tumorzellinokulation erhielten die Tiere systemisch PBS (Kontrollgruppe) oder Interleukin-1, Interferon-gamma und Tumor-Nekrose-Faktor-alpha in verschiedenen Kombinationen. Die Kombination von IL-1, TNFa und IFNg bzw. von IFNg und TNFa verringerte das Auftreten von zerebralen Metastasen signifikant gegenüber der Kontrollgruppe (∗ $p < 0{,}05$, log-rank-Test der Überlebenszeiten). Alle anderen getesteten Zytokinkombinationen unterschieden sich nicht von der Kontrollgruppe (◆ $p < 0{,}05$)

fach diskutierter lokaler Mangel an Zytokinen [1] unter besonderen Umständen, wie intrazerebralem Tumorwachstum, könnte also durch systemische Zytokinapplikation substituiert werden.

Die Befunde am Mausmodell lassen eine Kombination der untersuchten Zytokine mit aktiv-spezifischer Immuntherapie bei Patienten mit metastasiertem Melanom zur Prophylaxe von therapeutisch meist nicht kurierbaren Hirnmetastasen sinnvoll erscheinen.

Zusammenfassung

Das Auftreten experimentell induzierter syngener Melanommetastasen kann im Mausmodell durch Kombination von aktiv-spezifischer Immuntherapie mit den systemisch applizierten Zytokinen TNFa, IFNg und IL-1 verhindert werden. Die aktiv-spezifische Immuntherapie ist in diesem Modell der Mono- oder kombinierten Zytokintherapie überlegen.

Summary

Mice are protected from experimentally induced cerebral metastases by a combination of active-specific immunotherapy with cytokines TNF-α, IFN-γ, and IL-1. Active-specific immunotherapy in this model is more effective than single or multiple cytokine treatment.

Literatur

1. Mitchell MS (1989) Relapse in the central nervous system in melanoma patients successfully treated with biomodulators. J Clin Oncol 7:1701–1709
2. Staib L et al. (1992) Active-specific immunotherapy for solid tumors. In: Gall FP, Beger HG, Ungeheuer E (Hrsg) Chirurgisches Forum 1992 f. experimentelle u. klinische Forschung. Springer, Berlin Heidelberg, pp 253–257
3. Hofman FM, Hinton DR (1991) Cytokine interactions in the central nervous system. Regional Immunology 3:268–278
4. Mitchell MS (1991) Attempts to optimize active specific immunotherapy for melanoma. Int Rev Immunol 7:331–347

Dr. med. L. Staib, Allgemeinchirurgische Universitätsklinik, Steinhövelstraße 9, W-7900 Ulm

Summary

Mice are protected from experimentally induced cerebral metastases by a combination of active specific immunotherapy with cytokines TNF-α, IFN-γ, and IL-4. Active specific immunotherapy in this model is more effective than single or multiple cytokine treatment.

Literatur

1. Mitchell MS (1989) Relapse in the central nervous system in melanoma patients successfully treated with biomodulators. J Clin Oncol 7:1701–1709
2. Schlag P et al. (1992) Active specific immunotherapy for solid tumors. In: [illegible] HP, Rei[illegible] ger (eds) Hämodynamik [illegible] (Gesellschaft [illegible] Forum 1992 f. experimentelle u. klinische Forschung). Springer, Berlin Heidelberg, pp [illegible]
3. Gutman M, Fidler IJ (1991) Biology of metastasis in the central nervous system. [illegible]
4. Mitchell MS (1991) Attempts to optimize active specific immunotherapy for melanoma. Int Rev Immunol 7:331–347

Dr. med. [illegible], Allgemeine Chirurgische Universitätsklinik, Steinhövelstraße 9, W-7900 Ulm

Phänotypisierung und Funktionsanalyse von Lymphocyten bei Patienten mit colorectalem Carcinom

Phenotyping and Functional Analysis of Peripheral Blood Lymphocytes from Patients with Colorectal Carcinoma

B. Donnerstag[1], K. Henzel[1], E. Staib-Sebler[2], K. Holzer[2] und M. Lorenz[2]

[1]Zentrum der Biologischen Chemie, J.-W.-Goethe-Universität Frankfurt/M.
[2]Klinik für Allgemeinchirurgie, J.-W.-Goethe-Universität Frankfurt/M.

Einleitung

Neben der Proliferationsrate bestimmt der Immunstatus das Tumorwachstum. Bei Patienten mit einem Rezidiv eines colorectalen Carcinoms interessierte die langfristige Beeinflussung des Immunstatus durch Operation und/oder adjuvante bzw. palliative Therapie, im Hinblick auf die mögliche Applikation von Immunmodulatoren [1].

Material und Methoden

Tabelle 1. Einteilung der Patientengruppen nach kurativer Operation des Primärtumors oder von Lebermetastasen

Gruppe	N	Chemotherapie (5-FU und FA)[a]	Operationen	Lokalisation der nichtoperierten Metastasen
A	6	–	Leberresektion	–
B	3	adjuvant arteriell	Leberresektion Katheterimplantation	–
C	7	arteriell	Katheterimplantation	Leber
D	7	arteriell oder systemisch (palliativ)	Katheterimplantation	Leber Lunge

[a] (1000 mg 5-FU (kontinuierlich), 200 mg Folinsäure (Kurzzeitinfusion) 5d/28d)

Die analysierten Gruppen von Patienten nach kurativer Operation des Primärtumors oder Lebermetastasen sind in Tabelle 1 aufgeführt. Parallel dazu wurden periphere Blutlymphocyten (PBL) von 19 gesunden Kontrollpersonen auf ihre Funktion getestet (Abb. 1). Die Phänotypisierung wurde mit Hilfe der Flowcytometrie durchgeführt [2].

Chirurgisches Forum 1993
f. experim. u. klinische Forschung
Becker/Beger/Hartel (Hrsg.)

Dazu wurden folgende Parameter bestimmt: CD4, CD8, CD3, CD19, CD16, CD56, CD2, CD25 und HLA-DR. Die Markierung erfolgte mittels fluoreszenzkonjugierter monoklonaler Antikörper (Maus anti-human). Zur Funktionsanalyse wurden PBL mit nIL-2 für 5–7 Tage stimuliert und dann als Effektorzellen eingesetzt. Als Targetzellen dienten NK-Zell sensible (K562) oder resistente (Raji) Zellen. Bei beiden Zelltypen handelt es sich um kommerziell erhältliche Tumorlinien. Die cytotoxische Aktivität wurde mit einem Europiumassay mit Fluorescenz [3] ermittelt und der Effekt anhand der prozentualen Lyse der Targetzellen bestimmt.

Ergebnisse

Die Ergebnisse von Phänotypisierung und Funktionsanalyse der einzelnen Gruppen korrelieren gut. Verglichen mit den Werten der Kontrollpersonen (Abb. 1) sind die Werte der Gruppe A normal (Werte der Phänotypisierung im Normbereich, keine eingeschränkte NK-Zell Aktivität, spezifische T-Zell Aktivität). Patienten der Gruppe B zeigen teilweise leicht erniedrigte Werte bei der Phänotypisierung (CD4 und CD19), während eine normale cytotoxische Aktivität zu verzeichnen ist. Die Patienten der Gruppe C weisen erniedrigte CD4-, CD19- und CD3-Populationen bei der Phänotypisierung auf. Die Funktionsanalyse ergibt meist eine bis zu 50% eingeschränkte cytotoxische Aktivität mit NK-Zell-sensiblen Targetzellen, während sich die Aktivität mit NK-Zell-resistenten Rajizellen teilweise um mehr als 100% erhöht

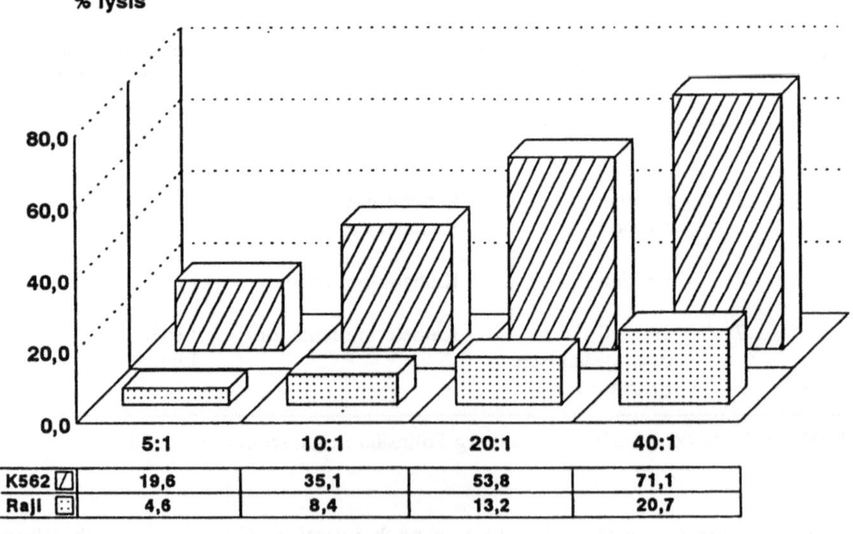

	5:1	10:1	20:1	40:1
K562	19,6	35,1	53,8	71,1
Raji	4,6	8,4	13,2	20,7

Abb. 1. Funktionsanalyse von Lymphocyten in der Kontrollgruppe (nicht erkranktes Kollektiv). *E/T Ratio* = Effektor : Target Ratio

zeigt (Tabelle 2). Da T-Lymphocyten der HLA-Restriktion unterliegen, auf den verwendeten Targetzellinien aber keine körpereigenen HLA-Antigene vorhanden sind, stellt sich die Frage nach der Spezifität der gemessenen Cytotoxizität. Die gemessene lytische Aktivität ist also nur die der nicht HLA-restringierten cytotoxischen T-Lymphocyten. Diese fällt beim Gesunden im Vergleich zur NK-Zell Aktivität niedrig aus (siehe Abb. 1). Ein Anstieg um 100% deutet auf eine massive Aktivierung der körpereigenen unspezifischen Abwehr hin. Verglichen mit klinischen Daten zeigte sich parallel zu diesem Anstieg häufig eine Progredienz des Tumors. Gruppe D zeigt bei der Phänotypisierung und Funktionsanalyse ein ähnliches Bild wie Gruppe C.

Tabelle 2. Funktionsanalyse von Lymphocyten eines Patienten der Gruppe C, Targetzellen: K562 und Raji, E/T Ratio = Effektor : Target Ratio

	E/T Ratio (Raji)				E/T Ratio (K562)			
Datum	5:1	10:1	20:1	40:1	5:1	10:1	20:1	40:1
27.03.1992	1	3	11	13	11	23	44	61
22.04.1992	0	0	0	0	0	2	2	4
29.05.1992	17	25	37	58	21	38	55	81
04.06.1992	0	0	0	6	1	3	7	12
30.06.1992	12	18	21	29	18	34	55	83
04.08.1992	6	19	34	73	19	47	68	100
30.09.1992	3	6	13	15	8	14	26	35
30.10.1992	4	10	13	26	8	14	30	52
17.11.1992	15	24	42	53	26	47	70	83
				(Zellyse in %)				

Diskussion

Die Korrelation des Immunstatus mit dem Krankheitsverlauf bei Patienten mit colorectalem Carcinom zeigte keine langfristige Beeinflussung durch Operation und adjuvante bzw. palliative Therapie. Da die Phänotypisierung von Lymphocyten des peripheren Blutes nicht notwendigerweise auf pathologische Veränderungen in anderen Organen hinweist [4], wurde zusätzlich die cytotoxische Aktivität ermittelt, die Rückschlüsse auf die Funktion zuläßt. Dabei zeigten sich nur geringe, durch regionale, aber auch systemische Chemotherapie (90% der untersuchten Patienten der Gruppe D) bedingte Effekte von 5-FU und Folinsäure auf das Immunsystem. Progredientes Tumorwachstum hingegen supprimiert die Lymphocyten-Proliferation [5] sowie die cytotoxische Funktion der NK-Zellen, kann aber auch zum Entgleisen der spezifischen cytotoxischen Abwehr führen, was dann in einer ungerichteten Aktivität der NK-Zellen resultiert (Tabelle 2).

Zusammenfassung

Bei 24 Patienten mit colorectalem Carcinom sollte der Krankheitsverlauf mit dem Immunstatus korreliert werden. Dabei wurden die Patienten in Gruppen unterteilt, um den Einfluß von Tumor und/oder Chemotherapie zu ermitteln. Es zeigte sich nur eine geringfügige Beeinflussung von Phänotypus und Funktion der Lymphocyten durch 5-FU und Folinsäure. Weiterhin ließen sich immunologische Parameter definieren, die mit einer Progredienz des Tumorwachstums korrelieren.

Summary

In 24 patients with colorectal carcinoma, the clinical course was compared with immunological functions. In order to investigate the influence of tumors and/or chemotherapy, we analyzed separate groups. Little influence on phenotypes and cytotoxic activity could be evaluated after the addition of 5-FU and folinic acid. Furthermore, it was possible to define immunological parameters correlating with the progression of tumor growth.

Literatur

1. Uchida A, Kariya Y, Okamoto N, Sugie K, Fujimoto T, Yagita M (1990) Prediction of postoperative clinical course by autologous tumor-killing activity in lung cancer patients. JNCI 82:1697–1701
2. Yoo Y-K, Heo DS, Hata K, Van Thiel DH, Whiteside TL (1990) Tumor-infiltrating lymphocytes from human colon carcinomas. Gastroenterol 98:259–269
3. Volgmann T, Klein-Struckmeier A, Mohr M (1989) A fluorescence-based assay for quantitation of lymphokine-activated killer cell activity. J Immunol Meth 119:45–51
4. Westermann J, Pabst R (1990) Lymphocyte subsets in the blood: a diagnostic window on the lymphoid system. Immunol Today 11:406–410
5. Richner J, Armbinder EP, Feuer EJ, Bekesi G (1992) Plasma immunosuppressive factors in patients with advanced colorectal cancer. Tumordiagn Ther 13:127–131

Dr. B. Donnerstag, Zentrum der Biologischen Chemie, Johann-Wolfgang- Goethe-Universität, Theodor-Stern-Kai 7, W-6000 Frankfurt am Main 70

Aktivierung von Monozyten und Lymphozyten durch in vitro Gentransfer und Expression von humanem Interleukin-2 (hIL-2) in menschlichen Tumorzellen

Activation of Monocytes and Lymphocytes by In Vitro Transfer and Expression of the Human Interleukin-2 Gene (hIL-2) in Human Tumor Cells

H.K. Schackert[1], A. Mehrabi[1], A. Buttler[2], G. Schackert[2] und Ch. Herfarth[1]

[1]Chirurgische Universitätsklinik (Dir.: Prof. Dr. Ch. Herfarth), Heidelberg
[2]Neurochirurgische Universitätsklinik (Dir.: Prof. Dr. St. Kunze), Heidelberg

Einleitung

Die unzureichende Immunabwehr gegen maligne Tumoren wurde unter anderem auf die geringe Immunogenität des tumorassoziierten Antigens und eine defekte T-Helferfunktion zurückgeführt. Das Konzept der "associate recognition" von Lake und Mitchison [1] fordert die Expression von mindestens zwei Antigenen auf der Zelloberfläche, um eine Immunantwort zu erzeugen. Im Tierexperiment wird dies bestätigt. Die Expression eines viralen Antigens [2] verbessert die Immunabwehr gegen die antigenen Strukturen der Tumorzelle. Andererseits wird eine defekte T-Helferfunktion im Rahmen der Immunabwehr gegen Tumoren mit der Produktion und Sekretion von Interleukin-2 durch die Tumorzelle umgangen [3].

Ziel dieser Arbeit war die Übertragung des letztgenannten Ansatzes in die humane Situation, um den in vitro Effekt von lokal sezerniertem humanen Interleukin-2 (hIL-2) versus extern zugeführtem hIL-2 bei der Aktivierung von Monozyten und Lymphozyten gegen Tumorzellen zu studieren. Dieser Ansatz impliziert die Frage nach den potentiellen Vorteilen einer lokalen Expression von hIL-2 nach Transfer des Gens in Tumorzellen versus systemischer Gabe von hIL-2 bei der Immuntherapie maligner Tumoren.

Material und Methoden

hIL-2 Konstrukt: Das menschliche IL-2 Gen (hIL-2-Gen) wurde in dem 542 bp HindIII-EcoRI DNA Fragment aus dem Vektor pBEH-IL-2 (Gabe von Harald S. Conradt, Gesellschaft für Biotechnologische Forschung Braunschweig) in den pUHD 10-1 Vektor (Deuschle, PNAS 1989) kloniert. Daraus resultierte pUHD 10-1-IL-2, in dem das hIL-2 Gen von einem CMV Promotor getrieben wird.

Chirurgisches Forum 1993
f. experim. u. klinische Forschung
Becker/Beger/Hartel (Hrsg.)

Zellinien: Die menschliche Coloncarcinomlinie KM 12, die Melanomlinie A 375 (beides Gaben von Isaiah J. Fidler, MD, Anderson Cancer Center, Houston, Texas) und die Glioblastomlinie T1115 (Gabe von Hans Fischer, Deutsches Krebsforschungszentrum Heidelberg) exprimieren das hIL-2 Gen nach Kotransfektion von pUHD 10-1-IL-2 mit pSV2neo (Southern, J. Mol. Appl. Genet., 1982) mittels Calcium-Präzipitation und nach G418 Selektion. Klon 2 der Glioblastomlinie T1115 produziert die höchste hIL-2 Menge mit 5.800 pg/10^5 Zellen/24 h (hIL-2 Elisa: Biermann, Bad Nauheim; 76 Picogramm = 1 Unit hIL-2) und wurde neben der ursprünglichen, nichttransfizierten T1115 Linie für die in vitro Untersuchungen verwendet.

Zytotoxizitätsassays: Im Monozyten-Zytotoxizitätsassay wurden ^{3}H-Thymidin-markierte Tumorzellen mit menschlichen Monozyten inkubiert, die nach Separierung über einen Ficollgradienten und durch Adhärenz an Plastik angereichert worden waren (Nachweis durch Peroxidase Färbung und Morphologie). Mononukleäre Zellen, die über den Ficollgradienten angereichert worden waren und an Plastik nicht adhärent waren, fanden als Effektorzellen im LAK Zellassay (Lymphokin aktivierte Killerzellen) Verwendung. Sowohl LAK Zellen als auch Monozyten wurden in 96 Lochplatten in einer Dichte von 200.000 Zellen pro Loch als Dreifachansatz ausgesät. Das Effektor-/Zielzellen-(Tumorzellen)Verhältnis betrug 20:1 mit Ausnahme des Kokultivationsexperimentes von Klon2 und T1115 (Verhältnis 10:1). Zellen wurden in RPMI 1640 Medium (Gibco, Eggenstein) inkubiert, das mit 10% fetalem Kälberserum, Gentamycin, nichtessentiellen Aminosäuren, $NaHCO_3$, HEPES, Vitaminen und 1-Glutamin angereichert war.

Menschliches rekombinantes IL-2, IFN-γ, TNF-α (alle Boehringer Mannheim) wurden in Medium verdünnt und dem Zytotoxizitätsassay zugeführt. Alle verwendeten Medien und Substanzen waren frei von Endotoxin, was mit dem Limulus amebocyte assay (Pyroquant, Walldorf; Sensitivität = 0,06 ng/ml) nachgewiesen wurde.

Tumorzellen wurden für 24 h mit 0,5 μCi/ml [^{3}H]-Thymidin (Amersham, Braunschweig; spezifische Aktivität 25 Ci/μmol) inkubiert, mehrfach gewaschen und im Verhältnis 20:1 (Effektor-/Zielzellen) mit den Effektorzellen inkubiert. Diese Koinkubation im Zytotoxizitätsassay erstreckte sich generell über 3 Tage. Die Stimulation der Effektorzellen erfolgte einerseits über einen 24 h-Zeitraum davor, und die Stimulanzien wurden danach aus der Kultur durch mehrfaches Waschen mit Medium entfernt. Andererseits wurden exogenes hIL-2 oder von Klon 2 produziertes endogenes hIL-2 als Stimulanzien über den Zeitraum von 3 Tagen mit Effektor- und Targetzellen inkubiert. 72 h nach der Kokultivierung von Effektor- und Zielzellen wurden die Kulturen dreimal mit PBS gewaschen und die adhärenten Zellen mit 0,2 ml 0,1N NaOH lysiert. Die Radioaktivität wurde in einem Betacounter (Wallac 1410 liquid scintillation counter) als cpm (counts per minute) gemessen. Die Berechnung der Zytotoxizität bei Klon 2 erfolgte nach der Formel: % Zytotoxizität = 100 × (cpm von Klon 2 Zellen allein – cpm von Klon 2 Zellen kokultiviert mit Effektorzellen)/(cpm von Klon 2 Zellen allein). Die Berechnung der Zytotoxizität bei T1115 erfolgte nach der Formel: % Zytotoxizität = 100 × (cpm von T1115 Zellen kokultiviert mit nichtaktivierten Effektorzellen – cpm von T1115 Zellen kultiviert mit aktivierten Effektorzellen)/(cpm von T1115 Zellen kokultiviert mit nichtaktivierten Effektorzellen). Die angegebenen Werte sind Mittelwerte und Standardabweichung aus Dreifachbestimmungen pro Ansatz.

Ergebnisse

LAK Zellen und Monozyten, die vor der Zugabe der Zielzelle T1115 über 24 h mit 100 U/ml hIL-2 stimuliert worden waren, bewirken eine 70%ige bzw. 67%ige Zytotoxizität gegen T1115 im anschließenden Dreitageassay. Im Vergleich dazu resultiert die dreitägige Inkubation unstimulierter LAK Zellen und Monozyten mit Klon 2 in einer 79%igen bzw. 80%igen Zytotoxizität. Die Spontanzytotoxizität beträgt weniger als 10% (Abb. 1).

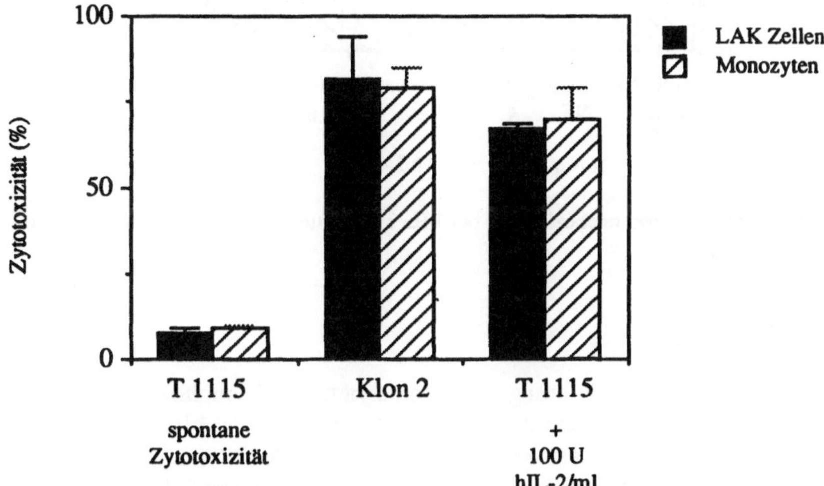

Abb. 1. hIL-2 vermittelte Aktivierung von Monozyten und LAK-Zellen

Ein separater Monozytenassay zeigt die Dosis-Wirkungsbeziehung der exogenen hIL-2 vermittelten Effektorzell-Zytotoxizität im Vergleich zu Klon 2 und zur 24stündigen Präinkubation der Monozyten mit 100 U/ml hIL-2/ml oder je 1.000 Units TNF-α und IFN-γ/ml (Abb. 2). Im LAK Zellassay sind die Resultate ähnlich. Die Stimulation mit 5 U, 10 U, 50 U und 100 U hIL-2/ml Medium über 3 Tage ergibt Zytotoxizitätswerte von 24%, 42%, 68% und 71%. Die Inkubation von Klon 2 mit nichtstimulierten LAK Zellen resultiert in einer 86%igen Zytotoxizität.

Die Kokultivierung von 10.000 T1115 Zellen mit 10.000 Klon 2 Zellen und nichtstimulierten Monozyten zeigt, daß sowohl Klon 2 (57% Zytotoxizität) als auch T1115 (53% Zytotoxizität) effektiv lysiert werden. Klon 2 alleine wird zu 54% lysiert. Die Zytotoxizitätswerte im LAK Assay unter Kokultivationsbedingungen betragen 50% für Klon 2 und 45% für T1115. Klon 2 alleine wird zu 55% lysiert.

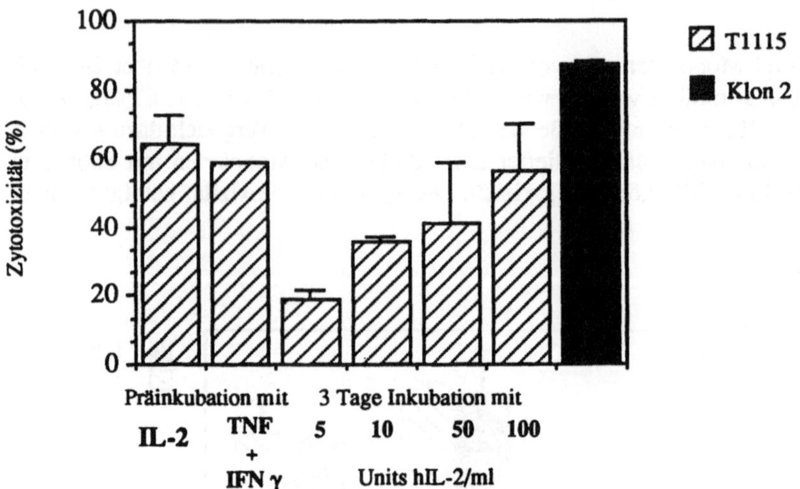

Abb. 2. Dosis-Wirkungsbeziehung der hIL-2 vermittelten Monozytenzytotoxizität

Diskussion

Die zytotoxische Aktivierung von Monozyten und Lymphozyten durch IL-2 ist bekannt [4]. Wir zeigen, daß die endogene Produktion von hIL-2 durch die Tumorzelle (Klon 2) eine starke Zytotoxizität der Effektorzelle (Monozyt oder Lymphozyt) bewirkt. Klon 2 Zellen im Zytotoxizitätstest produzieren pro 0,3 ml Ansatz in den ersten 24 h maximal 25,4 Units hIL-2/ml Medium. Die von Anfang an wirksame exogene hIL-2 Menge beträgt dagegen bis zu 100 Units/ml. Es muß jedoch davon ausgegangen werden, daß endogen produziertes und sezerniertes hIL-2 lokal im Bereich der Effektorzellen in hoher Konzentration vorliegt. Dies ist vermutlich der Grund für die Effektivität des von Klon 2 produzierten hIL-2, das nicht nur eine Zytotoxizität gegen Klon 2, sondern auch gegen kokultivierte T1115 Zellen vermittelt. Unsere Beobachtungen reihen sich in tierexperimentelle Untersuchungen ein, die bestätigen, daß die lokale Produktion von Zytokinen durch Tumorzellen die Immunabwehr effektiv aktiviert [3, 5]. Der Transfer und die Expression von Zytokingenen in menschlichen Tumoren gibt zur Hoffnung Anlaß, die potente immunstimulatorische Wirkung von hIL-2 unter Vermeidung der Nachteile der systemischen Gabe hoher Dosen hIL-2 [6] lokal entfalten zu können.

Zusammenfassung

Tumorzellen, die nach Gentransfer Zytokine produzieren, können eine Immunität vermitteln, die gegen den Tumor gerichtet ist. Untersuchungen in Tiermodellen zeigen, daß die Interleukin-2 Sekretion durch Tumorzellen die T-Helferfunktion umgeht, während Tumorzellen, die Interleukin-4 produzieren, weitgehend unabhängig von T-Zellen abgestoßen werden. Beide Zytokine erzeugen jedoch eine systemische Immunantwort gegen den ursprünglichen Tumor.

Diese Arbeit versucht, den Effekt des Zytokingentransfers auf die in vitro Zytotoxizität von menschlichen Monozyten und LAK Zellen zu studieren. Zu diesem Zweck wurde die menschliche Glioblastomlinie T1115 mit einem Plasmidvektor, der die menschliche Interleukin-2 cDNA enthält, und pSV2neo kotransfiziert. Klon 2 produziert 76 Units hIL-2/10^5 Zellen/24 h und wurde in den LAK und Monozytenassays verwendet. Die Kokultivierung von Klon 2 mit Effektorzellen erzeugt eine starke Zytotoxizität von Monozyten und LAK Zellen sowohl gegen Klon 2 als auch gegen T1115. Ähnliche Zytotoxizitätsraten können durch 100 Units/ml exogen zugeführten hIL-2 erreicht werden. Der Vorteil der lokalen Zytokinproduktion im Vergleich zur systemischen Gabe bei der Immuntherapie maligner Tumoren ist die hohe Aktivierung der Effektorzellen ohne systemische Nebenwirkungen. Die Daten tierexperimenteller Untersuchungen zusammen mit diesen in vitro Ergebnissen sind eine Basis für die potentielle Anwendung des Transfers von Zytokingenen in menschliche Tumorzellen als neue Behandlungsform der Immuntherapie maligner Tumoren.

Summary

Tumor cells engineered to produce cytokines after gene transfer can mediate antitumor immunity. Interleukin-2 production by tumor cells has been shown to bypass T-helper function in an animal model while tumor cells expressing interleukin-4 are predominantly rejected in a T-cell-independent manner. Both cytokines generate a systemic immune response against parent tumor cells.

In an attempt to study the effect of cytokine gene transfer on in vitro cytotoxicity of human monocytes and lymphokine-activated killer cells (LAK), human glioblastoma cell line T1115 was cotransfected with a plasmid containing the human interleukin-2 gene cDNA and pSV2neo. Clone 2 produces 76 U hIL-2/10^5 cells/24 h and was used in LAK and monocyte assays. Cocultivation of clone 2 cells and effector cells results in strong monocyte and LAK cell cytotoxicity against clone 2 and its parent cell line T1115. Similar cytotoxicity rates can be achieved by addition of 100 U hIL-2/ml medium. The advantage of local cytokine production over systemic application in immunotherapy of cancer is high activation of immune effector cells without systemic side effects. Data from animal experiments in conjunction with these in vitro results provide a rationale for potential use of cytokine gene transfer in human tumor cells as a modality for cancer immunotherapy.

Literatur

1. Lake P, Mitchison NA (1976) Associate control of the immune response to cell surface antigens. Immunol Commun 5:795–805
2. Schackert HK, Itaya T, Schackert G, Fearon E, Vogelstein B, Frost P (1989) Systemic immunity against a murine colon tumor (CT-26) produced by immunization with syngeneic cells expressing a transfected viral gene product. Int J Cancer 43:823–827

3. Fearon ER, Pardoll DM, Itaya T, Golumbek P, Levitsky HI, Simons JW, Karasuyama H, Vogelstein B, Frost P (1990) Interleukin-2 production by tumor cells bypasses T helper function in the generation of an antitumor response. Cell 60:397–403
4. Higashi N, Nishimura Y, Higuchi M, Osawa T (1991) Human monocytes in a long-term culture with interleukin-2 show high tumoricidal activity against various tumor cells. J Immunother 10:247–255
5. Golumbek PT. Lazenby AJ, Levitsky HI et al. (1991) Treatment of established renal cancer by tumor cells engineered to secrete interleukin-4. Science 254:713–716
6. Rosenberg SA, Lotze MT, Yang JC, Aebersold PA, Linehan WM, Seipp CA, White DE (1989) Experience with the use of high-dose interleukin-2 in the treatment of 652 patients with cancer. Ann Surg 210:474–485

Priv.-Doz. Dr. H.K. Schackert, Chirurgische Universitätsklinik, Im Neuenheimer Feld 110, W-6900 Heidelberg

Funktionelle Ergebnisse der freien Jejunuminterposition nach radikaler Resektion des Hypopharynx-Karzinomes

Functional Results of Free Jejunal Interposition After Radical Resection of Hypopharyngeal Cancer

J. Faß[1], J. Braun[1], H. Klimek[2], A. Tittel[1], J. Silny[3] und V. Schumpelick[1]

[1]Chirurgische Klinik, RWTH Aachen (Direktor: Prof. Dr. med. V. Schumpelick)
[2]Klinik für HNO, RWTH Aachen (Direktor: Prof. Dr. med. H. Schlöndorff)
[3]Helmholtz-Institut für Biomedizinische Technik, RWTH Aachen (Direktor: Prof. Dr. med. P. Rau)

Einleitung

In der chirurgischen Therapie des Hypopharynxkarzinomes hat heute die Ösophagolaryngektomie einen festen Stellenwert. Beim Ersatz der zervikalen Speiseröhre durch die Transplantation eines mikrovaskulär angeschlossenen autologen Jejunalsegmentes ist jedoch wenig über dessen Funktion bekannt. Erste Untersuchungen konnten zeigen, daß extrinsisch denervierte Dünndarmtransplantate viele Motilitätscharakteristika des Dünndarmes behalten [3, 4, 5].

Ziel der vorliegenden Studie sollte die Definition der Transportfunktion des interponierten Jejunalsegmentes beim Schluckakt und seiner spontanen Motilitätsbedingungen sein.

Methode

10 Patienten nach radikaler Resektion eines Hypopharynxkarzinomes mit freier Jejuninterposition wurden 6 Wochen und 6 bis 27 Monate postoperativ untersucht. Bei allen Patienten waren zum Zeitpunkt der Untersuchung ein locoregionäres Tumorrezidiv sowie eine Anastomosenstenose ausgeschlossen.

Als Funktionstests dienten die 8-Kanal-Perfusionsmanometrie (Sondendurchmesser: 3,6 mm, Meßpunktabstand: 5 cm), die Impedanzmetrie (Bestimmung der Bolustransportvorgänge, siehe [2]) und eine Ösophagusszintigraphie mit 99Tc-S-markiertem Haferschleim.

Zur Erfassung der subjektiven Beschwerden diente ein standardisiertes Interview.

Chirurgisches Forum 1993
f. experim. u. klinische Forschung
Becker/Beger/Hartel (Hrsg.)

Ergebnisse

Lediglich ein Patient mit 20 cm langem Interponat klagte über Dysphagie und gelegentliche Regurgitation.

Frühpostoperativ wurde bei 2 Patienten, spätpostoperativ bei allen Patienten im Jejuninterponat ein MMC nachgewiesen. Dabei war die Zyklusdauer verkürzt ($37,7 \pm 18,4$ min), die Phase 3 sowohl in ihrer Dauer ($7,1 \pm 2,5$ min) als auch Propagierungsgeschwindigkeit ($8,6 \pm 1,4$ cm/min) normal. In keiner Messung konnte nach der Nahrungsaufnahme eine Konvertierung zu einem "fed pattern" im Jejunuminterponat festgestellt werden (Abb. 1).

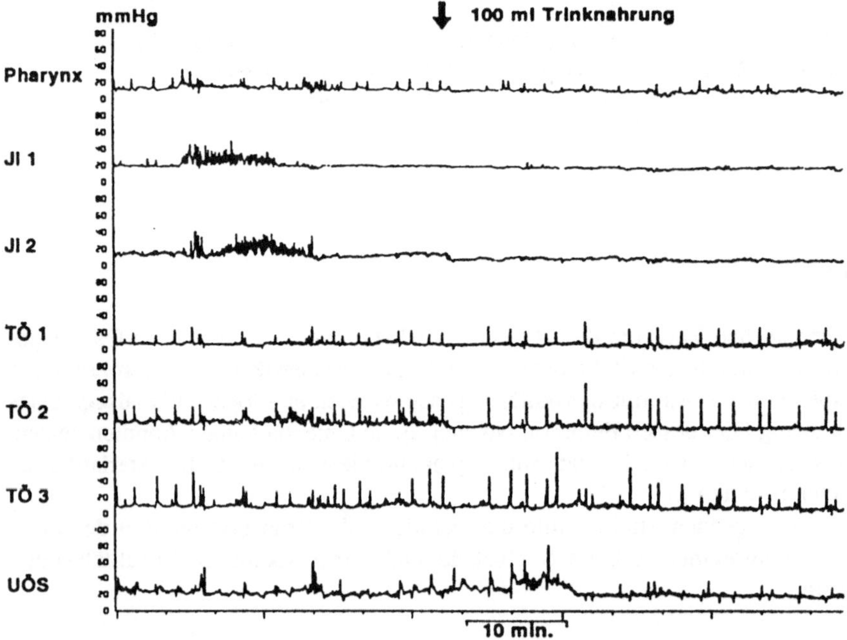

Abb. 1. Nüchternmotilität und postprandiales Muster nach Nahrungsreiz. Fortgeleitete Phase III in JI 1 und JI 2. Keine Konvertierung zum "fed pattern" nach Nahrungsreiz. *JI*, Jejunuminterponat; *TÖ*, tubulärer Ösophagus; *UÖS*, unterer Ösophagussphinkter

Bei keinem Patienten war der obere Ösophagussphinkter nachweisbar. Während des Schluckaktes nahm das Interponat nicht aktiv an der Propulsion teil, während der tubuläre Restösophagus ebenso wie der untere Ösophagussphinkter eine regelrechte Peristaltik zeigte (Abb. 2). Der Bolustransport erfolgte im Interponat passiv und wies für semisolide Testmahlzeiten eine signifikante Verzögerung auf (Abb. 3). Diese Befunde konnten ösophagusszintigraphisch durch Nachweis einer deutlichen Passageverzögerung im Jejunuminterponat bestätigt werden.

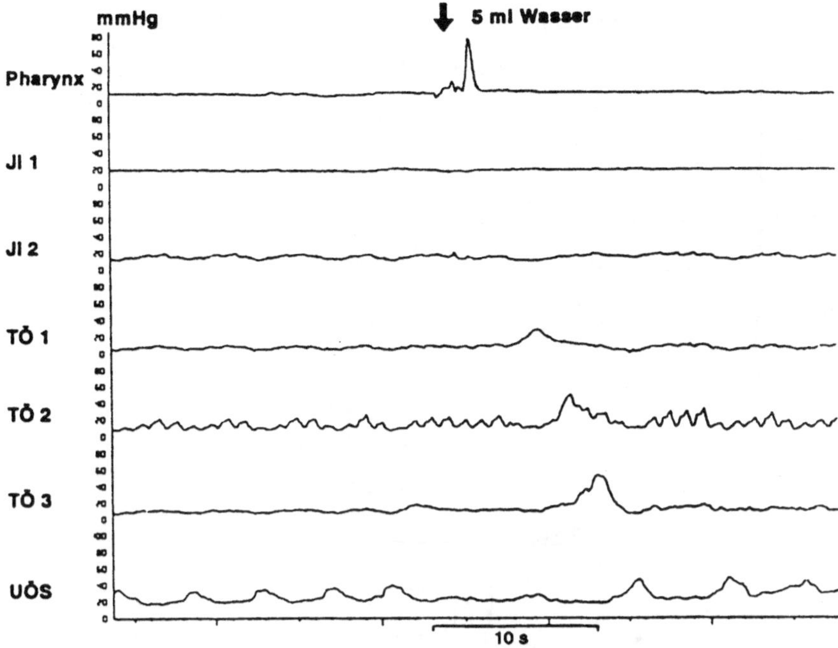

Abb. 2. Manometrische Darstellung eines Schluckaktes (5 ml Wasser). Das Jejunuminterponat zeigt keine aktive Transportfunktion. Normale Peristaltik in TÖ 1–3 und Funktion des UÖS: s. Abb. 1

Diskussion

Die freie Jejunuminterposition ergibt klinisch gute Ergebnisse, obwohl der transplantierte Darm vorwiegend als Platzhalter und nicht als aktives Transportorgan wirkt. Der Speisenbolus wird im Interponat vorwiegend durch die Beschleunigung des Gaumendruckes transportiert und findet im Restösophagus wieder ein intaktes Transportorgan vor.

Bei der Rekonstruktion sollte daher die Interponatslänge so kurz wie möglich gewählt werden, um das Auftreten einer Dysphagie zu vermeiden.

Die Erhaltung des interdigestiven Motilitätsmusters im extrinsisch denervierten Dünndarm und das Fehlen einer Konvertierung zum "fed pattern" weisen darauf hin, daß die Nüchternmotilität in ihrer Entstehung offensichtlich unabhängig und das postprandiale Motilitätsmuster abhängig vom extrinsischen Nervensystem ist. Dies entspricht auch der Beobachtung anderer Autoren [3, 4, 5]. Die Verkürzung der interdigestiven Zyklen im Interponat könnte durch die Ausschaltung dieses Segmentes aus dem Einflußbereich des duodenalen Schrittmachers resultieren [1].

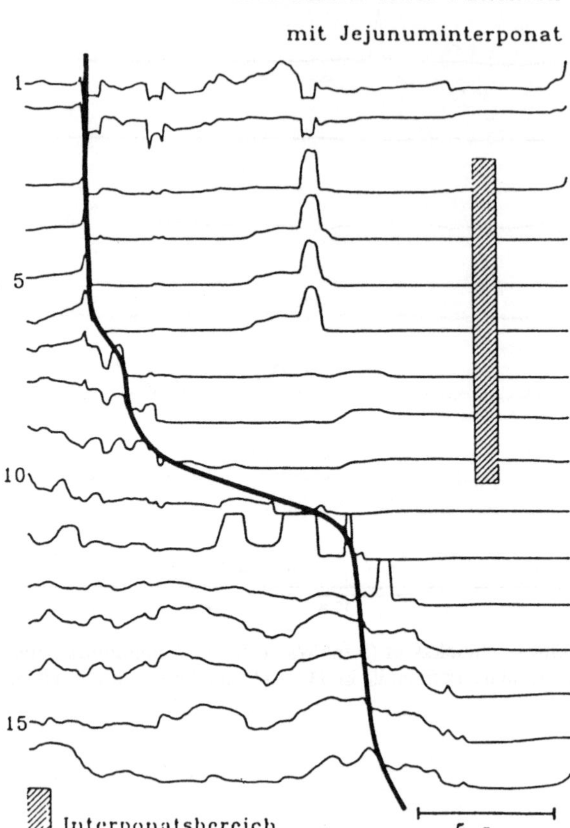

Abb. 3. Bolustransport (Kartoffelbrei) bei einem Patienten mit Jejunuminterponat gemessen mit der Impedanzmetrie: Deutliche Passageverzögerung im Interponat

Zusammenfassung

10 Patienten nach Rekonstruktion des zervikalen Ösophagus mittels freier Jejunuminterposition wurden 6 Wochen und 6 bis 27 Monate postoperativ manometrisch, szintigraphisch und mittels Impedanzmetrie funktionell untersucht.

Bei klinisch guter Schluckfunktion wurde im Jejunuminterponat keine aktive Teilnahme am Schluckakt gefunden, der Bolustransport für semisolide Nahrung war hier deutlich verzögert. Während die Nüchternmotilität im transplantierten Dünndarm weitgehend unverändert war, wurde eine Konvertierung zum "fed pattern" nach Nahrungsaufnahme nicht beobachtet. Wir schließen daraus, daß bei der Rekonstruktion die Interponatslänge so kurz wie möglich gehalten werden sollte.

Das interdigestive Muster des Dünndarmes ist in seiner Entstehung unabhängig, das "fed pattern" abhängig vom extrinsischen Nervensystem.

Summary

Ten patients who had undergone reconstruction of the cervical esophagus by free jejunal interposition were investigated using manometry, scintigraphy, and impedance measurement 6 weeks and 6–27 months after surgery. Although swallowing was clinically good, no active participation by the jejunal graft in deglutition was found. There was a marked delay in bolus transport for semisolid test meals. While interdigestive motility was nearly unaltered, no conversion to a fed pattern was observed in the jejunal segment after a meal. We conclude that the length of the jejunal graft for reconstruction of the cervical esophagus should be restricted to a minimum.

Interdigestive motility of the small bowel is not related to extrinsic innervation, whereas the fed pattern depends on it.

Literatur

1. Code CF, Szurszewski JH (1970) The effect of duodenal and mid small bowel transection on the frequency gradient of the pacesetter potential in the canine small intestine. J Physiol 207:281–289
2. Faß J, Silny J, Braun J, Heindrichs U, Dreuw B, Schumpelick V, Rau G (1989) Ein neues Verfahren zur quantitativen Bestimmung oesophagealer Motilitätsmuster mittels einer vielfachen Impedanzmessung. Langenbecks Arch Chir [Suppl] Forum 1989:139–144
3. Kerlin P, McCafferty GJ, Robinson DW, Theile D (1986) Function of a free jejunal "conduit" graft in the cervical esophagus. Gastroenterology 90:1956–1963
4. Quigley EMM, Spanta AD, Rose SG, Lof J, Thompson JS (1990) Long-term effects of jejunoileal autotransplantation on myoelectrical activity in canine small intestine. Dig Dis Sci 35:1505–1517
5. Sarr MG, Kelly KA (1981) Myoelectric activity of the autotransplanted canine jejunoileum. Gastroenterol 81:303–310

Dr. med. J. Faß, Chirurgische Klinik der RWTH Aachen, Pauwelsstraße 30,
W-5100 Aachen

Gastroösophageale Funktionsstörungen beim Endobrachyösophagus*

Gastroesophageal Function in Patients with Barrett's Esophagus

H.J. Stein[1], A.H. Hölscher[1], H. Feussner[1], T.R. DeMeester[2] und J.R. Siewert[1]

[1]Chirurgische Klinik und Poliklinik, Technische Universität München
(Direktor: Prof. Dr. med. J.R. Siewert)
[2]Department of Surgery, University of Southern California, Los Angeles, USA
(Chairman: Prof. Dr. T.R. DeMeester)

Einleitung

Als Endobrachyösophagus oder Barrett-Ösophagus wird heute allgemein der Ersatz des Plattenepithels in der distalen Speiseröhre durch Zylinderepithel als Folge von chronischem gastroösophagealen Reflux bezeichnet [1]. Die Gründe, warum es nur bei etwa 10%–20% der Patienten mit pH-metrisch nachgewiesenem Reflux zum Zylinderepithelersatz in der distalen Speiseröhre und dem damit verbundenen Risiko der malignen Entartung kommt, sind jedoch unklar. Als mögliche prädisponierende Faktoren werden eine verlängerte Expositionszeit und erhöhte Aggressivität des Refluates, ein inkompetenter unterer Ösophagussphinkter und eine gestörte peristaltische oder Clearance-Aktivität der tubulären Speiseröhre diskutiert [1, 2]. In der vorliegenden Studie verglichen wir ösophageale Säureexposition, Kompetenz des unteren Ösophagussphinkters, Clearance-Funktion der tubulären Speiseröhre und Magensaftsekretion bei Patienten mit Endobrachyösophagus, Patienten mit Refluxösophagitis ohne Endobrachyösophagus und normalen Probanden.

Methodik

Detaillierte gastroösophageale Funktionsdiagnostik, d.h. ambulante pH-Metrie der Speiseröhre, Manometrie des unteren Ösophagussphinkters und der tubulären Speiseröhre und Magensaftanalyse erfolgte bei 24 Patienten mit einem endoskopisch und bioptisch gesicherten Endobrachyösophagus und bei 24 Patienten mit Refluxösophagitis ohne Endobrachyösophagus, die nach dem "matched-pairs" Prinzip (Alter und Geschlecht) einander zugeordnet wurden. Als Kontrollgruppe für die pH-Metrie und Manometrie dienten 50 normale Probanden ohne Refluxsymptomatik oder Voroperationen im oberen Gastrointestinaltrakt.

Die ambulante 24-h pH-Metrie erfolgte mit einer kombinierten Glaselektrode, die 5 cm oberhalb des unteren Ösophagussphinkters plaziert wurde. Ösophageale Exposi-

* Unterstützt z.T. durch die Heidenhain Stiftung, Traunreuth.

Chirurgisches Forum 1993
f. experim. u. klinische Forschung
Becker/Beger/Hartel (Hrsg.)

tionszeit für pH < 2, pH < 3 und pH < 4 sind als % der Gesamtmeßzeit angegeben. Die Anzahl der Refluxepisoden und die Anzahl von Refluxepisoden mit einer Dauer über 5 min wurden für den Schwellenwert pH < 4 berechnet [3].

Der Ruhedruck des unteren Ösophagussphinkters wurde mittels Durchzugmanometrie gemessen. Die Clearance-Funktion der distalen Speiseröhre wurde durch die Kontraktionsamplitude und die Anzahl von propulsiven Kontraktionen bei 10 "wet swallows" mittels Standardmanometrie quantifiziert. Die Ergebnisse der Magensaftanalyse sind als basale, unstimulierte Säuresekretion (BAO) und als maximal stimulierbare Sekretionskapazität (MAO) dargestellt. Die Details der funktionellen Untersuchungen sind andernorts ausführlich beschrieben [3].

Der Vergleich der Ergebnisse der pH-Metrie, Manometrie und Magensaftanalyse zwischen Probanden und den beiden Patientengruppen erfolgte mittels Standardtests für nicht parametrische Daten. Ein p-Wert unter 0,05 wurde als signifikant betrachtet. Alle Daten sind als Mittelwert ± Standardfehler dargestellt.

Ergebnisse

Im Vergleich zu Patienten mit Refluxösophagitis hatten Patienten mit einem Endobrachyösophagus eine signifikant höhere Anzahl und längere Dauer von Refluxeppisoden in der ambulanten 24-h pH-Metrie der Speiseröhre. Die ösophageale Expositionszeit für pH < 2, pH < 3 und pH < 4 war bei den Patienten mit Endobrachyösophagus ebenfalls deutlich verlängert (Tabelle 1).

Tabelle 1. Ösophageales pH-Profil und Refluxpattern bei normalen Probanden, Patienten mit Refluxösophagitis und Patienten mit Endobrachyösophagus

	Probanden	Ösophagitis	Endobrachyösophagus
Anzahl Refluxepisoden	19,2 ± 2,2	49,2 ± 11,9[a]	110,4 ± 29,5[b]
Anzahl Refluxepisoden > 5 min	0,8 ± 0,3	5,2 ± 1,7[a]	14,9 ± 4,1[b]
% Zeit pH < 4	2,5 ± 0,6	13,1 ± 2,9[a]	22,5 ± 4,5[b]
% Zeit pH < 3	1,2 ± 0,2	3,9 ± 0,6[a]	11,2 ± 2,7[b]
% Zeit pH < 2	0,4 ± 0,2	2,4 ± 0,7[a]	4,8 ± 0,6[b]

Mittelwerte ± Standardfehler
[a]: p < 0,05 vs Probanden
[b]: p < 0,05 vs Ösophagitis

Die Durchzugsmanometrie zeigte bei Patienten mit Endobrachyösophagus einen signifikant niedrigeren Ruhdruck des unteren Ösophagussphinkters als bei normalen Probanden oder Patienten mit Refluxösophagitis (Tabelle 2). Der untere Ösophagussphinkter hatte einen Ruhedruck unter 6 mmHg bei 21/24 Patienten mit Endobrachyösophagus im Vergleich zu 10/24 Patienten mit Refluxösophagitis (p < 0,05).

In der Manometrie der tubulären Speiseröhre war die Anzahl von propulsiven Kontraktionen und die Kontraktionsamplitude in der distalen Speiseröhre bei Patienten mit Endobrachyösophagus signifikant erniedrigt (Tabelle 2). Im Vergleich zu den Patienten mit Refluxösophagitis ergab die Magensaftanalyse bei Patienten mit Endobrachyösophagus eine vermehrte basale (BAO) und stimulierte (MAO) Magensäuresekretion (Tabelle 2).

Tabelle 2. Ruhedruck im unteren Ösophagussphinkter (UÖS), Häufigkeit propulsiver Kontraktionen und Kontraktionsamplitude in der distalen Speiseröhre und Magensäuresekretion (BAO und MAO) bei normalen Probanden, Patienten mit Refluxösophagitis und Patienten mit Endobrachyösophagus

	Probanden	Ösophagitis	Endobrachyösophagus
Ruhedruck im UÖS (mmHg)	12,1 ± 2,1	8,9 ± 2,3[a]	4,2 ± 0,8[b]
Propulsive Kontraktionen (%)	88,8 ± 6,1	74,3 ± 5,5[a]	58,1 ± 6,1[b]
Kontraktionsamplitude (mmHg)	75,7 ± 7,9	55,2 ± 10,3[a]	37,2 ± 6,1[b]
BAO (mMol/h)	—	2,7 ± 0,4	6,3 ± 1,3[b]
MAO (mMol/h)	—	13,2 ± 3,1	23,4 ± 5,2[b]

Mittelwerte ± Standardfehler
[a]: $p < 0{,}05$ vs Probanden
[b]: $p < 0{,}05$ vs Ösophagitis

Diskussion

Die vorliegenden funktionellen Untersuchungen zeigen, daß im Vergleich zu Refluxpatienten ohne Endobrachyösophagus die zugrundeliegende gastroösophageale Refluxkrankheit bei Patienten mit Endobrachyösophagus einen schwereren Charakter hat. Insbesondere ist die Quantität und Qualität des Regurgitates bei Patienten mit Endobrachyösophagus eine andere als bei Patienten ohne Barrett-Mukosa. Dies scheint vor allem auf die Kombination eines inkompetenten unteren Ösophagussphinkters, einer gestörten Clearance-Funktion der tubulären Speiseröhre und einer vermehrten Sekretion von Magensäure zurückzuführen zu sein.

Wie schon in einer Untersuchung von Gillen et al. [4], zeigte die ambulante 24-h pH-Metrie der Speiseröhre in unserer Studie bei Patienten mit Endobrachyösophagus eine deutlich größere Anzahl und längere Dauer von Refluxperioden als bei Refluxpatienten ohne Zylinderzellersatz. Dies scheint in erster Linie auf einen erniedrigten Druck des unteren Ösophagussphinkters zurückzuführen zu sein. So konnte in der vorliegenden Studie eine Sphinkterinkompetenz, d.h. ein Ruhedruck unter 6 mmHg, bei 87,5% der Patienten mit Endobrachyösophagus nachgewiesen werden. Wird das Druckprofil des unteren Ösophagussphinkters mit mehreren radial orientierten Druckaufnehmern dreidimensional untersucht, kann eine Sphinkterinkompetenz sogar bei bis zu 95% der Patienten mit Endobrachyösophagus dokumentiert werden [3].

Bei Patienten mit einem inkompetenten unteren Ösophagussphinkters führt eine gestörte Clearance-Funktion der tubulären Speiseröhre zu einer verlängerten Kontaktzeit der Ösophagusmukose mit dem Regurgitat. Mittels simultaner Radiologie und Manometrie konnte gezeigt werden, daß die Propulsion eines Bolus im distalen Ösophagus und demzufolge die "Clearance" des Regurgitats von peristaltischen

Kontraktionen mit einer Mindestamplitude von 30–40 mmHg abhängt [3]. In unserer Studie war bei Patienten mit Endobrachyösophagus die Anzahl ineffektiver Kontraktionen vor allem in der distalen Speiseröhre erhöht. Dieser Verlust der ösophagealen Clearance-Funktion erklärt die große Anzahl von langen Refluxepisoden mit einer Dauer über 5 min und die damit verlängerte Refluxzeit bei Patienten mit Endobrachyösophagus. Ob eine gestörte Clearance-Funktion primär zum Zylinderzellersatz in der distalen Speiseröhre führt oder erst sekundär nach Entstehung eines Endobrachyösophagus auftritt, bleibt jedoch unklar.

Neben einer erhöhten Anzahl von Refluxepisoden und einer verlängerten Kontaktzeit des Refluates konnten wir bei Patienten mit Endobrachyösophagus auch eine erhöhte Expositionszeit für aggressivere pH Werte, d.h. pH < 2, dokumentieren. Eine gesteigerte Säuresekretion im Magen und ein Reflux großer Mengen hochkonzentrierter Säure in den Ösophagus könnte somit ebenfalls zur Entstehung eines Endobrachyösophagus beitragen. In unserer Untersuchung war die basale und stimulierte Magensäuresekretion bei Patienten mit Endobrachyösophagus signifikant erhöht und ein Zylinderzellersatz in der distalen Speiseröhre ist bei Patienten mit einem Zollinger-Ellison Syndrom beschrieben [1]. Gesteigerte Säuresekretion alleine reicht jedoch nicht aus, einen Zylinderzellersatz im Ösophagus hervorzurufen [1]. Vielmehr ist ein inkompetenter unterer Ösophagussphinkter die entscheidende Voraussetzung für den chronischen Reflux hochkonzentrierter Säure [1, 5]. Die chirurgische Rekonstruktion des inkompetenten unteren Ösophagussphinkters ist somit derzeit die einzige kausale therapeutische Alternative, um bei Patienten mit therapieresistentem Reflux die Entstehung eines Endobrachyösophagus und dem damit verbundenen Malignitätsrisiko zu verhindern [2, 5].

Zusammenfassung

Patienten mit Endobrachyösophagus haben im Vergleich zu Patienten mit Refluxösophagitis eine deutlich höhere Anzahl von Refluxperioden, Refluxepisoden mit einer Dauer > 5 min und eine erhöhte ösophageale Expositionszeit mit pH < 2, pH < 3 und pH < 4. Dies scheint durch die Kombination eines inkompetenten unteren Ösophagussphinkters, einer gestörten Clearance-Funktion der tubulären Speiseröhre und Hypersekretion von Magensäure verursacht zu sein.

Summary

Compared with patients with reflux esophagitis, patients with Barrett's esophagus are characterized by a markedly increased frequency of reflux episodes, reflux episodes lasting longer than 5 min, and a prolonged esophageal exposure time to pH < 2, pH < 3, and pH < 4. This appears to be secondary to a combination of an incompetent lower esophageal sphincter, a defective esophageal clearance function, and gastric acid hypersecretion.

Literatur

1. Stein HJ, Siewert JR (1993) Endobrachyösophagus – Pathogenese, Epidemiologie und maligne Degeneration. Dtsch Med Wschr (im Druck)
2. Iascone C, DeMeester TR, Little AG, Skinner DB (1983) Barrett's esophagus: Functional assessment, proposed pathogenesis, and surgical therapy. Arch Surg 118:543–549
3. Stein HJ, DeMeester TR, Hinder RA (1992) Outpatient physiologic testing and surgical management of foregut motility disorders. Cur Probl Surg 29:415–555
4. Gillen P, Keeling P, Byrne PJ, Hennessy TPJ (1987) Barrett's esophagus: pH profile. Br J Surg 74:774–776
5. Stein HJ, Barlow AP, DeMeester TR (1992) Complications of gastroesophageal reflux disease: Role of the lower esophageal sphincter, esophageal acid/alkaline exposure, and duodenogastric reflux. Ann Surg 216:35–43

Dr. med. H. Stein, Chirurgische Klinik und Poliklinik, Technische Universität München, Ismaninger Straße 22, W-8000 München 80

Postoperative Hemmung der Magenmotilität: Einfluß von Calcitonin Gene Related Peptide (CGRP) und spinalen Afferenzen bei der Ratte

Role of Calcitonin-Gene-Related Peptide (CGRP) and Spinal Afferents in the Postoperative Gastric Ileus in the Rat

T.T. Zittel*[,2] und H.E. Raybould[1]

[1]Departments of Physiology and Medicine, School of Medicine, Los Angeles, USA
[2]Center for Ulcer Research and Education, University of California, Los Angeles, USA

Einleitung

Abdominalchirurgische Eingriffe hemmen die Magenmotilität in der Regel für 24–48 h [1]. Bei der Ratte führen abdominalchirurgische Eingriffe ebenfalls zur Hemmung der Magenmotilität [2]. Erst kürzlich konnte gezeigt werden, daß Capsaicin-sensitive Afferenzen die postoperative Hemmung der Magenmotilität teilweise vermitteln [3]. Capsaicin-sensitive Afferenzen enthalten CGRP [4], und CGRP hemmt die Magenmotilität [5]. Ziel unserer Studie war, den Einfluß von CGRP und spinalen Afferenzen auf die postoperative Hemmung der Magenmotilität zu untersuchen.

Methodik

Männliche Sprague-Dawley Ratten (200–250 g) wurden mit Urethan (1,25 g/kg intraperitoneal) anästhesiert und mit einem intragastrischen und einem intravenösen (iv) Katheter versorgt. Der Pylorus wurde ligiert und der Magen mit warmer Kochsalzlösung (NaCl 0,9%) gespült. Der intragastrische Tonus wurde auf 5 cm Wassersäule standardisiert und die Magenmotilität für 30 min aufgezeichnet. Der abdominalchirurgische Eingriff bestand aus einer Unterbauchlaparotomie mit vorsichtiger Manipulation des Zökums für 1 min. Monoklonaler CGRP Antikörper (CGRP MAb, 2 mg in 1 ml als Bolus) wurde 1 h, $CGRP_{8-37}$ (CGRP Rezeptorantagonist, 10 nmol/300 μl/h) oder NaCl 0,9% (300 μl/h) 20 min vor dem abdominalchirurgischen Eingriff i.v. appliziert. Anschließend wurde die Magenmotilität für 1 h aufgezeichnet. In einem separaten Experiment wurde 14 Tage vor dem abdominalchirurgischen Eingriff das Ganglion coeliacum/Ganglion mesentericum superius mit Capsaicin, einem Neurotoxin, das zum funktionellen Ausfall afferenter C-Fasern führt, oder Vehikel vorbehandelt. Die Magenmotilität wurde mittels Redtech-Software, welche den Motilitätsindex (Fläche unter der Kurve) berechnet, analysiert. Die präoperative Magenmotilität wurde 100% gleichgesetzt.

* Gefördert durch DFG-Stipendium Zi 415/1-1.

Chirurgisches Forum 1993
f. experim. u. klinische Forschung
Becker/Beger/Hartel (Hrsg.)

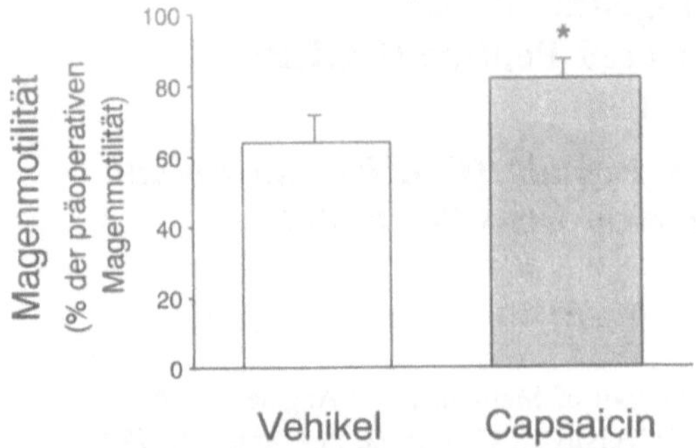

Abb. 1. Vorbehandlung des Ganglion coeliacum/Ganglion mesentericum superius mit Capsaicin (▩, n = 4) führt zu einer signifikanten Zunahme der postoperativen Magenmotilität im Vergleich zur Vorbehandlung mit Vehikel (□, n = 3). Postoperative Magenmotilität (0–60 min postoperativ) als % der präoperativen Magenmotilität. * $p < 0{,}05$)

Statistik

Alle Daten sind als Mittelwert ± Standardabweichung des Mittelwertes angegeben. Differenzen zwischen den verschiedenen Gruppen wurden mittels ANOVA (Varianzanalyse), gefolgt von Fisher's LSD (least significant difference) Test, analysiert. Eine Wahrscheinlichkeit von $p < 0{,}05$ wurde als signifikante Differenz gewertet.

Ergebnisse

Die alleinige Applikation von CGRP MAb, $CGRP_{8-37}$ oder NaCl 0,9% hatte keinen Einfluß auf die Magenmotilität. Während mit NaCl 0,9% vorbehandelte Ratten 1 h postoperativ noch eine reduzierte Magenmotilität aufwiesen, war bei mit CGRP MAb bzw. $CGRP_{8-37}$ vorbehandelten Ratten die Magenmotilität bereits nach 15 bzw. 35 min auf präoperatives Niveau zurückgekehrt (s. Tabelle 1). Capsaicin-Vorbehandlung des Ganglion coeliacum/Ganglion mesentericum superius führte zu einer signifikanten Zunahme der postoperativen Magenmotilität verglichen mit Vehikel-Vorbehandlung des Ganglion coeliacum/Ganglion mesentericum superius (s. Abb. 1).

Tabelle 1. Einfluß von CGRP MAb oder $CGRP_{8-37}$ auf die postoperative Magenmotilität

Zeit (min)	NaCl 0,9% (n = 7	CGRP MAb (n = 6)	$CGRP_{8-37}$ (n = 8)
0–5	41 ± 5	48 ± 5	52 ± 5
5–10	56 ± 6	67 ± 6[a]	67 ± 5[a]
15–20	75 ± 6	103 ± 6[b]	87 ± 6
35–40	84 ± 6	115 ± 7[b]	100 ± 6
55–60	86 ± 5	108 ± 6[b]	104 ± 5[a]

Postoperative Zeitsegmente, Angaben als % der präoperativen Magenmotilität.
[a]: $p < 0{,}05$ vs NaCl 0,9%, [b]: $p < 0{,}01$ vs NaCl 0,9%

Diskussion

Der abdominalchirurgische Eingriff führte zu einer anhaltenden Hemmung der Magenmotilität bei der Ratte. CGRP MAb, $CGRP_{8-37}$ oder Capsaicin-Vorbehandlung des Ganglion coeliacum/Ganglion mesentericum superius, welche spinale, CGRP-enthaltende Afferenzen funktionell ausschaltet, führten zu einer signifikanten Zunahme der postoperativen Magenmotilität. Die postoperative Hemmung der Magenmotilität kann somit durch Immunoneutralisation von CGRP, CGRP Rezeptorblockade oder funktionelle Ausschaltung von spinalen afferenten Fasern teilweise verhindert werden. Möglicherweise wird die postoperative Hemmung der Magenmotilität durch einen Reflex über das Ganglion coeliacum/Ganglion mesentericum superius vermittelt und beinhaltet die Freisetzung von CGRP aus spinalen Afferenzen auf Ganglion- oder Rückenmarksebene.

Zusammenfassung

Der abdominalchirurgische Eingriff führte zu einer anhaltenden Hemmung der Magenmotilität bei der Ratte. Immunoneutralisation von CGRP, CGRP Rezeptorblockade oder Capsaicin-Vorbehandlung des Ganglion coeliacum/Ganglion mesentericum superius führten zu einer signifikanten Zunahme der postoperativen Magenmotilität. Unsere Ergebnisse deuten auf eine Beteiligung von CGRP und spinalen Afferenzen bei der postoperativen Hemmung der Magenmotilität hin.

Summary

Abdominal surgery decreases gastric motility in the rat. This is partly reversed by calcitonin-gene-related peptide (CGRP) immunoneutralization, CGRP receptor antagonist, or capsaicin pretreatment of the celiac/superior mesenteric ganglion. Our data indicate that CGRP and spinal afferent fibers partly mediate postoperative gastric ileus.

Literatur

1. Livingston E, Passaro E (1990) Postoperative ileus. Dig Dis Sci 35:121–132
2. Dubois A, Weise V, Kopin I (1973) Postoperative ileus in the rat. Physiopathology, etiology and treatment. Ann Surg 178:781–786
3. Barquist E, Zinner M, Rivier J, et al. (1992) Abdominal surgery-induced delayed gastric emptying in rats: role of CRF and sensory neurons. Am J Physiol 262:G616–G620
4. Sternini C, Reeve J, Brecha N (1987) Distribution and characterization of CGRP immunoreactivity in the digestive system of normal and capsaicin-treated rats. Gastroenterol 93:852–862
5. Raybould H, Kolve E, Taché Y (1988) Central nervous system action of CGRP to inhibit gastric emptying in the conscious rat. Peptides 9:735–737

Dr. med. T.T. Zittel, CURE/VA Wadsworth, Building 115, Room 115, Los Angeles, CA 90073, USA

Elektromyographische Funktion des coloanalen Pouches

Electromyographic Function of the Coloanal Pouch

U. Hildebrandt, T. Zuther, W. Lindemann und K. Ecker

Abteilung für Allgemeine Chirurgie, Abdominal- und Gefäßchirurgie, Universitätskliniken des Saarlandes, Homburg

Einleitung

Nach Rektumresektion im distalen Drittel ist die Stuhlfrequenz oft stark erhöht. Die Konstruktion des coloanalen J-Pouches führt im Vergleich zur direkten coloanalen Anastomose zur signifikanten Reduktion der Stuhlfrequenz [1–3]. Unbeantwortet ist bisher, ob beim Colonpouch die günstige Funktion auf dem Kapazitätseffekt des künstlich geformten Äquivalents zur Ampulle beruht, oder ob es durch die operativen Veränderungen am Pouch zu einer elektrischen Aktivitätsänderung im Sinne quantitativer und/oder qualitativer Potentialänderungen der die glatte Muskulatur steuernden nervalen Impulse kommt. Mit Hilfe eines neuen direkten, elektromyographischen Ableitverfahrens an definierten Positionen des Colonpouches können die neuromuskulären Vorgänge postoperativ registriert werden.

Methode

Bei zehn untersuchten Patienten war wegen eines Rektumkarzinoms im distalen Drittel ein coloanaler Pouch konstruiert worden. Vor Ausführung der Anastomose wurden drei Elektrodenpaare in der Muscularis propria implantiert: Paar 1 am intakten Colon proximal des Pouches, Paar 2 am langen und Paar 3 am kurzen Schenkel des J-Pouches. Wir benutzten Stahlelektroden mit 0,8 mm Durchmesser. Das Modell 6500 der Firma Medtronic wird normalerweise in der Kardiochirurgie als temporäre Schrittmacherelektrode verwendet. Die Elektroden haben an der dem Leiter abgewandten Seite einen kurzen, spiralig gewickelten Polypropylen-Faden, der, wie ein Anker wirkend, die Dislokation der Elektroden verhindert. Der elektrische Kontaktbereich mißt 8 mm^2. Die drei Leiterpaare wurden durch die Bauchdecke nach außen geführt. Am 8. postoperativen Tag wurden über ein mit Vorverstärker ausgerüstetes Voltmeter der Firma Gould die verschiedenen Potentiale bipolar an den drei beschriebenen Positionen abgeleitet und parallel in analoger Form aufgezeichnet. Die Auswertung der Ergebnisse erfolgte hinsichtlich des zeitlichen Verlaufs, der Abhängigkeit von der Gabe des motilitätssteigernden Cisaprid (40 mg) sowie in Bezug auf Quantität und Qualität der gemessenen Potentiale.

Chirurgisches Forum 1993
f. experim. u. klinische Forschung
Becker/Beger/Hartel (Hrsg.)

Ergebnisse

Wegen der in der Literatur uneinheitlichen Terminologie zur Beschreibung der unterschiedlichen Formen von Potentialschwankungen bei elektromyographischen Untersuchungen am Gastrointestinaltrakt ist zunächst eine Begriffsbestimmung erforderlich:

Frexinos et al.:

SSB	= short spike burst	⟶	kurze neuromuskuläre Erregung, keine Propagation, lediglich örtliche Mischung des Coloninhaltes
LSB	= long spike burst	⟶	noch auf nähere Umgebung begrenzt, entstehende mechanische Kontraktionen verstärkt, keine Ausbreitung über mehrere cm
MLSB	= migrating LSB	⟶	über größere Distanz wandernde Erregungsfront mit entsprechendem Korrelat

Sarna et al.:

ECA	= electrical control activity basic electrical rhythm pacesetter potential	⟶	entspricht dem Summenpotential der spontanen Membrandepolarisation (Frequenz im Colon nach Fourier-Analyse 2–12/min)
ERA	= electrical response activity = spike potentials = Einzelspike	⟶	entsteht, wenn ECA bestimmte Potentialdifferenz überschreitet
CERA	= continuous ERA = LSB = contractile electrical complex	⟶	siehe LSB

Wir folgten der Nomenklatur von Sarna [4] mit der Ausnahme des MLSB, der zwar üblicherweise vor allem im Dünndarm auftritt, jedoch gelegentlich auch wie bei uns im distalen Colon bzw. im coloanalen Pouch identifiziert werden kann. Es wurde verzichtet, eine Aussage über die Colon-ECA zu treffen, da es im Colon im Gegensatz zum restlichen Magendarmtrakt kaum ein phase-locking zwischen benachbarten Zellen gibt. Das führt zu vom Zufall beeinflußten, gegenseitigen Auslöschphänomenen mit der Folge, daß die Frequenz des ECA ständig schwankt. (Erklärt wird das Phänomen mit einer vermuteten, verminderten Anzahl von gap-junctions zwischen Colonzellen.)

Durchschnittliche Verteilung und Häufigkeit der elektromyographischen Aktivität am coloanalen Pouch (n = 10):

A. In Ruhe, 8. postop. Tag, gleiche Tageszeit

	ERA	CERA	Ereignisse/min
Kanal 1	0,030	0,142	
Kanal 2	0,060	0,072	
Kanal 3	0,239	0,070	

B. Im Anschluß an Aktivierung mit Cisaprid (40 mg)

	ERA	CERA
Kanal 1	0,070	0,235
Kanal 2	0,118	0,088
Kanal 3	0,312	0,152

C. Migrating long spike burst

	Dauer (sec)		Ausbreitungsgeschwindigkeit (cm/sec)
Kanal 1	42,5	($\pm 8,8$)	fast zeitgleich
Kanal 2	38,0	($\pm 10,4$)	für Kanal 1–3
Kanal 3	36,2	($\pm 12,0$)	0,62 ($\pm 0,21$)

Abb. 1 faßt die Ergebnisse zusammen.

Diskussion

Es wird deutlich, daß die Frequenz der Einzelspikes (ERA) vom intakten Colon zum kurzen Schenkel der Pouchkonstruktion zunehmen. Dies bedeutet eine Steigerung von unkoordinierter, nicht der Propulsion dienenden elektrischen Aktivität, entsprechend einem niedrigen Ordnungsgrad.

Auf der anderen Seite zeigt sich eine Abstufung der gemessenen CERA mit höchsten Werten im zuführenden Colon und niedrigsten Werten an der coloanalen Anastomose. Die Ruheaktivität bzgl. der CERA ist im Pouchbereich nur unbedeutend stärker als an der Position 2, läßt sich jedoch durch motilitätsfördernde Medikamente deutlich steigern. Dies bedeutet eine Verringerung der zu koordinierten muskulären Propulsionsbewegungen führenden kontraktilen elektrischen Komplexe in Richtung auf den coloanalen Übergang und den kurzen Schenkel des J-Pouches.

Die Messung des MLSB als einem von einem Ableitungsort zum nächsten wandernden elektrischen Komplex zeigt eine Verkürzung der Erregungsdauer vom Colon zum Pouch.

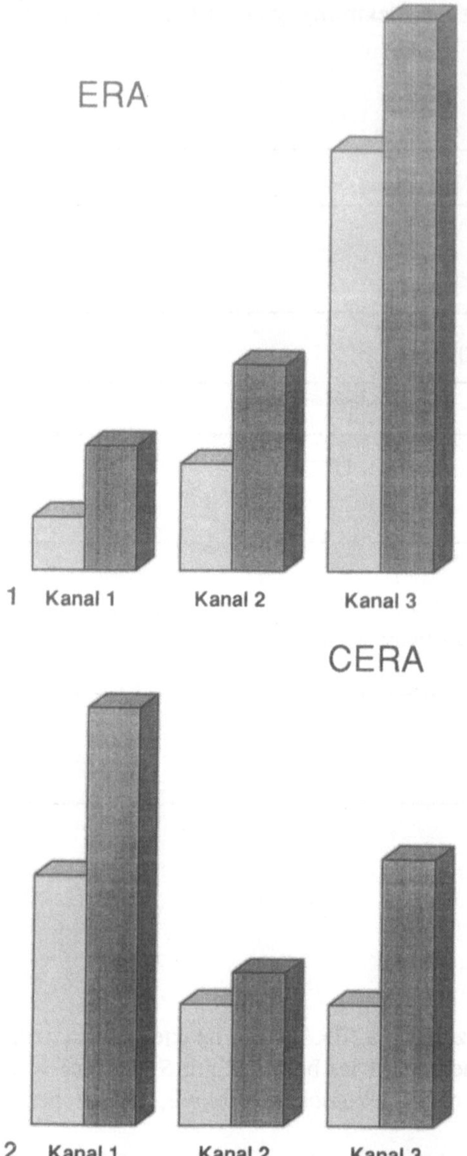

Abb. 1. Aktionen pro Minute für ERA und CERA: *linke Säule* in Ruhe, *rechte Säule* nach Cisaprid

Gleichzeitig besteht eine signifikante Änderung der Ausbreitungsgeschwindigkeit. Während die Erregungsfront zwischen dem Elektrodenpaar Kanal 1 und Kanal 3 und die damit einhergehende Peristaltik mit großer Geschwindigkeit wandert, kommt es zwischen Ableitungspunkt 2 und 3 zu einer deutlichen Verzögerung der Kontraktionswelle, d.h., die Peristaltik verläuft in der künstlichen Ampulle verlangsamt.

Zusammenfassung

Durch elektromyographische Untersuchungen am Colonpouch ist eine neuromuskuläre Aktivitätsveränderung im Sinne einer Motilitätsminderung nachweisbar. Dies konnte durch eine Zunahme unkoordinierter Einzelspikes und eine Abnahme der CERA, die lokale Kontraktionen bewirkt, nachgewiesen werden. Die Konstruktion des coloanalen Pouches bietet daher neben der durch das Volumen erzeugten Reservoirfunktion gleichzeitig eine verminderte Motilität. Aus diesen Befunden erklärt sich das funktionell bessere Ergebnis des coloanalen Pouches im Vergleich zu der konventionellen End-zu-End-Anastomose.

Summary

Electromyographic recordings demonstrated reduced action in the coloanal pouch. This is based on the increase of uncoordinated spike potentials and the decrease of continuous electrical response activity. Therefore, the construction of the coloanal pouch provides both an increased capacity and a reduced motor activity. These two factors explain the superior functional results compared to the straight coloanal anastomosis.

Literatur

1. Lewis WG, Holdsworth PJ, Stephenson BM, Pinan PJ, Johnston D (1992) Role of the rectum in the physiological and clinical results of coloanal and colorectal anastomosis after anterior resection for rectal carcinoma. Br J Surg 79:1082–1086
2. Lazorthes F, Fahes P, Chiotasso P, Lemozy J, Bloom E (1086) Resection of the rectum with construction of a colonic reservoir and coloanal anastomosis for carcinoma of the rectum. Br J Surg 73:136–138
3. Nicholls RJ, Lubowski DZ, Donaldson DR (1988) Comparison of colonic reservoir and straight coloanal reconstructions after rectal excision. Br J Surg 75:318–320
4. Sarna SK (1991) Physiology and pathophysiology of colonic motor activity. Dig Dis Sci 36:827–862

U. Hildebrandt, Abteilung für Allgemeine Chirurgie, Abdominal- und Gefäßchirurgie, Universitätskliniken des Saarlandes, W-6650 Homburg/Saar

Der Zusatz des Dipeptids Alanin-Glutamin zur parenteralen Ernährung verhindert die intestinale Atrophie und Dysfunktion im Rattenmodell

Alanine/Glutamine-Supplemented Parenteral Nutrition Prevents Gut Atrophy and Functional Alterations in Rats

J. Schröder, F. Fändrich, E. Schweizer und P. Schroeder

Klinik für Allgemeine Chirurgie und Thoraxchirurgie, Christian-Albrechts-Universität Kiel (Direktor: Prof. Dr. med. B. Kremer)

Einleitung

Eine "total parenterale Ernährung" führt zu einer Atrophie der Dünndarmschleimhaut und funktionellen Veränderungen [2, 5]. Die nicht essentielle Aminosäure Glutamin, die ein wesentliches Substrat im Stoffwechsel der intestinalen Schleimhautzellen darstellt, ist aufgrund der Instabilität von Glutamin nicht in den gebräuchlichen Infusionslösungen zur parenteralen Ernährung enthalten [1].

Im Tierexperiment soll die Hypothese überprüft werden , ob eine Substitution zur parenteralen Ernährung mit dem stabilen Dipeptid Alanin-Glutamin (Ala-Gln) die Atrophie und funktionelle Alteration verhindert.

Material und Methodik

Bei männlichen Wistar-Ratten (250–300 g) wurde nach 12stündigem Fasten in Äthernarkose ein PE 20-Katheter über die V. jugularis interna in die obere Hohlvene gelegt.

Die Kontrolltiere wurden bei freiem Zugang zur Ratten-Altromindiät (250 kcal/kg KG) 10 Tage enteral ernährt (Gruppe 1; n = 6). In der Gruppe 2 (n = 6) erhielten die Tiere eine isocalorische und isonitrogene parenterale Ernährung ohne Glutaminzusatz und in der Gruppe 3 (n = 6) eine Ernährung unter Substitution der Dipeptidlösung Ala-Gln (30% Gln-N). Die parenterale Ernährung erfolgte als Mischinfusion mit einer Kohlehydrat-, Fett- und Aminosäurelösung (62,5 ml, 250 kcal/kg KG, Gesamt-N = 0,5 g/kg).

Im Anschluß an die 10tägige Ernährung wurden morphologische Untersuchungen nach Clarke durchgeführt und die Zottenfläche nach Lorenz-Maeyer berechnet. In einer Rezirkulationsapparatur, modifiziert nach Menge, wurde die Eliminationsrate von Glukose und Wasser bestimmt. Die Bürstensaumenzymaktivität der alkalischen Phosphatase (aP) wurde nach Gutschmidt und die der Maltase nach Evers gemessen. Die statistische Analyse erfolgte mittels Student T-Test.

Chirurgisches Forum 1993
f. experim. u. klinische Forschung
Becker/Beger/Hartel (Hrsg.)

Ergebnisse

Aus der glutaminfreien parenteralen Ernährung resultiert eine signifikante Verminderung der Zottenhöhe und -fläche im Jejunum ($p < 0{,}01$) im Vergleich zur Kontrolle. Ala-Gln substituierte Tiere wiesen signifikant höhere und größere Zotten im Vergleich zur Gruppe 2 auf ($p < 0{,}01$), die sich nicht von denen der Kontrolle unterschieden. Eine Funktionseinschränkung mit signifikant verminderter Glucose- und Wasserresorption lag bei Tieren unter glutaminfreier Ernährung im Vergleich zur Kontrolle und zu den substituierten Tieren vor ($p < 0{,}01$). Unter Ala-Gln-Zusatz bestand kein Unterschied der Resorptionskapazität zwischen Gruppe 3 und der Kontrolle. Die Aktivität der aP und der Maltase war durch die parenterale Ernährung signifikant gegenüber der Kontrolle herabgesetzt ($p < 0{,}01$). Unter Ala-Gln-Zusatz bestand eine Aktivitätsminderung der aP gegenüber der Kontrolle ($p < 0{,}01$) und eine signifikante Erhöhung gegenüber der Gruppe 2 ($p < 0{,}01$). Die Maltase normalisierte sich unter Ala-Gln und war gegenüber der Gruppe 2 signifikant erhöht (s. Tabelle 1).

Tabelle 1. Morphologische und funktionelle Ergebnisse

Gruppe	1	2	3
Morphologie			
– Zottenhöhe (μm)	396 ± 29	297 ± 30[a]	377 ± 32[b]
– Zottenfläche (cm^2)	0,50 ± 0,06	0,26 ± 0,04[a]	0,42 ± 0,05[b]
Resorptionskapazität			
– Glc (μmol/cmxh)	8,75 ± 1,25	5,27 ± 0,52[a]	8,31 ± 0,69[b]
– Wasser (ml/cmxh)	0,22 ± 0,06	0,11 ± 0,02[a]	0,19 ± 0,02[b]
Enzymaktivität			
– aP (U/g)	208 ± 16[c]	57 ± 21[a]	156 ± 20[b]
– Maltase (U/g)	9,5 ± 1,7	4,9 ± 1,3[a]	8,0 ± 0,9[b]

[a] s Gruppe 1 vs 2, $p < 0{,}01$
[b] s Gruppe 2 vs 3, $p < 0{,}01$
[c] s Gruppe 1 vs 3, $p < 0{,}01$

Gruppe 1: Ausschließlich enteral ernährt (n = 6)
Gruppe 2: Total parenterale Ernährung (n = 6)
Gruppe 3: Parenterale Ernährung, Zusatz von Ala-Gln (n = 6)

Diskussion

Die nicht essentielle Aminosäure Glutamin ist in Dünndarmepithelzellen, in der Niere und im Immunsystem ein wesentliches Substrat für die Bereitstellung von Stickstoff und Kohlenstoff zur Nukleinsäuresynthese [1]. Eine Ursache der Atrophie der Dünndarmschleimhaut bei einer parenteralen Ernährung, verbunden mit funktionellen Veränderungen, mit einer Suppression der lokalen Abwehr und einer erhöhten Permeabilität für Bakterien und Makromoleküle, mag die unzureichende Versorgung mit Glutamin sein [1, 2, 5]. Die Aminosäure ist aufgrund ihrer Instabilität nicht in den gebräuchlichen Lösungen zur parenteralen Ernährung enthalten [3]. Die Entwicklung von Dipeptiden wie Glycin-Glutamin oder Alanin-Glutamin macht heute einen klinischen Einsatz möglich.

Im Rattenmodell verhindert eine Substitution von Glutamin in Form des Dipeptids Alanin-Glutamin die Atrophie der Dünndarmschleimhaut, normalisiert die Resorption von Glukose und Wasser sowie die Bürstensaumenzymaktivität. Alverdy et al. [1] konnten zeigen, daß Glutamin im Rattenmodell eine Suppression der lokalen Abwehr vermeidet.

Ein klinischer Einsatz von Glutamin in Form des Dipeptids erscheint möglich. Therapeutische Ansatzpunkte ergeben sich bei Funktionsstörungen des Dünndarms nach Operationen, Bestrahlung, Transplantation und zur Aufrechterhaltung der intestinalen Barrierefunktion, um eine Translokation von Bakterien und Makromolekülen zu vermeiden [3, 4, 5].

Zusammenfassung

Eine parenterale Ernährung führt im Tiermodell der Ratte im Vergleich zu einer enteral ernährten Kontrollgruppe zu einer Atrophie der Dünndarmschleimhaut, zu einer verminderten Resorption von Glukose und Wasser und zu einer reduzierten Aktivität der Bürstensaumenzyme alkalische Phosphatase und Maltase. Die intestinale Dysfunktion kann durch den Zusatz des Dipeptids Alanin-Glutamin zur parenteralen Ernährung verhindert werden.

Summary

Total parenteral nutrition in rats causes villous atrophy, diminished resorption of glucose and water, and a decreased activity of villous enzymes compared with an enterally fed control group. Addition of alanine/glutamine to parenteral nutrition solutions prevents intestinal atrophy and functional alterations.

Literatur

1. Alverdy JA, Aoys A, Weiss-Carington P, Burke DA (1992) The effect of glutamine-enriched TPN on gut immune cellularity. J Surg Res 52:34–38
2. Illig KA, Ryan CK, Hardy DJ, Rhodes J, Locke W, Sax HC (1992) Total parenteral nutrition-induced changes in gut mucosal function: atrophy alone is not the issue. Surgery 112:631–637
3. Klimberg SV, Salloum RM, Kasper M, Plumley DA, Dolson DJ, Hautamaki RD, Mendenhall WR, Bova FC, Bland KI, Copeland EM, Souba WW (1992) Oral glutamine accelerates healing of the small intestine and improves outcome after whole abdominal radiation. Arch Surg 125:1040–1045
4. Parry-Billings M, Baigrie RJ, Lamont PM, Morris PJ, Newsholme EA (1992) Effects of major and minor surgery on plasma glutamine and cytokine levels. Arch Surg 127:1237–1240

5. Schroeder P, Schweizer E, Blömer A, Deltz E (1992) Glutamine prevents mucosal injury after small bowel transplantation. Transplant Proc 24:1104

Dr. med. J. Schröder, Abteilung für Allgemeine Chirurgie und Thoraxchirurgie, Universitätskliniken Kiel, Arnold-Heller-Straße 7, W-2300 Kiel

Können Nahrungsmittelproteine auch über den Dickdarm resorbiert werden?

Can Food Proteins Be Absorbed from the Colon?

P. Kremer, W. Saß und J. Seifert

Experimentelle Chirurgie der Klinik für Allgemeine Chirurgie und Thoraxchirurgie, Christian-Albrechts-Universität Kiel

Einleitung

Während vornehmlich der mittlere und untere Dünndarmabschnitt für die Resorption von Eiweiß verantwortlich ist, hat nach heutigen Erkenntnissen der Dickdarm beim Menschen, aber auch bei Tieren, die Aufgabe der Wasser- und Elektrolytregulation des Verdauungstraktes. In der Literatur finden sich jedoch einige wenige Hinweise, daß auch der Dickdarm in der Lage ist, Nahrungsmittel- und bakterielle Proteine zu resorbieren [2, 3] und sich immunologisch damit auseinanderzusetzen [4]. Deswegen sollte mittels eines tierexperimentellen Versuchsansatzes der Frage nachgegangen werden, ob, wieviel und in welcher Form Fremdproteine resorbiert werden können, welche in das Colon descendens verabreicht worden waren.

Methodik

^{123}Jod markiertes 20% humanes Serumalbumin (HSA) wurde als Testprotein verwendet. Davon bekamen Kaninchen (n = 5) 5 ml in Äthernarkose in das Colon descendens verabreicht. Kontrolltiere erhielten nur ^{123}Jod. Bei allen Tieren wurden in regelmäßigen Abständen über 24 h Serumproben entnommen und die resorbierte Radioaktivität in einem Szintillationszähler gemessen. Um die Verteilung von intaktem radioaktiv markiertem HSA, Bruchstücken von HSA und abgespaltener Markierung zu untersuchen, wurden mit dem Serum radiochromatographische Trennungen mit Sephadex G25 durchgeführt und im Anschluß daran mit einem hochspezifischen Antiserum (Anti-HSA) die Identität von HSA im Serum und am Ende des Versuches auch in der Lymphe der Kaninchen nachgewiesen. Dazu wurde bei einem Teil der Tiere in Äthernarkose eine Drainage eines abdominalen Lymphgefäßes durchgeführt.

Ergebnisse

Kaninchen, die radioaktiv markiertes HSA in das Colon descendens verabreicht bekamen, zeigen im Blut einen langsameren Anstieg der Radioaktivität, der bis zur 6. Stunde ein Maximum aufweist (s. Tabelle 1). In den darauffolgenden 18 h fällt

Chirurgisches Forum 1993
f. experim. u. klinische Forschung
Becker/Beger/Hartel (Hrsg.)

die Konzentration der Radioaktivität im Blut wieder auf Werte ab, die in der zweiten Stunde nach Applikation beobachtet wurden. Der halbmaximale Wert ist bei den ^{123}J-HSA-Tieren nach 20 h erreicht. Ganz anders stellt sich die Resorption der Jodmarkierung bei den Kontrolltieren dar. Das Maximum wird schon nach 1 h erreicht und nach weiteren 5 h der halbmaximale Wert.

Tabelle 1. Radioaktivität im Serum (cpm) von Versuchs- und Kontrolltieren. Während Versuchstiere radioaktiv markiertes menschliches Serumalbumin (^{123}J-HSA) in das Colon descendens verabreicht bekamen, war es bei den Kontrolltieren nur die radioaktive Markierung ohne das Protein

	30 min	1 h	3 h	6 h	8 h	20 h	24 h
Kontrolltiere	7.648	11.328	9.875	8.567	6.277	976	116
123J (x ± sx)	±810	±980	±760	±850	±650	±120	±108
Versuchstiere	--	871	3.183	4.120	3.811	2.916	1.819
123J-HSA (x ± sx)		±189	±406	±553	±952	±1.179	±740

Die radiochromatographische Auftrennung des Serums ergab, daß am Ende des Versuches, also 24 h nach der Verabreichung von ^{123}J-HSA noch 14% der Radioaktivität an makromolekulares HSA gebunden war. Bei den Kontrolltieren, denen ^{123}Jod appliziert worden war, fanden sich 2% an makromolekularen Strukturen gebunden. Das liegt innerhalb der Fehlerbreite der Trennmethode. Die immunologische Identifizierung mit Hilfe von spezifischem Anti-HSA zeigt eindeutige Präzipitationslinien mit dem Serum und der Lymphe von Tieren, die ^{123}J-HSA in das Colon descendens verabreicht bekommen hatten. Bei keinem der Kontrolltiere konnten solche Präzipitationslinien beobachtet werden.

Tabelle 2. Radiochromatographische Trennung der resorbierten Radioaktivität mittels Sephadex G-25 nach Applikation von ^{123}J-HSA bei Versuchstieren und ^{123}Jod bei Kontrolltieren. Die makromolekularen und mikromolekularen Fraktionen (cpm) wurden integriert anhand der Simpsonschen Näherungsformel

	Makromolekular	Mikromolekular	Relation
Kontrolltiere 123J (x ± sx)	420 ± 25	17.231 ± 1.176	2%
Versuchstiere 123J-HSA (x ± sx)	1.947 ± 103	13.805 ± 989	14%

Die Berechnung der insgesamt über die Beobachtungszeit resorbierten Menge und deren Verteilung in makro- und mikromolekular ist in der Abb. 1 dargestellt. Daraus ergibt sich, daß innerhalb von 24 h 100 mg HSA resorbiert worden sind, davon 10% in der großmolekularen Form.

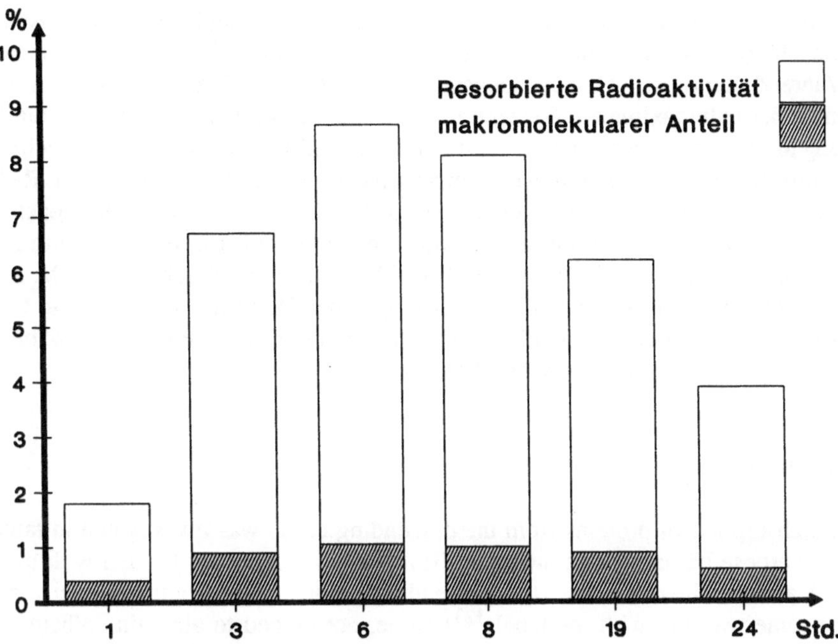

Abb. 1. Resorptionsraten nach Gabe von 5 ml ^{123}J-HSA in das Colon descendens. Die schraffierten Flächen entsprechen dem prozentualen Anteil an makromolekular resorbiertem ^{123}J-HSA, die nicht schraffierten Flächen dem prozentualen Anteil an ^{123}J-HSA-Bruchstücken oder ^{123}J-Markierung

Diskussion

Die Untersuchungen zeigen, daß der Dickdarm nicht ausschließlich ein Organ der Wasser- und Elektrolytregulation ist, sondern, daß dort auch Proteine aufgenommen werden können und damit auch eine immunologische Auseinandersetzung in diesem Organ zu erwarten ist. Schon frühere Untersuchungen am Menschen deuten darauf hin, daß durch den Dickdarm Proteine resorbiert werden können. So fand man nach rektal verabreichter Streptokinase beim Menschen Antikörper, die belegen, daß entweder der Dickdarm Streptokinase resorbiert hat oder sich das lymphatische Gewebe des Dickdarmes vor Ort mit der Streptokinase auseinandergesetzt hat [1]. Wenn auch über die Resorptionsmechanismen von Makromolekülen aus dem Dickdarm noch wenig bekannt ist, sollte bei ausgedehnten Dickdarmresektionen daran gedacht werden, daß damit auch eine Beeinträchtigung der Antigenresorption und nachfolgenden immunologischen Abwehrreaktionen verbunden sein kann.

Zusammenfassung

Bei Kaninchen wurde die Resorption von Protein aus dem Dickdarm untersucht. Dazu wurde humanes Serumalbumin verwendet, welches mit dem radioaktiven Isotop

^{123}Jod markiert war und das den Tieren in das Colon appliziert wurde. Kontrolluntersuchungen wurden mit ^{123}Jod durchgeführt, das nicht an Albumin gebunden war. Während markiertes Albumin langsam resorbiert wird mit einem Maximum nach 6 h und einer halbmaximalen Konzentration nach 20 h, wird das ^{123}Jod, also die Markierung allein, wesentlich schneller resorbiert und eliminiert. Das Maximum wird bei den Kontrolltieren nach 1 h und der halbmaximale Wert wird nach 5 h erreicht. Radiochromatographische Untersuchungen zeigen, daß 14% der resorbierten Radioaktivität bei den Versuchstieren an das großmolekulare, nicht degradierte Serumalbumin gebunden und der Rest an HSA-Bruchstücke. Das Albumin wurde durch spezifische Antiseren in Serum und Lymphe identifiziert. Damit ist der Dickdarm nicht nur ein Organ der Wasser- und Elektrolytregulation, sondern auch ein Ort der Proteinresorption und der nachfolgenden immunologischen Folgereaktion.

Summary

The absorption of proteins from the descending colon was investigated in rabbits. For this purpose human serum albumin (HSA) was radioactively labeled with the isotope ^{123}I and administered into the descending colon. Control animals were treated in the same way but with the label ^{123}I alone, not tagged to albumin. Whereas labeled albumin is slowly absorbed with a maximum concentration 6 h after administration and with a half-maximum concentration after 20 h, the label alone is rapidly absorbed and eliminated. The maximum for the control animals was found 1 h after administration and the half-maximum value after 5 h. Radiochromatographic separation showed that 14% of the absorbed radioactivity is tagged to high molecular undegraded albumin and the rest to HSA fragments. Albumin was identified by specific antiserum in serum and lymph fluid of animals which were treated with albumin. These results show that the colon is not only an organ of water and electrolyte regulation, but also a place of protein absorption and subsequent immunological reactions.

Literatur

1. Bachmann F (1968) Development of antibodies against perorally and rectally administered streptokinase in man. J Lab Med 72:228–238
2. Reattig HJ (1983) Die lokale Immunisierung mit inaktivierten Mikroorganismen. Bundesgesundheitsblatt 26:263–276
3. Warshaw AL, Bellini CA, Walker WA (1977) The intestinal mucosal barrier to intact antigenic protein. Difference between colon and small intestine. Am J Surg 133:55–58
4. Worthington BS, Enwonwu C (1975) Absorption of intact protein by colonic cells of the rat. Dig Dis 20:750–763

Dr. P. Kremer, Experimentelle Chirurgie der Klinik für Allgemeine Chirurgie und Thoraxchirurgie, Universität Kiel, Michaelisstraße 5, W-2300 Kiel 1

Bioverfügbarkeit von Vitamin A nach experimenteller Gastrektomie

Effect of Total Gastrectomy on Bioavailability of Vitamin A

R. Schindler[1], E. Schweizer[2] und P. Schroeder[2]

[1]Institut für Humanernährung, Christian-Albrechts-Universität, Kiel
[2]Klinik für Allgemein- und Thoraxchirurgie, Christian-Albrechts-Universität, Kiel

Einleitung

Die totale Gastrektomie führt gewöhnlich zu einer Beeinträchtigung der Ernährungssituation des Patienten. Diesem Mangelzustand kann eine Malassimilation von Nährstoffen zugrunde liegen. Ursachen für eine Störung der insbesondere für die Protein- und Fettresorption entscheidenden intraluminalen Verdauungsvorgänge sind eine ungenügende Anreicherung der Ingesta mit Verdauungssekreten, eine verkürzte Verweildauer des Speisebreies im Intestinum und eine bakterielle Fehl- oder Überbesiedlung des Darms [1].

Da unklar ist, wie sich einzelne Methoden zur Wiederherstellung der Nahrungspassage auf die Fettassimilation auswirken, haben wir unter Verwendung des oralen Vit. A-Belastungstests den Einfluß verschiedener Rekonstruktionsverfahren auf die Bioverfügbarkeit von Lipiden untersucht [2].

Methoden und Material

In einem genehmigten Tierversuch wurden 30 männliche Lewis-Ratten 5 Studiengruppen zugewiesen. 6 scheinoperierte Tiere dienten als Kontrollen, die übrigen wurden in Äthernarkose gastrektomiert. Die Wiederherstellung der Nahrungspassage erfolgte in zwei Gruppen durch Oesophagojejunostomie (Roux-Y) und in den beiden übrigen Gruppen durch Dünndarminterposition nach Longmire-Gütgemann (Interponat). Jeweils 6 Tiere mit Roux-Y-Schlinge bzw. mit Interponat erhielten zusätzlich noch einen Pouch. Um den Funktionszustand des Darms zu prüfen, wurde den Tieren am 90. postoperativen Tag Vit. A-Ester (30 μg/g KG), gelöst in Olivenöl, appliziert. Blutentnahmen für die Vit. A-Bestimmung erfolgten vor Gabe des Bolus und 2, 4, 6 und 8 h danach. Als relatives Maß für die über 8 h aufgenommene Vit. A-Menge wurde die Fläche unter der Resorptionskurve (AUC_{0-8}) nach der Trapezoidregel ermittelt.

Chirurgisches Forum 1993
f. experim. u. klinische Forschung
Becker/Beger/Hartel (Hrsg.)

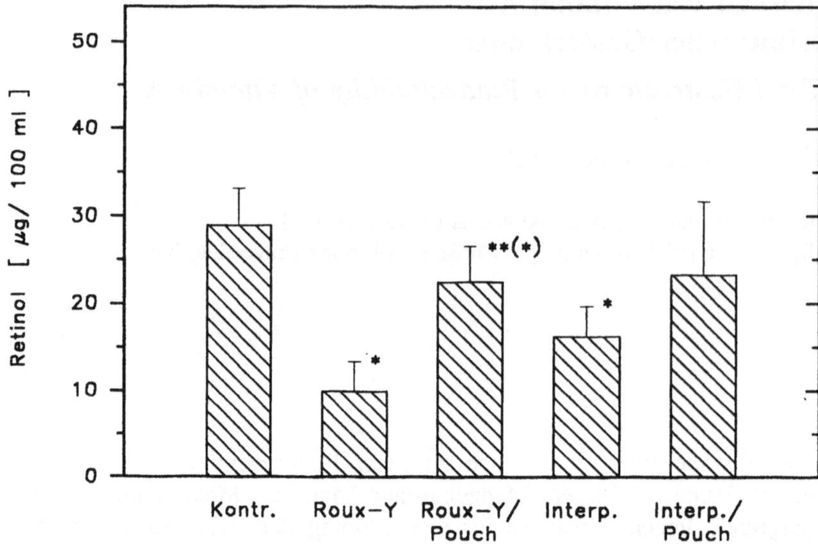

Abb. 1. Nüchternwerte des Plasmaretinols am 90. postoperativen Tag. Mittelwerte ± Standardabweichung, 6 Tiere in jeder Gruppe. Die Studiengruppe der Tiere mit Interponat/Pouch-Rekonstruktion bildet hier mit n = 2 eine Ausnahme. Unterschiede für die Abnahme des Plasmaretinols für Tiere mit Roux-Y bzw. Interponat gegen Scheinoperierte * $p < 0{,}01$; für Tiere mit Roux-Y/Pouch gegen Scheinoperierte ** $p < 0{,}05$; für Tiere mit Roux-Y/Pouch gegen Tiere mit Roux-Y *** $p < 0{,}01$ (Student t-Test)

Ergebnisse

Gegen Ende des Beobachtungszeitraums wurden alle Tiere einem Vit. A-Belastungstest unterzogen. Eine Ausnahme bildeten die Tiere mit Interp./Pouch-Rekonstruktion. Mit ca. 30% war die Überlebensrate dieser Tiere unerwartet niedrig.

Um zunächst Auskunft über die Vit. A-Versorgung extrahepatischer Gewebe zu erhalten, wurden die Nüchternwerte des Plasmaretinols bestimmt (Abb. 1). Im Vergleich zu den Kontrollen wurden nach Gastrektomie im Serum signifikant niedrigere Retinolkonzentrationen nachgewiesen. Weiterhin fällt auf, daß sowohl eine Pouch-Anlage (Roux-Y vs. Roux-Y/Pouch, $p < 0{,}01$) als auch der Erhalt der Duodenalpassage sich günstig auf das Plasmaretinol auswirkten. Als Ursache für den Abfall des Retinols wurde eine Fettresorptionsstörung aufgrund der Ergebnisse des Vit. A-Tests ausgeschlossen (Abb. 2). Wie ein Vergleich der entsprechenden AUC_{0-8}-Werte für die Kontrollen und für Tiere mit Roux-Y-, Roux-Y/Pouch- und Interponat-Rekonstruktionen ergibt, unterscheiden sich diese nur unwesentlich voneinander (524,7 ± 144,3; 606,1 ± 528,7; 518,8 ± 208,5; 1048,5 ± 504,3 µg Vit. A × 100 ml^{-1} × h^{-1}). Eine Ausnahme bilden die Tiere mit Jejunuminterposition. Diese zeichnen sich gegenüber den anderen Tieren durch größere AUC_{0-8}-Werte aus.

Die in den Lebern nachgewiesenen, recht umfangreichen Vit. A-Reserven bestätigen weiterhin, daß die Abnahme des Plasmaretinols nach Gastrektomie nicht auf einen Vit. A-Mangel zurückzuführen ist (935,3 ± 181,7; 654,9 ± 322,7; 568,8 ± 201,6;

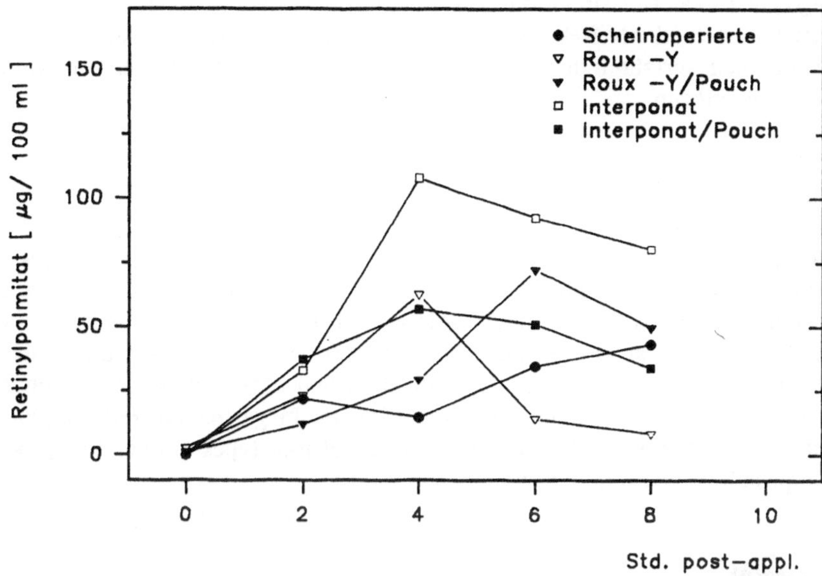

Abb. 2. Vergleichende Darstellung der postprandialen Konzentrationsverläufe des Retinylpalmitats. Medianwerte von jeweils n = 6 Tieren. Die Studiengruppe der Tiere mit Interponat/Pouch-Rekonstruktion bildet hier ebenfalls mit n = 2 eine Ausnahme

623,7 ± 265,0 μg Frischgew.). Diese Untersuchungen ergaben zusätzlich, daß in den Lebern der Scheinoperierten die höchsten und in den Tieren mit Roux-Y/Pouch-Rekonstruktion die niedrigsten Konzentrationen vorlagen ($p < 0{,}01$). Auch der Unterschied zwischen den Kontrollen und den Tieren mit Interponat erwiesen sich als statistisch signifikant (935,3 vs. 623,7 μg/g; $p < 0{,}05$).

Diskussion

Der Umfang der Vit. A-Reserven dient als Maß für eine den Bedarf langfristig übersteigende Vit. A-Zufuhr. Entsprechend deuten niedrige Vit. A-Konzentrationen der Leber darauf hin, daß unmittelbar nach Magenentfernung erwartungsgemäß ein zeitlich begrenzter Funktionsverlust des Intestinaltraktes und/oder ein Mehrbedarf an Vit. A vorgelegen hat.

Daß sich die Serumretinolkonzentration trotz gefüllter Vit. A-Speicher am 90. postoperativen Tag noch immer nicht erholt hatte, wird mit einer unzureichenden Mobilisierung des Vitamins durch die Leber erklärt. Als Ursache hierfür ist ein Proteinmangelzustand nicht auszuschließen.

Zusammenfassung

In einer Studie an Ratten wurde unter Verwendung des Vit. A-Belastungstests geprüft, welchen Einfluß unterschiedliche Methoden zur Wiederherstellung der Nahrungspassage nach totaler Gastrektomie auf die intestinale Fettresorption haben. Wie der Vergleich verschiedener Rekonstruktionsarten ergab, sind die aufwendigen chirurgischtechnischen Verfahren der risikoloseren Roux-Y-Technik in dieser Hinsicht nicht eindeutig überlegen.

Summary

The aim of the study was to examine the influence of several techniques for reconstruction of the gastrointestinal tract on compensatory changes that follow total gastrectomy. We used the vitamin A tolerance test to determine whether fat absorption is still impaired at day 90 after initial operation. The results indicate that gastrectomy can significantly affect the circulation and tissue levels of vitamin A, despite a sufficient oral bioavailability of this vitamin. In gastrectomized rats, however, no difference was observed between the effects of four types of operative procedures on the postabsorptive plasma vitamin A response.

Literatur

1. Becker HD, Caspary WF (1980) Postgastrectomy and postvagotomy syndromes. Springer, Berlin Heidelberg New York
2. Merkle P, Schlag P, Krause F (1976) Zur Frage der agastrischen Dystrophie nach Gastrektomie. Chirurg 47:380

Dr. R. Schindler, Institut für Humanernährung der Christian-Albrechts-Universität, Düsternbrooker Weg 17, W-2300 Kiel

Ist die Bildung eines Ersatzmagens nach totaler Gastrektomie anzustreben? Szintigraphische und klinische Untersuchungen beim Jejunumpouch

Should a Gastric Substitute Be Reconstructed after Total Gastrectomy? Scintigraphic and Clinical Evaluation in Patients with a Jejunal Pouch

A. Stier, A.H. Hölscher und J.R. Siewert

Chirurgische Klinik und Poliklinik, Technische Universität, Klinikum rechts der Isar, München

Einleitung

Nach totaler Gastrektomie sind eine Reihe von Rekonstruktionsverfahren zur klinischen Anwendung gekommen. Bei der Wiederherstellung der Intestinalpassage ist es ein wesentliches Therapieziel, den Verlust der Reservoirfunktion des Magens durch die Bildung eines Magenersatzes auszugleichen, auch im Hinblick darauf, die Lebensqualität des gastrektomierten Patienten zu verbessern [1, 2]. Dieses Prinzip wird durch die Ösophagojejunoplikatio aufgegriffen: Nach dem Verschluß des Duodenalstumpfes wird eine doppelläufige Jejunumschlinge als Pouch mit dem distalen Ösophagus anastomosiert; die galleführende Schlinge wird nach Roux-Y etwa 40 cm weiter distal implantiert. Dabei kann die im Vergleich zur einfachen intramediastinalen Ösophagojejunostomie zeitlich aufwendigere Pouchbildung durch den Einsatz von Klammernahtgeräten abgekürzt werden [3].

Füllungsvermögen und Entleerungsverhalten bestimmen die Funktion des Jejunumpouches. Damit ist unter Verwendung der alimentären Szintigraphie meßbar, ob tatsächlich eine Reservoirfunktion durch dieses Interponat übernommen werden kann. Das Entleerungsverhalten des Pouches wird der mit gleicher Methodik gemessenen Transitzeit der Ösophagojejunostomie gegenübergestellt und mit klinischen Erhebungen korreliert.

Material und Methodik

2 Gruppen mit jeweils 15 Patienten wurden mindestens 6 Monate nach totaler Gastrektomie untersucht. In der einen Gruppe befanden sich die Patienten, die aufgrund eines Magenkarzinoms im mittleren oder distalen Drittel total reseziert wurden. Die Intestinalpassage war immer als Ösophagojejunoplikatio unter Verwendung automatischer Nähapparate (Premium-CEEA, CIA 90) ausgeführt worden [3]. Die Patienten der anderen Gruppe waren aufgrund eines Karzinoms am gastroösophagealen Übergang grundsätzlich transmediastinal erweitert reseziert und mit einer einfa-

Chirurgisches Forum 1993
f. experim. u. klinische Forschung
Becker/Beger/Hartel (Hrsg.)

chen End-zu-Seit-Ösophagojejunostomie rekonstruiert worden. Hinsichtlich der TNM-Klassifikation waren beide Gruppen vergleichbar: Das T_2-Stadium wurde bei keinem Patienten überschritten; kein resezierter Lymphknoten war tumorbefallen; der Tumor war vollständig entfernt worden. Damit wurden ausschließlich R0-resezierte Patienten in die Studie aufgenommen, bei denen sich aufgrund der zu erwartenden günstigen Prognose der Mehraufwand einer Ersatzmagenbildung vorteilhaft auf die postoperative Lebensqualität auswirken konnte. Die an der Klinik selbst durchgeführten Restaging-untersuchungen kurz vor Eintritt in die Studie hatten bei keinem Patienten ein Tumorrezidiv ergeben. In der Endoskopie war vor allem eine mechanische Behinderung im Anastomosenbereich ausgeschlossen worden.

Hinsichtlich der Alters- und Geschlechtsverteilung waren beide Gruppen vergleichbar. Die Gruppe mit Jejunumpouch setzte sich aus 9 Männern und 6 Frauen mit einem Durchschnittsalter von 60,9 Jahren, die ohne Pouch aus 10 Männern und 5 Frauen mit einem Durchschnittsalter von 63,2 Jahren zusammen. Die Kontrollgruppe umfaßte insgesamt 12 magengesunde, nicht operierte Probanden (7 Männer, 5 Frauen) mit einem Durchschnittsalter von 55,7 Jahren.

Die szintigraphische Untersuchung wurde bei jedem Patienten morgens nach einer 12stündigen Nüchternphase in sitzender Position standardisiert durchgeführt. Die Testmahlzeit sollte von allen Patienten gleichermaßen gut toleriert werden und durfte zum einen wegen des vergleichsweise kleinen Jejunumpouch nicht volumenbelastend und zum anderen wegen der veränderten postoperativen Stoffwechselsituation nicht reich an Fettsäuren sein. Daher wurde als solide Testmahlzeit ein Pfannkuchen aus 60 g Mehl (Aurora Fertiggericht) verabreicht, der mit 100 μBq 99 M Tc-Albures markiert worden war. Die Aktivität erfaßte eine dorsal positionierte Großfeldkamera, die zum Beginn der Nahrungsaufnahme gestartet und auf den Jejunumpouch zentriert wurde. Der Aktivitätsverlauf wurde über einen Zeitraum von 60 min kontinuierlich in Einzelbildern von je 90 sek Dauer aufgezeichnet. Aus mehreren übereinander projezierten Einzelbildern konnten anschließend die Regions of interest (ROI) – Ösophagus, Pouch und abführende Schlinge – festgelegt werden. Die prozentuale Aktivitätsveränderung innerhalb dieser ROI pro min wurde graphisch dargestellt.

Darüberhinaus wurde jeder Patient zu seinen aktuellen Beschwerden befragt. Auf einen standardisierten Fragebogen konnte er überwiegend postprandial auftretende Symptome, wie Völlegefühl, Übelkeit und Meteorismus, aber auch Fragen zu seinem Allgemeinbefinden, wie Appetit, Müdigkeit und körperliche Leistungsfähigkeit, nach dem Schweregrad des Auftretens auf einer Skala von 1 bis 6 einschätzen. Dieser aus der Gesamtsumme gebildete individuelle Score wurde in Beziehung zu seinem Entleerungsverhalten gesetzt.

Ergebnisse

Die physiologische, solide Magenentleerung ist durch eine durchschnittlich 9,2 min dauernde sogenannte "lag phase" ausgezeichnet, in der aufgrund der Speisebreidurchmischung keine Entleerung stattfindet. Daran schließt sich eine annähernd linear verlaufende, abfallende Entleerungskurve an. Nach 1 h sind individuell unterschiedlich zwischen 37 und 69% der gesamten Testmahlzeit in das Duodenum übergetreten.

Eine lag phase wird nach totaler Gastrektomie bei keinem Patienten mehr beobachtet. Beim Jejunumpouch ist die Transitzeit sowohl nach 30 wie nach 60 min signifikant langsamer als bei der Ösophagojejunostomie. Beide Entleerungsmuster bleiben gegenüber der physiologischen Magenentleerung signifikant beschleunigt (Tabelle 1). Extreme Passagezeiten – verzögerte mit einer prozentualen Abnahme von höchstens 20% und beschleunigte mit einer Abnahme von mindestens 80% innerhalb der Untersuchungszeit – wurden bei 4 Patienten in der Pouchgruppe und bei 6 in der Jejunostomiegruppe gemessen, wobei nur 1 Patient mit und 3 Patienten ohne "Ersatzmagen" eine beschleunigte Passage aufwiesen. Ein erneuter Aktivitätsanstieg innerhalb der Ösophagusregion während der zweiten Untersuchungshälfte im Sinne eines intestinoösophagealen Refluxes wurde bei 3 Jejunostomie- und 1 Pouchpatienten nachgewiesen.

Tabelle 1. Durchschnittliche Entleerungszeit (angegeben als prozentuale Aktivität nach 30 und 60 min) und der durchschnittliche postprandiale Score

	n	A%/30min	A%/60min	Score	n (Score<3)
Jejunumpouch	15	61 ± 22	39 ± 25	2,8	10
Ösophagojejunostomie	15	48 ± 27	28 ± 24	3,7	4
Kontrollgruppe	12	75 ± 19	54 ± 17		

10 von 15 Patienten mit Jejunumpouch beurteilten ihre Situation 6 Monate nach der Operation, gemessen an den durchschnittlichen Scorepunkten, als überwiegend gut (Score von 2,2), 3 immerhin noch als befriedigend (3,4) und 2 als unbefriedigend (4,7). In der Gruppe ohne Pouch waren 4 Patienten mit einem Durchschnittsscore von 2,6 zufrieden, 7 Patienten empfanden ihre Situation als befriedigend (3,5) und 4 klagten über gehäuft auftretende postprandiale Beschwerden (4,6) (Tabelle 2). Die extremen Entleerungsmuster beider Gruppen (insgesamt 10 von 30) korrelierten gut mit den klinischen Angaben der Patienten.

Tabelle 2. Durchschnittliche Scorepunkte für häufig genannte postprandiale Beschwerden und die Anzahl der Patienten (mit/ohne Pouch), bei denen diese Symptome verstärkt auftraten (Score > 4)

	Jejunumpouch	Jejunostomie	n (Score>4)
Völlegefühl	2,4	2,9	3/5
Übelkeit	2,1	3,0	2/4
Schwindel	1,9	2,4	1/3
Bauchschmerzen	2,6	3,3	3/6
Fehlendes Hungergefühl	3,1	3,3	7/8

Der postoperative Gewichtsverlauf zeigte bei 7 der Pouch- und 3 Jejunostomiepatienten einen Anstieg des Entlassungsgewichtes 6 Monate zuvor von mindestens 2 kg. Ein postoperativ fehlendes Hungergefühl wurde in beiden Gruppen häufig beobachtet, bei insgesamt 7 Pouch- und 8 Jejunostomiepatienten.

Diskussion

Erwartungsgemäß übernimmt nach totaler Gastrektomie der Jejunumpouch insoweit eine Ersatzmagenfunktion, als er im Vergleich zur Ösophagojejunostomie die Passage der Testmahlzeit signifikant verzögern kann. Dafür spricht auch die höhere Anzahl von Pouchpatienten mit einem guten Scoredurchschnitt und der bessere postoperative Gewichtsverlauf [1, 2, 4]. Beides korreliert gut mit den szintigraphisch gemessenen Entleerungsmustern, denn nur die 4 Patienten dieser Gruppe mit extrem verzögerter oder beschleunigter Entleerung haben einen Score größer 3,5 und verzeichnen auch keinen Anstieg ihres Körpergewichtes.

Insgesamt werden extrem veränderte Entleerungsmuster häufiger bei der einfachen Jejunostomie beobachtet; hier treten Sturzentleerungen und Stase gleichmäßig häufig auf und bestimmen mehr als ein Drittel des Patientengutes. Eine nicht mechanisch bedingte verzögerte Transitzeit hingegen wird innerhalb der Pouchgruppe dreimal häufiger als eine Passageverzögerung beobachtet. Die beschleunigte Entleerung verursacht den Patienten beider Gruppen schwerwiegendere Beschwerden als die Stase, der alle betroffenen Patienten durch diätetische Veränderungen offenbar besser entgegenwirken können.

Ein Reflux der soliden Testmahlzeit in den Ösophagus wurde bei der Jejunostomie häufiger gemessen als beim Jejunumpouch. In der Frühphase der Entleerung innerhalb der ersten 60 min ist dieser Reflux mehr auf die Plikatio als Antirefluxbarriere und auf das Fehlen des unteren Ösophagussphincters bei der einfachen Jejunostomie als auf die Roux-Y-Ableitung zurückzuführen. Insgesamt wird der intestinoösophageale Reflux jedoch nur bei 13% aller 30 untersuchten Patienten beobachtet.

Die beiden Rekonstruktionsverfahren haben keinen erkennbaren Einfluß auf die postoperative Entwicklung des fehlenden Hungergefühls, das über die Hälfte aller gastrektomierten Patienten dieser Studie beklagen.

Zusammenfassung

Die Entleerung einer soliden, radioaktiv markierten Testmahlzeit aus einem Jejunumpouch verläuft 6 Monate nach totaler Gastrektomie signifikant langsamer als die bei einfacher Ösophagojejunostomie. Gemessen an den postprandialen Symptomen, die in einem Score individuell erfaßt wurden, sind 73% aller Patienten mit einem Ersatzmagen überwiegend beschwerdefrei im Vergleich zu 27% ohne Magenersatz. Daher sollte, sofern die Tumorlokalisation keine transmediastinale Resektion erforderlich macht und das Tumorstadium eine günstige Prognose erwarten läßt, zur Verbesserung der postoperativen Lebensqualität eine Ersatzmagenbildung in Form einer Ösophagojejunoplikatio durchgeführt werden.

Summary

Six months after total gastrectomy, the emptying pattern of a solid radioactively labeled test meal is significantly slower in the case of a jejunal pouch in comparison to a simple esophagojejunostomy. Indicated by an individual score, 73% of all patients with gastric replacement had no major postprandial symptoms, compared with 27% without gastric replacement. Depending on tumor localization and staging and also on the type of resection, an esophagojejunoplicatio with pouch should be performed to improve the quality of life.

Literatur

1. Roder JD, Herschbach P, Henrich G, Böttcher K, Siewert JR (1992) Lebensqualität nach totaler Gastrektomie wegen Magenkarzinom – Ösophagojejunoplikatio mit Pouch versus Ösophagojejunostomie ohne Pouch. Dtsch Med Wochenschr 117:241–247
2. Vestweber KH, Troidl H (1989) Lebensqualität nach Magenoperationen. Chirurg 60:450–453
3. Siewert JR, Böttcher K (1992) Ösophagojejunoplikatio in Stapler-Technik. Ergebnisse einer kontrollierten Studie. Langenbecks Arch Chir 377:186–189
4. Herfarth C, Schlag P, Buhl K (1987) Surgical procedures for gastric substitution. World J Surg 11:689–698

Dr. A. Stier, Chirurgische Klinik und Poliklinik, TU München, Klinikum rechts der Isar, Ismaninger Straße 22, W-8000 München 80

Neue tierexperimentelle Studien zur Adhäsionsprophylaxe

New Experimental Studies on the Prevention of Adhesions

K.-H. Treutner, P. Bertram, M. Klimaszewski und V. Schumpelick

Chirurgische Klinik, Medizinische Fakultät, Rheinisch-Westfälische Technische Hochschule, Aachen

Einleitung

Postoperative, intraabdominelle Adhäsionen werden auch nach primär komplikationslosen Eingriffen häufig zum Problem. Bei der operativen Therapie des Ileus finden sich in 44–66% der Fälle Adhäsionen als Ursache. Bei 93% dieser Patienten findet sich in der Vorgeschichte eine Laparotomie, wobei in 38% lediglich eine Appendektomie durchgeführt wurde. Auch wenn die Adhäsionen nicht zum Ileus führen, so stellen sie doch bei der Zunahme von Relaparotomien aufgrund höherer Lebenserwartung und erweiterter Indikationsstellung ein wachsendes intraoperatives Problem und Komplikationsrisiko dar [2]. In der vorliegenden Studie sollten deshalb Substanzen zur Adhäsionsprophylaxe untersucht werden.

Methodik

Die Untersuchungen wurden an 120 weiblichen Chincilla-Bastard Kaninchen mit einem durchschnittlichen Ausgangsgewicht von 3160 g durchgeführt. Alle Tiere wurden in Allgemeinnarkose (Rompun + Ketamin i.v.) laparotomiert. Mit einem speziellen Instrumentarium aus einem Stempel und einer Bank wurden standardisierte Läsionen der Serosa von Ileum, Appendix und Bauchdecke gesetzt (10 cm^2, 400 p, 280er Schleifpapier) [3]. Vor dem schichtgerechten Verschluß der Bauchhöhle erhielten alle Tiere, außer denen der Kontrollgruppe (I), 1 ml pro 100 ml Körpergewicht der verschiedenen Prüfsubstanzen intraperitoneal verabreicht (Tabelle 1).

Nach 10 Tagen wurden die Tiere euthanasiert (Narcoren i.v.) und die Adhäsionsflächen mittels Digitizer, Personalcomputer und spezieller Software objektiv vermessen [3]. Zudem wurden licht- und elektronenmikroskopische Untersuchungen durchgeführt.

Ergebnisse

Von den 120 Tieren verstarben 7 aufgrund von Narkoseproblemen oder mußten wegen Pilzinfektionen vorzeitig euthanasiert werden. Die Ergebnisse der Adhäsionsvermessung (Tabelle 2) und die Auswertung der mikroskopischen Präparate zeigte einen po-

Chirurgisches Forum 1993
f. experim. u. klinische Forschung
Becker/Beger/Hartel (Hrsg.)

sitiven Zusammenhang zwischen der Ausdehnung der Adhäsionen und dem Ausmaß von Fibrinablagerungen und Bindegewebsneubildungen. Die statistische Auswertung mittels t-Test und Wilcoxon-Test zeigte einen signifikanten Unterschied zwischen den Gruppe V und VI ($p < 0,05$), die Vergleiche aller anderen Gruppen gegeneinander zeigte sonst hochsignifikante Differenzen ($p < 0,01$). Toxische Effekte oder eine Beeinträchtigung der Wundheilung wurden nicht beobachtet.

Tabelle 1. Einteilung der Gruppen: * die Dosis ist angegeben pro 100 g Körpergewicht, das applizierte Volumen betrug immer 1 ml pro 100 g Körpergewicht

Gruppe	n	Substanz und Dosis*	Handelsname
I	20	- - - Kontrolle - - -	- - -
II	20	1 ml NaCl 0,9%	- - -
III	20	0,25 ml Taurolidin 2%	Taurolin
IV	20	0,5 E Plasmin + 300 E DNAse	Fibrolan
V	20	2000 IE Streptokinase + 500 IE Streptodornase	Varidase
VI	20	50% TCDO	Oxoferin

Tabelle 2. Ergebnisse der einzelnen Gruppen im Hinblick auf die Adhäsionsflächen in mm^2 mit SD (Standard Deviation – Standardabweichung) und SEM (Standard Error of Mean – Standardabweichung des Mittelwertes)

Gruppe	n	Minimum	Maximum	Mittel	SD	SEM
I	19	1183,7	2939,4	1998,3	541,1	124,1
II	18	976,9	1775,1	1367,9	246,9	58,2
III	19	639,9	1297,1	1012,2	208,9	47,9
IV	19	482,2	950,8	673,5	144,7	33,2
V	19	0	663,7	360,4	192,2	44,1
VI	19	0	599,9	239,9	197,3	45,3

Diskussion

Das hier angewandte Tiermodell konnte seine Eignung für eine standardisierte Überprüfung von Substanzen zur Adhäsionsprophylaxe beweisen [3]. Die Applikation von Flüssigkeit allein (NaCl 0,9%) kann, wahrscheinlich aufgrund der Distanzierung der Läsionen, die Adhäsionsfläche verkleinern. Durch Taurolidin lassen sich bessere Ergebnisse erzielen, zumindest beim vorliegenden Versuch ohne Peritonitis sind jedoch die Substanzen von größerer Effektivität, die Einfluß auf den Abbau von Fibrin haben (Plasmin + DNAse und Streptokinase/-dornase) [4]. Die geringsten Verwachsungsflächen fanden sich nach der Applikation von TCDO, das wahrscheinlich über

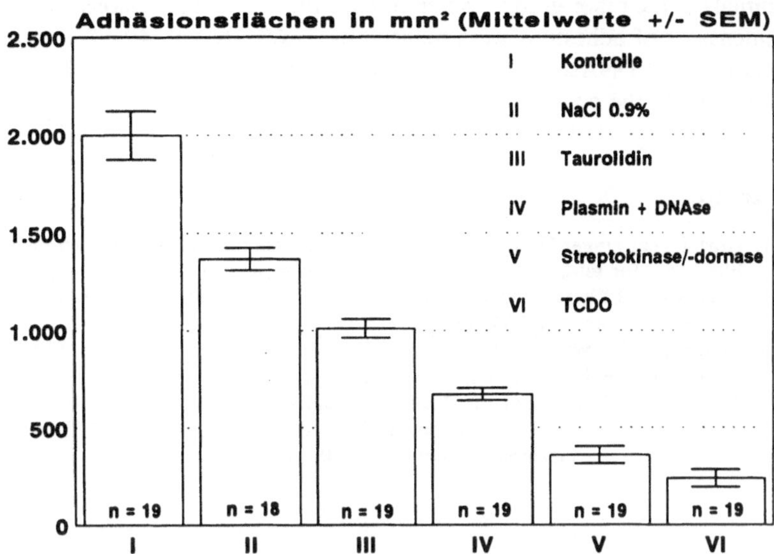

Abb. 1. Mittelwerte der Adhäsionsflächen pro Gruppe in mm^2 ± SEM (Standard Error of Mean – Standardabweichung des Mittelwertes)

eine Erhöhung des lokalen pO_2 und eine Aktivierung der Makrophagen wirkt [1]. Hieraus ergibt sich als Vorteil gegenüber den Substanzen, die in das Gerinnungssystem eingreifen, daß keine erhöhte Gefahr der postoperativen Nachblutung befürchtet werden muß (Abb. 1).

Zusammenfassung

In der Untersuchung sollten Substanzen zur Prophylaxe postoperativer, intraabdomineller Adhäsionen geprüft werden. Bei 120 Kaninchen in 6 Gruppen (n = 20) wurden standardisierte Serosaläsionen gesetzt. Die Kontrollgruppe erhielt keine Medikation, den Tieren der anderen Gruppen wurden 5 verschiedene Substanzen intraperitoneal appliziert. Nach 10 Tagen wurden die Verwachsungsflächen objektiv vermessen. Das Ausmaß der Adhäsionen konnte um 31,6% (NaCl), 49,4% (Taurolidin), 66,3% (Plasmin + DNAse), 82% (Streptokinase/-dornase) bzw. 88% (TCDO) gegenüber der Kontrollgruppe reduziert werden. Die Unterschiede waren signifikant.

Summary

The underlying study evaluates the effect of various substances in the prevention of postoperative intra-abdominal adhesions. One hundred and twenty rabbits in six groups ($n = 20$) underwent standardized lesions of the serosa. The controls received no medication, whereas five different substances were intraperitoneally administered to the animals in the other groups. After 10 days the areas of adhesions were measured. The dimensions of adhesions were reduced by 31.6% (NaCl), 49.4% (taurolidine), 66.3% (plasmin and DNAse), 82% (streptokinase/-dornase), and 88% (TCDO), respectively, compared to the controls. These differences were all significant.

Literatur

1. Hinz J, Hautzinger H, Stahl K-W (1986) Rationale for and results from randomised, double-blind trial for tetrachlorodecaoxygen anion complex in wound healing. Lancet I:825–828
2. Menzies D, Ellis H (1990) Intestinal obstruction from adhesions – how big is the problem? Ann R Coll Surg Engl 72:60–63
3. Treutner K-H, Winkeltau G, Lerch MM, Stadel R, Schumpelick V (1989) Postoperative, intraabdominelle Adhäsionen – Ein neues standardisiertes und objektiviertes Tiermodell und Testung von Substanzen zur Adhäsionsprophylaxe. Langenbecks Arch Chir 374:99–104
4. Vipond MN, Whawell SA, Thompson JN et al. (1990) Peritoneal fibrinolytic activity and intraperitoneal adhesions. Lancet 335:1120–1122

Dr. med. K.-H. Treutner, Chirurgische Klinik, RWTH, Pauwelsstraße 30, W-5100 Aachen

Bedeutung von Scoringsystemen bei der Diagnose der akuten Appendizitis

Importance of Scoring Systems for the Diagnosis of Acute Appendicitis

C. Franke[1], Q. Yang[2], H. Böhner[1], P. Verreet[1] und C. Ohmann[2]

[1]Klinik für Allgemein- und Unfallchirurgie, Heinrich-Heine-Universität, Düsseldorf
[2]Funktionsbereich Theoretische Chirurgie, Heinrich-Heine-Universität, Düsseldorf

Einleitung

Die Diagnose einer akuten Appendizitis stellt immer noch ein schwieriges Problem dar. Dies wird durch die immer noch hohe Rate perforierter Appendices und durch den hohen Anteil negativer Appendektomien belegt [1]. Wichtigste Voraussetzung für die Diagnose der akuten Appendizitis ist eine standardisierte und strukturierte Anamnese und klinische Untersuchung. Darüber hinaus gibt es zahlreiche diagnostische Hilfsmittel, wie z.B. Speziallabor, Röntgen, Ultraschall, die den Diagnoseprozeß sinnvoll unterstützen können. In den letzten Jahren sind mit der computerunterstützten Diagnose und mit den Scoringsystemen weitere vielversprechende Entscheidungshilfen hinzugekommen [2].

Diagnostische Scoringsysteme haben in den Originalpublikationen gute Ergebnisse gezeigt und scheinen für eine Diagnoseunterstützung bestens geeignet [3, 4]. Leider fehlen bisher adäquate prospektive Evaluierungen. Wir haben daher eine Evaluierungsstudie durchgeführt, bei der wir überprüft haben, ob publizierte Scores bei unserem Krankengut die Diagnosefindung bei akuter Appendizitis unterstützen können.

Methodik

Zwei publizierte Scores für die Diagnose einer akuten Appendizitis (Alvarado-Score, Lindberg-Score) wurden auf einer prospektiven Datenbank getestet. Diese Datenbank wurde im Rahmen einer konzertierten europäischen Aktion an sechs deutschen Kliniken aufgebaut. In die Studie wurden innerhalb eines definierten Zeitraumes (3/89–12/89) alle Patienten mit akuten Bauchschmerzen, die innerhalb einer Woche vor Krankenhausaufenthalt aufgetreten waren und denen kein Trauma zugrunde lag, eingebracht.

Anamnese und klinischer Befund wurden mit Hilfe eines speziell entwickelten Fragebogens standardisiert und strukturiert erfaßt. Für die Entlassungsdiagnose wurden der Verlauf, Spezialuntersuchungen und ggf. eine Operation (Histologie) herangezogen. Insgesamt wurden 1254 Patienten untersucht. Die fünf häufigsten Diagnosen

Chirurgisches Forum 1993
f. experim. u. klinische Forschung
Becker/Beger/Hartel (Hrsg.)

waren: Unspezifische Bauchschmerzen 39,7%, akute Appendizitis 16,8%, Dyspepsie 7,8%, akute Gallenwegserkrankungen 6,9% und Ileus 3,7%.

Beschreibung der Scores

Alvarado-Score [3]: Schmerzwanderung (rechter unterer Quadrant: 1, sonstige: 0), Appetitlosigkeit (ja: 1, nein: 0), Übelkeit und Erbrechen (ja: 1, nein: 0), Druckschmerz im rechten unteren Quadrant (ja: 2, nein: 0), Loslaßschmerz (ja: 1, nein: 0), Temperaturerhöhung > 37,3°C (ja: 1, nein: 0), Leukocytose > 10000 (ja: 2, nein: 0), Linksverschiebung im Blutbild (ja: 1, nein: 0).

Lindberg-Score [4]: Geschlecht (männlich: +8, weiblich: –8), Leukocyten (< 9000: –14, 9000–14000: +2, > 14000: +10), Schmerzdauer (< 24 h: +3, 24–48 h: = 0, > 48 h: –12), Schmerzzuwachs (ja: +3, nein: –5), erneutes Auftreten des Schmerzes (ja: +7, nein: –9), Erbrechen (ja: +7, nein: –5), Verschlimmerung durch Husten (ja: +4, nein: –11), Loslaßschmerz (ja: +5, nein: –10), Abwehrspannung (ja: +13, nein: –4), Schmerzen außerhalb des rechten unteren Quadranten (ja: –6, nein: +4).

In den Originalpublikationen wurden mit Hilfe von Schwellenwerten drei verschiedene Gruppen entsprechend dem weiteren therapeutischen Vorgehen definiert.

- hohes Risiko (Operation): Lindberg-Score > 0, Alvarado-Score > 7
- mittleres Risiko (stationäre Überwachung): Lindberg-Score –26–0, Alvarado-Score 5–6
- niedriges Risiko (Entlassung): Lindberg-Score < –26, Alvarado-Score < 4

Die beiden Scores wurden auf unserer Datenbank getestet, der Anteil der Patienten mit akuter Appendizitis in den drei Gruppen – Operation, Überwachung, Entlassung - bestimmt und die Ergebnisse mit den Literaturergebnissen verglichen.

Ergebnisse

Aufgrund des Lindberg-Scores wurden 196 Patienten der Gruppe Operation, 354 Patienten der Gruppe Überwachung und 704 Patienten der Gruppe Entlassung zugeordnet (Alvarado-Score: 62, 196, 996). Der Anteil der Patienten mit akuter Appendizitis betrug beim Lindberg-Score in der Gruppe Operation 47%, in der Gruppe Überwachung 17% und in der Gruppe Entlassung 8% (Alvarado-Score: 71%, 43%, 8%).

Diese Ergebnisse waren erheblich schlechter als in den Originalpublikationen (siehe Abb. 1 und 2).

Aufgrund unserer Daten hätte eine Entscheidung für eine Operation (hohes Risiko) anhand der Scores zu einer primären negativen Laparotomierate von 53% beim Lindberg-Score und 29% beim Alvarado-Score geführt. Umgekehrt würden beim Lindberg-Score 27% der Patienten, beim Avlarado-Score 39% der Patienten mit einer akuten Appendizitis der Gruppe mit niedrigem Risiko (Entlassung) zugeordnet.

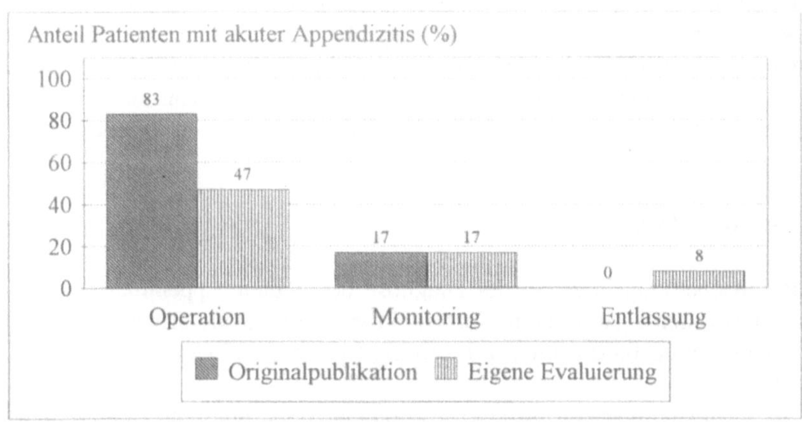

Abb. 1. Vorhersagewert des Lindberg-Scores bei akuter Appendizitis. Vergleich zwischen publizierten Daten und eigener Evaluierung (n = 1254)

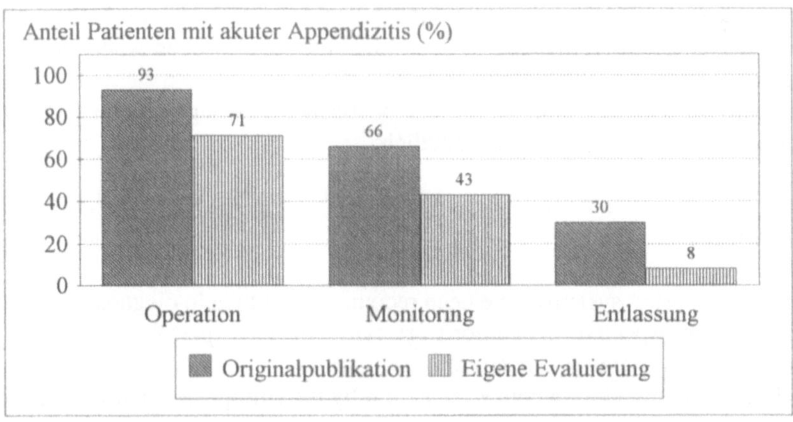

Abb. 2. Vorhersagewert des Alvarado-Scores bei akuter Appendizitis. Vergleich zwischen publizierten Daten und eigener Evaluierung (n = 1254)

Diskussion

Unterschiedliche Ursachen müssen für die schlechten Ergebnisse der computerunterstützten Diagnose diskutiert werden [5]. Geographische Variationen bei der akuten Appendizitis wurden in der Literatur beobachtet und negative Einflüsse dieser Unterschiede auf die Richtgkeit von diagnostischen Entscheidungshilfen berichtet. Ein weiteres Problem resultiert aus den Variationen der Terminologie, der Definitionen und der klinischen Untersuchungen. Scores, die an einem Zentrum entwickelt und getestet werden (z.B. Lindberg-Score, Alvarado-Score), führen bekanntermaßen zu besseren Ergebnissen wegen des besonderen Engagements der Untersucher und wegen der Vergleichbarkeit von Terminologie und Definitionen. Hinzu kommen methodische Fehler, wie z.B. die gleichzeitige Verwendung eines Datensatzes für die Entwicklung und die Testung eines Scores (Reklassifikation), die überoptimistische Ergebnisse erzeugen können. Diese und andere Gründe sind verantwortlich dafür, daß die unabhängige Testung eines schwedischen (Lindberg) und eines amerikanischen Scores (Alvarado) auf einer multizentrischen Datenbank zu unbefriedigenden Ergebnissen geführt hat.

Zusammenfassung

Als Entscheidungshilfe bei der Diagnose der akuten Appendizitis sind verschiedene Scoring-Systeme empfohlen worden. Prospektive Evaluierungen sind jedoch selten. In einer Studie haben wir zwei Scoring-Systeme auf einer prospektiven Datenbank getestet.

Im Rahmen einer konzertierten Aktion der EG wurden die Anamnese und der klinische Befund bei akuten Bauchschmerzen standardisiert und strukturiert aufgezeichnet. Zwei Scoring-Systeme wurden auf einer prospektiven Datenbank, die in der EG-Studie erarbeitet wurde (n = 1254), getestet. Im Gegensatz zu den Originalarbeiten waren die Scores deutlich seltener in der Lage, Patienten mit einer akuten Appendizitis zu bestimmen. Ihre Anwendung hätte zu negativen Appendektomieraten von 53% und 29% (Lindberg-Score, Alvarado-Score) und zu unterlassenen Appendektomien in 27% und 39% geführt.

Somit ist die Anwendung von diagnostischen Scoring-Systemen für die Diagnose der akuten Appendizitis wenig nützlich.

Summary

Different scoring systems have been recommended to help diagnose acute appendicitis. However, prospective evaluations are rare. We have performed a study to evaluate two scoring systems prospectively.

In the framework of a concerted action by the European Community, a standardized anamnestic and clinical evaluation was developed for acute abdominal pain. Two scoring systems (Lindberg and Alvarado) were tested on the prospective database collected in the EC study (n = 1254). In contrast to the original data, the scores were not able to identify patients with acute appendicitis, and its application would have led to negative appendectomies in 53% and 29% of cases and failure to identify appendicitis in 27% and 39% of cases, respectively (Lindberg and Alvarado scoring systems). Therefore, the diagnostic scores tested are not useful in diagnosing acute appendicitis.

Danksagung

Dem Bundesministerium für Forschung und Technologie wird für seine Unterstützung (MEDWIS-Projekt A 70) gedankt.

Literatur

1. de Dombal FT (1979) Diagnose und Operationsindikation bei der akuten Appendizitis. Wie viele Irrtümer sind unvermeidlich? Chirurg 50:291–296
2. Adams ID, Chan M, Clifford PC, Cooke WM, Dallos V, de Dombal FT, Edwards MH, Hancock DM, Hewett DJ, McIntyre N, Somerville PG, Spiegelhalter DJ, Wellwood J, Wilson DH (1986) Computer-aided diagnosis of acute abdominal pain: a multicentre study. Br Med J 293:800–804
3. Alvarado A (1986) A practical score for the early diagnosis of acute appendicitis. Ann Emerg Med 15:79–86
4. Lindberg G, Fenyö G (1988) Algorithmic diagnosis of appendicitis using Bayes' theorem and logistic regression. Bayesian Statistics 3:665–668
5. Ohmann C, Kraemer M (1992) Evaluierung von Entscheidungsunterstützungssystemen bei der Diagnose von akuten Bauchschmerzen. Eine Analyse publizierter Systeme. Biometrie Informatik Med Biol 23:107–111

Dr. C. Franke, Klinik für Allgemein- und Unfallchirurgie, Heinrich-Heine-Universität, Moorenstraße 5, W-4000 Düsseldorf

Literatur

1. de Dombal FT (1979) Diagnose und Operationsindikation bei der akuten Appendizitis. Wie viele Irrtümer sind unvermeidlich? Chirurg 50:291–296
2. Adams ID, Chan M, Clifford PC, Cooke WM, Dallos V, de Dombal FT, Edwards MH, Hancock DM, Hewett DJ, McIntyre N, Somerville PG, Spiegelhalter DJ, Wellwood J, Wilson DH (1986) Computer aided diagnosis of acute abdominal pain: a multicentre study. Br Med J 293:800–804
3. Alvarado A (1986) A practical score for the early diagnosis of acute appendicitis. Ann Emerg Med 15:557–564
4. Lindberg G, Fenyö G (1988) Algorithmic diagnosis of appendicitis using Bayes' theorem and logistic regression. Bayesian Statistics 3:665–668
5. Ohmann C, Kraemer M (1992) Evaluierung von Entscheidungsunterstützungssystemen bei der Diagnose von akuten Bauchschmerzen. Eine Analyse gebräuchlicher Verfahren. Informatik Med Biol 23:103–113

Dr. C. Franke, Klinik für Allgemeine und Unfallchirurgie, Heinrich-Heine-Universität, Moorenstraße 5, W-4000 Düsseldorf

Die chronische Abstoßungsreaktion eines Nierentransplantates im Rattenmodell ist durch Retransplantation in das Empfängertier reversibel

Characteristics of Chronic Rejection Are Reversible in a Rat Kidney Allograft Model After Retransplantation into the Donor Strain

S.G. Tullius[1], U.W. Heemann[1], G. Schmidbauer[2] und N.L. Tilney[1]

[1]Surgical Research Laboratory, Harvard Medical School und Chirurgische Abteilung Brigham and Woman's Hospital, Boston, USA
[2]Chirurgische Abteilung, Universitätsklinikum, Gießen

Einleitung

Die chronische Abstoßungsreaktion stellt ein herausragendes Problem der Transplantationschirurgie dar. Während es im ersten Jahr post transplantationem zu einem Transplantatverlust von 2%–3% durch irreversible akute Abstoßungsreaktion kommt, folgt in jedem weiteren Jahr ein Transplantatverlust von ca. 6%–7% durch chronische Abstoßungsreaktion [1]. Die bisher zu diesem Thema vorliegenden Arbeiten haben zumeist deskriptiven Charakter und beschreiben in erster Linie das histologische und funktionelle Geschehen. Ein persistierendes entzündliches perivaskuläres Infiltrat mit Glomerulo- und Nephrosklerose entwickelt sich einhergehend mit einem zunehmenden Funktionsverlust. Als pathophysiologische Grundlage wird eine multifaktorielle Ursache diskutiert [2]. Sowohl Alloantigen abhängige, als auch Alloantigen unabhängige Faktoren scheinen eine Rolle zu spielen. Die vorliegende Arbeit diente zur Differenzierung dieser Faktoren.

Material und Methoden

Zeichen der chronischen Abstoßungsreaktion entwickeln sich progressiv in Nierentransplantaten in einer Spender-Empfängerkombination von Fisher (F-344, $RT1^{lvl}$), nach Lewis ($RT1^{l}$) Ratten. Zur Prävention einer initial auftretenden akuten Absoßung wurde Cyclosporin A (1,5 mg/kg/d × 10 d) verabreicht. Lewis Ratten wurden intra transplantationem einseitig und 10 Tage später kontralateral nephrektomiert. Nierenallotransplantate (A) (n = 20) wurden nach 4, 8, 12 und 16 Wochen in ein Tier des

Chirurgisches Forum 1993
f. experim. u. klinische Forschung
Becker/Beger/Hartel (Hrsg.)

Spenderstammes (F-344) retransplantiert, und 4, 8, 16 und 20 nach der Retransplantation histologisch und immunohistologisch aufgearbeitet. Isotransplantate (I) (n = 8), zu entsprechenden Zeitpunkten retransplantiert und histologisch untersucht, sowie nicht retransplantierte A (n = 28) und I (n = 12) dienten als Kontrolle. Die Nierentransplantationen wurden unter mikrochirurgischen Bedingungen orthotop mittels End-zu-End Anastomose von Nierengefäßen und Ureter durchgeführt. Alle Eingriffe wurden unter Äthernarkose, die Operationen unter zusätzlicher Verabreichung von Chloralhydrat, vorgenommen. Histologisch wurden Transplantatnieren und Lymphknoten mit Hämatoxilin-Eosin, Thionin, sowie Benzidine, einer spezifischen Färbung für Makrophagen und Granulocyten, aufgearbeitet. Makrophagen (ED-1), Granulocyten (MOM) und T-Lymphozyten (OX-19), sowie die Expression von ICAM-1 in den Transplantatnieren wurde immunohistologisch mit der APAAP Methode angefärbt. Die Bindung von Lymphozyten auf Nieren und Lymphknoten wurde mittels eines von Stamper und Woodruff beschriebenen in-vitro Adhäsionsassays untersucht [3].

Ergebnisse

Der Zeitraum von 12 Wochen post transplantationem (p.t.) stellte eine Zäsur für die Reversibilität aufgetretener chronischer Läsionen dar. Nicht retransplantierte A zeigten bis zu diesem Zeitpunkt geringe bis moderate sklerotische Veränderungen. Ab der 16. Woche p.t. kam es bei diesen Tieren zu einer progressiven Sklerosierung von Glomeruli und Gefäßen, interstitieller Fibrosierung, sowie zu einer zunehmenden tubulären Atrophie. Zu diesem Zeitpunkt verstarben die Tiere gehäuft in der Urämie. A, die 4 oder 8 Wochen p.t. retransplantiert wurden und 8 oder 12 Wochen später histologisch untersucht wurden, wiesen nur geringe Veränderungen im Vergleich mit nicht retransplantierten A auf. Im Gegensatz dazu zeigten A, die nach der 12. Woche retransplantiert wurden, histologische Zeichen der chronischen Abstoßung, die von nicht retransplantierten A des Vergleichsbeobachtungszeitraumes nicht zu unterscheiden waren.

Immunohistologisch fand sich eine Makrophageninfiltration bei nicht retransplantierten A in der 12. Woche p.t. (c. 31 Zellen/Gesichtsfeld (Z/G)), mit einem Gipfel in der 16. Woche p.t. (c. 92 Z/G) und einem anschließenden Rückgang nach 24 bzw. 32 Wochen p.t. auf Werte von c. 20 Z/G. A, die nach 4 oder 8 Wochen retransplantiert wurden, wiesen nur eine geringe Makrophageninfiltration (15–20 Z/G) auf. A, nach der 12. Woche retransplantiert, zeigten eine intensive Makrophageninfiltration mit einer maximalen Ausprägung in der 24. Woche (52 Z/G). Die Infiltration von Makrophagen in Glomeruli von nicht retransplantierten A hatte ihren Gipfel in der 16. Woche p.t. (c. 7 Zellen/Glomeruli (Z/GL)). A, die vor der 12. Woche retransplantiert wurden, zeigten nur eine geringe Infiltration der Glomeruli (2 Z/GL). Im Gegensatz dazu wiesen nach der 12. Woche retransplantierte A eine ausgeprägte Makrophageninfiltration mit einem Gipfel 24 Wochen p.t. (c. 11 Z/GL) auf. Retransplantierte, sowie nicht retransplantierte I hatten eine geringe, wenngleich über den Beobachtungszeitraum ansteigende Makrophageninfiltration.

T-Lymphozyten infiltrierten nicht retransplantierte A zunehmend über den Beobachtungszeitraum mit einem Gipfel in der 32. Woche p.t.. A, die vor der 12. Woche p.t.

retransplantiert wurden, zeigten eine zunehmende, gleichwohl geringer ausgeprägte Infiltration von T-Lymphozyten, als nicht retransplantierte oder nach der 12. Woche retransplantierte A.

Der Zeitraum von 12 Wochen p.t. schien ebenso eine Zäsur für das Bindungsverhalten von Lymphozyten unbehandelter, sowie transplantierter Tiere auf nicht retransplantierten oder retransplantierten A darzustellen. Lymphozyten adhärierten spezifisch auf nicht retransplantierten A, die zwischen der 8. und der 24. Woche p.t. untersucht wurden. A, die nach der 12. Woche retransplantiert wurden, hatten ein vergleichbares Adhäsionsmuster der Lymphozyten. Im Gegensatz dazu zeigten A, die vor der 12. Woche retransplantiert wurden, ein unspezifisches Adhäsionsmuster.

Diskussion

Makrophagen scheinen eine entscheidende Rolle im Rahmen der chronischen Rejektion zu spielen. Morphologische Veränderungen erscheinen parallel zu einem zeitlichen und quantitativen Auftreten dieser Zellpopulation. In dem hier vorgestellten Modell waren Zeichen des chronischen Abstoßungsprozesses bis zu einem kritischen Zeitpunkt (hier: 12 Wochen p.t.) durch Retransplantation in ein Tier des Empfängerstammes reversibel. Eine Retransplantation nach diesem Eingriff verzögerte die Ausprägung der Zeichen des chronischen Abstoßungsprozesses, eine Reversibilität war jedoch nicht mehr möglich.

Zelluläre und histologische Zeichen traten bei nach der 12. Woche retransplantierten Tieren mit einer 8 wöchigen Latenz auf. Die nach diesem Zeitpunkt auftretende progrediente Zellinfiltration, sowie zunehmende Sklerosierung und Fibrosierung war durch Retransplantation nicht mehr umkehrbar.

Ähnliche Ergebnisse wurden in einem akuten Abstoßungsmodell beschrieben, in dem Herzallotransplantate in unbehandelten Ratten in 7 Tagen abgestoßen wurden. Die Zeichen des akuten Abstoßungsprozesses waren durch Retransplantation bis zum 5. Tag p.t. in ein Tier des Spenderstammes reversibel. Die zu diesem Zeitpunkt vorliegende massive Zellinfiltration war per se nicht in der Lage, das Organ abzustoßen [4].

In dem von uns untersuchten chronischen Modell lassen eine kontinuierliche Zellinfiltration, sowie gering ausgeprägte histologische Veränderungen bei A, die vor der 12. Woche retransplantiert wurden, an dem Einfluß von Faktoren, die unabhängig von der immunologischen Herausforderung des genetisch differenten Empfängers sind, denken. Insgesamt liegen den frühen Veränderungen der chronischen Abstoßung wahrscheinlich Alloantigen bedingte Ursachen zugrunde, die nach Retransplantation in ein Tier des Spenderstammes reversibel sind. Später auftretende histologische Veränderungen dagegen sind irreversibel. Alloantigen unabhängige Faktoren, wie die Dauer von warmer und kalter Ischämiezeit, Perfusionsschaden, sowie eine Diskrepanz zwischen Körpergewicht und funktionierendem Organparenchym [5] können den Prozeß beeinflussen und eine zunehmende Bedeutung erlangen.

Zusammenfassung

Die chronische Abstoßungsreaktion zeichnet sich für einen großen Anteil später Transplantatverluste verantwortlich und stellt ein vordringliches Problem der Transplantationschirurgie dar. Nur wenige Informationen liegen bisweilen über die pathophysiologischen Mechanismen vor. Es gibt Vermutungen, daß sowohl antigenabhängige, als auch -unabhängige Faktoren einen Einfluß haben. In einem Rattenmodell, in dem es zur progredienten Ausprägung der für die chronische Abstoßungsreaktion typischen histologischen und funktionellen Veränderungen kommt, wurden F-344 Nierenallotransplantate (A) in LEW Empfänger transplantiert. Die Nieren wurden nach 4, 8, 12 und 16 Wochen in ein Tier des Empfängerstammes retransplantiert und nach weiteren 4, 8, 12 und 16 Wochen histologisch und immunohistologisch aufgearbeitet. Ferner wurde das Bindungsverhalten von Lymphozyten in einem in-vitro Adhäsionsassay untersucht. Nicht-retransplantierte A wurden als Kontrolle verwandt.

Zwölf Wochen post transplantationem (p.t.) stellte eine Zäsur für die Reversibilität der chronischen Läsionen dar. A, die nach 4 oder 8 Wochen retransplantiert wurden und 8 Wochen später histologisch untersucht wurden, zeigten nur geringe Veränderungen, während nicht-retransplantierte A, 12 Wochen p.t. moderate und 16 Wochen p.t. ausgeprägte Zeichen im Sinne einer Glomerulosklerose und Tubulusatrophie zeigten. A, die 12 Wochen oder später retransplantiert wurden, zeigten histologische Veränderungen, die vergleichbar mit nicht-retransplantierten A waren. Immunhistologische Untersuchungen und das Bindungsverhalten von Lymphozyten bestätigten die histologischen Untersuchungen.

Diese Ergebnisse zeigen, daß die chronische Abstoßungsreaktion im Rattenmodell, bei Retransplantation in ein Tier des Empfängerstammes, bis zu einem kritischen Zeitpunkt rückbildungsfähig ist. Alloantigen-abhängige Faktoren scheinen eine entscheidende Rolle in der Frühphase zu spielen. Progrediente sklerotische Veränderungen machen eine Reversibilität zu einem späteren Zeitpunkt unmöglich. Eine kontinuierliche Zellinfiltration mit einhergehenden gering ausgeprägten histologischen Veränderungen lassen gleichzeitig an dem Einfluß von alloantigen-unabhängigen Faktoren denken.

Summary

Chronic rejection represents a major problem in organ transplantation contributing to the destruction of a significant proportion of grafts regardless of organ source. Pathophysiological mechanisms are only poorly understood and seem to be multifaced. Alloantigen-dependent and -independent factors might be involved. In a rat kidney allograft model, where changes of chronic rejection occur progressively, Lewis rats served as recipients of F-344 kidneys. Allografts were retransplanted orthotopically using microsurgical technique into the donor strain 4, 8, 12, and 16 weeks after grafting and harvested 4, 8, 12, and 16 weeks thereafter. Nonretransplanted allografts harvested at comparable time intervals served as controls. Histological, immunohistological, and lymphocyte binding studies were performed.

Twelve weeks after transplantation seemed to be a critical time period for the reversibility of chronic lesions. Nontransplanted allografts developed moderate signs of sclerosis of glomeruli, interstitium, and vessels 12 weeks after transplantation. This process increased by week 16; tubular atrophy had advanced, and animals were beginning to die by this time. In contrast, allografts retransplanted 4 or 8 weeks after grafting and harvested 8 weeks thereafter did not show comparable histological features. Allografts retransplanted 12 weeks after their original grafting or later showed histological signs comparable to nonretransplanted allografts. Immunohistological staining and lymphocyte binding patterns supported these findings.

These results show that characteristics of chronic rejection are reversible up to a critical point (< 12 weeks p.O.) if the host immunological drive is stopped. Alloantigen-dependent factors seem to be dominant in the early period of the process. Progressive sclerosis occurring thereafter was irreversible. Continuous cell infiltration and minor histological changes in allografts retransplanted before 12 weeks suggest the influence of alloantigen-independent factors.

Literatur

1. Häyry P, Mennander A, Yilmaz S, et al. (1992) Towards understanding the pathophysiology of chronic rejection. Clin Invest 70:780–790
2. Hancock WW, Whitley DW, Tullius SG et al. (in press) Cytokines, adhesion molecules and the pathogenesis of chronic rejection of rat renal allografts. Transplant (in press)
3. Stamper HB, Woodruff JJ (1976) Lymphocyte homing into lymph nodes: In vitro demonstration of the selective affinity of recirculating lymphocytes for high-endothelial venules. J Exp Med 144:828–833
4. Kupiec-Weglinski JW, Araujo JL, Topwik E et al. (1985) Host-graft relationship: the system nature of allograft rejection. Surgery 98,2:259–265
5. Olsen JL, Hostetter TH, Rennke HG et al. (1982) Altered glomerular permselectivity and progressive sclerosis following extreme ablation of renal mass. Kidney Int 22,2:112–126

Diese Arbeit wurde unterstützt aus Mitteln eines USPHS Fonds RO1 A1 19071-18. Dr. Tullius ist Empfänger eines DFG Stipendiums (Tu 63/1-1).

Dr. S. Tullius, Surgical Research Laboratory, Harvard Medical School, Building E, Boston, MA., 02115, USA

Nierentransplantation bei Kindern unter 2 Jahren – Ergebnisse und Indikationen von 93 Transplantationen zwischen 1965 und 1992

Renal Transplantation in Children Under 2 Years of Age – Results of 93 Transplants Performed Between 1965 and 1992

C. Troppmann, A.J. Matas, J.S. Najarian und R.W. Grüßner

Department of Surgery, University of Minnesota Hospital and Clinics, Minneapolis, USA

Einleitung

Die Nierentransplantation hat sich im Verlauf der vergangenen zwei Jahrzehnte als Therapie der Wahl zur Behandlung der terminalen Niereninsuffizienz bei Erwachsenen und Adoleszenten durchgesetzt. Verbesserungen der operativen Technik und der postoperativen Nachsorge, sowie Fortschritte in der Organpräservation und Immunsuppression haben bei diesen Patienten zu einer 1-Jahr Transplantatfunktionsrate von über 90% geführt [3]. Im Gegensatz hierzu ist die Nierentransplantation zur Behandlung des chronischen Nierenversagens bei Kindern vor allem in Hinsicht auf die langfristigen Konsequenzen der Immunsuppression umstritten [1, 2]. Wir berichten hier über unsere Erfahrungen mit Nierentransplantationen bei Kindern unter zwei Jahren, welche an unserem Zentrum im Verlauf der vergangenen drei Jahrzehnte durchgeführt wurden.

Patienten und Methodik

Zwischen dem 1.1.1965 und dem 31.7.1992 wurden 93 konsekutive Nierentransplantationen an Kindern unter zwei Jahren vorgenommen. Hierbei handelte es sich um 88 Erst- und 5 Zweittransplantate. Die Transplantatnieren stammten in 77 Fällen von Lebendspendern (83%, 76 Verwandte, 1 nichtverwandter Spender) sowie in 16 Fällen (17%) von Leichenspendern. Das Durchschnittsalter zum Zeitpunkt der Transplantation betrug 1,7 Jahre [(SE: ± 0,05 Jahre, Spannweite 6 Monate–2 Jahre]. 57 Transplantatempfänger waren männlich (61%), 36 weiblich (39%). Die häufigste Ursache der terminalen Niereninsuffizienz waren hypoplastische Nieren [21 Patienten (23%)] und obstruktive Uropathien [19 Patienten (20%)], gefolgt von kongenitalem nephrotischen Syndrom [n = 9 (10%)] und Oxalose [n = 9 (10%)]. 72 Patienten (77%) waren vor Transplantation dialysepflichtig. Die durchschnittliche Anzahl der HLA-Mismatches betrug 1,5 (± 0,1) für die AB-Antigene und 0,8 (± 0,6) für die DR-Antigene. Die maximale PRA (panel reactive antibodies) in Prozent vor Transplantation betrug 4,0% (± 1,4), die durchschnittliche PRA 1,1% (± 0,2). Präoperative Vorbereitung und tech-

Chirurgisches Forum 1993
f. experim. u. klinische Forschung
Becker/Beger/Hartel (Hrsg.)

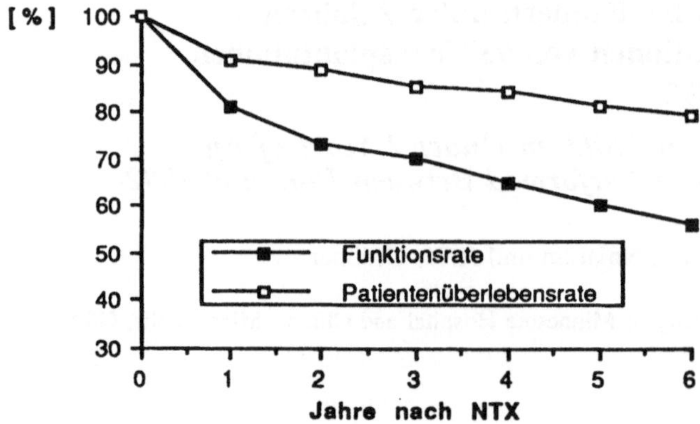

Abb. 1. Funktions- und Patientenüberlebenszeiten von n = 88 Erstnierentransplantaten

nische Einzelheiten des in allen Fällen intraabdominell vorgenommenen Eingriffs sind andernorts publiziert [3]. Während des untersuchten Zeitraums änderte sich die Immunsuppression: Zwischen 1965 und 1984 wurde als Erhaltungstherapie Prednison (0,25 mg/kg/die) und Azathioprin (2,5 mg/kg/die) gegeben. Zur Induktionstherapie wurden zusätzlich 30 mg/kg/die Antilymphoblastenglobulin (ALG) für 14 Tage verwendet. In allen Fällen wurden zur Desensibilisierung vor Transplantation drei bis fünf spenderunspezifische Bluttransfusionen unter gleichzeitiger Azathiopringabe (1,5 mg/kg/die) gegeben, ferner wurde zum Zeitpunkt der Transplantation eine Splenektomie vorgenommen. Seit 1984 entfällt die Splenektomie, wird ALG zur Induktion niedriger dosiert (20 mg/kg/die) und Ciclosporin A (CSA) (5 mg/kg/die) wird sequentiell ab dem 12. postoperativen Tag (triple-drug Erhaltungstherapie) gegeben.

Akute Abstoßungsepisoden wurden bioptisch diagnostiziert und anschließend mit Kortikoiden (2 mg/kg/die Prednison mit anschließender stufenweiser Dosisreduktion) behandelt. ALG für 10–14 Tage wurde bei steroidresistenten Abstoßungen verwendet.

Die Transplantatfunktionsraten und die Patientenüberlebensraten wurden mit der Lifetable-Schätzer Methode berechnet und unter Verwendung des Gehan-Tests statistisch verglichen.

Ergebnisse

Die Ersttransplantatfunktionsraten und Patientenüberlebensraten für Nierentransplantate sind in Abb. 1 dargestellt. Es fand sich ein signifikanter Unterschied bei dem Vergleich zwischen den Nieren von Verwandten- und hirntoten Organspendern zugunsten der Verwandtennieren (Abb. 2). Im Hinblick auf immunsuppressive Therapie zeigte sich, daß die CSA-Erhaltungstherapie sowohl bei Verwandten- als auch Leichennieren zu signifikant besseren Funktionsraten führten (Abb. 3). Gegenwärtig (31.12.92) sind 55 (60%) Transplantate funktionstüchtig und 69 (75%) aller Empfänger am Leben.

Insgesamt kam es zu 38 Transplantatverlusten: In 14 Fällen (37%) handelte es sich um chronische, in 5 Fällen (13%) um akute Abstoßungen. Ein Rezidiv der Grund-

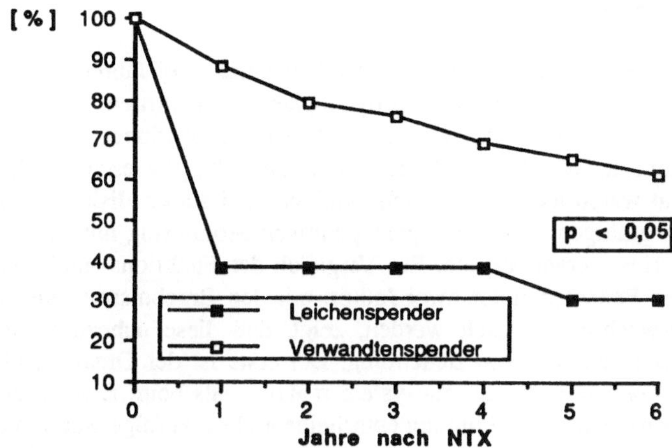

Abb. 2. Erstnierentransplantatfunktionsraten nach Spenderquelle

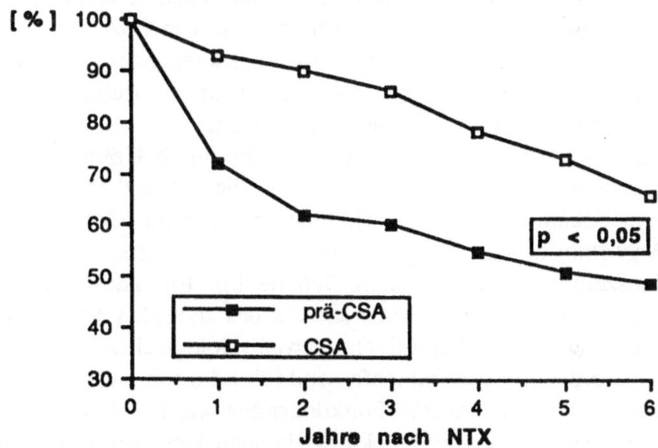

Abb. 3. Immunosuppression und Erstnierentransplantatfunktionsraten: Prä-CSA- versus CSA-Ära

erkrankung führte bei 6 Patienten (16%) zum Transplantatverlust. 8 Kinder (21%) starben mit einem funktionstüchtigen Transplantat; technische Komplikationen [n = 3 (8%)] sowie andere Ursachen [n = 5 (13%)] machten die verbleibenden Fälle aus.

Die häufigste Todesursache bei den 20 Empfängern, die während des Nachbeobachtungszeitraumes starben, waren Infektionen in 9 Fällen (45%); dies schließt vier Todesfälle aufgrund einer fulminanten Sepsis nach Splenektomie ein (alle ereigneten sich vor 1984 mit routinemäßiger Splenektomie vor Transplantation). Fünf Kinder (25%) verstarben an einem Rezidiv der Grunderkrankung (Oxalose). Seit 1983 sind 64 (70%) aller analysierten Transplantationen durchgeführt worden; lediglich vier dieser Patienten sind zwischenzeitlich gestorben.

Diskussion

Nierentransplantationen bei Kindern unter zwei Jahren zur Therapie der chronischen Urämie ist in der gegenwärtigen Literatur umstritten; in diesem Zusammenhang wird auf die höhere Rate an technischen Komplikationen, die niedrige Transplantatfunktionsrate und höhere Patientenmortalität hingewiesen [1, 2]. In unserem Patientengut waren technische Komplikationen bei standardisiertem operativen Vorgehen und sorgfältigem intra- und postoperativen Monitoring nur in 3% für einen Transplantatverlust verantwortlich. Ein Vergleich der Funktions- und Überlebensraten von unseren Patienten unter zwei Jahren mit den Ergebnissen, die bei älteren Kindern oder Erwachsenen erzielt werden, zeigt, daß diese nahezu identisch sind. Hierbei sind zwei Faktoren von Bedeutung. Der erste ist der Organspender: da bei pädiatrischen Empfängern das Immunsystem reaktiver als beim Erwachsenen ist [2], ist eine gute Gewebeübereinstimmung entscheidend. Demzufolge waren die Langzeitergebnisse für Nieren von Verwandtenspendern signifikant besser als für die von hirntoten Spendern. Der zweite Faktor ist die Immunsuppression, die seit der Einführung von CSA zu wesentlich besseren Ergebnissen geführt hat; dies gilt sowohl für die Verwandten- als auch Leichennieren mit einer 1-Jahr Funktionsrate von über 90%. Im Laufe des letzten Jahrzehnts, insbesondere seit Verwendung von CSA, ist die durch infektiöse Komplikationen bedingte Mortalität stark zurückgegangen, nicht zuletzt auch aufgrund der Entwicklung von potenten Medikamenten zur Behandlung von viralen Infektionen und weniger nephrotoxischen Antibiotika.

Ein weiterer wichtiger Aspekt ist die durch Urämie verursachte Wachstums- und allgemeine Entwicklungsretardierung, die hinlänglich bei chronisch dialysierten Kindern dokumentiert ist [4, 5]. Eine erfolgreiche Nierentransplantation führt zu einer Wachstumsakzelerierung mit teilweiser Kompensation der bis zu dem Transplantationszeitpunkt aufgetretenen Defizite [3]. Ein günstiger Einfluß der normalisierten Nierenfunktion auf die Entwicklung des zentralen Nervensystems mit nachfolgender Verbesserung von kognitiven neurophysiologischen Testscores ist ebenfalls beschrieben worden [3]. Zusammenfassend führt die Nierentransplantation bei Kindern unter 2 Jahren zu vergleichbaren Funktionsraten wie bei Erwachsenen. Nierentransplantation von Verwandten resultiert kurz- als auch langlebig in signifikant besseren Ergebnissen als die Leichennierentransplantation bei Kindern unter 2 Jahren und ist somit als Therapie der Wahl des chronischen Nierenversagens auch in dieser Altersgruppe anzusehen.

Zusammenfassung

93 Nierentransplantationen bei Kindern unter zwei Jahren wurden retrospektiv analysiert. 77 Nieren stammten von Lebendspendern und 16 Nieren von hirntoten Organspendern. 1- und 6-Jahres Funktionsraten von 88 Ersttransplantaten betrugen 81% beziehungsweise 56% (Patientenüberlebensrate 91% und 79%). Nierentransplantate von Verwandtenspendern hatten signifikant bessere Funktionsraten als Leichennieren. Die Nierentransplantation bei unter 2-jährigen führt zu vergleichbaren Funktions- und Patientenüberlebensraten wie bei Erwachsenen und ist somit – insbesondere bei

Verwendung von Lebendspendern – als Therapie der Wahl zur Behandlung der chronischen Niereninsuffizienz in dieser Altersgruppe anzusehen.

Summary

We retrospectively studied 93 renal transplants in children under 2 years of age. Seventy-seven kidneys were procured from living donors and 16 from cadaveric donors. One- and 6 year graft survival rates in 88 primary transplants were 81% and 56%, respectively (patient survival rates, 91% and 79%). Grafts from living donors had a significant better survival rate than cadaveric kidneys. Renal transplantation in children under 2 years of age has similar results to those of adults and is therefore considered to be the treatment of choice for chronic renal failure in this age category, especially when using living relatives as donors.

Literatur

1. Moel DI, Butt KMH (1981) Renal transplantation in children less than 2 years of age. J Pediatr 99:535
2. Fine RN (1988) Renal transplantation to the infant and young child and the use of pediatric cadaver kidneys for transplantation in pediatric and adult recipients. Am J Kid Dis 12:1
3. Najarian JS, Frey DJ, Matas AJ (1990) Renal transplantation in infants. Ann Surg 212:353
4. Polinsky MS, Kaiser BA, Stover BA (1987) Neurologic development of children with severe chronic renal failure from infancy. Pediatr Nephrol 1:157
5. Bird AK, Semmler CJ (1986) The early development and neurological sequelae of children with kidney failure treated with CAPD/CCPD. Pediatr Res 20:446a

Dr. med. C. Troppmann, Department of Surgery, University of Minnesota Hospital and Clinics, 420 Delaware Street SE, Box 458, Minneapolis, Minnesota, USA

In situ Cytokinproduktion bei steroidsensitiver Lebertransplantatabstoßung: Analyse der Proteinsynthese und Genexpression mittels kompetitiver PCR

In Situ Cytokine Production During Steroid-Sensitive Liver Allograft Rejection: Analysis of Protein Synthesis and Gene Expression Using Competitive Polymerase Chain Reaction

C.D. Heidecke[1], K. Deutsch[2], S. Westerholt[1], D. Volk[3], W.W. Hancock[4] und J. Adolf[1]

[1]Chirurgische Klinik, TU München, München
[2]Medizinische Klinik, TU München, München
[3]Institut für Medizinische Immunologie, Charité, Berlin
[4]Dept. of Pathology and Immunology, Monash Medical School, Prahran, Australia

Einleitung

Die orthotope Lebertransplantation (OLT) stellt mittlerweile ein etabliertes Verfahren bei akutem Leberversagen und beim Endstadium chronischer Lebererkrankungen dar. Akute Abstoßungsreaktionen und Sepsis sind in der frühpostoperativen Phase die häufigsten Komplikationen. Cytokine sind an der Pathogenese der Transplantatrejektion und anderer Dysfunktionen beteiligt. Die Kinetik und die präzise Bedeutung der einzelnen Cytokine in situ sind jedoch nicht hinreichend definiert. Um die lokale Immunregulation der Transplantatabstoßung und den Einfluß immunsuppressiver Medikamente zu charakterisieren, wurde Leberbiopsiematerial von OLT-Patienten während und nach Abstoßungsepisoden immunhistochemisch und molekularbiologisch auf die Produktion von Cytokinen untersucht.

Methodik

Patienten: 37 Patienten wurden zwischen 4/91 und 11/92 orthotop lebertransplantiert. Die Basisimmunsuppression bestand aus Cyclosporin A, Methylprednisolon und Azathioprin. Innerhalb der ersten 30 postoperativen Tage fand sich bei 11 Patienten eine bioptisch gesicherte, akute Abstoßungsreaktion Grad I–II (30%) mit klinischen oder laborchemischem Korrelat. Kontrollbiopsien wurden nach ca. 7 Tagen entnommen. Alle Abstoßungen waren steroidempfindlich (3 × 1 g Methylprednisolon). Bei einer Patientin trat später eine Rerejektion auf, die eine OKT3 Therapie erforderlich machte.

Gewebeproben: Leberstanzzylinder wurden wöchentlich oder bei Verdacht auf Abstoßung entnommen, in drei Portionen geteilt und sofort in flüssigem Stickstoff mit und ohne Gefriereindeckmedium eingefroren bzw. in Formalin fixiert und konventionell aufgearbeitet. 8 Probenserien (Rejektion und nach Therapie) standen für die

Chirurgisches Forum 1993
f. experim. u. klinische Forschung
Becker/Beger/Hartel (Hrsg.)

Immunhistologie zur Verfügung und 7 zur molekularbiologischen Untersuchung. Als Kontrollen dienten 7 Proben von Patienten, die keine Rejektion hatten.

Immunhistologie: Serielle Cryostatschnitte (4 μm) wurden zur Lokalisation von Zytokinen in Aceton fixiert und nach Inkubation mit einem Panel von Antikörpern (Ab) einer Peroxidase-Antiperoxidase-Färbung unterzogen (Spezifität und Quelle der Abs [1]). Zytokin- und Endothel-Färbung wurde semiquantitativ anhand der Anfärbung intra- und extrazellulärer (Zytokine in und um mononukleäre Zellen) bzw. kontinuierlicher (Endothelium) Strukturen ausgewertet.

PCR: Lebergewebe von 5–10 mg wurde unter flüssigem Stickstoff zermösert und die mRNA unter Anwendung der Guanidin-Thiocyanat-Methode isoliert. cDNA wurde mit der SuperScript reversen Transcriptase und Oligo dT Primern synthetisiert. Unter Verwendung eines Kontrollfragments wurde eine kompetitive PCR mit den respektiven 5' und 3' Primern für Actin, γ-IFN, IL-10, TNF-α und IL-6 wie im Maussystem beschrieben ([2], Manuskript für humane kompetitive PCR in Vorbereitung) durchgeführt.

(Semi)Quantifizierung: Zur Angleichung der cDNA Mengen wurden sämtliche Proben für Actin gegen das Kontrollfragment quantifiziert und entsprechend verdünnt, bis alle Proben das gleiche Verhältnis zum eingesetzten Kontrollfragment hatten. Danach wurden IL-10 und γ-IFN jeweils mit und IL-6 und TNF-α ohne Kontrollfragment amplifiziert. Zur Quantifizierung wurden die PCR Produkte elektrophoretisch getrennt, unter UV-Licht durch Ethidium Bromid Färbung sichtbar gemacht und fotographiert. Die Negative wurden densitometrisch quantifiziert.

Ergebnisse

Zum Zeitpunkt der akuten Transplantatabstoßung fand sich ein deutliches periportales Infiltrat bestehend aus T-Lymphozyten und Makrophagen. 10 bis 20% der portalen mononukleären Zellen (MNC) exprimierten Proliferationsmarker wie IL-2R (CD25) und Ki-67. Ferner waren immunhistochemisch 10 bis 20% der MNC positiv für IL-2 und 20 bis 30% positiv für γ-IFN (Tabelle 1), während proinflammatorische Zytokine wie IL-1, IL-6 und IL-8 an 20 bis 50% der MNC und fokal an Sinusoidalzellen nachweisbar waren. Nach Kortikoid-Stoßtherapie waren das MNC-Infiltrat unterschiedlich stark zurückgegangen und die Proliferationsmarker sowie die T-Zell-Zytokine immunhistochemisch nicht mehr nachweisbar (Tabelle 1). An den Kontrollproben ließ sich keine T-Zell-Aktivierung nachweisen. Die proinflammatorischen Zytokine waren auf 10 bis 20% der portalen Zellen reduziert. Bei den Kontrollpatienten ohne Abstoßung war in situ keine T-Zell-Aktivierung nachweisbar.

Auf mRNA-Ebene ließ sich zum Zeitpunkt der Transplantatabstoßung in allen Fällen eine wenigstens doppelt so starke Genexpression für γ-IFN nachweisen wie nach Therapie (Tabelle 1). Umgekehrt war IL-10 mRNA in 5 von 7 Patienten nach Abstoßungstherapie wenigstens doppelt so stark exprimiert wie zum Zeitpunkt der

Rejektion, während bei 2 Patienten die IL-10 Genexpression unverändert blieb. IL-6 mRNA war während der Abstoßung deutlich stärker exprimiert als nach Therapie.

Tabelle 1. Immunhistologie und Genexpression von Zytokinen an Lebertransplantatbiopsien während und nach steroidsensitiver Abstoßungsreaktion

Marker	Proteinebene akute Abstoßung	nach Therapie
IL-2R (CD25)	10–20% portale MNC	negativ
Ki-67	10–20% portale MNC	negativ
IL-2	10–20% portale MNC	negativ
IFN-γ	20–30% portale MNC	negativ
IL-10	n.d.	n.d.
IL-6	20–50% portale MNC + fokal Sinusoidalzellen	10–20% portale MNC + fokal Sinusoidalzellen
Marker	**mRNA-Ebene akute Abstoßung**	**nach Therapie**
IL-2 (CD25)	n.d.	n.d.
Ki-67	n.d.	n.d.
Il-2	n.d.	n.d.
IFN-γ	+ – +++	negativ – +
IL-10	negativ – +	(+) – ++
IL-6	+ – ++	negativ – +

Diskussion

Die Ergebnisse zeigen, daß während akuter Lebertransplantatabstoßung in situ eine T-Zellaktivierung und klonale Expansion alloreaktiver T-Zellen stattfindet. Dies ließ sich sowohl auf Proteinebene wie auf mRNA-Ebene, wo als immunregulatorisches Zytokin γ-IFN in allen Proben nachweisbar war, dokumentieren. IL-2 mRNA ließ sich bislang nicht nachweisen, was möglicherweise an der extrem kurzen Halbwertszeit liegen mag. Zu ähnlich negativen Ergebnissen bezüglich der IL-2 Genexpression sind auch andere gekommen [3]. Im Gegensatz zu diesen Autoren konnten wir erstmals zeigen, daß TH1 Zytokine (IL-2 und γ-IFN) an der Pathogenese der Transplantatabstoßung beteiligt sind und nach erfolgreicher Abstoßungstherapie dramatisch downreguliert worden sind. Umgekehrt konnten wir bei den meisten Patienten nach Abstoßungstherapie eine deutlich vertärkte Genexpression von IL-10 zeigen, eines Zytokins, das über Antigen präsentierende Zellen die Zytokin-Produktion von TH1 Zellen hemmt [4]. Es kann spekuliert werden, daß neben weiteren Faktoren das Schicksal des Lebertransplantats bezüglich des Auftretens von Abstoßungsreaktionen von der Zytokinexpression von TH1 und TH2 Klonen in situ reguliert wird.

Proinflammatorische Zytokine konnten im Blut vermehrt während akuter Abstoßungsepisoden nach Nieren- und Lebertransplantation nachgewiesen werden [1, 5]. In situ konnten Transkripte für IL-1β, TNF-α und IL-6 in Transplantaten mit und ohne Abstoßung nachgewiesen werden [3]. Unsere Ergebnisse zeigen, daß IL-6 auf Proteinebene und mRNA Ebene während der Abstoßungsepisode vermehrt exprimiert wird, während dies für TNF-α nicht so eindeutig ausfiel (Ergebnisse nicht gezeigt). Diese Zytokine könnten somit die globale Zellularität der Transplantate regulieren, deren Rolle bezüglich ihrer aktuellen Beteiligung an der Pathogenese von Abstoßungsreaktionen bedarf weiterer Untersuchungen.

Zusammenfassung

Während der akuten Lebertransplantatabstoßung kommt es zur in situ T-Zell-Aktivierung mit Expression von Aktivierungsantigenen an MNC und Zytokin-Produktion auf Protein- und mRNA-Ebene. Nach Kortisonstoßtherapie wird die T-Zell-Aktivierung in situ abgeschaltet. Parallel hierzu wird IL-10 verstärkt exprimiert. Die proinflammatorischen Zytokine werden unterschiedlich stark exprimiert.

Summary

Acute liver allograft rejection is associated with increased mononuclear cell (MNC) graft cellularity and in situ T cell activation both at the protein and at the mRNA levels. Following steroid pulse therapy, T cell activation is switched off while IL-10 gene expression is enhanced. Proinflammatory mediators are expressed at different levels during and after rejection.

Literatur

1. Tsuchida A, Salem H, Thomson N, Hancock WW (1992) Tumor necrosis factor production during human renal allograft rejection is associated with depression of plasma protein C and free protein S levels and decreased intragraft thrombomodulin expression. J exp Med 175:81–90
2. Platzer C, Richter G, Überla K, Müller M, Blöcker H, Diamantstein T, Blankenstein T (1992) Analysis of cytokine mRNA levels in IL4 transgenic mice by quantitative PCR. Eur J Immunol 22:1179–1184
3. Martinez OM, Krams SM, Sterneck M, Villanueva JC, Falco DA, Ferrel LD, Lake J, Roberts JP, Ascher NL (1992) Intragraft cytokine profile during human liver allograft rejection. Transplantation 53:449–456
4. Fiorentino DF, Zlotnik A, Vieira P, Mosmann TR, Howard M, Moore KW, O'Garra A (1991) IL-10 acts in the antigen-presenting cell to inhibit cytokine production by Thl cells. J Immunol 146:3444–3451
5. Imigawa DK, Millis JM, Olthoff KM, Derus LJ, Chia D, Sugich LR, Ozawa M, Dempsey RA, Iwaki Y, Levy PJ, Terasaki PI, Busuttil RW (1990) The role of tumor necrosis factor in allograft rejection: I. Evidence that elevated levels of tumor necrosis factor-alpha predict rejection following orthotopic liver transplantation. Transplantation 50:219–225

Dr. C.D. Heidecke, Chirurgische Klinik, Technische Universität München, Ismaninger Straße 22, W-8000 München 80

Mindert die HLA-Übereinstimmung zwischen Spender und Empfänger das Risiko der akuten Abstoßung nach Lebertransplantation?

Does HLA Compatibility Between Donor and Recipient Reduce the Risk of Acute Rejection Following Liver Transplantation?

W.O. Bechstein, G. Blumhardt, G. Schneider und P. Neuhaus

Chirurgische Klinik und Poliklinik, Universitätsklinikum Rudolf Virchow, Freie Universität Berlin (Direktor: Prof. Dr. P. Neuhaus)

Einleitung

Während der Vorteil einer möglichst guten Übereinstimmung der HLA-Merkmale zwischen Spender und Empfänger für das Transplantatüberleben nach Nierentransplantation durch eine Reihe internationaler Studien als erwiesen angesehen werden kann [1, 2], wird die Bedeutung des HLA-Systems für die Lebertransplantation kontrovers beurteilt [3, 4, 5]. Ziel dieser Untersuchung war es, die Häufigkeit des Auftretens einer akuten Abstoßungsreaktion nach Lebertransplantation in Abhängigkeit der Übereinstimmung der Merkmale des HLA-Systems zwischen Spender und Empfänger zu ermitteln.

Methoden

Im Zeitraum von September 1988 bis März 1992 wurden 245 konsekutive orthotope Lebertransplantationen (OLT) bei Erwachsenen durchgeführt. Bei 17 (7%) von 245 OLT handelte es sich um eine Retransplantation (Rezidiv der Grundkrankheit, initiale Nichtfunktion des Transplantats, und chronische Abstoßung). Akute, irreversible Abstoßung führte lediglich zweimal zur Retransplantation. Retransplantationen wurden von der Auswertung ausgeschlossen, somit verblieben 228 konsekutive Ersttransplantationen. Die HLA-A, HLA-B und HLA-DR Antigene wurden bei den Empfängern serologisch mit Hilfe kommerziell erhältlicher Antikörper (Dynal, A.S., Oslo, Norwegen) durch das Typisierungslabor der Abt. für Transfusionsmedizin (Leiter: Prof. Eckstein) im Rahmen der präoperativ vorbereitenden Untersuchungen bestimmt. Die HLA-A, HLA-B und HLA-DR Antigene der Spender wurden durch verschiedene, meist Eurotransplant angeschlossene, Typisierungslabors bestimmt. Die Nomenklatur des WHO-Reports des 10. HLA-Workshops fand Berücksichtigung. Nichtübereinstimmung der HLA-Antigene, ohne Berücksichtigung von Subspezifitäten ("split"-Antigene), wurde als mismatch bezeichnet. Es wurden nur akute Abstoßungsreaktionen in die Auswertung einbezogen, die innerhalb der ersten 90 Tage

Chirurgisches Forum 1993
f. experim. u. klinische Forschung
Becker/Beger/Hartel (Hrsg.)

nach Transplantation auftraten, histologisch gesichert waren und eine Behandlung mit Steroid-Bolus Therapie (3 × 500 mg Methylprednisolon i.v.) oder OKT3 (5 mg, 5–10 Tage i.v.) erforderlich machten. Die Basisimmunsuppression bestand in der Regel aus einer Vierfach-Induktions-Therapie (ATG, Cyclosporin, Azathioprin und Prednisolon) und wurde nach 7 Tagen als Dreifach-Immunsuppression unter Weglassen von ATG fortgeführt. Einige Patienten erhielten einen Interleukin-2-Rezeptor Antikörper (BT 563, Biotest, Dreieich) im Rahmen einer Phase II Studie anstelle von ATG, während andere Patienten Tacrolimus (FK 506, Fuijsawa, München) und Prednisolon im Rahmen einer Phase III Studie erhielten. Die Abstoßungsraten in den einzelnen Gruppen wurden mit Hilfe des Chi-Quadrat Tests verglichen.

Ergebnisse

Insgesamt traten im Verlauf der ersten 90 postoperativen Tage bei 70 (31%) von 228 Patienten Abstoßungsreaktionen auf, die mit Steroidbolustherapie behandelt wurden. Bei 27 von 228 Patienten (12%), die alle zuvor Steroidbolustherapie erhalten hatten, erfolgte eine zusätzliche Behandlung mit OKT3 wegen persistierender Abstoßung. Daten über die Nichtübereinstimmung bezüglich der Einzel-loci HLA-A und HLA-B konnten für 161 (70%) Spender-Empfängerkombinationen vollständig ermittelt werden, für den HLA-DR locus nur für 121 (53%) Spender-Empfänger-Kombinationen (Tabelle 1). Betrachtet man die Anzahl der mismatches in Bezug auf die Einzel-loci, so zeigt sich kein unterschiedlich häufiges Auftreten von Abstoßungsreaktionen in den einzelnen Gruppen (Tabelle 1). Es wurde daher im nächsten Schritt die Anzahl der mismatches unter gleichzeitiger Berücksichtigung der Merkmalsausprägungen zweier HLA-loci analysiert (Tabelle 2). Die Fälle mit 0 bzw. lediglich 1 mismatch waren dabei so selten, daß sie sich einer statistischen Analyse entzogen. Mit Ausnahme der Gruppe mit 2 mismatches der HLA-A/HLA-DR Kombinationen ließ sich in allen Gruppen ein deutlicher Trend des gehäuften Auftretens von akuten Abstoßungsreaktionen bei Zunahme der Nichtübereinstimmungen der HLA-Merkmalskombinationen nachweisen, jedoch ohne statistische Signifikanz. In den Gruppen mit kompletter Nichtübereinstimmung (4 von 4 möglichen mismatches) lag die Abstoßungshäufigkeit regelmäßig sowohl über der durchschnittlichen Abstoßungshäufigkeit im Gesamtkollektiv (36%–45% gegenüber 31%) als auch über der Abstoßungsfrequenz der jeweiligen Gruppen, für die keine kompletten Angaben verfügbar waren.

Zusammenfassung

Mit Hilfe einer retrospektiven Analyse der Daten von 228 konsekutiven primären Lebertransplantationen bei Erwachsenen wurde ein möglicher Zusammenhang zwischen HLA-Merkmalsübereinstimmung und der relativen Häufigkeit des Auftretens einer akuten, histologisch gesicherten und behandelten Abstoßungsreaktion während der ersten 90 postoperativen Tage untersucht. Nichtübereinstimmung der HLA-

Tabelle 1. Anzahl der HLA-mismatches und Auftreten von Abstoßungsreaktionen nach Lebertransplantation (n = 228)

	Anzahl der mismatches			
	0	1	2	keine Angabe
HLA-A				
n OLT	7	67	87	67
n Rej (%)	1 (14)	25 (37)	30 (34)	14 (21)
HLA-B				
n OLT	3	34	124	67
n Rej (%)	1 (33)	6 (18)	39 (32)	24 (36)
HLA-DR				
n OLT	6	44	71	107
n Rej (%)	2 (33)	15 (34)	22 (31)	31 (29)

Abkürzungen: Anzahl mismatches – Anzahl der Nichtübereinstimmungen zwischen Spender und Empfänger HLA-Merkmalen, n OLT – Anzahl der Lebertransplantationen, n Rej (%) – Anzahl der Lebertransplantationen mit mindestens einer histologisch gesicherten und behandelten Abstoßungsreaktion (% bezogen auf Gesamtzahl der Lebertransplantation mit x mismatches in der jeweiligen Gruppe)

Tabelle 2. Anzahl der HLA-A/HLA-B, HLA-A/HLA-DR und HLA-B/HLA-DR mismatches und Auftreten von Abstoßungsreaktionen nach nach Lebertransplantation (n = 228)

	Anzahl der mismatches					
	0	1	2	3	4	keine Angabe
HLA-A/HLA-B						
n OLT	2	1	20	60	67	78
n R (%)	1 (50)	0	2 (10)	17 (28)	26 (39)	24 (31)
HLA-A/HLA-DR						
n OLT	2	4	21	50	40	111
n R (%)	1 (50)	0	8 (38)	12 (24)	18 (45)	31 (28)
HLA-B/HLA-DR						
n OLT	2	1	14	47	53	111
n R (%)	1 (50)	0	4 (28)	15 (32)	19 (36)	31 (28)

Abkürzungen: Anzahl mismatches – Anzahl der Nichtübereinstimmungen zwischen Spender und Empfänger HLA-Merkmalen, n OLT – Anzahl der Lebertransplantationen, n R (%) – Anzahl der Lebertransplantationen mit mindestens einer histologisch gesicherten und behandelten Abstoßungsreaktion (% bezogen auf Gesamtzahl der Lebertransplantation mit x mismatches in der jeweiligen Gruppe)

Antigene, ohne Berücksichtigung von Split-Antigenen, wurde als mismatch bezeichnet. Wurden die jeweiligen mismatches von HLA-A, HLA-B und HLA-DR isoliert betrachtet, so zeigte sich kein Unterschied bezüglich des Auftretens einer akuten Abstoßungsreaktion. Bei Analyse der Merkmalskombinationen von zwei HLA-loci zeigte sich (mit Ausnahme der Gruppe mit 2 mismatches der HLA-A/HLA-DR Kombination) in allen Gruppen ein deutlicher Trend des gehäuften Auftretens von akuten Abstoßungsreaktionen bei Zunahme der Nichtübereinstimmung der HLA-Merkmalskombinationen. Aufgrund der kleinen Zahlen und fehlenden statistischen Signifikant sollte jedoch zum jetzigen Zeitpunkt noch nicht von der bisherigen Organverteilung der Transplantatlebern ohne Berücksichtigung der HLA-Übereinstimmung abgerückt werden.

Summary

A potential relationship between HLA compatibility and the occurrence of acute, histologically proven and treated rejection episodes during the first 90 days after surgery was analyzed retrospectively in a sample of 228 consecutive primary liver transplants in adult recipients. Non-compatibility of HLA antigens, not considering split antigens, was denoted as mismatch. When mismatches of HLA-A, HLA-B and HLA-DR loci were analyzed separately, no difference in the occurrence of acute rejection episodes could be observed. However, when combinations of two HLA loci were analyzed, there was a clear trend in all groups towards an increasing occurrence of acute rejection episodes as the number of HLA mismatches increased, with the exception of only one group of two mismatches in the HLA-A/HLA-DR combination. Because of the small numbers and the lack of statistical significance, the current practice of allocating organs for liver grafts without taking HLA compatibility into account should not be abandoned.

Literatur

1. Opelz G (1987) Effect of HLA-Matching in 10000 cyclosporine treated cadaver kidney transplants. Transplant Proc 19:641–646
2. Takemoto S, Terasaki PI, Cecka JM, Cho YW, Gjertson DW, for the UNOS scientific renal transplant registry (1992) Survival of nationally shared, HLA-matched kidney transplants from cadaveric donors. N Engl J Med 327:834–839
3. Markus BH, Duquesnoy RJ, Gordon RD, Fung JJ, Vanek M, Klintmalm G, Bryan C, Thiel D, Starzl TE (1988) Histocompatibility and liver transplant outcome. Does HLA exert a dualistic effect? Transplantation 46:372–377
4. Steinhoff G (1990) Major histocompatibility complex antigens in human liver transplantation. J Hepatol 11:9–15
5. Lauchart W, Hunke M, Pichlmayr R (1990) Effect of HLA-compatibility on human liver allograft rejection episodes. HPB Surgery 2 [Suppl]:32

Dr. W.O. Bechstein, Chirurgische Klinik und Poliklinik, Universitätsklinikum Rudolf Virchow, Augustenburger Platz 1, 1000 Berlin 65

Korrelation morphometrischer Parameter in der Nullbiopsie mit der frühen Transplantatfunktion nach Lebertransplantation

Correlation of Morphometric Parameters in the Time Zero Biopsy with the Early Function of the Transplant After Liver Transplantation

K. Datsis[1], A. Sakata[2], W.J. Hofmann[2], G. Otto[1] und Ch. Herfarth[1]

[1]Chirurgische Universitätsklinik Heidelberg
[2]Pathologisches Institut, Universität Heidelberg

Einleitung

Die primäre Nichtfunktion des Transplantates ist nach wie vor eine der wichtigsten Frühkomplikationen nach Lebertransplantation. Die Entscheidung zur Retransplantation muß möglichst rasch erfolgen. Sie unterliegt neben klinischen und laborchemischen Kriterien vor allem dem subjektiven Urteil des Chirurgen. Morphologische Parameter aus der nach Reperfusion vom transplantierten Organ gewonnenen Biopsie (sogenannte Nullbiopsie) könnten zusätzliche Kriterien über den Zustand des Transplantates zu einem sehr frühen Zeitpunkt liefern [1, 2]. Die vorliegende Untersuchung sollte klären, ob Volumenverschiebungen der Hepatozyten- und Sinusoidfraktion und/oder die Granulozytenzahl im Leberläppchen, die in tierexperimentellen Untersuchungen bereits als veränderliche Größe ermittelt wurden [3, 4], solche prognostisch relevanten Parameter darstellen und eventuell einen Beitrag in der pathophysiologischen Erklärung des Transplantatversagens liefern können.

Material und Methode

Aus 143 Lebertransplantaten wurden als Untersuchungsgruppe diejenigen Transplantate ausgewählt, die nach Ersttransplantation ein primäres Transplantatversagen zeigten (n = 5). Ein primäres Transplantatversagen wurde bei sehr starkem Transaminasenanstieg und bei fehlender Syntheseleistung der Leber mit frühzeitig (Tag 0–2) erforderlicher Retransplantation diagnostiziert. Als Kontrollgruppe dienten Transplantate, die einem Transplantat aus der Untersuchungsgruppe vorausgingen bzw. nachfolgten und in der Folgezeit eine gute Transplantatfunktion zeigten (n = 10). Bei allen Transplantaten wurde 1 h nach Reperfusion eine Leberbiopsie gewonnen. Die Biopsie wurde sofort in Formalin fixiert und routinemäßig aufgearbeitet. Mit dem Punktzählverfahren nach Weibel und Gomez [5] wurden durch Auszählen von insgesamt 10 intralobulären Feldern pro Biopsie das Volumen und die Oberfläche der Hepatozyten und der Sinusoide, bezogen auf das Gesamtvolumen, ermittelt. Außerdem wurde die Zahl der nekroseassoziierten und nicht-nekroseassoziierten Granulozyten pro mm^3 Leberläppchenvolumen in der Peripherie, in der Mitte und im Zentrum der

Chirurgisches Forum 1993
f. experim. u. klinische Forschung
Becker/Beger/Hartel (Hrsg.)

Lobuli bestimmt. Die statistische Auswertung erfolgte mit dem Kruskal-Wallis-Test und dem u-Test nach Wilcoxon-Mann-Whitney bei Signifikanzschranken von $p = 0{,}05$.

Ergebnisse

Die Relativvolumina der Hepatozyten und Sinusoide und die relativen Oberflächen dieser Strukturen zeigten keine signifikanten Unterschiede zwischen der Untersuchungs- und Kontrollgruppe (Tabelle 1). Die Zahl der Granulozyten im Leberläppchen war jedoch in der Untersuchungsgruppe gegenüber der Kontrolle signifikant erhöht. Dieser Unterschied war alleine durch die nekroseassoziierten Granulozyten bedingt, da die nicht-nekroseassoziierten Granulozyten in beiden Gruppen auf einem konstant niedrigen Niveau lagen (Tabelle 1, Abb. 1). Bei der topographischen Verteilung der nekroseassoziierten Granulozyten in der Untersuchungsgruppe war eine zentrale Akzentuierung der Veränderungen als Trend, nicht jedoch als signifikanter Unterschied zu beobachten (Tabelle 1, Abb. 1).

Diskussion

Dem primären Transplantatversagen gehen in der Nullbiopsie keine signifikanten Veränderungen der relativen Volumina und der relativen Oberflächen von Hepatozyten- und Sinusoidfraktion voraus. Parenchymschäden stellen somit zumindest keine frühen Veränderungen beim Transplantatversagen dar und sind daher auch als Ursache des Transplantatversagens unwahrscheinlich. Ein Anstieg der intralobulären Granulozyten in einer reperfundierten Leber, dem ein allmählicher Abfall folgt, wurde von uns bereits tierexperimentell beobachtet [3, 4] und stellt wahrscheinlich das morphologische Korrelat der intravitalmikroskopischen Granulocytenadhärenz dar [6]. Dieser

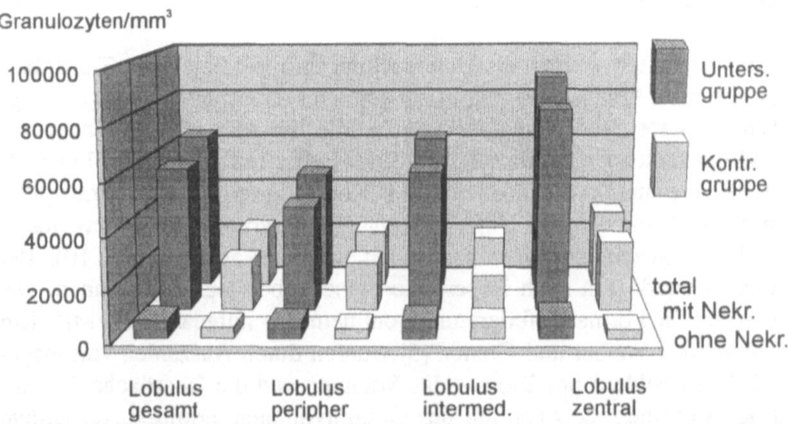

Abb. 1. Granulozyten pro mm^3 Läppchenvolumen in Nullbiopsien aus Lebertransplantaten mit (Untersuchungsgruppe) und ohne (Kontrollgruppe) späterem primärem Transplantatversagen

Tabelle 1. Morphometrische Parameter aus der Nullbiopsie von Transplantatlebern mit späterem primären Transplantatversagen (Untersuchungsgruppe) bzw. unauffälligem postoperativen Verlauf (Kontrollgruppe); Mittelwerte und Standardabweichung

	Untersuchungsgruppe (n = 5)	Kontrollgruppe (n = 10)
rel.Hepatozytenvol. (%)	$83,8 \pm 1,5$	$82,5 \pm 3,1$
rel.Sinusoidvolumen (%)	$16,2 \pm 1,5$	$17,5 \pm 3,1$
Hepatozytenoberfl./ Gesamtvol.(mm^2/mm^3)	$233,7 \pm 11,6$	$228,8 \pm 13,2$
Sinusoidoberfl./ Gesamtvol.(mm^2/mm^3)	$75,2 \pm 9,2$	$72,5 \pm 7,0$

	Untersuchungsgruppe			Kontrollgruppe		
Granulozyten/mm^3	ohne Nekr.	mit Nekr.	total	ohne Nekr.	mit Nekr.	total
Gesamtläppchen	6939 ±4202	56776*[1] ±45115	63716** ±44262	4266 ±2567	19447* ±12994	23714** ±12997
Läppchenperipherie	6082 ±4334	41488§ ±39141	47571§§ ±38755	3773 ±3522	18907§ ±18754	22680§§ ±19058
Läppchenmitte	7409 ±5522	55391# ±43663	62800## ±44704	6262 ±4337	13836# ±13805	20099## ±13321
Läppchenzentrum	8573 ±4995	80055¶ ±64676	88628¶¶ ±62152	3704 ±2280	27477¶ ±21396	31182¶¶ ±20493

[1] Zwischen Werten mit gleichen Symbolen besteht ein signifikanter Unterschied ($p < 0,05$; U-Test nach Wilcoxon-Mann-Whitney)

Anstieg ist in Organen mit einem späteren primären Transplantatversagen signifikant größer und kann somit als früh zur Verfügung stehender prognostischer Parameter betrachtet werden. Die gegenüber der Kontrollgruppe vermehrten Granulozyten sind dabei immer mit hepatozellulären Nekrosen assoziiert. Zusammen mit der zumindest tendenziellen zentrolobulären Akzentuierung dieser Veränderungen könnte dies für einen hypoxischen Schaden im Rahmen von Mikrozirkulationsstörungen sprechen.

Zusammenfassung

Bei morphometrischen Untersuchungen der Nullbiopsie zeigten sich keine signifikanten Unterschiede der relativen Volumina und Oberflächen-Volumenverhältnisse von Hepatozyten und Sinusoiden zwischen der Untersuchungsgruppe aus 5 transplantierten Lebern mit einem primären Transplantatversagen im Verlauf der ersten 2 postoperativen Tage und der Kontrollgruppe aus 10 transplantierten Lebern mit einem unauffälligen postoperativen Verlauf. Die Granulozytenzahl pro Leberläppchenvolumen war jedoch in den Nullbiopsien aus den Transplantaten mit einem späteren primären Transplantatversagen signifikant erhöht. Diese Erhöhung wurde durch Granulozyten verursacht, die mit hepatozellulären Nekrosen assoziiert waren, und war in den zentralen Läppchenarealen akzentuiert. Die Granulozytenzahl im Leberläppchen in der Nullbiopsie stellt somit einen prognostischen Parameter für das primäre Transplantatversagen nach Lebertransplantation dar, wobei den mit Nekrosen assoziierten Granulozyten die entscheidende Rolle zukommt. Ob die Nekrosen Ursache oder Folge der Granulozytenakkumulation sind, muß weiter untersucht werden.

Summary

Morphometric analysis of the time zero biopsy from five transplanted livers with a primary nonfunction during the course of the next 2 days showed no significant differences in the relative volumes and surface to volume ratios of hepatocytes and sinusoids compared with time zero biopsies from ten transplanted livers with a normal and stable course. Numbers of granulocytes per lobular volume, however, were significantly increased in the time zero biopsies from livers with a subsequent primary nonfunction. This difference was due to an increase in granulocytes associated with hepatocyte necrosis and was more pronounced in the centrolobular areas. Thus, numbers of granulocytes within the hepatic lobule might be of prognostic value in predicting primary non-function of the transplant. Furthermore, granulocyte sticking alone after reperfusion does not seem to have an impact on prognosis unless it occurs in association with hepatocyte necrosis. Whether hepatocyte necrosis is the cause or the consequence of the increase of granulocytes has yet to be elucidated.

Literatur

1. Kakizoe S, Yanaga K, Starzl TE, Demetris AJ (1990) Evaluation of protocol before transplantation and after reperfusion biopsies from human orthotopic liver allografts: considerations of preservation and early immunological injury. Hepatology 11:932–941
2. Gaber LW, Gaber OA, Tolley EA, Hathaway DK (1992) Prediction by postrevascularization biopsies of kadaveric kidney allografts of rejection, graft loss, and preservation nephropathy. Transplantation 53:1219–1225
3. Manner M, Kraus T, Hofheinz H, Roy K, Hofmann WJ, Otto G (1992) Wirkung der Eicosanoide auf den Reperfusionsschaden nach experimenteller Lebertransplantation. Langenbecks Arch Chir [Suppl] Chir Forum, S 135–138
4. Otto G, Hofheinz H, Hofmann WJ, Manner M (1991) Questionable role of leukocyte sticking in the pathogenesis of preservation damage. Transplant Proc 23:2385–2386
5. Weibel ER, Gomez DM (1962) A principle for counting tissue structures on random sections. J Appl Physiol 17:343–348
6. Marzi I, Knee J, Menger M, Bühren V, Harbauer G, Trentz O (1990) Intravitalmikroskopische Untersuchungen zur Granulozytenadhärenz und Mikrozirkulation an der orthotop transplantierten Rattenleber. Langenbecks Arch Chir [Suppl] Chir Forum, S 373–377

Dr. med. K. Datsis, Chirurgische Universitätsklinik, Zimmer 224, Im Neuenheimer Feld 154, W-6900 Heidelberg

Mikrozirkulationsstörungen nach Lebertransplantation in Abhängigkeit von der Temperatur der Ausspüllösung

Effect of Temperature of Rinse Solution on Microcirculatory Impairment After Liver Transplantation

S. Post[2], M. Rentsch[1], P. Palma[1], A.P. Gonzalez[1], G. Otto[2] und M.D. Menger[1]

[1]Institut für Chirurgische Forschung, Ludwig-Maximilians-Universität, München
[2]Chirurgische Universitätsklinik, Heidelberg

Einleitung

Störungen der Transplantatfunktion nach Leberkonservierung sind nicht nur von Ischämiezeit und verwendeter Konservierungslösung abhängig, sondern auch von der Lösung, mit der das Organ unmittelbar vor Reperfusion ausgespült wird. So wurde nachgewiesen, daß eine spezielle Ausspüllösung, die unter anderem Antioxidantien und Adenosin enthält (sog. "Carolina rinse" = CR), die Ausprägung des Reperfusionsschadens der transplantierten Leber vermindert [1]. Bei Ausspülung mit Ringer-Laktat (RL) – wie sie häufig noch bei der klinischen Lebertransplantation zur Anwendung kommt – wurde kürzlich im Rattenmodell über eine Verlängerung der Überlebenszeit durch Anwärmung der Ausspüllösung berichtet [2]. Mittels intravitaler Fluoreszenzmikroskopie (IVM) sollte nun erstmals für RL und CR der Einfluß der Temperatur der Ausspüllösung auf Störungen der mikrovaskulären Perfusion und hepatozellulären Funktion analysiert werden.

Methodik

Bei 35 männlichen Lewis-Ratten (190–280 g) wurde in Äthernarkose eine syngene, orthotope Lebertransplantation mit arterieller Revaskularisation durchgeführt [3]. Bei konstanten Konservierungsbedingungen (24 h in UW-Lösung) unterschieden sich vier experimentelle Gruppen lediglich in Art und Temperatur der verwendeten Ausspüllösung: RL 4°C (RL4, n = 12), RL 37°C (RL37, n = 8), CR 4°C (CR4, n = 7), CR 37°C (CR37, n = 8).

30–90 min nach Reperfusion wurde die Unterfläche des linken Leberlappens zur Intravitalmikroskopie ausgelagert. Der technische Aufbau mit modifiziertem Leitz Orthoplan Mikroskop, Auflicht-Beleuchtung, hochempfindlicher Videokamera und Videoaufnahme-Einheit wurde bereits früher detailliert beschrieben [4]. Die Fluoreszenz-Kontrastierung des Lebergewebes und der zellulären Blutbestandteile erfolgte durch intravenöse Injektion von Natrium-Fluoreszein (2–4 μmol/kg) und Rhodamin G (0,1 μmol/kg). In Einzelbild-Analyse der intravitalmikroskopischen Video-

Chirurgisches Forum 1993
f. experim. u. klinische Forschung
Becker/Beger/Hartel (Hrsg.)

aufnahmen wurde "off-line" die Perfusionsverteilung mit relativen Anteilen nicht-perfundierter Azini bzw. Sinusoide quantifiziert [3, 4].

Als Maß der Transplantatfunktion diente der Galleflu während der ersten 90 min Reperfusion, der mittels eines zuvor eingelegten Choledochus-Katheter bestimmt wurde.

Die statistische Analyse der Daten erfolgte durch Varianzanalyse, für intravitalmikroskopische Parameter im hierarchischen ("nested") Design. Nicht normal verteilte Daten (Shapiro-Wilk-Statistik mit $p < 0,05$ in mindestens einer Gruppe) gingen nach Rang-Transformation in die Berechnungen ein. Multiple Mittelwertvergleiche gegen dieselben Kontrollwerte (Gruppe RL4) wurden durch Anwendung des Dunnett-Test ausgeführt. Alle Werte sind als Mittelwerte ± Standardfehler des Mittelwertes (SEM) angegeben. Die Berechnungen erfolgten mit den SAS-Prozeduren GLM und UNIVARIATE, Version 6.04 (SAS Institute, Cary, USA) für Personal Computer.

Ergebnisse

In der Referenzgruppe zeigten sich nach 30 bis 90 min Reperfusion massive Alterationen der Mikrozirkulation mit Störungen der azinären und sinusoidalen Perfusion: 17,9 ± 2,6% der Azini und innerhalb perfundierter Azini 21,1 ± 1,5% der Sinusoide waren nicht perfundiert. Diese Mikrozirkulationsstörungen gingen mit Einschränkungen der hepatozellulären exkretorischen Funktion einher: Der Galleflu lag bei 1,0 ± 1,2 ml/90 min/100 g Leber (frühe Untersuchungen an nicht transplantierten Tieren unter identischen Versuchsbedingungen hatten 10fach höhere Werte ergeben [5]).

Durch Anwärmung der Ausspüllösung auf 37°C ließ sich eine signifikante Verbesserung der mikrovaskulären Perfusion und hepatozellulären Exkretion erzielen: Der Anteil nicht perfundierter Azini lag nur noch bei 7,4 ± 1,6%, derjenige nicht-perfundierter Sinusoide bei 14,5 ± 1,3%, der Galleflu war auf 3,9 ± 0,8 ml/90 min/100 g verbessert ($p < 0,05$ gegen RL4 für sämtliche Werte).

Ähnliche, tendenziell sogar noch deutlichere Effekte ließen sich im Vergleich mit RL4 durch Einsatz von Carolina Rinse (4°C) erzielen: 5,2 ± 1,2% nicht-perfundierte Azini, 11,4 ± 1,0% nicht-perfundierte Sinusoide, 3,7 ± 0,6 ml/90 min/100 g Galleflu (alle $p < 0,05$ gegen RL4). Durch zusätzliche Erwärmung von CR auf 37°C waren keine Effekte zu erzielen, die weit über die in den Gruppen RL37 und CR4 beobachteten hinausgingen: 6,6 ± 1,9% nicht-perfundierte Azini, 8,5 ± 1,1% nicht-perfundierte Sinusoide, 4,9 ± 1,1 ml/90 min/100 g Galleflu (alle $p < 0,05$ gegen RL4). Somit zeigten die beiden unterschiedlichen Ansatzpunkte der Modifikation des Reperfusionsschadens (Anwärmung und speziell zusammengesetzte Ausspüllösung) im verwendeten Modell weder additive noch potenzierende Effekte.

Zusammenfassung

Bei 35 orthotopen Lebertransplantationen an der Ratte mit Konservierung für 24 h in UW Lösung wurde das Transplantat unmittelbar vor Reperfusion mit zwei verschiedenen Ausspüllösungen (Ringer-Laktat und Carolina Rinse (CR)) bei jeweils zwei verschiedenen Temperaturen (4°C und 37°C gespült. Mittels *in vivo* Fluoreszenzmikroskopie wurde im Vergleich zu kalter Ringerlösung in allen drei weiteren Versuchsgruppen (warme Ringer, kalte und warme CR) 1 h nach Reperfusion eine signifikante Reduktion der azinären und sinusoidalen Perfusionsausfälle beobachtet. Parallel dazu verbesserte sich der Gallefluß während der ersten 90 min nach Reperfusion. Sowohl durch Anwärmung der Ausspüllösung als auch durch Verwendung von CR kann somit eine erhebliche Verbesserung der mikrovaskulären Perfusion und exkretorischen hepatozellulären Funktion erreicht werden. Während Anwärmung für RL als Ausspüllösung den Reperfusionsschaden des Transplantats erheblich vermindert, scheinen die protektiven Effekte von CR weitgehend temperaturunabhängig zu sein.

Summary

Following cold preservation for 24 h in University of Wisconsin (UW) solution, 35 orthotopic liver transplantations were performed in the rat. Immediately before reperfusion the grafts were rinsed with one of two different rinse solutions (Ringer's lactate or Carolina Rinse, CR) using two different temperatures (4°C and 37°C, respectively). Quantitative assessment by in vivo fluorescence microscopy 1 h after reperfusion verified significant improvement of both acinar and sinusoidal microvascular perfusion after rinse with either warm Ringer's lactate, cold CR, or warm CR when compared with cold Ringer's lactate. In addition, bile flow during the first 90 min after reperfusion was found to be markedly lower after cold Ringer's rinse compared with all other experimental groups. We conclude that both warming of the rinse solution and application of CR may improve microvascular perfusion and excretory hepatocellular function. While warming of Ringer's rinse may attenuate reperfusion injury of the graft, the positive effects of CR seem to be exerted independently of the temperature of the rinse solution.

Literatur

1. Gao W, Takei Y, Marzi I, Lindert KA, Caldwell-Kenkel JC, Currin RT, Tanaka Y, Lemasters JJ, Thurman RG (1991) Carolina rinse solution – a new strategy to increase survival time after orthotopic liver transplantation in the rat. Transplantation 52:417–424
2. Takei Y, Gao WS, Hijioka T, Savier E, Lindert KA, Lemasters JJ, Thurman RG (1991) Increase in survival of liver grafts after rinsing with warm Ringer's solution due to improvement of hepatic microcirculation. Transplantation 52:225–230
3. Post S, Menger MD, Rentsch M, Gonzalez AP, Herfarth C, Messmer K (1992) The impact of arterialization on hepatic microcirculation and leukocyte accumulation after liver transplantation in the rat. Transplantation 54:789–794
4. Menger MD, Marzi I, Messmer K (1991) In vivo fluorescence microscopy for quantitative analysis of the hepatic microcirculation in hamsters and rats. Eur Surg Res 23:158–169

5. Post S, Gonzalez AP, Palma P, Rentsch M, Stiehl A, Menger MD (1992) Assessment of hepatic phagocytic activity by in vivo microscopy after liver transplantation in the rat. Hepatology 16:803–809

Dieses Forschungsvorhaben wurde durch die Deutsche Forschungsgemeinschaft (He 368/7, Me 900/1-2) und den Forschungsschwerpunkt Transplantation Heidelberg unterstützt.

Priv.-Doz. Dr. med. S. Post, Chirurgische Universitätsklinik, Kirschnerstraße 1, W-6900 Heidelberg

Konservierungsschäden humaner Gallengänge nach kalter Ischämie – Analyse mit einem neuen in vitro Modell

Preservation Damage of Human Bile Ducts After Cold Ischemia – Analysis with a New In Vitro Model

M. Knoop[1], N. Schnoy[2], H. Keck[1] und P. Neuhaus[1]

[1]Chirurgische Klinik und Poliklinik, Universitätsklinikum Rudolf Virchow, Freie Universität, Berlin
[2]Institut für Pathologie, Universitätsklinikum Rudolf Virchow, Freie Universität, Berlin

Einleitung

Die Inzidenz anastomosenunabhängiger Gallengangsläsionen nach humaner Lebertransplantation, sog. "ischemic type biliary lesions", zeigte in einer retrospektiven Studie der Mayo Klinik eine positive Korrelation nur mit der Dauer der kalten Ischämiezeit des Transplantates [1]. Wenn die kalte Ischämiezeit 13 h überschritt, kam es zu einem drastischen Anstieg intrahepatischer Gallengangsstrikturen. Andere Faktoren, die ebenfalls derartige Läsionen verursachen könnten, wie Thrombose der A. hepatica, ABO Inkompatibilität sowie chronische Abstoßung, waren im Patientengut nicht vorhanden.

Während der Leberentnahme wird das Leberparenchym via A. hepatica und Pfortader mit University of Wisconsin-Lösung (UW) zwar perfundiert und konserviert, im Gallengangssystem dagegen verbleibt unverändert Galle. Daher wird in den meisten Zentren nach Spenderhepatektomie das Gallengangssystem mittels einer in den distalen D. choledochus eingeführten Sonde mit UW-Lösung ausgespült [2]. Dadurch wird Galle zwar aus großen, zentralen Gängen entfernt, kleine, periphere Gänge dagegen werden unverändert mit Galle konserviert.

In dieser Studie untersuchten wir den Einfluß von Galle und UW-Lösung auf humane Gallengänge in einem in vitro Modell, das eine Simulation der klinischen Organkonservierung mit prolongierten kalten Ischämiezeiten erlaubt.

Material und Methoden

Während zehn konsekutiver Multiorganentnahmen (Spenderalter 19–51 J.; medianes Alter 47 J.; 3 weibl., 7 männl.) inklusive Pankreas wurden Segmente des distalen, redundanten D. choledochus nach Leberperfusion mit UW-Lösung, Hepatektomie und Ausspülen des Gallengangssystems über den geöffneten distalen D. choledochus asserviert. Bei der zuvor routinemäßig durchgeführten Cholezystektomie wurde Blasengalle gewonnen. Die Gallengangssegmente wurden nach Entnahme sofort 12, 24, 48 und 72 h lang in UW-Lösung plus 50% Galle oder in reiner Galle hypotherm auf Eis

Chirurgisches Forum 1993
f. experim. u. klinische Forschung
Becker/Beger/Hartel (Hrsg.)

bei 4°C konserviert (Tabelle 1). Nach dem jeweiligen Intervall wurden die Proben in Formalin (5%) fixiert, bis zur H&E Färbung standardisiert weiterverarbeitet und lichtmikroskopisch untersucht.

Tabelle 1. Art der Gallengangskonservierung in Abhängigkeit von Gallengangslokalisation und hypothetischem Gallegehalt nach Spülung mit UW-Lösung über den distal offenen D. choledochus nach Spenderhepatektomie

Abschnitt im Gallengangsystem	Verhältnis Galle/ Konservierungsmedium	In vitro Simulation
D. choledochus	0 : 1	100% UW-Lösung
großer, zentraler Gallengang	1 : 1	50% UW-Lösung + 50% Galle
kleiner, peripherer Gallengang	1 : 0	100% Galle

Ergebnisse

Eine Konservierung von 12 h in UW-Lösung führte zu einer exzellenten Erhaltung sämtlicher Schichten der Gallengangswand (Tabelle 2). Nach 48 h in UW-Lösung waren epitheliale Zellkerne normal gestaltet, während das Cytoplasma bereits hydropisch geschwollen war. Dieser Befund war nach 72 h mit Vakuolisierung des Cytoplasmas ausgeprägter. Die Gallengangswand war zu allen Untersuchungszeitpunkten intakt.

Tabelle 2. Übersicht der histologischen Ergebnisse nach 12–72 h kalter Ischämie in verschiedenen Lagerungsmedien

Kalte Ischämiezeit	UW-Lösung	UW-Lösung + Galle 1 : 1	Reine Galle
12 h	intakte Mucosa u. Gangwand	subtotale Nekrose von Epithel u. Gangwand	totale Nekrose
24 h	intakte Mucosa u. Gangwand	totale Nekrose	totale Nekrose
48 h	hydropisches Epithel, intakte Wand	totale Nekrose	totale Nekrose
72 h	hydropisches Epithel, Vakuolisierung, intakte Wand	totale Nekrose	totale Nekrose

Nach 12 h Konservierung in UW-Lösung plus 50% Galle kam es zu einer vollständigen Desquamation des Epithels mit schattenhafter Kernfärbung sowie zur

Nekrose intramuraler Drüsen und Endothelien, so daß zu diesem Zeitpunkt bereits eine subtotale Nekrose sämtlicher Schichten vorlag. Nach 24 h war eine Totalnekrose sämtlicher epithelialer und mesenchymaler Strukturen mit ödematöser Dissoziation der nur noch schattenhaft vorhandenen Kollagenfasern eingetreten.

Nach 12 h Lagerung in reiner Galle kam es zu einer Totalnekrose des Gallengangs (Tabelle 2).

Diskussion

Die Resultate zeigen, daß UW-Lösung ein ausgezeichnetes Medium zur kalten Konservierung von Gallengangsepithel darstellt. Lagerung in Galle dagegen führt zur Nekrose von Mucosa und Wandstrukturen. Die Gallengangsproben wurden während der Multiorganentnahme in situ mit kalter UW-Lösung perfundiert, so daß die extrahepatischen Gallengänge eine vergleichbare physiologische Kondition wie die tatsächlich transplantierten intrahepatischen Gallengänge aufwiesen.

Sogenannter "early sludge" neben Lebertransplantation, eine visköse Masse aus nekrotischen Epithel- sowie Kollagenfaserresten, wurde als faßbarer Ausdruck des Konservierungsschadens im Gallengangsystem interpretiert [3]. Die hier beobachteten Läsionen nach kalter Ischämie produzierten dieses nekrotische Material, das in den ersten Tagen nach Lebertransplantation auftritt. Die Destruktion der Gallengänge nach 12 h Konservierung in Galle adressiert das klinische Problem der Konservierung peripherer Gallengänge, die nicht durch Spülung über den distalen D. choledochus erreicht werden. Periphere Gallengänge humanen Ursprungs sind für eine Konservierungsstudie nicht verfügbar, wie der redundante Anteil des D. choledochus, der hier verwendet wurde. Ob die pathologischen Veränderungen des distalen D. choledochus repräsentativ für intrahepatische Läsionen unter gleichen Versuchsbedingungen sind, bleibt offen. Auch Tiermodelle tragen nicht zur Klärung der humanen Pathologie bei, da speziesspezifische Unterschiede beobachtet wurden [4, 5].

Die Verwendung konzentrierter Blasengalle, die bei der Cholezystektomie des Transplantates gewonnen wird, hat sicherlich den Schaden, den intraluminale Lebergalle verursacht hätte, prononciert; das Prinzip einer chemisch-toxischen Schädigung des Gallengangepithels durch Gallenbestandteile während kalter Ischämie dürfte jedoch gültig sein.

Aus den Ergebnissen läßt sich ableiten, daß bei der zur Zeit üblichen Praxis der Gallengangskonservierung ein von zentral nach peripher progredienter Konservierungsschaden auftritt, der über Reparationsvorgänge zu symptomatischen Strikturen und Dilatationen im Gallengangsystem führt. Bei der Konservierung des Lebertransplantates ist daher die Spülung und Instillation der erreichbaren zentralen Gallengänge mit UW-Lösung wichtig. Eine medikamentös induzierte Cholerese und Cholekinese zur Konzentrationsminderung der Galle auch in peripheren Gängen könnte eine wichtige Ergänzung im Management des Organspenders darstellen. Ob weniger visköse Konservierungsmedien als UW-Lösung bzw. der Zusatz von zellprotektiven Substanzen eine morphologisch bessere Konservierung während kalter Ischämie bewirken können, wird mit dem hier vorgestellten Modell weiter erarbeitet.

Zusammenfassung

Prolongierte kalte Ischämiezeiten des Transplantates sind für intrahepatische biliäre Läsionen nach Lebertransplantation verantwortlich gemacht worden. Wir untersuchten den Konservierungsschaden an humanen D. choledochus-Segmenten, die bei Multiorganentnahme asserviert und auf Eis mit UW-Lösung, Blasengalle oder eine 1:1 Mischung aus beiden für 12–72 h gelagert wurden. Reine UW-Lösung konservierte den Gallengang exzellent bis zu 72 h, während die Präsenz von Galle zur raschen Autolyse sämtlicher Wandschichten führte. Dieses Resultat unterstreicht die Bedeutung einer Spülung und Füllung des Gallengangsystems mit UW-Lösung bei der Spenderhepatektomie. Das hier verwandte in vitro Modell ermöglicht weitere Untersuchungen zur Optimierung der Gallengangkonservierung.

Summary

It has been suggested that prolonged cold ischemic times produce ischemic-type biliary lesions after human liver transplantation. We investigated the preservation damage to human specimens of the distal common bile duct that were collected during multiorgan retrieval and stored on ice for 12–72 h in University of Wisconsin (UW) solution, bladder bile, or in a 1:1 mixture of both. UW solution produced an excellent preservation for up to 72 h while the presence of bile led to a rapid autolysis of duct walls. These results indicate the importance of thoroughly rinsing and filling the biliary tree with UW solution during donor hepatectomy. The in vitro model used allows further research to be made into better methods of preserving the biliary system.

Literatur

1. Sanchez-Urdazpal L, Gores GJ, Ward EM, Maus TP, Wahlstrom HE, Moore SB, Wiesner RH, Krom RAF (1992) Ischemic-type biliary complications after orthotopic liver transplantation. Hepatology 16:49–53
2. Belzer FO, D'Alessandro A, Hoffmann R, Kalayoglu M, Sollinger H (1992) Management of the common duct in extended preservation of the liver. Transplantation 53:1166–67
3. McMaster P, Herbertson B, Cusick C, Calne RY, Williams R (1978) Biliary sludging following liver transplantation in man. Transplantation 25:56–62
4. McMaster P, Walton RM, White DGD, Medd RK, Syrakos TP (1980) The influence of ischemia on the biliary tract. Br J Surg 67:321–324
5. Syrakos TP, White DGD, McMaster P, Marni A, Alfani D (1979) Damage to the biliary tract during preservation. Transplantation 28:166–171

Dr. med. M. Knoop, Chirurgische Klinik und Poliklinik, Universitätsklinikum Rudolf Virchow, Augustenburger Platz 1, 1000 Berlin 65

Einfluß der Dünndarmtransplantation und chronischen Abstoßung auf die Morphologie und Funktion der intestinalen Muskulatur

Effect of Small-Bowel Transplantation and Chronic Rejection on the Morphology and Function of Intestinal Smooth Muscle

P.F. Heeckt[1,*], A.J. Bauer[3], W.M. Halfter[2], K.K.W. Lee[1] und W.H. Schraut[1]

[1]Department of Surgery, University of Pittsburgh School of Medicine, Pittsburgh, USA
[2]Department of Neurobiology, University of Pittsburgh School of Medicine, Pittsburgh, USA
[3]Department of Medicine/Division of Gastroenterology and Hepatology, University of Pittsburgh School of Medicine, Pittsburgh, USA

Einleitung

Die Dünndarmtransplantation ist seit Einführung effektiver Immunsuppressiva klinisch möglich geworden und gewinnt zunehmend als definitive Therapie des Kurzdarmsyndroms an Bedeutung. Mit der erfolgreichen Unterdrückung akuter Abstoßung durch Cyclosporin (CsA) und FK 506 kommt es zu langzeitigem Transplantatüberleben. Damit treten chronische Abstoßung und zunehmende gastrointestinale Motilitätsstörungen des Transplantats in den Vordergrund [1]. Die vorliegende Studie wurde durchgeführt, um die bisher unbekannten Auswirkungen der Dünndarmtransplantation, gefolgt von chronischer Abstoßung, auf die Morphologie und Funktion der intestinalen Muskulatur zu untersuchen.

Methodik

Einzeitige, orthotope Dünndarmtransplantation wurde entweder an syngenen ACI zu ACI (n = 6) oder allogenen ACI zu LEW Rattenpaaren (n = 6) durchgeführt. Alle operierten Tiere erhielten eine kombinierte Anästhesie mit Methoxyfluran (Inhalation) und Pentobarbital (50 mg/kg KG intraperitoneal). Temporäre Immunsuppression mit CsA (15 mg/kg KG Tag 0–6 täglich i.m., 7–28 einmal alle 2 Tage) in der allogenen Kombination war von chronischer Abstoßung gefolgt [2], die am 90. postoperativen Tag noch klinisch stumm war (normales Körpergewicht und Stuhlgang), aber histopathologisch offensichtliche Veränderungen wie Wandverdickung, Mesenterialfibrose und obliterative Arteriopathie bei noch normaler Schleimhaut aufwies. In syngenen Transplantaten traten erwartungsgemäß solche Veränderungen nicht auf. Die Morphologie der Dünndarmmuskulatur wurde 90 Tage nach Transplantation durch immunhistochemische Methoden untersucht. Zur Messung der mechanischen Muskelfunktion wurden gleichzeitig ca. 4 × 10 mm große Streifen zirkulärer Muskulatur aus dem proximalen

* Unterstützt durch die Deutsche Forschungsgemeinschaft (He 2043/1-1).

Chirurgisches Forum 1993
f. experim. u. klinische Forschung
Becker/Beger/Hartel (Hrsg.)

Jejunum in ein mit oxygenierter Krebslösung bei 37.5°C kontinuierlich perfundiertes Organbad eingebracht und an einen isometrischen Kraftaufnehmer gekoppelt. Spontane mechanische Muskelkontraktionen und Dosis-Wirkungskurven mit ansteigenden Konzentrationen von Bethanechol wurden aufgezeichnet und analysiert. Zur näheren Bestimmung der zellulären Funktion wurden direkte elektrische Ableitungen an zirkulären Muskelzellen mit intrazellulär eingebrachten Mikroelektroden (20–60 MΩ) im physiologischen Organbad durchgeführt. Hierbei wurde das Ruhemembranpotential, sowie die Amplitude und Frequenz spontaner langsamer Depolarisation (slow waves) bestimmt [3]. Als Kontrolle dienten in allen Experimenten normale ACI-Ratten gleichen Alters.

Ergebnisse

Immunhistochemische Färbungen der glatten Muskulatur des Jejunums mit Rhodamin-markiertem Phalloidin (Molecular Probes Co., Eugene, Oregon/USA) zeigte eine signifikante Verdickung der intestinalen Muskulatur der allogenen, chronisch abstoßenden Transplantate. Die mittlere Dicke der zirkulären und longitudinalen Muskelschichten normaler Ratten betrug $53,6 \pm 4,6$ und $40,1 \pm 2,4$ μm. Bei chronischer Abstoßung fand sich eine Zunahme auf $178,9 \pm 38,9$ und $99,7 \pm 14,6$ μm. Die Transplantate in der syngenen Kombination zeigten ebenfalls eine Dickenzunahme der Ring- und Längsmuskulatur auf $80,2 \pm 9,7$ und $64 \pm 5,6$ μm (Mittelwert $\pm$ S.E.M., $p <$ 0,001), die jedoch deutlich weniger ausgeprägt war (Abb. 1a). Die Auszählung der einzelnen Zellschichten anhand der mit Bisbenzimide (Molecular Probes Co., Eugene, Oregon/USA) gefärbten Zellkerne ergab eine signifikante Hyperplasie der Ring- und Längsmuskulatur der chronisch abstoßenden Transplantate und proportional zur Gesamtdicke auch der syngenen Transplantate (Abb. 1b). Vorläufige Ergebnisse elektronenmikroskopischer Analysen der zirkulären Muskulatur deuten auf eine zusätzliche Muskelhypertrophie der chronisch abstoßenden Transplantate. Die mittlere Fläche der einzelnen Muskelzelle vergrößert sich um etwa das 1,7-fache von $88,4 \pm 17,1$ μm^2 auf $146,9 \pm 32$ μm^2. Ob es auch nach syngener Transplantation zu einer Hypertrophie kommt, läßt sich derzeit noch nicht mit Sicherheit sagen.

Die parasympathomimetische Substanz Bethanechol (Carbamyl-β-Methylcholin) verursachte eine konzentrationsabhängige (0,1–300 μM), zum Muskelquerschnitt relative Zunahme der Kontraktionskraft (Gramm/mm^2/min). Trotz erheblicher Verdickung der Muskelschicht leisteten chronisch abstoßende Transplantate nur noch 23% der maximalen Kontraktionskraft normaler Tiere bei einer Bethanechol Konzentration von 300 μM und wiesen eine um 60% geringere Spontanaktivität auf. Syngene Transplantate erreichten die gleiche maximale Kontraktionskraft wie normale Dünndärme bei allerdings um 77% erhöhter Spontanaktivität (Abb. 2). Die geringste Dosis, bei der eine Kontraktion ausgelöst wurde (Schwellenwert) und die halbmaximale Konzentration (EC_{50}) betrugen 0,65 und 17,1 μM im normalen Dünndarm gegenüber 4,8 und 13,3 μM während chronischer Abstoßung (n.s.), sowie 2,63 und 11,1 μM in syngenen Transplantaten (n.s.).

Intrazelluläre Ableitungen zirkulärer Muskelzellen ergaben eine signifikante Verminderung des Ruhemembranpotentials in chronisch abstoßenden Transplantaten von

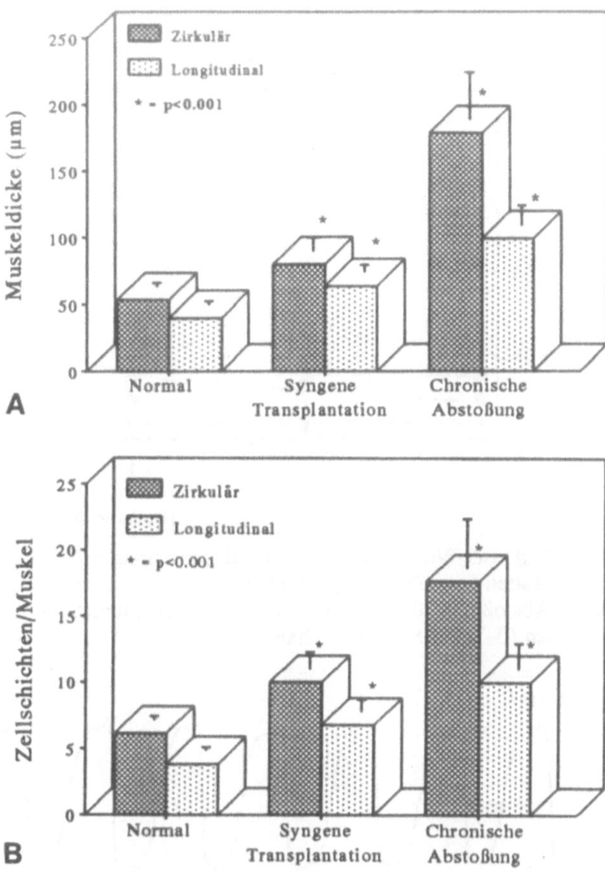

Abb. 1A. Die Muskeldicke der zirkulären und longitudinalen intestinalen Muskulatur normaler Ratten (n = 12) nimmt nach syngener Dünndarmtransplantation (n = 6) und bei chronischer Abstoßung nach allogener Transplantation (n = 6) signifikant zu (90 Tage post transplantationem). **B** Proportional zur Zunahme der Muskeldicke kommt es zu einer Hyperplasie beider Muskelschichten

$-69,6 \pm 0,95$ mV (normal) auf $-65,5 \pm 0,92$ ($p < 0{,}01$). Die Amplitude spontaner langsamer Depolarisationen (slow waves) war ebenfalls signifikant von $20,3 \pm 0,45$ mV (normal) auf $14,5 \pm 0,9$ vermindert ($p < 0{,}0001$) (Abb. 3). Es kam zusätzlich zu einer leichten Abnahme der slow wave Frequenz, die jedoch nicht signifikant war: $29,8 \pm 0,97$ (normal) gegenüber $27,3 \pm 1,1$ ($p > 0{,}05$). Intrazelluläre Ableitungen syngener Transplantate zeigten keinen signifikanten Unterschied zum normalen Dünndarm.

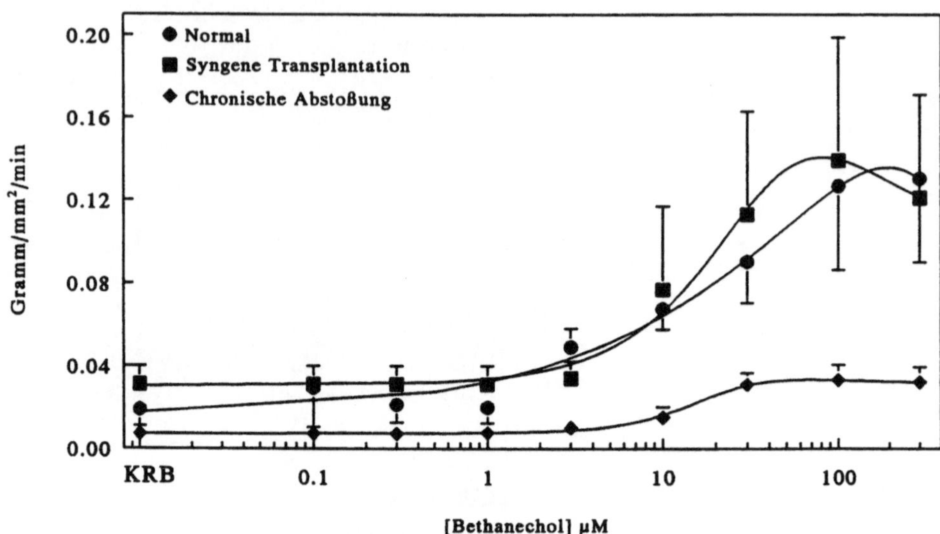

Abb. 2. Dosis-Wirkungs Kurven der Kontraktionskraft zirkulärer, intestinaler Muskulatur normaler Ratten (n = 7), 90 Tage nach syngener Dünndarmtransplantation (n = 6) und bei chronischer Abstoßung 90 Tage nach allogener Transplantation (n = 6) unter ansteigenden Konzentrationen (0–300 μM) von Bethanechol

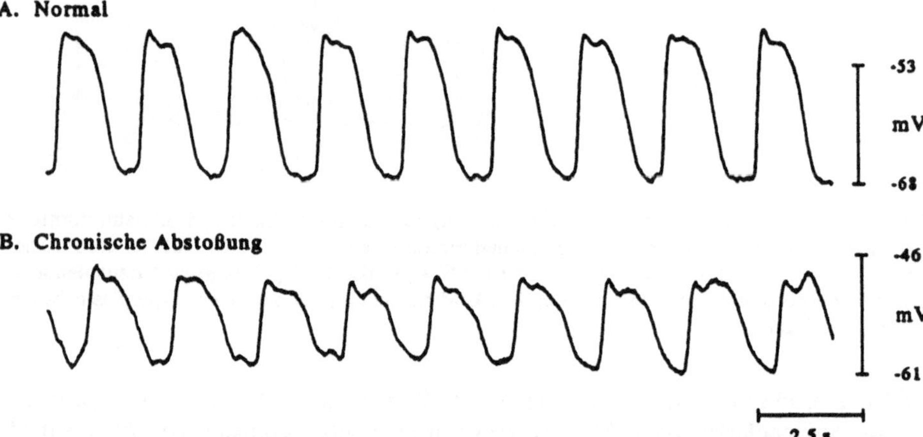

Abb. 3A. Intrazelluläre Ableitung von slow waves einer normalen, zirkulären, intestinalen Muskelzelle. **B** Signifikante Abnahme des Ruhemembranpotentials und der slow wave Amplitude bei chronischer Abstoßung des Dünndarmtransplantates

Zusammenfassung

Der Einfluß der Dünndarmtransplantation auf die Morphologie und Funktion der Muskulatur des Intestinaltransplantates wurde in einem vollallogenen, chronisch abstoßenden Rattenmodell und in syngen transplantierten Ratten untersucht. In beiden

Fällen kam es zu einer signifikanten Verdickung der glatten Muskulatur, die durch Hypertrophie und Hyperplasie der Muskelzellen verursacht wurde und bei chronischer Abstoßung sehr ausgeprägt war. Funktionell kam es während der chronischen Abstoßung zur Verminderung der mechanischen Kontraktionskraft sowie zur Abnahme der Amplitude intrazellulär abgeleiteter slow waves und des Ruhemembranpotentials intestinaler Muskelzellen. Diese schwerwiegenden Veränderungen in Folge einer chronischen Abstoßung sind bereits im Stadium klinischer Symptomlosigkeit nachzuweisen.

Summary

We evaluated the effects of small-bowel transplantation and chronic rejection on the morphology and function of intestinal smooth muscle in a fully allogeneic rat model of chronic rejection and in syngeneic transplants. Both experimental conditions led to a significant thickening of the intestinal musculature, which was most pronounced in chronic rejection. This was due to a marked degree of hyperplasia and hypertrophy of the smooth muscle cell. In these grafts contractile force as well as intracellularly recorded resting membrane potentials and slow wave amplitudes were significantly decreased. These profound morphologic changes and functional impairments of intestinal smooth muscle are detected in chronically rejecting small-bowel grafts prior to clinical graft failure.

Literatur

1. Todo S, Tzakis AG, Abu-Elmagd K (1992) Intestinal transplantation in composite visceral grafts or alone. Ann Surg 216:223–234
2. Langrehr JM, Banner B, Lee KWL, Schraut W: Clinical course, morphology and treatment of chronically rejecting small bowel allografts. Transplantation (in press)
3. Bauer AJ, Reed JB, Sanders KM (1985) Slow wave heterogeneity within the circular muscle wall of the canine gastric antrum. J Physiol (London) 366:221–232

Dr. P.F. Heeckt, University of Pittsburgh, School of Medicine, Department of Surgery, 497 Scaife Hall, Pittsburgh, PA 15261, USA

Bereits in der Frühphase einer akuten Abstoßungsreaktion kommt es zur Paralyse des transplantierten Dünndarmes

Graft Paralysis Occurs During Early Stage Rejection of Jejunal Allograft

H. Pernthaler[1], A. Kreji[2], R. Plattner[1], M. Kofler[1], G. Pfurtscheller[1] und R. Margreiter[1]

[1]I. Universitätsklinik für Chirurgie, Abteilung für Transplantationschirurgie, Innsbruck
[2]Pathologisches Institut, Universität Innsbruck

Einleitung

Die Bedeutung der Motilität für die resorptive Funktion des Dünndarmes sowie auch zu seiner Selbstreinigung ist unbestritten. Einige experimentelle Untersuchungen des transplantierten Dünndarmes im isogenen oder autologen Modell haben gezeigt, daß der migratorische myoelektrische Komplex (MMC) durch Denervierung und Ischämie zwar gestört wird, aber nach einer Erholungsphase am Transplantat wieder auftritt [1].

Die vorliegende Studie widmet sich der Frage, ob die akute Abstoßungsreaktion einen Einfluß auf die Darmmotilität bewirkt.

Material und Methoden

In Äther-Inhalationsnarkose wurden von Lewis Spendern nach in-situ Perfusion 10 cm proximales Jejunum entnommen und in Eiswasser gelagert. In mikrochirurgischer Technik wurde das Darmsegment Brown Norway Ratten ohne Resektion von Eigendarm 1 cm unterhalb der Treitz'schen Flexur interponiert, die Gefäße wurden mit der infrarenalen Aorta bzw. V. cava, der Darm E/E anastomosiert (Gruppe 1, n = 14). Als Kontrolltiere dienten isogene Empfängertiere (Gruppe 2, n = 5). Am Transplantat und am folgenden Eigendarm wurden jeweils drei bipolare Elektroden fixiert, diese durch einen subkutanen Tunnel zur Interskapularregion geführt und von dort über einen Teflonschlauch und eine dünne Glasröhre aus dem Käfig geleitet, so daß sich die Tiere frei bewegen konnten.

Je zwei Tiere der Gruppe 1 wurden vom 5. bis 11. postoperativen Tag mit einer Überdosis Äther getötet und der Dünndarm zur histologischen Untersuchung entnommen. Die elektromyographischen Untersuchungen wurden nach 12 stündiger Nüchternphase ab Tag 5 oder 6 bis zur vorgesehenen Darmentnahme an alternierenden Tagen durchgeführt. In der Gruppe 2 wurde die Elektromyographie an alternierenden Tagen ab Tag 5 aufgezeichnet, die Tiere nach der letzten Untersuchung am Tag 11 ge-

Chirurgisches Forum 1993
f. experim. u. klinische Forschung
Becker/Beger/Hartel (Hrsg.)

opfert. Die interdigestive Phase wurde durch Fütterung von 3 g Rattenfutter beendet, die myoelektrischen Aufzeichnungen über 15 min fortgesetzt.

Ergebnisse

Ab Tag 5 wurden an den Transplantaten 26 (7,4%) von 351 und am Eigendarm 25 (25,5%) von 296 regelmäßige MMCs beobachtet. Nach Fütterung zeigten die Transplantate wie auch der Eigendarm postprandiale Aktivitätsmuster. Ab Tag 8 war am transplantierten Darm der Gruppe 1 keine aktive Phase des MMC nachweisbar, wohl aber am Eigendarm derselben Gruppe und an beiden Darmsegmenten der Gruppe 2. Die Nahrungsaufnahme zeigte ab diesem Tag keine myoelektrische Reaktion an den Transplantaten der Gruppe 1. Histologisch fanden sich in den Transplantaten der Gruppe 1 am Tag 7/8 als Zeichen einer frühen Abstoßungsreaktion lediglich Rundzellinfiltrate in der Mukosa und nur vereinzelt am Plexus submucosus. Im Bereiche des Plexus myentericus sowie auch der Muscularis propria waren erst ab Tag 9 Infiltrate zu erkennen.

Diskussion

Der transplantierte Darm der Ratte zeigt in unserem Modell bereits ab dem 5. postoperativen Tag MMCs, so daß sich histologisch faßbare Abstoßungszeichen erst nach Wiedereinsetzen der Darmmotorik zeigen [2]. Die beobachtete Unregelmäßigkeit der MMCs scheint für ein Dünndarmtransplantat typisch und durch die extrinsische Denervation sowie den anoxischen Schaden bedingt zu sein [1].

Das Fehlen der myoelektrischen Aktivität in der Nüchternphase sowie nach Nahrungsaufnahme als Folge einer fortschreitenden akuten Abstoßungsreaktion ist wohl als myoelektrisches Korrelat zum paralytischen Ileus zu sehen. Zum Unterschied vom heterotopen Allotransplantat im Hundemodell zeigen unsere Versuchstiere beim Auftreten der Paralyse histologisch eine erhaltene Darmarchitektur mit einem Rundzellinfiltrat in der Mukosa und Submukosa [3].

Als Ursache für die abstoßungsbedingte Darmparalyse wird eine Aktivierung von Hemmneuronen angenommen, da die Infiltration der für die Motilität bedeutsamen Strukturen erst nach dem Auftreten der Paralyse zu beobachten ist.

Von den klinischen Folgen einer Abstoßungsreaktion abgesehen, könnte die Überwachung der Darmmotorik eine hilfreiche Maßnahme zur Früherkennung einer akuten Abstoßungsreaktion nach Dünndarmtransplantation sein.

Zusammenfassung

Der Einfluß der akuten Abstoßungsreaktion auf die myoelektrische Aktivität eines orthotop transplantierten Dünndarmsegmentes wurde im Rattenmodell (Lewis/Brown Norway, n = 14) untersucht. Als Kontrollgruppe dienten isogene Empfänger (Lewis/Lewis, n = 5). In beiden Gruppen wurde der Eigendarm der Empfängertiere belassen und ebenso elektromyographisch untersucht. Ab dem 5. Tag waren an den Transplantaten und am Eigendarm MMCs zu beobachten, die nach Gabe von Futter durch postprandiale Aktivität ersetzt wurden. Ab dem Tag 8 wurden an den Allotransplantaten in der Nüchternphase keine aktiven Phasen des MMC registriert. Im Gegensatz zum Eigendarm und zu den Kontrolltieren bewirkte die Nahrungsaufnahme keine myoelektrische Reaktion. Dieser elektromyographisch verifizierte paralytische Ileus war in einer histologisch frühen Phase der Abstoßungsreaktion ohne Infiltration des Plexus myentericus oder der Muscularis zu beobachten. Die Überwachung der Darmmotorik könnte deshalb zur Früherkennung einer Abstoßungsreaktion eines Dünndarmtransplantates herangezogen werden.

Summary

The impact of rejection on myoelectric activities of an orthotopic jejunal allograft was studied in a rat model (Lewis/Brown Norway, $n = 14$), with Lewis rat recipients serving as controls ($n = 5$). Electrodes were placed on grafts and recipients' native bowel. Migration myoelectric complexes (MMC) were detectable from day 5 onwards in grafts and native bowel and were replaced by postprandial activities after food intake. From day 8 onwards allografts did not generate active phases of the MMC or react to food intake, in contrast to the native bowel and controls. This electromyographically diagnosed paralytic ileus was observed at a histologically early stage of rejection without infiltration of the plexus myentericus or muscular layer. Apart from its clinical significance, monitoring of graft motility could be helpful in diagnosing acute graft rejection.

Literatur

1. Quighley EMM, Spanta AD, Ropse SG, Lof J, Thompson JS (1990) Long term effects of jejunoileal autotransplantation on myoelectrical activity in canine small intestine. Dig Dis Sci 35:1505–1517
2. Grant D, Zhong R, Hurlbut D, Garcia B, Cheng H, Lamont D, Wang P, Stiller C, Duff J (1991) A comparison of heterotopic and orthotopic intestinal transplantation in rats. Transplantation 51:948
3. Dennison AR, Collin J, Watkins RM, Millard PR, Morris PJ (1987) Segmental small intestinal allografts in the dog. Transplantation 44:474–8

Dr. H. Pernthaler, I. Universitätsklinik für Chirurgie, Anichstraße 35,
A-6020 Innsbruck

Wachstumsverhalten und Regulationsmechanismen von syngen und allogen transplantierten Nebennierenrindengeweben an der Ratte. Grundlagen eines klinischen Transplantationsmodells*

Growth and Regulation of Syngeneic and Allogeneic Grafts of Adrenal Cortical Cells: A Study of Cell Transplantation in the Rat

G.F.W. Scheumann[1], W.F.A. Hiller[1], Th. Schürmeyer[2], S. Schröder[3] und H. Dralle[1]

[1]Klinik für Abdominal- und Transplantationschirurgie, Medizinische Hochschule Hannover, Hannover (Direktor: Prof. Dr. R. Pichlmayr)
[2]Abteilung für Klinische Endokrinologie, Medizinische Hochschule Hannover, Hannover (Direktor: Prof. Dr. A. von zur Mühlen)
[3]Universitätskliniken Hamburg-Eppendorf, Institut für Pathologie, Hamburg (Direktor: Prof. Dr. Helmchen)

Einleitung

Der künstliche Hormonersatz nach vollständiger operativer Entfernung oder Funktionsverlust der Nebennierenrinden ist ein bislang nicht befriedigend gelöstes Problem. Im Rahmen primärer und sekundärer adrenocorticaler Insuffizienzen konnte nachgewiesen werden, daß auch bei mehrfach fraktionierter Substitution und individueller Anpassung der Steroiddosis Addisonkrisen, aber auch inadäquat hohe Steroidspiegel mit zum Teil manifesten Cushingsyndromen auftreten können [1]. Die durch mangelhafte Regulationsmechanismen bedingte fehlende endogene Streßreserve bedeutet für die Patienten bei Infektionen, Unfällen, Operationen, Dehydratationen und ausgeprägten emotionalen Streßzuständen eine erhebliche Gefährdung [2]. Aber auch subklinisch verlaufende Steroidmangelzustände führen zu belastenden somatischen und psychischen Beschwerden wie Müdigkeit, Muskelschwäche bis zur muskulären Paralyse, Hypotonie, Hyperpigmentierung, Gewichtsverlust, Hypogonadismus sowie Wahrnehmungsdefiziten bis zur Ausbildung eines psychoorganischen Syndroms. Daher gerinnt die Suche nach einem adäquaten Organersatz nach primären und sekundären adrenocorticalen Insuffizienzen eine besondere Bedeutung. Als Voraussetzung einer möglichen klinischen Anwendung einer Nebennierenrindentransplantation bzw. Autotransplantation ist die Analyse im Tiermodell notwendig.

* Diese Arbeit wurde von der Deutschen Forschungsgemeinschaft unterstützt (KennNr.: Sche-358/1-1).

Chirurgisches Forum 1993
f. experim. u. klinische Forschung
Becker/Beger/Hartel (Hrsg.)

Material und Methoden

Die Genehmigung nach §8 Abs. 1 des Tierschutzgesetzes (BgBl.I S. 1319) AZ.504-42502-91/425 wurde durch die Bezirksregierung erteilt, alle Eingriffe erfolgten in Allgemeinnarkose auf Ketamin- und Hypnorm-Basis. Die Nebennierenrinde von syngenen und allogenen Ratten wurde durch Kollagenase-Digestion und definierte Dichtezentrifugation mittels eines Percollgradienten von sämtlichen Markzellen getrennt und unter die Nierenkapsel transplantiert [5]. Im Anschluß wurde durch einen, für Nebennierenrindenzellen spezifischen, Dichtegradienten eine hochreine Suspension endokriner Zellen erstellt. Die Eliminierung von Blut- und Bindegewebszellen wurde durch zytologische Präparate nach immunzytochemischer Färbung kontrolliert. Nach bilateraler Adrenalektomie erfolgten Funktionskontrollen durch Messung des Corticosteronspiegels und nach 8 Wochen die histologische Untersuchung des Transplantates. Die Corticosteronbestimmung erfolgt mit Radioimmunassay Technik mit einer Doppelbestimmung aus 10 μl Rattenserum. Für die hochfrequente episodische Corticosteronmessung (n = 144/24 h) wurde den Ratten in Narkose ein Jugulariskatheter implantiert, den die Tiere zur Gewöhnung und zum Streßabbau für 5 Tage vor Versuchsbeginn trugen. Dann wurden bei freier Beweglichkeit der Tiere über 24 h jeweils alle 10 min Proben entnommen und sofort zur Messung weiterverarbeitet.

Ergebnisse

Syngenetische zelluläre Transplantationen zeigten bereits nach 24 h eine ausreichende Funktionsaufnahme mit Werten bis 0,2 $\eta g \times (24\ h \times gKG)^{-1}$ Corticosteron. Nach 15 Tagen wurden mit Werten von 0,45 $\eta g \times (24\ h \times gKG)^{-1}$ $(0,45 \pm 0,05)$ etwa 90% der unstimulierten Steroid-Tagesleistung eines normalen Tieres $(0,5 \pm 0,05)$ synthetisiert. In

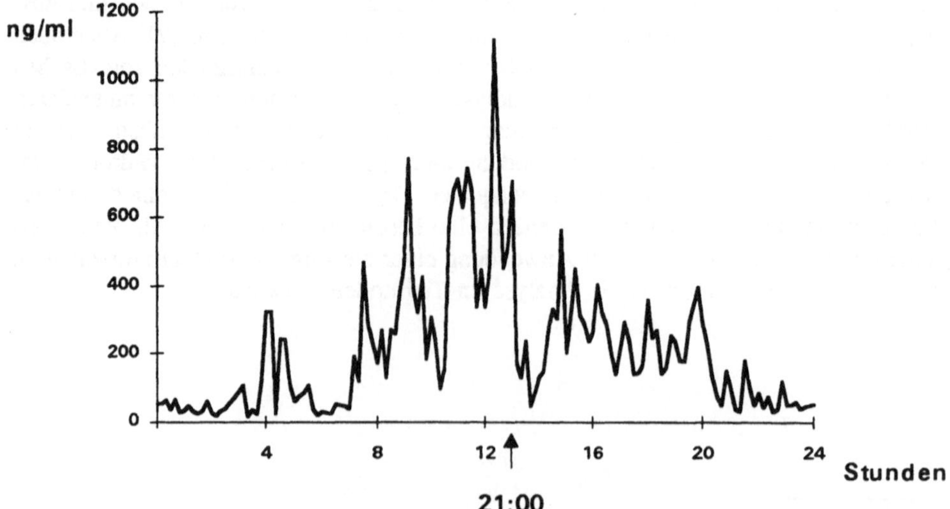

Abb. 1. Episodische Corticosteronsekretion über 24 h bei einer Lewis Ratte (n = 144 Proben)

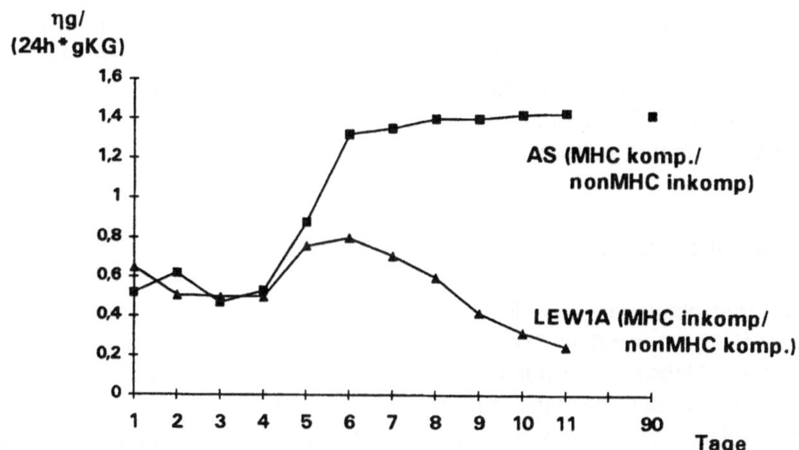

Abb. 2. Corticosteronsekretion bei Zelltransplantationen von Lewis Nebennierenrindenzellen auf MHC-kompatible/Non-MHC inkompatible Empfänger (AS), sowie MHC-inkompatible/-Non-MHC kompatible Empfänger (LEW 1A)

der Analyse der hochfrequenten episodischen Corticosteronmessung wurde eine Halbwertszeit von Corticosteron in der Ratte von 15 min ermittelt. Darüber hinaus konnte ein episodisches Sekretionsmuster des Corticosterons nachgewiesen werden, das prinzipiell der pulsatilen Sekretion von Cortisol beim Menschen gleicht. Auch beim Versuchstier wird die dominierende Abhängigkeit der Sekretionsspitzen von der metabolischen und sozialen Aktivität deutlich (bei den nachtaktiven Tieren liegt das Sekretionsmaximum gegen 21 Uhr) (siehe Abb. 1). Die allogene Transplantation von Nebennierenrindengewebe zeigte eine deutliche Abhängigkeit des Abstoßungsverhaltens vom Grad der Histoinkompatibilität. Empfänger von MHC-inkompatiblen Transplantaten stießen das Transplantat bereits am 5. Tag ab (Rückgang der täglichen Corticosteronsekretion um über 20%). Im Gegensatz dazu reagierten Ratten mit einer Inkompatibilität im Non-MHC Bereich (Lewis Ratten auf AS Ratten, beide $RT1^{\ell}$) bei Transplantationen hochreiner Zellsuspensionen in einem Zeitraum von 90 Tagen nicht mit einer Abstoßung (siehe Abb. 2).

Schlußfolgerungen

Es konnte ein reproduzierbares Transplantationsmodell für allogene und syngene Nebennierenrindenzelltransplantationen bei der Ratte etabliert werden. Die große Ähnlichkeit zum menschlichen Steroidsystem ermöglicht grundlegende Untersuchungsmöglichkeiten zu Regulationsmechanismen der Nebenniere und zu einer möglichen klinischen Anwendung der Nebennierentransplantation. In wieweit hier die Bedeutung und die Expression des MHC-Komplexes (RT^1-Komplex) dem anderer endokriner Zellen, wie etwa den Inselzellen, gleicht [3], muß durch weiterführende Untersuchungen zur MHC-Expression und zum Abstoßungsverhalten von Nebennierenrindenzellen untersucht werden. Im klinischen Bereich berichteten Hurst et al. 1922 erstmals über eine gelungene Allotransplantation mit einer einwandfreien Funktion über mehr als 11 Monate ohne jede Immunsuppression [4]. Inwieweit solche singulären Erfolge auf ein besonderes immunologisches Verhalten der Nebennierenrindenzellen zurückzuführen sind, wird darüber entscheiden, ob solche Toleranzen reproduzierbar und in klinischen Projekten etablierbar sind.

Zusammenfassung

Die Transplantation von Nebennierenrindengewebe ist eine potentielle Therapie bei lebenslang notwendiger Steroidsubstitution wegen bilateraler Adrenalektomie oder primärer Nebennierenrindeninsuffizienz. Voraussetzung einer möglichen klinischen Anwendung der Nebennierentransplantation ist die Analyse im Tiermodell. Die Nebennierenrinde von syngenen und allogenen Ratten wurde durch Kollagenase-Digestion und definierte Zentrifugation von sämtlichen Markzellen getrennt und unter die Nierenkapsel transplantiert. Nach bilateraler Adrenalektomie erfolgten Funktionskontrollen durch Messung des Corticosteronspiegels. Syngenetische zelluläre Transplantationen zeigten bereits nach 15 Tagen 90% der unstimulierten Steroid-Tagesleistung eines normalen Tieres. Darüber hinaus konnte ein episodisches Sekretionsmuster des Corticosterons nachgewiesen werden, das prinzipiell der pulsatilen Sekretion von Cortisol beim Menschen gleicht. Die allogenen Transplantationen von Nebennierenrindengewebe zeigte eine deutliche Abhängigkeit der Abstoßung von der RT1-Antigenstruktur. Transplantierte Ratten mit Inkompatibilität des RT1- (MHC)-Komplexes stießen das Transplantat bereits am 5.–7. Tag nach Transplantation ab. Im Gegensatz dazu reagierten Ratten mit einer Inkompatibilität im Non-MHC Bereich, aber kompatiblen RT1 Antigenen, über einen Zeitraum von 90 Tagen nicht mit einer Abstoßung. Schlußfolgernd konnte ein reproduzierbares Transplantationsmodell von Nebennierenrindenzellen bei der Lewis Ratte etabliert werden. Die große Ähnlichkeit zum menschlichen Steroidsystem ermöglicht grundlegende Untersuchungen zu Regulationsmechanismen der Nebenniere und zu einer möglichen klinischen Anwendung der Nebennierenrindentransplantation.

Summary

Transplantation of adrenal cortical tissue is a potential therapy for patients undergoing bilateral adrenalectomy or suffering from Addison's disease. A main question is whether or not the graft is competent to provide a substitute for the patient in a complete physiological way. We have developed an animal model which allows transplantation of syngeneic and allogeneic adrenal cortex cells in the rat and the investigation of their growth and regulation mechanisms. The technique of preparation, purification, and transplantation was carried out essentially as described previously. Episodic steroid secretion and stress reaction in grafts were monitored by blood samples from a central intravenous catheter every 10 min. Twenty-four-hour steroidogenesis was monitored by 24 h urine samples. We demonstrated that 15 days after transplantation syngeneic grafts showed 90% of the total steroid amount of normal animals. The episodic steroid secretion is basically comparable to humans. Steroid secretion in allogeneic cell transplantation showed a clear dependence on the degree of histoincompatibility. Rats with grafts incompatible at the major histocompatibility complex (MHC) but compatible at non-MHC-antigens, lost the competence of steroidogenesis within 5–7 days. Rats with compatible MHC-antigens, but incompatible non-MHC-antigens, showed a normal steroid secretion for more than 90 days. In conclusion, this model may be useful to investigate regulation mechanisms in normal adrenal cortical cells as well as in adrenal cortical cell transplants.

Literatur

1. Allolio B, Winkelmann W, Fricke U, Heesen D, Kaulen D (1978) Cortisol Plasmakonzentrationen bei Patienten mit primärer Nebennierenrinden-Insuffizienz unter einer Substitutionstherapie mit Cortisonacetat. Verh Dtsch Ges Innere Med 84:1456–1458
2. Brabant EG (1989) Endokrinologische Notfälle. In: Hesch RD (Hrsg) Endokrinologie. Urban & Schwarzenberg, pp 1305–1315
3. Hiller WFA, Steiniger B, Klempnauer J (1993) The role of histocompatibility antigens in transplantation os isolated islets of Langhans in the rat. Diabetes 42: in press
4. Hurst AF (1922) Addison's disease treated by suprarenal grafting. Brit Med J 1:268
5. Scheumann GFW, Hiller W, Schröder S, Schürmeyer T, Klempnauer J, Dralle H (1989) Adrenal cortex transplantation after bilateral total adrenalectomy in the rat. Henry Ford Hosp Med J 38:154–156

Dr. med. G.F.W. Scheumann, Klinik für Abdominal- und Transplantationschirurgie, Medizinische Hochschule Hannover, Konstanty Gutschow-Straße 8, W-3000 Hannover 61

transplantation syngeneic grafts showed 90% of the total steroid amount of normal animals. The episodic steroid secretion is basically comparable to humans. Steroid secretion in allogeneic cell transplantation showed a clear dependence on the degree of histocompatibility. Rats with grafts incompatible at the major histocompatibility complex (MHC) but compatible at non-MHC antigens, lost the competence of steroidogenesis within 5-7 days. Rats with compatible MHC antigens, but incompatible non-MHC-antigens, showed a normal steroid secretion for more than 20 days. In conclusion, this model may be useful to investigate regulation mechanisms in normal adrenal cortical cells as well as in adrenal cortical cell transplants.

Literatur

1. Allolio B, Winkelmann W, Fricke U, Heesen D, Kaulen D (1979) Cortisol-Plasmakonzentrationen bei Patienten mit primärer Nebennierenrinden-Insuffizienz unter Substitutionstherapie mit Cortisonacetat. Dtsch Med Wochenschr 104:1356-1360
2. Brodish DG (1985) Endokrinologie. In: Dutch RH (Hrsg) Endokrinologie. Urban & Schwarzenberg, pp 1308-1313
3. Hiller WFA, Schlager R, Klempnauer J (1989) The role of histocompatibility antigens in transplantation of isolated islets of Langerhans in the rat. Diabetes 38 Suppl
4. Hurst AF (1923) Addison's disease treated by suprarenal grafting. Brit Med J 1:63
5. Scheumann GFW, Schmidt G, Stichtenoth D, Klempnauer J, Pichlmayr R (1989) Adrenal cortical cell function after bilateral total adrenalectomy in the rat. Henry Ford Hosp Med J 37:130-134

Dr. med. G.F.W. Scheumann, Klinik für Abdominal- und Transplantationschirurgie, Medizinische Hochschule Hannover, Konstanty-Gutschow-Straße 8, W-3000 Hannover 61

Bakterielle Flora und entzündliche Leberveränderungen nach biliodigestiver Roux-Y Anastomose – Eine tierexperimentelle Studie an der Ratte

Bacterial Flora and Hepatic Inflammation Following Biliodigestive Roux-Y Anastomosis – An Experimental Study in the Rat

G. Arlt[1], Ch. Peiper[1], U. Bolder[2], H. Wolf[1] und V. Schumpelick[1]

[1]Chirurgische Klinik, RWTH, Aachen (Direktor: Prof. Dr. V. Schumpelick)
[2]Chirurgische Klinik, Städtische Kliniken, Dortmund (Leiter: Prof. Dr. D. Löhlein)

Einleitung

Die Ursache entzündlicher Veränderungen der Gallengänge und der Leber nach Anlage einer biliodigestiven Anastomose wird vielfach in der Aszension von Keimen aus dem Dünndarm vermutet [1, 2]. Klinische Untersuchungen haben gezeigt, daß bei über 90% der Patienten mit einer Roux-Y Hepatikojejunostomie das proximale Jejunum bakteriell fehlbesiedelt ist [1]. Tierexperimentell wurde dieser Befund bestätigt. Im Keimspektrum fand sich eine Vermehrung der Bacteroides-Stämme und Clostridien. Im distalen Anteil der Roux-Schlinge wurden regelhaft höhere Keimzahlen beobachtet als im proximalen Abschnitt [2]. Bei der Anlage einer biliodigestiven Roux-Y Anastomose gilt daher die allgemeine Empfehlung, eine ausreichend lange, refluxfreie Roux-Y Schlinge zu verwenden. Ziel der vorliegenden Studie war es, die bakterielle Flora und assoziierte Entzündungen der Leber bei biliodigestiven Roux-Y Anastomosen mit und ohne enterobiliären Reflux zu untersuchen.

Material und Methoden

Der Versuch wurde an 85 Sprague-Dawley Ratten mit einem mittleren Gewicht von 400 ± 50 g durchgeführt. Die operative Technik entsprach der bei [3] beschriebenen Methode. Im Gegensatz zu dem vorangegangenen Versuch erfolgten die Eingriffe unter sterilen Bedingungen. Im einzelnen ergaben sich folgende Op.-Gruppen:

Chirurgisches Forum 1993
f. experim. u. klinische Forschung
Becker/Beger/Hartel (Hrsg.)

Gruppen mit biliodigestiver Roux-Y Anastomose	
10 cm anisoperistaltische Schlinge (obligater Reflux)	n = 15
3 cm isoperistaltische Schlinge (fakultativer Reflux)	n = 15
10 cm isoperistaltische Schlinge (kein Reflux)	n = 15
Vergleichsgruppen mit blinder Roux-Y Schlinge	
10 cm anisoperistaltische Schlinge	n = 10
3 cm isoperistaltische Schlinge	n = 10
10 cm isoperistaltische Schlinge	n = 10
Scheinoperierte Kontrollen	n = 10

Nach 4 Monaten wurde die Keimanalyse aus dem proximalen Anteil der Roux-Schlingen vorgenommen. Die quantitative Keimanalyse erfolgte mit einer 10er Verdünnungsreihe bis 10^{-9} bezogen auf 100 mg Darmgewicht und 1 ml Lösungsmittel. Zur Differenzierung dienten entsprechende Nährmedien und das API-System. Für jede Op.-Gruppe wurden Median und Standardabweichung berechnet. Die Signifikanzen wurden mit dem Wilcoxon Test für unverbundene Stichproben errechnet.

Für die Beurteilung entzündlicher Leberveränderungen wurde eine Probe aus dem zentralen Leberparenchym nach HE und PAS gefärbt. Die Quantifizierung der entzündlichen Veränderungen erfolgte mit einer eigenen Modifikation des Leber-Histologie-Scores von Lichtman et al. [4]. Die scheinoperierten Kontrolltiere lieferten die Normalwerte für die Anzahl der Portalfelder bei 100facher Vergrößerung, die Zahl der Gallengänge pro Portalfeld bei 400facher Vergrößerung sowie das Vorhandensein von PAS-positiven Makrophagen im Portalfeld bei 400facher Vergrößerung und den Nachweis für Leberzellnekrosen bei 100facher Vergrößerung. Der Score sah folgende Punkteverteilung vor:

	Norm	+ 1 SD	+ 2 SD	
Zahl der Portalfelder	0	1	2	Pkt.
Zahl der Gallengänge	0	1	2	Pkt.
		nein	ja	
PAS-positive Makrophagen		0	2	Pkt.
Parenchymnekrosen		0	2	Pkt.
total		0 bis 8 Pkt.		

Für die Op.-Gruppen wurden Mittelwert und Standardabweichung berechnet. Die Signifikanz-Analyse erfolgte mit dem t-Test für unverbundene Stichproben.

Ergebnisse

In den anisoperistaltischen Schlingen war die Keimzahl gegenüber allen anderen Gruppen signifikant ($p < 0,05$) erhöht ($2,5$–$2,8 \times 10^9$ versus 9×10^4–$1,7 \times 10^7$). Die Keimzahl in Schlingen mit Galleﬂuß lag immer über der Vergleichsgruppe ohne Gallengangsanastomose. Hierfür war vornehmlich eine Vermehrung der gallensäurenspaltenden Spezies verantwortlich. Dekonjugierende Spezies fanden sich signifikant ($p < 0,05$) häufiger bei Tieren mit Gallengangsanastomosen als bei den Ratten mit einer blinden Schlinge (10^6 versus 10^2). Die Keimzahl am proximalen Ende der Roux-Schlinge war bei kurzer biliodigestiver Schlinge höher ($1,7 \times 10^7$) als bei langer refluxfreier Schlinge ($2,0 \times 10^6$).

Zeichen der schweren Cholangitis bestanden zum Zeitpunkt der Nachuntersuchung in vergleichbarer Häufigkeit bei allen Tieren mit selbstfüllender Schlinge (Score 6,1 und 5,4). Tiere mit isoperistaltischer biliodigestiver Roux-Schlinge zeigten geringere Entzündungen der intrahepatischen Gallengänge. Es ergab sich jedoch kein signifikanter Unterschied zwischen kurzen (Score 3,0) und langen Schlingen (Score 2,6). Bei allen Ratten mit isoperistaltischen blinden Schlingen fanden sich unauffällige Verhältnisse in der Leberhistologie (Score 0,77 und 0,83).

Schlußfolgerung

Nach Anlage einer biliodigestiven Roux-Y Anastomose wird das Keimspektrum in der Roux-Schlinge zugunsten gallensäurenspaltender Spezies verschoben. Es besteht jedoch keine direkte Korrelation zwischen der Keimdichte in der proximalen Roux-Schlinge und den konsekutiven entzündlichen Leberveränderungen. Auch bei einer langen refluxfreien Roux-Schlinge treten entzündliche Veränderungen an den intrahepatischen Gallengängen auf. Histologisch gleichen diese Veränderungen den Läsionen beim experimentellen Blindsacksyndrom [3]. Demnach müssen andere Mechanismen als die direkte Keimaszension – zumindest bei dieser Tierspezies – für die beobachteten entzündlichen Veränderungen der intrahepatischen Gallengänge verantwortlich gemacht werden.

Zusammenfassung

In einer tierexperimentellen Studie an 85 Ratten wurden Keimspektrum und entzündliche Leberveränderungen nach Anlage biliodigestiver Roux-Y Anastomosen mit obligatem (selbstfüllende Schlinge), fakultativem (kurze selbstentleerende Schlinge) und ohne Reflux (lange selbstentleerende Schlinge) untersucht. Zum Vergleich dienten entsprechend operierte Tiere ohne Gallengangsanastomose und scheinoperierte Kontrollen. Bei Tieren mit biliodigestiver Anastomose zeigte sich eine Verschiebung des Keimspektrums zugunsten gallensäurenspaltender Spezies. Schwere entzündliche Leberveränderungen fanden sich bei allen selbstfüllenden Schlingen mit und ohne Gallengangsanastomose. Bei den selbstentleerenden biliodigestiven Schlingen fanden sich geringere Leberentzündungen ohne Unterschied zwischen solchen mit fakultativem Reflux oder ohne Reflux.

Summary

In an experimental study on 85 rats, bacterial flora and hepatic inflammation following biliodigestive Roux-Y anastomosis with obligate (self-filling loop), facultative (short self-emptying loop), or without reflux (long self-emptying loop) were investigated. Animals with comparable blind loops and sham-operated animals served as controls. Animals with biliodigestive anastomosis showed a shift towards a bile acid deconjugating flora. Severe hepatic inflammation was present in all self-filling loops with and without biliary anastomosis. In self-emptying biliary loops, mild inflammation was found, regardless of the presence or absence of reflux.

Literatur

1. Arlt G, Bolder U, Bares R, Schumpelick V (1990) Erhöhte Gallensäurenretention bei biliodigestiven Roux-Y Anastomosen im Tierexperiment. Langenbecks Arch Chir 375:283–288
2. Hölscher AH, Chapman N, Siewert JR, Blümel G, Ruckdeschl G (1987) Bakteriologische Fehlbesiedlung als obligate Folge der Rouxschen Schlingenbildung. Langenbecks Arch Chir [Suppl] Chir Forum, pp 103–107
3. Lichtman SN, Sartor RB, Keku J, Schwab JH (1990) Hepatic inflammation in rats with experimental small intestinal bacterial overgrowth. Gastroenterology 98:414–423
4. Nielsen ML, Justesen T, Lenz K, Nielsen OV, Jensen L (1977) Bacterial flora of the small intestine and bile acid metabolism in patients with hepatico-jejunostomy Roux-en-Y. Scand J Gastroenterol 12:977–982

Dr. G. Arlt, Chirurgische Klinik, Medizinische Fakultät, RWTH Aachen,
Pauwelsstraße 30, W-5100 Aachen

Der Einfluß verschiedener Vagotomieverfahren auf die Freisetzung von Cholecystokinin beim Hund

The Influence of Different Methods of Vagotomy on the Secretion of Cholecystokinin in Dogs

F. König, H. Köhler, R. Nustede und A. Schafmayer

Klinik und Poliklinik für Allgemeinchirurgie, Universität Göttingen (Direktor: Prof. Dr. med. H.-J. Peiper)

Einleitung

Nach Vagotomien kommt es häufig zu Postvagotomiesyndromen und gelegentlich zur Ausbildung eines Dumpingsyndroms [1]. Verantwortlich dafür sind eine veränderte Motorik und möglicherweise auch eine veränderte Freisetzung gastrointestinaler Hormone. Ziel unserer Studie war es, den Einfluß verschiedener Vagotomieverfahren am selben Tier auf die nahrungsstimulierte Cholecystokininausschüttung zu untersuchen.

Material und Methodik

6 Hunden wurde nach einer nächtlichen Fastenperiode von 12 h ein standardisiertes Futter verabreicht. Während einer Basalperiode und nach Nahrungsapplikation wurden in 15 minütigen Abständen Blutproben aus einer peripheren Vene zur radioimmunologischen Bestimmung von Cholecystokinin entnommen. Die Messung von Cholecystokinin erfolgte mittels eines von uns entwickelten hochsensitiven und spezifischen Radioimmunoassays. Es wurde dann jeweils am selben Tier nacheinander zunächst eine selektiv proximale Vagotomie (SPV), eine gastrale Vagotomie (SGV) und eine trunkuläre Vagotomie (TV) über einen transthotakalen Zugang vorgenommen, wobei somit bei fortschreitendem Versuchsverlauf zentralere Vagusfasern durchtrennt wurden. Die oben genannten Fütterungstests zur Hormonbestimmung wurden jeweils 6 Wochen postoperativ durchgeführt.

Ergebnisse

Die basalen und postprandialen Cholecystokinin-Konzentrationen vor und nach den verschiedenen nacheinanderfolgenden Vagotomieverfahren sind in Abb. 1 aufgezeigt.

Die postprandialen postoperativen Cholecystokinin-Konzentrationen sind im Vergleich zu den präoperativen Cholecystokinin-Konzentrationen bei allen Vagotomieverfahren signifikant erhöht, wobei die höchsten Cholecystokinin-Spiegel nach Durchtrennung trunkulärer Vagusfasern gemessen wurden.

Chirurgisches Forum 1993
f. experim. u. klinische Forschung
Becker/Beger/Hartel (Hrsg.)

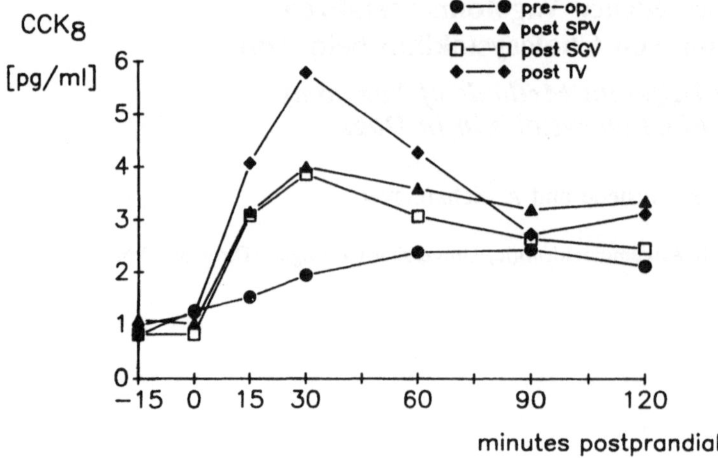

Abb. 1. Einfluß verschiedener Vagotomieverfahren auf die postprandialen CCK-Plasmaspiegel bei Hunden. *SPV*, selektiv proximale Vagotomie; *SGV*, gastrale Vagotomie; *TV*, trunkuläre Vagotomie

Diskussion

In verschiedenen experimentellen Studien wurden sowohl stimulierende [2] als auch hemmende [5] Einflüsse des Nervus vagus auf die CCK-Sekretion beschrieben. Möglicherweise werden bei der Vagotomie Nervenfasern durchtrennt, die die CCK-Zelle hemmen. Eine veränderte CCK-Sekretion nach Vagotomie könnte aber auch Folge indirekter Mechanismen sein. Cholecystokinin stimuliert physiologischerweise die postprandiale exokrine Pankreassekretion und führt zur Gallenblasenkontraktion. Eine verminderte exokrine Pankreasenzymsekretion, eine verminderte Galleproduktion und eine verminderte Gallenblasenkontraktion wurde nach Vagotomie gefunden [4]. Es gibt Hinweise dafür, daß CCK beim Menschen [3] über einen negativen Rückkopplungsmechanismus an der Regulation der exokrinen Pankreasenzymsekretion beteiligt ist. Demzufolge könnte eine verminderte exokrine Pankreasenzymsekretion nach Vagotomie zu einer vermehrten CCK-Sekretion führen. Zusätzlich verändert eine Vagotomie die Magenentleerung. Nach einer selektiv proximalen Vagotomie wurde eine verzögerte Magenentleerung für flüssige Nahrungsbestandteile nachgewiesen [1]. Eine deshalb erhöhte Konzentration entsprechender Nahrungsbestandteile im Duodenum könnte die CCK-Zelle intensiver stimulieren.

Zusammenfassung

6 Hunde wurden nacheinander einer selektiv proximalen, einer gastralen und einer trunkulären Vagotomie unterzogen. Basale und postprandiale Cholecystokinin (CCK)-Konzentrationen im peripheren Blut wurden mittels Radioimmunoassay gemessen. Nach allen verschiedenen Vagotomieverfahren, besonders nach trunkulärer Vagoto-

mie, fand sich postoperativ eine erhöhte postprandiale CCK-Sekretion. Als mögliche Ursachen werden einerseits die Durchtrennung vagaler, die CCK-Zelle hemmende Fasern und andererseits eine veränderte Pankreasenzymsekretion und Magenentleerung diskutiert.

Summary

In six dogs, a selective proximal vagotomy, gastric vagotomy, and truncal vagotomy were performed successively. Basal and postprandial cholecystokinin (CCK) concentrations in the peripheral blood were measured in radioimmunoassay. After all the different types of vagotomy, especially after truncal vagotomy, an increased postprandial secretion of CCK was found compared with secretion in the healthy animal. Possible causes are the cutting of vagal fibers, which might inhibit the secretion of CCK cells, and the changed gastric and pancreatic secretion.

Literatur

1. Becker HD, Caspary WF (1973) Postgastrectomy and postvagotomy syndromes. Springer, Berlin Heidelberg New York
2. Cantor P, Holst JJ, Knuthen S, Rehfeld JF (1986) The effect of vagal stimulation of the release of cholecystokinin in anaesthetized pigs. Scand J Gastroenterol 21:1069–1072
3. Dlugosz J, Fölsch UR, Czaikowki A, Gabryelewicz A (1988) Feedback regulation of stimulated pancreatic enzyme secretion during intraduodenal perfusion of trypsin in man. Eur J Clin Invest 18:267–272
4. Holle F, Andersson S (1974) Vagotomy, latest advances. Springer, Berlin Heidelberg New York
5. Hopman WPM, Jansen J, Lamers C (1984) Plasma CCK response to a liquid meal in vagotomized patients. Ann Surg 200:693–697

Dr. F. König, Klinik und Poliklinik für Allgemeinchirurgie, Universität Göttingen, Robert-Koch-Straße 40, W-3400 Göttingen

Intravenöses Kontrastmittel verstärkt die Trypsinogen-Aktivierung und erhöht Pankreaszellnekrosen und Mortalität bei experimenteller Pankreatitis

Intravenous Contrast Medium Increases Trypsinogen Activation, Acinar Cell Necrosis, and Mortality in Experimental Pancreatitis

Th. Foitzik[1], K. Lewandrowski[3], C. Fernandez-del Castillo[2], D.W. Rattner[2], A.L. Warshaw[2] und Ch. Herfarth[1]

[1]Chirurgische Universitätsklinik, Heidelberg
[2]Department of Surgery, Massachusetts General Hospital and Harvard Medical School, Boston, USA
[3]Department of Pathology, Massachusetts General Hospital and Harvard Medical School, Boston, USA

Einleitung

Um die hohe Letalität der schweren akuten Pankreatitis (AP) zu begrenzen, müssen Patienten mit nekrotisierender Verlaufsform rechtzeitig therapeutischen Maßnahmen zugeführt werden, die bei Patienten mit ödematöser AP nicht gerechtfertigt sind. Zur Evaluation von Pankreasnekrosen gilt die kontrastverstärkte Computertomographie (CECT) derzeit als beste Methode. Da der Nachweis ischämischer Areale in der Frühphase der AP Rückschlüsse auf den weiteren Krankheitsverlauf zuläßt, wird die Durchführung eines CECT als initiales Staging von Patienten mit AP propagiert [1, 2]. Untersuchungen an der Niere haben gezeigt, daß intravenöses Kontrastmittel (KM) in einer Dosierung, wie sie zur Darstellung des Pankreas im CECT benötigt wird, vorbestehende ischämische Läsionen aggravieren kann [3]. Da die schwere AP durch Perfusionsstörungen charakterisiert ist [4], liegt der vorliegenden Studie die Frage zugrunde, ob der Verlauf der AP durch die Gabe von intravenösem KM in der Frühphase der Erkrankung beeinflußt wird. An einer schweren Form der AP an der Ratte wird der Effekt von ionischem und nicht-ionischem KM auf die Trypsinogen-Aktivierung, Pathomorphologie des Pankreas und Mortalität untersucht.

Methodik

Induktion einer akut nekrotisierenden Pankreatitis durch intraduktale Infusion von 0,5 ml Glykodeoxycholsäure (10 mmol/l) über 10 min, sowie anschließend intravenöse Infusion von 5 μg/kg Caerulein über 6 h. Nach 7 h Randomisation der 54 Versuchstiere in 3 Gruppen und intravenöse Infusion von 2 ml/kg NaCl 0,9% (Gruppe A, n = 18), ionischem KM (Iothalmat meglumin) (Gruppe B, n = 18) oder nicht-ionischem KM (Iopamidol) (Gruppe C, n = 18) über 1 min. Vor und nach Gabe

Chirurgisches Forum 1993
f. experim. u. klinische Forschung
Becker/Beger/Hartel (Hrsg.)

der Testsubstanzen (6.–9. h) Flüssigkeitssubstitution mit Ringer-Laktat (6 ml/kg/h), kontinuierliche Aufzeichnung von mittlerem arteriellen Druck und Urinausscheidung, sowie Bestimmung von Hämatokrit und Trypsinogen-Aktivationspeptiden (TAP) im Plasma (ELISA). Nach 24 h Autopsie der überlebenden Versuchstiere, Bestimmung von TAP im Aszites sowie morphometrische Untersuchung des Pankreas (K.L.).

Ergebnisse (Tabelle 1, 2)

Vor Administration der Testsubstanzen zeigten sich keine Unterschiede in den aufgezeichneten Parametern zwischen den drei Versuchsgruppen. *Nach Injektion der Testsubstanzen* blieben Blutdruck und Herzfrequenz unverändert, während die Urinausscheidung in Gruppe B (ionisches KM) und Gruppe C (nicht-ionisches KM) signifikant anstieg. Das ionische KM (ca. 1400 mOsm/kg) bewirkte eine stärkere Diurese als das nicht-ionische KM (ca. 680 mOsm/kg). Die Urinausscheidung der Kontrastmittel-Tiere blieb für 2 h erhöht. Nicht signifikant unterschied sich die zwischen der 7. h (Injektion der Testsubstanzen) und 24. h (Versuchsende) gesammelte Urinmenge im Vergleich der 3 Versuchsgruppen. Die Messungen von Blutdruck, Herzfrequenz, Hämatokrit und Plasma-TAP nach Injektion der Testsubstanzen ergaben keine Unterschiede zwischen den 3 Versuchsgruppen (Tabelle 1). Der Hämatokrit fiel in allen Gruppen bis zum Versuchsende kontinuierlich ab (6. h: 52%$\pm$0,8; 7. h: 47%$\pm$0,9; 9. h: 43%$\pm$0,8; 24. h: 32% $\pm$ 1,2). Die höchsten TAP-Werte im Plasma wurden vor Injektion der Testsubstanzen gemessen. Während der 24-h Versuchszeit verstarben 4 der 18 Kontrolltiere (Testsubstanz NaCl 0,9%) und je 10 der 18 Tiere in den beiden KM-Gruppen (4/18 vs 20/36; $p < 0{,}05$). Bei den überlebenden Tieren zeigten sich signifikante Unterschiede in den im Aszites gemessenen Trypsinogen-Aktivationspeptiden und im Ausmaß der Pankreaszellnekrosen (Tabelle 2).

Tabelle 1. Mittlerer arterieller Druck (MAP), Hämatokrit (Hkt), Urinausscheidung (UO) und Trypsinogen-Aktivationspeptide (TAP) im Plasma 1 h vor und nach Injektion von Kochsalz (NaCl), ionischem (ION) oder nicht-ionischem (NON) Kontrastmittel (Mittelwert ± SEM)

	vor Testsubstanz-Gabe		
	NaCl	ION	NON
MAP [mmHg]	109 ± 3,8	106 ± 2,9	107 ± 5,3
UO [ml/h]	0,5 ± 0,1	0,5 ± 0,1	0,5 ± 0,1
Hkt [%]	46 ± 0,8	47 ± 0,8	46 ± 0,9
TAP [nmol/l]	3,5 ± 0,5	3,6 ± 0,9	3,3 ± 0,7
	nach Testsubstanz-Gabe		
	NaCl	ION	NON
MAP [mmHg]	105 ± 4,6	102 ± 7,4	101 ± 5,5
UO [ml/h]	0,5 ± 0,1	1,9 ± 0,2[a,b]	1,2 ± 0,1[a,b]
Hkt [%]	41 ± 0,9[a]	43 ± 0,8[a]	41 ± 1,0[a]
TAP [nmol/l]	1,8 ± 0,3	2,1 ± 0,7	1,9 ± 0,5

[a] $p < 0{,}05$; verglichen mit Werten vor Testsubstanz-Gabe (gepaarter t-Test)
[b] $p < 0{,}05$; ION und NON *versus* SAL und ION *versus* NON (ungepaarter t-Test)

Tabelle 2. Mortalität, Trypsinogen-Aktivationspeptide (TAP) im Aszites und Pankreaszellnekrosen nach 24 h (Mittelwerte ± SEM)

	Gruppe A (NaCl 0,9%)	Gruppe B (ionisches KM)	Gruppe C (nicht-ion. KM)
Mortalität	4 / 18[a]	10 / 18	10 / 18
Aszites-TAP [pmol/l]	9,0 ± 2,4[b]	17,3 ± 5,6	17,7 ± 7,1
Nekrose [0–4 Pkte]	2,46 ± 0,07[c]	2,81 ± 0,1	2,59 ± 0,1

[a–c] $p < 0{,}05$; Kontroll-Gruppe (A) *versus* Kontrastmittel-Gruppen (B + C)
([a] χ-Test, [b] Mann Whitney U-Test, [c] t-Test)

Zusammenfassung

Die vorliegende Studie untersucht an einem Tiermodell der akut nekrotisierenden Pankreatitis Effekte von ionischem und nicht-ionischem Kontrastmittel (KM) auf die Trypsinogen-Aktivierung, Pathomorphologie des Pankreas und Mortalität. Hintergrund der Untersuchung ist die Frage, ob intravenöses Kontrastmittel, wie es in der Frühphase der akuten Pankreatitis (AP) zur Evaluation von Pankreasnekrosen mittels Computertomographie (CECT) eingesetzt wird, den Verlauf der Erkrankung beeinflußt. Nach Applikation von 2 ml/kg ionischem wie nicht-ionischem KM bei Ratten mit schwerer nekrotisierender Pankreatitis waren Trypsinogen-Aktivationspeptide im Aszites, Pankreaszellnekrosen und Mortalität im Vergleich zu Kontrolltieren, denen anstelle von KM Kochsalz injiziert worden war, signifikant erhöht. Demnach verschlechtert intravenöses KM in der Frühphase der schweren Pankreatitis in diesem Tiermodell den weiteren Krankheitsverlauf. Da KM die Blutzellenaggregation fördert und die Sauerstofffreisetzung aus den Erythrozyten herabsetzen kann [5], wird die bei schwerer AP verminderte Perfusion und Oxygenation des Pankreas [4] durch das KM möglicherweise weiter verschlechtert. Die sich im CECT abzeichnenden Areale verminderter Perfusion könnten sich infolge der KM-Gabe vergrößern oder zu manifesten Nekrosen transformiert werden. Die Ergebnisse der vorliegenden Untersuchung stellen somit den Einsatz der kontrastverstärkten Computertomographie in der Frühphase der akuten Pankreatitis in Frage.

Summary

Contrast-enhanced computer tomography (CECT) is used to demonstrate ischemic areas or pancreatic necrosis in acute pancreatitis (AP). In order to evaluate possible adverse effects of the contrast medium (CM) on the course of the disease, we studied the impact of ionic and nonionic intravenous CM on trypsinogen activation, pathomorphology of the pancreas, and survival in a model of severe acute AP in the rat. Trypsinogen activation peptides (TAP) in ascites, acinar cell necrosis, and mortality were significantly increased in animals that had received 2 ml/kg of either ionic or nonionic CM, as compared to animals given saline as the test solution. Our results indicate that intravenous CM can accentuate the severity of necrotizing pancreatitis when given early in the course of the disease. Since CM has been shown to increase red cell aggregation and impair oxygen release from the red cell, it may further compromise already decreased pancreatic perfusion in severe AP, thereby converting borderline ischemia to irreversible necrosis. With this in mind, CECT performed soon after hospital admission in order to demonstrate poorly perfused pancreatic tissue and to predict areas of necrosis may depict a self-fulfilling prophecy. The use of CECT early in acute pancreatitis should, therefore, be reconsidered and perhaps be avoided.

Literatur

1. Nordestgaard AG, Wilson SE, Williams RA (1986) Early computerized tomography as a predictor of outcome in acute pancreatitis. Am J Surg 152:127–132
2. Bradley EL, Murphy F, Ferguson C (1989) Prediction of pancreatic necrosis by dynamic pancreatography. Ann Surg 210:495–504
3. Deray G, Baumelou B, Martinez F, Brillet G, Jacobs C (1991) Renal vasoconstriction after low and high osmolar contrast agents in ischemic and non-ischemic canine kidney. Am J Nephrol 36:93–96
4. Bassi DG, Foitzik T, Kollias N, Fernandez-del Castillo C, Warshaw AL, Rattner DW (1992) Pancreatic perfusion in experimental pancreatitis. Evaluation by means of reflectance spectroscopy. Pancreas 7:A733
5. Aspelin P (1979) Effect of ionic and non-ionic contrast media on red cell deformability in vitro. Acta Radiol Diagn 20:1–12

Dr. Th. Foitzik, c/o Prof. Warshaw, Massachusetts General Hospital, 15 Parkman Street, WACC 336, Boston, MA 02114, USA

Parenchymprotektive Wirkung von hyperonkotischen Dextranen nach verzögertem Therapiebeginn bei nekrotisierender Pankreatitis der Ratte

Pancreas-Protecting Effect of Hyperoncotic Dextrans After Delayed Onset of Therapy in Necrotizing Pancreatitis of the Rat

K. Huch[1], J. Schmidt[1], H.P. Sinn[2], W. Schratt[1], E. Klar[1] und H.J. Buhr[1]

[1]Chirurgische Klinik, Universität Heidelberg (Direktor: Prof. Dr. Ch. Herfarth)
[2]Pathologisches Institut, Universität Heidelberg (Direktor: Prof. Dr. H.F. Otto)

Einleitung

In der Pathogenese der akuten nekrotisierenden Pankreatitis spielt die Mikrozirkulationsstörung des Pankreas eine zentrale Rolle. Eine Verbesserung der Pankreasperfusion kann zur Limitierung der morphologischen Veränderungen führen. Ein Therapieregime stellt die isovolämische Hämodilution mit Dextran 60 (6%, 60.000 D) in der Frühphase der Verringerung der Kapillarperfusion, 30 min nach Induktion der akuten Pankreatitis, dar [1]. Auch die Applikation von hyperonkotischem ultrahochmolekularem Dextran (10%, 500.000 D) zum gleichen Zeitpunkt resultierte in einer Reduktion der Mortalität und in einer Limitierung der azinären Nekrosen [2].

Die folgende Untersuchung sollte folgendes prüfen: Erstens, welchen Effekt haben die untersuchten Dextrane nach deutlich längerem therapiefreien Intervall (180 min), und zweitens, welchen Einfluß hat das Molekulargewicht auf die therapeutische Wirkung der eingesetzten Kolloide?

Material und Methodik

Narkose, Instrumentierung und Pankreatitisinduktion erfolgten gemäß einem neuen Therapiemodell, welches kürzlich charakterisiert wurde [3].

Narkose und Instrumentierung: Nach intraperitonealer Injektion von Pentobarbital (10 mg/kg) und Ketamin (40 mg/kg) wurden bei 30 nüchternen Dextran-resistenten Wistar-Ratten (dxdxPh-) Katheter in die rechte V. jugularis interna (Infusion) und in die linke A. carotis communis (Blutentnahme) implantiert. Nach Oberbauchlaparotomie wurde die Duodenalschlinge mobilisiert und der bilio-pankreatische Gang nach transpapillärer Kanülierung drainiert [3].

Chirurgisches Forum 1993
f. experim. u. klinische Forschung
Becker/Beger/Hartel (Hrsg.)

Pankreatitisinduktion: Nach Rekanülierung erfolgte eine Zeit- (2,5 min), Druck- (30 mmHg) und Volumen- (0,2–0,25 ml) kontrollierte Infusion von verdünnter (10 mmol/l) Glycodeoxycholsäure. Nach dem Bauchdeckenverschluß wurde zusätzlich mit einer intravenösen supramaximalen Stimulation mit Caerulein (30 μg/kg/6h) begonnen. Im Anschluß daran erwachten die Tiere aus der Narkose unter kontinuierlicher i.v.-Gabe von Morphin (0,1 mg/kg) in RL (2 ml/h) als Basisinfusion.

Behandlungsgruppen und Auswertung: 180 und 240 min nach der Pankreatitisinduktion wurde die Therapie mit Bolusinfusionen von A: Ringerlösung (*RL*, 12 ml/kg, n = 10), B: 10% Dextran 70.000 Dalton (*DEX-70*, 4 ml/kg, n = 10) und C: 10% Dextran 500.000 Dalton (*DEX-500*, 4 ml/kg, n = 10) über je 5 min durchgeführt.

Nach Abschluß der Beobachtungsphase von 9 h wurden die überlebenden Tiere getötet und das Pankreas in gepuffertem Formalin (6%) fixiert. Die histologische Auswertung erfolgte nach morphometrischen Gesichtspunkten (Zeiss Planimetrie). Hierzu wurden sämtliche Nekroseareale in Flachschnitten aus dem Kopf- und Schwanzbereich der Pankreata mit vollständigem Verlust der Kernfärbbarkeit bei 200facher Vergrößerung in einem Punktzählverfahren quantifiziert.

Ergebnisse

Mortalität: Innerhalb der 9-stündigen Beobachtungsphase starben 60% (6/10) der Tiere in der *RL*-Kontrollgruppe gegenüber 10% (1/10, $p < 0{,}03$, Fisher's exact test) in der Gruppe *DEX-70* und 20% (2/10, $p = 0{,}8$) in der Gruppe *DEX-500*.

Azinäre Pankreasnekrosen: Darüberhinaus bewirkte die Verwendung von *DEX-70* und *DEX-500* eine signifikante Reduktion der Parenchymnekrose im Pankreas (*RL* vs. *DEX-70* $p < 0{,}01$, *RL* vs. *DEX-500* $p < 0{,}02$, t-Test) (s. Abb. 1).

Diskussion

Die Progression der akuten ödematösen Pankreatitis zur nekrotisierenden Form wird wahrscheinlich durch eine drastische Perfusionsminderung der Azini unterhalten. Dafür spricht eine Protektion der Pankreasmorphologie bei experimenteller Pankreatitis durch Verbesserung der Mikroperfusion des Pankreas mittels Hämodilution mit hochmolekularen Dextranen (60.000 D) [1] und durch hyperonkotische ultrahochmolekulare Dextrane (500.000 D) jeweils 30 min nach Pankreatitis-Induktion [3].

Die vorliegende Studie zeigt, daß die Gabe von hyperonkotischen Dextranen auch noch nach einem wesentlich längeren therapiefreien Intervall von 3 h zu einer Reduktion der azinären Nekrosen führt und mit einer signifikanten Senkung der Mortalitätsrate einhergeht. Da in den Fällen mit letalem Verlauf der Tod meist schon innerhalb der ersten 6–7 h des Experiments eintrat, entspricht ein dreistündiges Therapiefreies Intervall in dieser experimentellen Situation einem deutlich längeren Intervall unter klinischen Bedingungen.

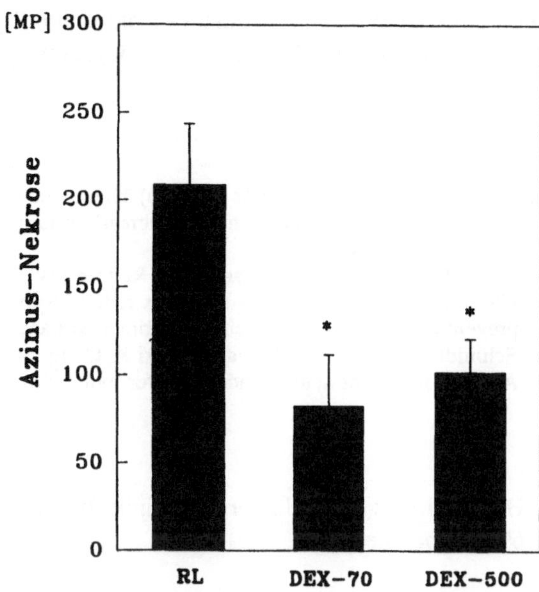

Abb. 1. Azinäre Pankreasnekrosen in den verschiedenen Therapiegruppen (Abkürzungen s. Text, *MP* = Meßpunkte)

Signifikante Differenzen in der Wirkung der beiden hyperonkotischen Dextrane unterschiedlichen Molekulargewichts ließen sich nicht feststellen. Folgende Wirkmechanismen gelten als wahrscheinlich: Verbesserung der mikrovaskulären Perfusion des Pankreas durch Verminderung der Blutviskosität, Hemmung der Leukozyten-Endothel-Interaktion und der Reduktion der intravasalen Gerinnung.

Zusammenfassung

Bei experimenteller nekrotisierender Pankreatitis bewirken hyperonkotische hoch- (70.000 D) und ultrahochmolekulare (500.000 D) Dextrane auch nach einem therapiefreien Intervall von 3 h eine deutliche Verbesserung der Überlebensrate und eine signifikante Reduktion der entstehenden Pankreasnekrosen. Entsprechend der in früheren Studien nachgewiesenen Verbesserungen der Pankreasmikrozirkulation mittels Hämodilution mit Dextran 60 gilt als wahrscheinlicher Mechanismus eine Steigerung der Blutfluidität.

Summary

Hyperoncotic high (70 kDa) and ultrahigh molecular (500 kDa) dextrane leads to an improvement of the survival rate and a significant reduction of pancreatic necrosis, even if given 3 h after induction of pancreatitis. We believe that the mechanism of action consists in an improvement of blood fluidity, a reduction of plasmatic hypercoagulability, and an inhibition of leukocyte-endothelium interaction.

Literatur

1. Klar E, Herfarth C, Messmer K (1990) Therapeutic effect of isovolemic hemodilution with dextran 60 on the impairment of pancreatic microcirculation in acute biliary pancreatitis. Ann Surg 211:346–353
2. Schmidt J, Fernandez-del Castillo C, Rattner DW, Lewandrowski K, Warshaw AL (1993) Ultrahigh-molecular dextran solutions reduce trypsinogen activation, lower mortality and prevent acinar necrosis in acute experimental pancreatitis. Am J Surg (in press)
3. Schmidt J, Rattner DW, Lewandrowski K, Compton CC, Knoefel WT, Warshaw AL (1992) A better model of acute pancreatitis for evaluating therapy. Ann Surg 215:44–56

K. Huch, Chirurgische Universitätsklinik, Im Neuenheimer Feld 110,
W-6900 Heidelberg

Gibt es eine akute, exokrine Pankreasinsuffizienz?

Acute Exocrine Pancreatic Insufficiency: Does It Exist in Man?

F. Pfeffer, M. Büsing, H.D. Becker und U.T. Hopt

Abteilung für Allgemeinchirurgie, Chirurgische Universitätsklinik, Tübingen

Einleitung

Während die physiologischen Grundlagen der exokrinen Pankreassekretion weitgehend bekannt sind, gibt es bislang wenig Erkenntnisse zum Verhalten der exokrinen Funktion während akuter Pankreatitis beim Menschen, insbesondere in der Frühphase der Erkrankung. Tierexperimentell konnte eine deutliche Einschränkung der exokrinen Funktion in verschiedenen Pankreatitismodellen nachgewiesen werden [3, 4]. Auf den Modellcharakter der Transplantatpankreatitis für die genuine Pankreatitis wurde erst kürzlich hingewiesen [1]. Die frühpostoperative Transplantatpankreatitis bietet die einzigartige Möglichkeit, die exokrine Pankreasfunktion beim Menschen kontinuierlich, vom Beginn der Erkrankung an, zu untersuchen.

Ziel dieser Untersuchung war es, den Einfluß der akuten Transplantatpankreatitis auf die exokrine Funktion beim Menschen zu evaluieren.

Patienten und Methodik

Untersucht wurde eine konsekutive Serie von 12 Typ I-Diabetikern, bei denen im Zeitraum zwischen März 1990 und März 1991 eine kombinierte Pankreas-Duodenal-Nieren-Transplantation durchgeführt wurde (Alter: 28–51 J., Diabetesdauer vor Operation 7–34 J., Ischämiezeit 9–16 h). Die Ableitung des Pankreassekretes erfolgte hierbei mittels Blasendrainagetechnik über eine Anastomose zwischen Spenderduodenum und Empfängerharnblase. Während der ersten 6 Wochen nach Operation wurde das Pankreassekret über einen intraoperativ in den Ductus pancreaticus plazierten Katheter perkutan drainiert. Dies erlaubte das direkte Monitoring der exokrinen Sekretion. Anhand eines prospektiven Protokolls wurden präoperativ und unmittelbar nach Reperfusion beginnend, bis zum 14. Tag die Pankreasenzyme (Lipase, P-Amylase) im Serum, sowie Volumen und Enzymgehalt des Pankreassekretes bestimmt.

Aufgrund des makroskopischen Befundes am Ende der Operation, der histologischen Befunde von Pankreasbiopsien, sowie des klinischen Verlaufes wurde eine Einteilung in 3 Schweregrade der Transplantatpankreatitis entsprechend der genuinen Pankreatitis vorgenommen.

Grad I war charakterisiert durch einen geringen Ischämie-/Reperfusionsschaden, ohne makroskopische bzw. mikroskopische Veränderungen des Pankreas. Im klinischen Verlauf traten keine längerdauernden Beschwerden auf. Unter Grad II wurden

Chirurgisches Forum 1993
f. experim. u. klinische Forschung
Becker/Beger/Hartel (Hrsg.)

Patienten mit milder, ödematöser Verlaufsform der Transplantatpankreatitis zusammengefaßt. Makroskopisch zeigten sich bereits intraoperativ "Kalkspritzer" des Pankreas, mikroskopisch konnten subkapsuläre und peripankreane Fettgewebsnekrosen, sowie vereinzelte Azinuszellnekrosen festgestellt werden. Der klinische Verlauf war durch eine verlängerte lokale Beschwerdedauer gekennzeichnet. Patienten mit schwerer, nekrotisierender Verlaufsform der Transplantatpankreatitis zeigten bereits intraoperativ schwere makroskopische Veränderungen mit inhomogener Reperfusion und massiven "Kalkspritzern". Histologisch fanden sich ausgedehnte Azinuszellnekrosen. Der klinische Verlauf war durch langdauernde Schmerzsymptomatik und wiederholt notwendige lokale Nephrektomien charakterisiert.

Ergebnisse

Pankreassekretion

Nach den obengenannten Kriterien wurde die Transplantatpankreatitis ihrem Verlauf entsprechend bei 4 Patienten in Grad I, und bei 6 Patienten in Grad II eingestuft. Lediglich bei 2 Patienten fand sich eine schwere Verlaufsform entsprechend Grad III der Transplantatpankreatitis. Diese Verteilung entspricht in etwa der unseres gesamten Patientengutes von zwischenzeitlich 69 Patienten.

In Abhängigkeit vom Schweregrad der Pankreatitis zeigte sich eine unterschiedliche Beeinträchtigung der exokrinen Funktion. Bei Grad I setzte die Pankreassekretion bereits intraoperativ ein. Die Flußrate lag am ersten Tag im Median bei 13,6 ml/h (7,5–35,4). Das Maximum lag im Median am 5. Tag bei 25 ml/h (12,5–43,7). Nach

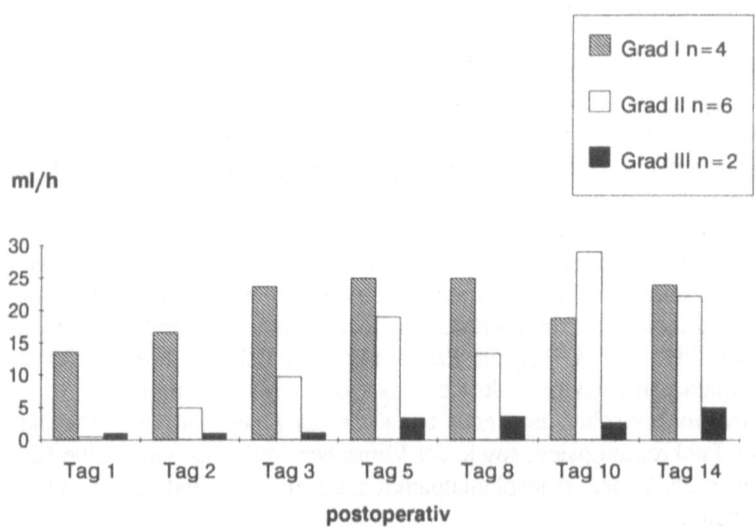

Abb. 1. Exokrine Pankreassekretion nach kombinierter Pankreas-/Nieren-Transplantation (KPNT) über den Pankreasgangkatheter im Median. *Grad I:* leichter Ischämie-/Reperfusionsschaden; *Grad II:* ödematöse Pankreatitis; *Grad III:* schwere, nekrotisierende Pankreatitis

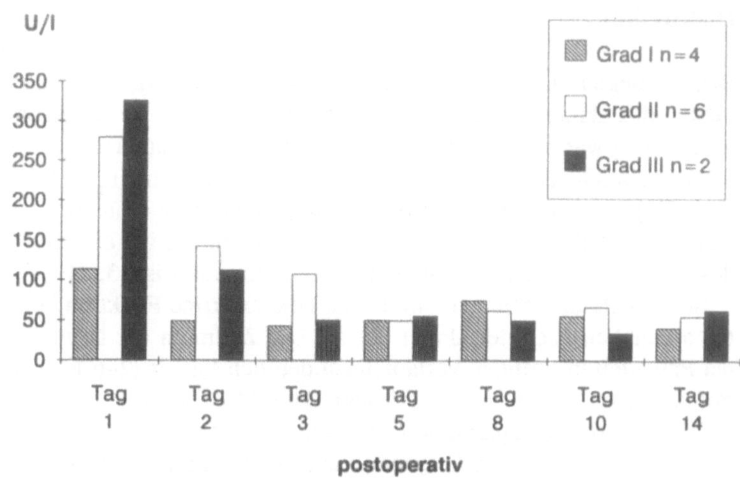

Abb. 2. Serumamylaseverlauf nach KPNT, unterteilt nach Schweregraden im Median

anschließendem Abfall der Sekretionsrate stabilisierte sich die exokrine Funktion bei allen Patienten bis zum 14. Tag, die Sekretionsrate lag im Median bei 23,9 ml/h (22,8–29,1). Die exokrine Sekretion der Patienten mit Grad II der Transplantatpankreatitis war durch ein verzögertes Einsetzen der exokrinen Funktion gekennzeichnet. Lediglich 2 von 6 Patienten produzierten intraoperativ kurzzeitig Pankreassekret. Im weiteren Verlauf sistierte der Sekretfluß bei allen Patienten passager. Am 3. Tag war bei 5 von 6 Patienten eine geringe Sekretion mit im Median 9,75 ml/h (0,2–20,8) zu verzeichnen. Bis zum 10. Tag hatte sich die exokrine Funktion soweit erholt, daß das Niveau der Sekretionsrate mit im Median 25,6 ml/h (10–37,5) über der von Grag I lag. Bis zum 14. Tag reduzierte sich die Flußrate und lag mit einem Median von 22,2 ml/h (8,3–37,2) in etwa im Niveau von Grad I.

Demgegenüber war bei den 2 Patienten mit Grad III während des gesamten Beobachtungszeitraumes keine nennenswerte Sekretion nachweisbar.

Die Enzyme im Pankreassekret zeigten einen analogen Verlauf wie das Sekretvolumen.

Pankreasenzyme im Serum

Betrachtet man den Amylaseverlauf im Serum, so findet sich lediglich in der Frühphase der Erkrankung ein deutlicher Unterschied des Enzymanstieges, in Abhängigkeit von der Schwere der Transplantatpankreatitis. Am ersten postoperativen Tag fanden sich in der Gruppe mit schwerer, nekrotisierender Verlaufsform die höchsten Enzymanstiege, im Median 326 U/l gegenüber 114 U/l bei Grad I und 279 U/l bei Grad II. Nach raschem Abfall der Enzymkonzentration erreichten die Serumwerte von Grad III bereits am 3. Tag postoperativ das Niveau von Grad I. Demgegenüber fiel ein längerandauernder Enzymanstieg bis zum 5. Tag bei Transplantatpankreatitis Grad II auf. Während des weiteren Beobachtungszeitraumes waren bei allen 3 Gruppen mäßiggradige Enzymanstiege ohne nennenswerte Unterschiede festzustellen.

Diskussion

Bislang liegen nur wenige Untersuchungen zur exokrinen Pankreassekretion bei Patienten mit akuter Pankreatitis vor. Insbesondere das Verhalten in der Frühphase der Erkrankung war beim Menschen bislang nicht näher untersucht. Anhand eines sondenlosen PABA-Tests konnte bisher lediglich gezeigt werden, daß die Pankreassekretion 3–10 Tage nach Beginn der Erkrankung pathologisch erniedrigt ist [2]. In verschiedenen Tiermodellen konnte jedoch gezeigt werden, daß die exokrine Sekretionsfähigkeit des Pankreas während der akuten Phase vermindert ist [3, 4].

In allen Untersuchungen erholte sich die exokrine Funktion bei den meisten Patienten allmählich nach der akuten Phase. Der Zeitraum der Normalisierung war hierbei bei Patienten mit milder Verlaufsform deutlich kürzer (2–6 Monate) als bei Patienten mit schwerer, nekrotisierender Pankreatitis (2–4 Jahre) [4].

Die Pankreastransplantation zur Behandlung des Typ I-Diabetes mittels Blasendrainagetechnik und perkutaner Drainage des Pankreassekretes durch einen Pankreasgangkatheter stellt ein ideales Verfahren zum exakten Monitoring der exokrinen Pankreassekretion dar. Auf den Modellcharakter der postoperativ in unterschiedlichen Schweregraden auftretenden Transplantatpankreatitis wurde bereits kürzlich verwiesen [1]. Abhängig vom Schweregrad der Pankreatitis kommt es zu einer unterschiedlichen Beeinträchtigung der Pankreassekretion. Während bei Pankreata mit geringem Ischämie-/Reperfusionsschaden bereits intraoperativ Pankreassekret sezerniert wird und sich die Funktion rasch bis zum 3. Tag erholt, kommt es bei Patienten mit ödematöser Pankreatitis zu einem verzögerten Einsetzen der Funktion bis zum 5. Tag und einer Stabilisierung nach 10–14 Tagen. Diese Ergebnisse stehen im Einklang mit den Ergebnissem die Tyden et al. [5] bei seinen Patienten nach Pankreastransplantation beschrieben hat. Demgegenüber stehen die Patienten mit schwerer, nekrotisierender Transplantatpankreatitis, bei denen während des gesamten Beobachtungszeitraumes keine nennenswerte exokrine Funktion zu verzeichnen ist.

Es scheint somit der Schluß erlaubt, daß in Analogie zu den bislang vorliegenden tierexperimentellen Ergebnissen, im Rahmen einer akuten Pankreatitis eine mäßiggradige Schädigung des Organs zu einer passageren, aber vollständig reversiblen Störung der physiologischen exokrinen Sekretionsmechanismen führt. Im Gegensatz hierzu ist die schwere, nekrotisierende Verlaufsform durch einen langdauernden, nahezu kompletten Verlust der exokrinen Sekretion, ohne vollständige restitutio ad integrum gekennzeichnet.

Hinsichtlich des Enzymverlaufs im Serum bestätigt sich die von der genuinen Pankreatitis bekannte Tatsache, daß sich normalerweise der Schweregrad der Entzündung nicht in der Höhe der Enzymfreisetzung im Serum widerspiegelt. Lediglich unmittelbar nach Einsetzen der Erkrankung zeigen sich deutliche Unterschiede in Abhängigkeit zum Schweregrad der Pankreatitis.

Zusammenfassung

In einer prospektiven Studie an 12 Typ I-Diabetikern mit kombinierter Pankreas-Duodenal-Nierentransplantation und passagerer Ableitung des Pankreassekretes über einen Pankreasgangkatheter, wurde der Einfluß der akuten Pankreatitis auf die exokrine Sekretion untersucht. Über 14 Tage wurden das Volumen des Pankreassekretes, sowie die Pankreasenzyme im Serum (P-Amylase, Lipase) bestimmt. Unterteilt nach 3 Schweregraden – leichter Ischämie-/Reperfusionsschaden, milde ödematöse Pankreatitis und schwere nekrotisierende Pankreatitis – zeigte sich eine unterschiedlich ausgeprägte Störung der Pankreassekretion in der Frühphase der Erkrankung. Eine mäßiggradige Schädigung des Organes resultierte in einer passageren, aber vollständig reversiblen Störung der physiologischen exokrinen Sekretionsmechanismen. Demgegenüber war die schwere, nekrotisierende Pankreatitis durch einen permanenten, nahezu kompletten Verlust der exokrinen Sekretion ohne nennenswerte Regeneration gekennzeichnet.

Summary

The effect of acute pancreatitis on pancreatic exocrine function was investigated in a prospective study of 12 diabetic patients after combined pancreas/kidney transplantation with temporary drainage of the pancreatic duct via catheter. For 14 days, pancreatic secretions as well as enzyme concentrations in serum (p-amylase, lipase) were measured. Graft damage was classified into three groups: mild ischemia/reperfusion damage, edematous pancreatitis, and severe necrotizing pancreatitis. According to the severity of graft damage, a characteristic impairment of pancreatic secretion was seen in the early postoperative course after transplantation. Edematous pancreatitis caused an almost total, but completely reversible acute insufficiency of exocrine secretory mechanisms for a few days. In contrast, severe necrotizing pancreatitis resulted in a permanent and almost complete lack of exocrine secretion, without regeneration of the acinar cell system.

Literatur

1. Büsing M, Hopt UT, Quacken M, Becker HD, Morgenroth K (1992) Morphological studies of graft pancreatitis following pancreas transplantation. Br J Surg (in press)
2. Mitchell CJ, Playforth MJ, Kelleher J, McMahon MJ (1983) Functional recovery of the exocrine pancreas after acute pancreatitis. Scand J Gastroenterol 18:5–8
3. Murayama KM, Drew JB, Nahrwold DL, Jochl RJ (1990) Acute edematous pancreatitis impairs pancreatic secretion in rats. Surgery 107:302–10
4. Niederau C (1989) Pankreassekretion während und nach akuter Pankreatitis. Z Gastroenterol 27:41–45
5. Tyden G, Brattström C, Häggmark A, Groth CG (1987) Studies on the exocrine secretion of segmental pancreatic grafts in human. Surg Gynecol Obstet 164:404–8

F. Pfeffer, Abteilung für Allgemeinchirurgie, Chirurgische Universitätsklinik, Hoppe-Seyler-Straße 3, W-7400 Tübingen

Octreotide bei akuter Pankreatitis: Ergebnisse einer unizentrischen prospektiven Studie mit drei verschiedenen Octreotide-Dosierungen

Octreotide in the Treatment of Acute Pancreatitis: Results of an Unicentric Prospective Trial with Three Different Octreotide Dosages

M. Binder[1], M. Büchler[1], W. Uhl[1], H. Friess[1], H.J. Dennler[2] und H.G. Beger[1]

[1]Abteilung für Allgemeine Chirurgie, Universität Ulm
[2]Klinische Forschung, Sandoz AG, Nürnberg

Die schwere akute Pankreatitis (AP) hat, trotz verbesserter diagnostischer und therapeutischer Konzepte international eine hohe Morbidität und Letalität, letztere bis zu 50% [1]. Was die Therapie der AP anbelangt, so gibt es bis heute keine spezifische Behandlung dieser Erkrankung. Studien mit Proteasen-Inhibitoren, wie die Hoffnungsträger Aprotinin und Gabexate mesilate, zeigten im klinischen Einsatz keinen positiven Effekt auf den Verlauf der AP [2].

Obgleich die Pathogenese der AP nicht aufgeklärt ist, zählt die Hyperstimulation der exokrinen Sekretion zu einem der wesentlichen Konzepte. Mit Octreotide wurde ein langwirksames Analogon des nativen Somatostatins synthetisiert, das hochwirksam die basale und stimulierte Pankreassekretion hemmt und subkutan appliziert werden kann.

Ziel der vorliegenden Arbeit war es, in einer klinischen Phase I/II Studie, bei Patienten mit mittelschwerer und schwerer akuter Pankreatitis, die Wertigkeit von Octreotide zu untersuchen.

Methoden

Um zu gewährleisten, daß Patienten mit mittelschwerer und schwerer akuter Pankreatitis in die Studie aufgenommen wurden, haben wir 14 Einschlußkriterien definiert (Tabelle 1).

Nach Randomisierungsplan erhielten je 8 Patienten:

a) 3 × 100μg Octreotide/Tag s.c. über einen Zeitraum von 10 Tagen
b) 3 × 200μg Octreotide/Tag s.c. über einen Zeitraum von 10 Tagen
c) 3 × 500μg Octreotide/Tag s.c. über einen Zeitraum von 10 Tagen

Die Patienten wurden nach der 10tägigen Therapie mit Octreotide weitere 21 Tage nachbeobachtet, so daß die Gesamtstudiendauer 31 Tage betrug.

Chirurgisches Forum 1993
f. experim. u. klinische Forschung
Becker/Beger/Hartel (Hrsg.)

Tabelle 1. Einschlußkriterien der Studie

I. Obligatorische Kriterien

- Erste deutliche Symptome der akuten Pankreatitis dürfen nicht länger als 96 bis maximal 168 h zurückliegen.
- Die Serumamylase oder die Serumlipase muß mehr als das Dreifache des Normalwertes innerhalb der letzten 96 h betragen.
- Deutlicher Spontanschmerz im Oberbauch während dieser Zeit.
- Der Patient gibt seine Einwilligung zur Teilnahme an der Studie.

II. Fakultative Kriterien
(mindestens 4 müssen zum Zeitpunkt des Therapiebeginns erfüllt sein)

- Lokale Abwehrspannung
- Subileus/Ileus
- Kreislaufschock
- Anurie
- Leukozyten > 12000/mm^3
- Blutzucker > 150 mg/dl
- $pO_2 < 60$ mmHg
- Hypocalcämie < 2 mmol/l
- Kreatinin > 200 μmol/l
- Charakteristischer Befund einer mittelschweren oder schweren Pankreatitis in Sonographie und/oder CT

Zur Beurteilung der Wirksamkeit wurden Anzahl und Schweregrad eintretender Komplikationen mit einem Score-System erfaßt [2] (Tabelle 2). Zur statistischen Auswertung wurden die ausgewählten Komplikationen bei Aufnahme des Patienten, und die neu hinzutretenden Komplikationen während des 31tägigen Untersuchungszeitraumes bewertet und die Punktsummen ermittelt. Zur Kennzeichnung des Therapieerfolges wurde die Punktsumme für die neu hinzukommenden Komplikationen von der Punktsumme des Aufnahmetages subtrahiert. Negative Punktedifferenzen kennzeichnen eine Verschlechterung der Situation des Patienten, positive Differenzen bedeuten einen Therapieerfolg.

Patienten

Es wurden 24 Patienten in die Studie aufgenommen. Davon waren 10 (42%) männliche und 14 (58%) weibliche Patienten. Bei 12 (50%) Patienten, mit einem durchschnittlichen Alter von 69 Jahren, lag eine biliäre Ätiologie zugrunde. Bei 9 Patienten wurde anamnestisch ein Alkoholabusus festgestellt, in dieser Gruppe war das Durchschnittsalter 41 Jahre. Weitere 2 Patienten hatten ein traumatisch geschädigtes Pankreas, bei einem Patienten war kein ätiologischer Faktor eruierbar. Das mittlere Alter aller Patienten war 57 Jahre (Range 22–88 Jahre). Der mittlere Ranson-Score betrug 3,4 (Range 1–10). Die drei Gruppen waren hinsichtlich Geschlechtsverteilung, Alter und Schweregrad der akuten Pankreatitis vergleichbar.

Tabelle 2. Ausgewählte Komplikationen und deren Gewichtung bei der Berechnung der Punktsummen [2]

Organkomplikationen	Punkte
Schock	4
Sepsis	4
pulmonale Insuffizienz	3
renale Insuffizienz	3
Peritonitis	3
Hämorrhagie (GI- und/oder abdominelle Blutung)	3
Ileus/Subileus	1
Metabolische Komplikationen	**Punkte**
Hypocalcämie	2
Gerinnungsstörung	2
Ikterus	1
Hyperglykämie	1
Enzephalopathie	1
Metabolische Azidose	1

Die Letalität wird mit 30 Punkten bewertet. Dies entspricht der Punktsumme aller Komplikationen zusammen +1.

Eine historische Kontrollgruppe [2], bestehend aus 108 Patienten mit akuter Pankreatitis, wies eine Geschlechtsverteilung von 66 (61%) männlichen Patienten und 42 (39%) weiblichen Patienten auf. Das mittlere Alter war 49 Jahre (Range 18–89 Jahre), der mittlere Ranson-Score lag bei 3,7 (Range 1–9).

Ergebnisse

Die bei Aufnahme der 24, mit Octreotide behandelten, Patienten vorhandenen und die im Verlauf neu hinzutretenden Komplikationen sind in der Abb. 1 dargestellt. 2 Patienten der Octreotide-behandelten Gruppe verstarben, dies entspricht einer Letalität von 8,3%. In der historischen Kontrollgruppe lag die Letalität bei 14,8%.

Die Komplikationsscores bei Aufnahme der Patienten waren im Mittel in allen Octreotide-Gruppen und in der Kontrollgruppe gleich (Abb. 2). Positive mittlere Punktedifferenzen zwischen Aufnahme- und Verlaufskomplikationsscore, und damit Therapieerfolge, lagen in den Octreotide-Gruppen mit den Dosierungen $3 \times 200 \mu g$ $(+3,0)$ und $3 \times 500 \mu g$ $(+1,0)$ vor. In der Niedrigdosis Octreotide-Gruppe und in der Kontrollgruppe wurden mittlere Scores von $-1,0$ und $-2,1$ ermittelt.

Die Therapie mit Octreotide war nebenwirkungsarm und wurde gut toleriert. 7 Patienten berichteten über ein Brennen an der Injektionsstelle, das wenige Minuten nach Injektion aufhörte. Dieses Phänomen wird auf das Lösungsmittel der Prüfsubstanz zurückgeführt [3]. Ein Patient entwickelte am 8. Behandlungstag (die Prüfsubstanz wurde abgesetzt) ein temporäres allergisches Exanthem für 2 Tage.

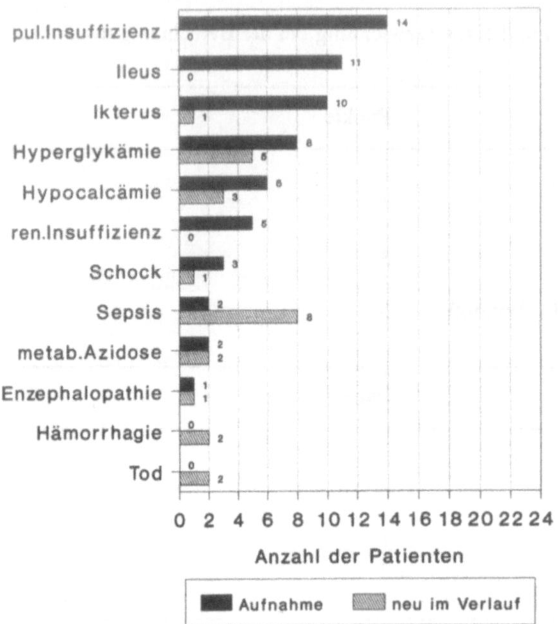

Abb. 1. Bei Aufnahme und im Verlauf neu eingetretene Komplikationen bei den 24 mit Octreotide behandelten Patienten mit mittelschwerer und schwerer akuter Pankreatitis

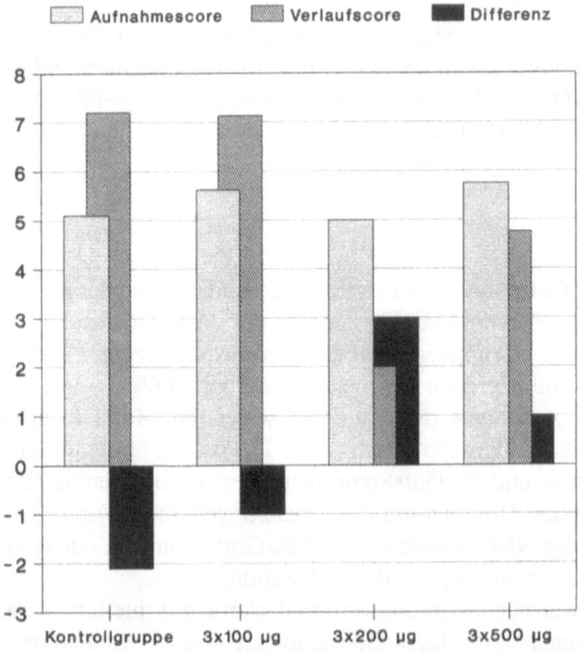

Abb. 2. Mittlere Komplikationsscore bei Aufnahme, Verlauf und als Punktedifferenz

Diskussion

Die Mortalität bei der akuten ödematösen Pankreatitis liegt heute unter 1%, dagegen versterben bei der schweren Verlaufsform 10–50% der Patienten trotz Anwendung moderner Intensivtherapiemaßnahmen [1]. Die Rationale für den Einsatz sekretionsinhibitorisch wirkender Substanzen ergibt sich daraus, daß – entgegen tierexperimentellen Ergebnissen – beim Menschen in der Frühphase der AP ein unverändertes Sekretionsverhalten nachgewiesen werden konnte [4]. Frühere klinische Studien mit dem nativen Somatostatin bei der humanen AP hatten angesichts mangelnder statistischer Power keinen positiven Effekt der Substanz auf den Verlauf der AP, wie Carballo et al. [5] in einer Meta-Analyse zeigen konnten.

Mit Octreotide liegt heute ein langwirksames, hochpotentes synthetisches Analogon des Somatostatins vor, das hochwirksam die basale und stimulierte Pankreassekretion hemmt. Ein weiterer wesentlicher Vorteil des Analogons ist die subcutane Applikationsmöglichkeit.

In unserer kausalen Therapie der mittelschweren und schweren akuten Pankreatitis mit Octreotide konnten wir eine dosisabhängige positive Beeinflussung des komplizierten Krankheitsverlaufes erreichen. Diese Ergebnisse der vorliegenden Studie unterstützen die Aussagen von Carballo et al. [5] und rechtfertigen eine kontrollierte Prüfung der Substanz an einem großen Patientenkollektiv.

Zusammenfassung

In dieser klinischen Phase I/II-Studie bei 24 Patienten mit mittelschwerer und schwerer akuter Pankreatitis konnte ein positiver Effekt von hochdosiertem Octreotide, ein potenter Pankreassekretionshemmer, auf die Komplikationsrate der akuten Pankreatitis gezeigt werden. Diese Ergebnisse rechtfertigen die Prüfung dieser Substanz an einem großen Patientenkollektiv in einer randomisierten, doppelblinden, kontrollierten Multizenterstudie.

Summary

Twenty-four patients with severe acute pancreatitis were treated with octreotide, a potent inhibitor of exocrine secretion, in a clinical phase I/II study. The complication rate was lower in the group of patients receiving octreotide in a high dosage.

These findings are promising and need to be validated in a randomized, double-blind, controlled multicentric trial.

Literatur

1. Beger HG, Büchler M (eds) Acute pancreatitis. Research and clinical management. Springer, Berlin Heidelberg New York London Paris Tokyo 1987

2. Büchler M, Malfertheiner P, Uhl W, Schölmerich J, Stockmann F, Adler G, Gaus W, Rolle K, Beger HG and the German Pancreatitis Study Group (1993) Gabexate mesilate in human acute pancreatitis. Gastroenterology (in press)
3. Büchler M, Friess H, Klempa I, Hermanek P et al. (1992) Role of octreotide in the prevention of postoperative complications following pancreatic resection. Am J Surg 163:125–131
4. Dominguez-Munoz JE, Pieramico O, Büchler M, Malfertheiner P (1992) Interdigestive exocrine pancreatic function and motilin release in the early phase of acute pancreatitis in humans. Dig 52:78
5. Carballo F, Dominguez E, Farnandez-Calvet L, Martinez-Pancorbo C, Garcia A, De la Morena J (1991) Is somatostatin useful in the treatment of acute pancreatitis? – A meta-analysis. Digestion 49:12–13

Dr. med. M. Binder, Abteilung für Allgemeinchirurgie, Universität Ulm,
Steinhövelstraße 9, W-7900 Ulm

Hemmung der exokrinen Pankreassekretion durch das Somatostatin-Analog SMS 201-995 (Sandostatin). Eine klinisch experimentelle Studie bei Patienten nach Duodenopankreatektomie

Suppression of Exocrine Pancreatic Secretion by the Somatostatin Analog SMS 201-995 (Sandostatin). A Clinical Study in Patients Following Duodenopancreatectomy

Th. Bömmer[1], I. Klempa[1], J. Menzel[1], I. Baca[1] und H. Fink[2]

[1] Klinik für Allgemein- und Gefäßchirurgie, Zentralkrankenhaus, Bremen
(Direktor: Prof. Dr. med. I. Klempa)
[2] Institut für Laboratoriumsmedizin, Zentralkrankenhaus Bremen
(Direktor: Prof. Dr. med. R. Haeckel)

Einleitung

Die partielle Duodenopankreatektomie nach Whipple ist das Standardverfahren bei der operativen Behandlung des Pankreaskopf- und Gallengangscarcinoms in kurativer Absicht. Trotz weltweit berichteter guter Erfahrungen mit geringer Morbidität und Mortalität bleiben die Komplikationsmöglichkeiten an der pancreatico-jejunalen Anastomose ein Problem [5]. Die tryptische Aktivität des Restpankreas kann zur Anastomoseninsuffizienz beitragen oder auch zur Ausbildung einer postoperativen Pankreatitis. Die Hemmung dieser tryptischen Aktivität ist deshalb ein logisches Konzept. Die Ergebnisse, die bei der Anwendung von z.B. Atropin, Glucagon und Calcitonin erzielt wurden, blieben allerdings enttäuschend. Die Hemmung der exokrinen Pankreassekretion durch Somatostatin hingegen ist ein sowohl experimentell als auch klinisch belegtes effektives Konzept [2, 3, 4].

Das SMS 201-995 ist ein synthetisch hergestelltes Somatostatin-Analog, das gegenüber dem natürlichen Hormon eine Reihe von Vorteilen zu bieten scheint. Es handelt sich um ein zyklisches Peptid aus 8 Aminosäuren (Octreotid), das auf molarer Basis wesentlich potenter wirkt als das natürliche Hormon. Es hat bei der i.v. oder s.c. Gabe eine etwa 50fach längere Halbwertszeit. Die klinische Wirksamkeit auf die verschiedenen Zielorgane beträgt 6–8 h. Im Gegensatz zum Somatostatin, das kontinuierlich intravenös verabreicht werden muß, genügt beim SMS die dreimal tägliche Gabe einer Einzeldosis i.v. oder s.c.

Die klinischen Erfahrungen mit dem SMS 201-995, die von Büchler et al. 1992 publiziert wurden, berichten von einer signifikanten Senkung der Komplikationsrate in der Pankreaschirurgie [1]. In einer klinisch experimentellen Studie untersuchten wir das Ausmaß der Hemmung der exokrinen Pankreasfunktion durch SMS 201-995

Chirurgisches Forum 1993
f. experim. u. klinische Forschung
Becker/Beger/Hartel (Hrsg.)

nach Stimulation des Pankreasrestes durch Sekretin bei Patienten nach Duodenopankreatektomie.

Methodik

Im Zeitraum vom 01.01.1992 bis zum 30.09.1992 haben wir bei insgesamt 14 Patienten die Hemmung der exokrinen Pankreassekretion durch SMS 201-995 nach partieller Duodenopankreatektomie untersucht. Die Operation war bei allen Patienten in kurativer Intention erfolgt, entweder wegen eines Pankreaskopf- oder eines Gallengangscarcinoms (12 bzw. 2 Fälle). Vor Fertigstellung der Pancreatico-Jejunostomie wurde ein dünner Silikonkatheter mit einem inneren Durchmesser von 2 mm in den Ductus wirsungianus der Restdrüse plaziert und via Jejunum durch die Bauchdecke nach außen geleitet (Abb. 1) [3]. Am 5. postoperativen Tag, noch vor Wiederaufnahme der oralen Nahrungszufuhr, wurde das Restpankreas mit Sekretin (25 E/h) über insgesamt 3 h maximal stimuliert. 60 min nach Versuchsbeginn wurden einmalig 100 μg SMS 201-995 subcutan appliziert.

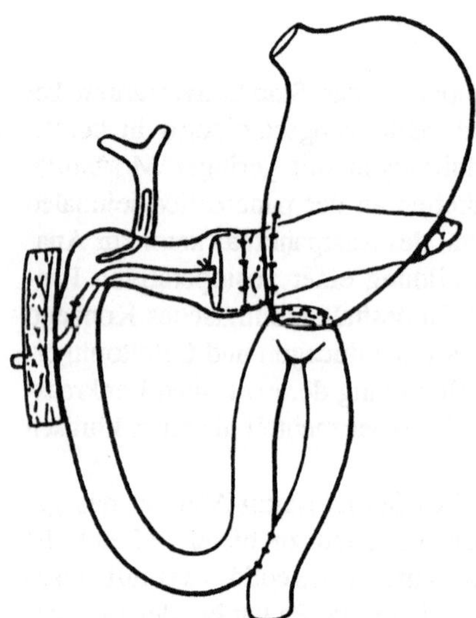

Abb. 1. Rekonstruktion der Oberbaucheinheit nach partieller Duodenopankreatektomie. Silikon-Katheter zur Pankreasdrainage in situ

Die exokrine Sekretionsleistung der Restdrüse wurde in Intervallen von jeweils 30 min bestimmt. Hierzu wurden das sezernierte Volumen und die Amylase- und Lipasekonzentration im Sekret bestimmt. Die Ausschüttung von Amylase bzw. Lipase wurde bestimmt nach der Formel

$$\frac{\text{Enzymkonzentration/l} \times \text{Volumen}}{1000}.$$

Die Bestimmung von Amylase und Lipase im Serum erfolgte zu Untersuchungsbeginn und dann nach 30, 90 und 150 min.

Die statistische Auswertung erfolgte wegen der kleinen Stichprobe (n < 15) mit dem U-Test nach Mann und Whitney bei einseitiger Fragestellung. Als signifikant wurde ein Ergebnis betrachtet, wenn $p < 0{,}05$.

Ergebnisse

Bei insgesamt 14 Patienten waren die Daten nur in 10 Fällen auswertbar. In 4 Fällen lag eine Dislokation bzw. Occlusion des Pankreaskatheters vor. Die Stimulation mit Sekretin führte zu einer kräftigen Steigerung des sezernierten Volumens auf $19,2 \pm 5,4$ ml in den ersten 30 min und auf $36,6 \pm 8,3$ ml für die zweiten 30 min. Analog verhielt sich die Amylase- bzw. die Lipaseausschüttung: Für die ersten 30 min betrug diese für Amylase $1,03 \pm 0,4$ kU. Danach kam es zu einer Steigerungsrate für die Amylaseausschüttung auf $2,12 \pm 0,5$ kU. Der Wert für die Lipaseausschüttung für die ersten 30 min betrug $2,91 \pm 0,23$ kU. Der Wert 60 min nach Stimulation für die Lipaseausschüttung betrug $5,46 \pm 1,7$ kU.

Nach subcutaner Gabe von 100 μg SMS 201-995 fand sich ein sofort einsetzender und dramatischer Abfall von sezerniertem Volumen, Amylase- und Lipaseausschüttung. Hierbei fanden sich die nachfolgenden Werte. 30 min nach Beginn der Hemmung fanden sich noch $0,46 \pm 0,21$ kU für die Amylase, $1,78 \pm 0,83$ kU für die Lipase und $18,8 \pm 8,68$ ml für das Volumen. Die weiteren Werte betrugen 60, 90 und 120 min nach Beginn der Hemmung für die Amylase $0,12 \pm 0,07$ kU, $0,13 \pm 0,08$ kU und $0,13 \pm 0,07$ kU; für die Lipase $0,66 \pm 0,02$ kU, $0,60 \pm 0,02$ kU und $0,54 \pm 0,03$ kU; für das Volumen $12,1 \pm 5,4$ ml, $14,6 \pm 5,0$ ml und $17,4 \pm 7,2$ ml.

Wird die Sekretionsleistung des stimulierten Pankreasrestes mit der Situation nach Gabe von SMS 201-995 verglichen, so ergibt sich eine hochsignifikante Hemmung ($p < 0{,}01$) aller drei untersuchten Parameter (Volumen, Amylase- und Lipaseausschüttung) über den gesamten Untersuchungszeitraum, wobei die Erfassung – wie beschrieben – in jeweils 30minütigen Sammelperioden erfolgte. In den letzten 30 min des Untersuchungszeitraumes fand sich gegenüber den beiden Sammelperioden davor ein geringer Anstieg für das Volumen und die Amylaseausschüttung, nicht hingegen für die Lipase. Dieser Anstieg erreicht jedoch bei weitem nicht Signifikanzniveau.

Diskussion

Das Somatostatin-Analog SMS 201-995 (Sandostatin) hemmt die stimulierte exokrine Sekretion des Pankreas bei subcutaner Applikation in einer Dosierung von 100 μg. Die Hemmung erstreckt sich über den gesamten Untersuchungszeitraum von 2 h.

Ein Maximum der Sekretionshemmung des Pankreasrestgewebes findet 60 min nach Gabe von SMS statt. Durchschnittlich verringert sich die sezernierte Pankreassekretmenge von $36,6 \pm 8,3$ ml auf $12,1 \pm 5,4$ ml 60 min nach SMS-Gabe. Dieses entspricht einer Hemmung der Pankreassekretmenge von 67%.

Der maximale Amylaseausstoß von $2,12 \pm 0,5$ kU wird 60 min nach Stimulation erreicht. Nach Gabe von SMS verringert sich der Amylaseausstoß auf $0,12 \pm 0,07$ kU

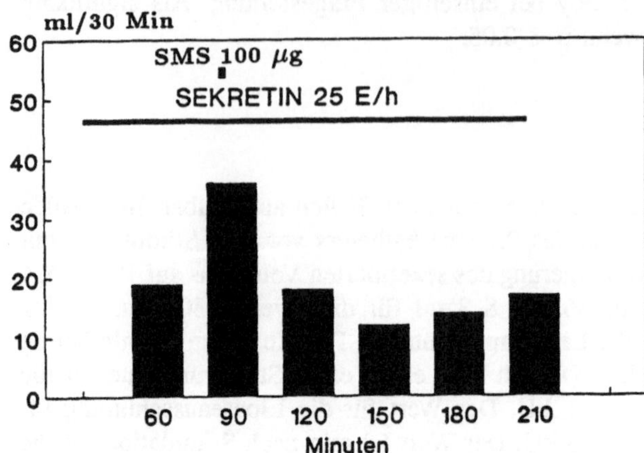

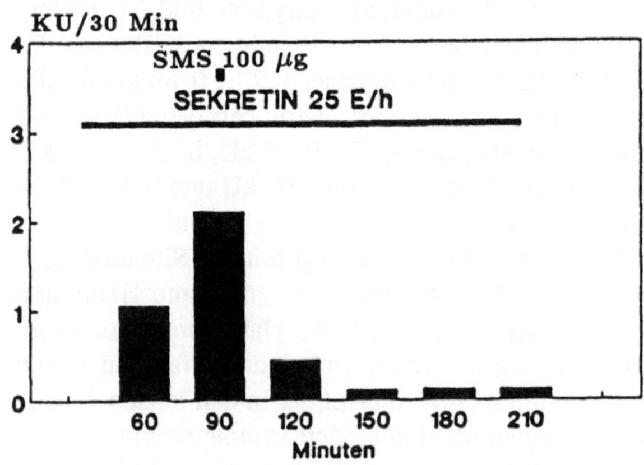

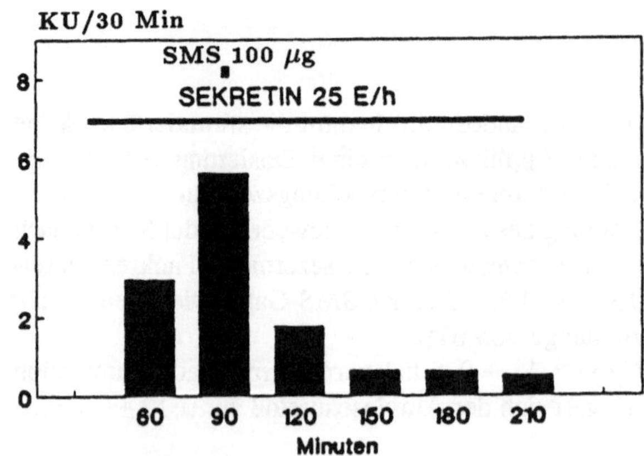

Abb. 2. Exokrine Funktion der Restdrüse nach Stimulation mit Sekretin und Hemmung mit SMS 201-995 (Sandostatin)

60 min nach SMS-Applikation. Die Hemmung des Amylaseausstoßes beträgt demnach 95%.

Auch beim Lipaseausstoß zeigt sich ein ähnliches Verhalten wie oben beschrieben. Der höchste Lipaseausstoß mit $5,46 \pm 1,7$ kU wurde ebenfalls 60 min nach Stimulation mit Sekretin gemessen. Der Lipaseausstoß verringert sich kontinuierlich über den gesamten Testzeitraum, so daß 120 min nach SMS Applikation ein Minimum des Lipaseausstoßes von $0,54 \pm 0,03$ kU gemessen wurde. Danach beträgt die Hemmung des Lipaseausstoßes 91%.

Zusammenfassung

Wie in einer klinischen Studie gezeigt werden konnte, läßt sich mit SMS 201-995 (Sandostatin) die Komplikationsrate in der Pankreaschirurgie senken. In dieser Studie untersuchten wir die Wirkung von SMS 201-995 auf die exokrine Pankreasfunktion bei Patienten nach einer Whipple'schen Operation. Nach Stimulation des Pankreasrestes fand sich unter SMS 201-995 eine hochsignifikante Reduktion der exokrinen Tätigkeit (Volumen, Anmylase, Lipase). Dies ist möglicherweise eine Erklärung für die günstigen klinischen Effekte der Substanz.

Summary

As was shown in a clinical trial, SMS 201-995 (Sandostatin) is effective in reducing the rate of perioperative complications in pancreatic surgery. In this study the effects of SMS 201-995 on the exocrine pancreatic function were investigated in patients after Whipple's procedure. After stimulation of the pancreatic remnant, we found a highly significant reduction in exocrine output (volume, amylase, lipase) after SMS 201-995 was given subcutaneously. This may be a possible explanation for the beneficial clinical effects.

Literatur

1. Büchler M, Frieß H, Klempa I (1992) Role of octreotide in the prevention of postoperative complications following pancreatic resection. Am J Surg 163:125–131
2. Creutzfeldt W, Lembcke B, Fölsch UR (1987) Effect of somatostatin analogue on pancreatic secretion in humans. Am J Med 82:49–52
3. Klempa I, Baca I, Menzel J, Schuszdiarra V (1991) Auswirkung von Somatostatin auf die basale und stimulierte exokrine Pankreassekretion nach partieller Duodenopankreatektomie. Chirurg 62:293–296
4. Solomon ET (1987) Effect of somatostatin on exocrine pancreas. In: Reichlin S (ed) Somatostatin basic and clinical status. Plenum, New York
5. Warshaw AL, Swanson RS (1988) Pancreatic cancer in 1988: possibilities and probabilities. Ann Surg 208:541–544

Dr. Th. Bömmer, Klinik für Allgemein- und Gefäßchirurgie, Zentralkrankenhaus, St.-Jürgen-Straße, W-2800 Bremen

Können Reperfusionsschäden bei Lebertransplantation durch die Applikation von PAF-Antagonisten oder Aprotinin verringert werden?

Is It Possible to Reduce Reperfusion Injury During Liver Transplantation by Application of Platelet-Activating Factor Antagonists or Aprotinin?

J. Hauss[1], K. Oldhafer[1], H.U. Spiegel[2] und R. Pichlmayr[1]

[1]Abteilung Abdominal- und Transplantationschirurgie, Medizinische Hochschule Hannover
[2]Chirurgische Universitätsklinik, Münster

Einleitung

Das Ausmaß des sogenannten Reperfusionsschadens beeinflußt den klinischen Verlauf nach Lebertransplantation entscheidend. Stets sind primär die den Sinusoidalraum auskleidenden Zellen (Sinusendothelzellen, Kupffer'sche Sternzellen) betroffen, die arterielle und portalvenöse Sinusoidaldurchblutung wird gestört. Ein empfindlicher Angriffspunkt im Bereich der Sinusoidalwand scheint der Aufhängeapparat der Endothelzellen an der extrazellulären Matrix zu sein, der zum größten Teil aus Proteoglykanen besteht, die wiederum für Proteinasen eine Zielstruktur darstellen [1]. Als pharmakologischer Therapieansatz erschien daher der Einsatz von Proteinase-Inhibitoren beim Transplantatempfänger vor und während der Reperfusionsphase sinnvoll [2]. In der vorliegenden experimentellen Studie wurde überprüft, ob durch die Applikation eines PAF-Antagonisten (WEB 2170) oder von Aprotinin beim Empfängertier Störungen der Leberhämodynamik vermieden bzw. zelluläre Schädigungen verringert werden können.

Methodik

Insgesamt wurden 3 Gruppen von jeweils 7 Schweinen (KG: 20–30 kg) in Neuroleptanästhesie transplantiert, Spender- und Empfängertier stammten jeweils aus dem gleichen Wurf; die Tierversuche waren genehmigt (Nr. 504-42502-90/405). Das Versuchsmodell wurde dem Ablauf einer klinischen orthotopen Lebertransplantation angepaßt [3]. Neben der Volumensubstitution erhielt das Empfängertier eine Vollbluttransfu-

Chirurgisches Forum 1993
f. experim. u. klinische Forschung
Becker/Beger/Hartel (Hrsg.)

sion (400 ml), die bei der Spenderoperation entnommen wurde. Immunsuppressiva und Steroide wurden nicht appliziert, da diese Substanzen den Reperfusionsschaden beeinflussen können [4]. Die Arterialisierung des Transplantates wurde mit einem thorakalen Aortensegment standardisiert, um vergleichende Messungen der arteriellen Leberdurchblutung zu ermöglichen. Die kalte Ischämiezeit betrug $5{,}9 \pm 0{,}5$ h, die Schwerkraftperfusion erfolgte mit kalter HTK-Lösung (Bretschneider) über die Pfortader ($p = 15$ mmHg) und die Aorta abdominalis ($p = 120$ mmHg). Bei der Empfängeroperation wurde ein heparinisierter passiver cavo-porto-jugulärer Y-Bypass verwendet, der Spendergallengang wurde zunächst geschient. Zur Vermeidung von postoperativen Magenentleerungsstörungen wurde eine Seit/Seit-Gastrojejunostomie angelegt. 6 h nach Revaskularisation erfolgte in gleicher Narkose eine geplante Relaparotomie mit erneuter Kontrolle des vollständigen Meßprogramms. Der Gallengang wurde anschließend mit einer Seit/Seit Choledocho-Choledochostomie anastomosiert. Katheter in der mittleren V. hepatica und in der A. carotis wurden belassen, subkutan nach dorsal getunnelt, ausgeleitet und fixiert.

Der PAF-Antagonist WEB 2170 wurde 7 Tieren kontinuierlich (0,1 mg/kg KG/h) während der anhepatischen Phase bis 6 h nach Revaskularisation appliziert, in der Aprotinin-Gruppe ($n = 7$) wurde nach der Hepatektomie ein Bolus von 20.000 KIU/kg KG gegeben, gefolgt von einer kontinuierlichen Infusion von 7.500 KIU/kg KG/h bis 6 h nach Reperfusion. Als wesentliche Parameter wurden die Enzymanstiege, der Gewebe-pO_2 der Leber – gemessen mit der Mehrdrahtoberflächenelektrode nach Kessler und Lübbers [5] – sowie die Druck- und Flußverhältnisse der Pfortader, Leberarterie und Lebervene kontrolliert. Am 5. postoperativen Tag wurden die Tiere nach erneuter Laparotomie und komplettem Untersuchungsprogramm in tiefer Narkose durch Applikation von 40 ml KCl 7,45% getötet.

Ergebnisse

Trotz der relativ langen Narkosedauer von durchschnittlich 10 h (Transplantation, Relaparotomie nach 6 h) wurden die Eingriffe in der Regel problemlos toleriert. 17 von insgesamt 21 Tieren wurden planmäßig am 5. postoperativen Tag getötet. Zwei Tiere aus der Kontrollgruppe und jeweils ein Tier aus beiden Therapiegruppen verstarben vorzeitig an kardialen ($n = 2$), pulmonalen ($n = 1$) bzw. hepatischen ($n = 1$) Komplikationen. Die maximalen Anstiege der Leberenzyme (GOT, GLDH) im Serum am 1. postoperativen Tag wurden in beiden Therapiegruppen reduziert, die Unterschiede waren jedoch nur in der Aprotinin-Gruppe signifikant (Tabelle 1). Die gepoolten pO_2-Histogramme der Leber waren in der Kontrollgruppe nach Freigabe der portalen Reperfusion deutlich linksverschoben mit zahlreichen hypoxischen Werten (42% > 10 mmHg), nach der Arterialisation fand sich ein markanter Rechtsshift (MW des gepoolten pO_2-Histogramms: 75,6 mmHg). Diese Effekte wurden sowohl durch die Applikation des PAF-Antagonisten als auch durch Aprotinin fast aufgehoben. Hämodynamisch fiel in allen Gruppen 1 h nach Reperfusion eine starke Erhöhung des arteriellen Flusses auf, verbunden mit einem drastischen Abfall des arteriellen und portal-venösen Gefäßwiderstandes. Nach 6 h waren sowohl in der Kontrollgruppe als auch in der WEB 2170-Gruppe die arteriellen Flußraten noch weiter angestiegen, während diese in der Aprotiningruppe konstant blieben.

Tabelle 1. Maximaler Anstieg der GOT und GLDH im Serum am 1. postoperativen Tag ($x + s_x$)

	Kontrollgruppe	WEB 2170	Aprotinin
GOT (U/l)	697 ± 121	526 ± 69	464 ± 82[a]
GLDH (U/l)	41 ± 15	24 ± 10	15 ± 5[a]

[a] Signifikanzniveau $p \leq 0{,}05$

Zusammenfassung

In einem Lebertransplantationsmodell am Schwein wurde überprüft, ob durch die Applikation eines PAF-Antagonisten (WEB 2170) oder von Aprotinin beim Empfängertier der sogenannte Reperfusionsschaden verringert werden kann. Als wesentliche Parameter wurden die Enzymanstiege im Serum, der Gewebe-pO_2 der Leber sowie die Druck- und Flußverhältnisse der Pfortader, Leberarterie und Lebervene kontrolliert. Die Enzymanstiege im Serum waren in beiden Versuchsgruppen geringer, die Unterschiede waren in der Aprotinin-Gruppe signifikant. Bei der Messung des Gewebe-pO_2 und der hämodynamischen Parameter fiel nur auf, daß bei allen Kontrolltieren zunächst eine Gewebehypoxie, anschließend eine ausgeprägte "reaktive Hyperoxygenierung" der Leber nach der Arterialisierung resultierte. Diese Effekte wurden deutlich durch die Applikation von Aprotinin, weniger markant durch Gabe des PAF-Antagonisten reduziert,

Summary

In a pig liver transplantation model we investigated whether reperfusion injury can be reduced by administering a platelet (PAF) activating antagonist (WEB 2170) or aprotinin to the recipient. As important parameters, maximal serum enzyme release was measured, tissue pO_2 of the liver was controlled with a multiwire surface electrode and hemodynamics were monitored by recording flow and pressure changes in the portal vein, hepatic artery and hepatic vein. Serum enzyme (GOT, GLDH) release was lowered in both groups, the differences being significant only in the aprotinin group. As far as the measurements of tissue pO_2 and hemodynamic parameters were concerned, it was shown that in all control animals at first liver tissue became hypoxic; this reaction was followed by a distinct "reactive hyperoxygenation" of the liver after arterialization. These effects were markedly reduced by application of aprotinin; the influence of the PAF antagonist was minor.

Literatur

1. Holloway CMB, Harvey PRC, Strasberg SM (1990) Viability of sinusoidal lining cells in cold-preserved rat liver allografts. Transplantation 49:225–229
2. Oldhafer KJ, Schüttler W, Wiehe B, Hauss J, Pichlmayr R (1991) Treatment of preservation/reperfusion liver injury by the protease inhibitor aprotinin after cold ischemic storage. Transpl Proc 23:2380–2381
3. Hauss J, Spiegel H-U, Oldhafer K, Pichlmayr R (1992) Entwicklungen der experimentellen Leberchirurgie und Lebertransplantation. In: Kronberger L (Hrsg) Experimentelle Chirurgie. Enke Verlag, S 146–156
4. Kawano K, Kim Y, Goto S, Nagai T, Ehashira T, Yamanaka Y, Kobayashi M (1990) Evidence that azathioprine, as well as cyclosporine, ameliorates warm ischemia in the rat. Transplantation 49:1002–1003
5. Hauss J, Schönleben K, Spiegel H-U (1982) Therapiekontrolle durch Überwachung des Gewebe-pO_2. Verlag Hans Huber, Bern

Gefördert durch die Volkswagen-Stiftung (I/65850).

Prof. Dr. J. Hauss, Abteilung für Abdominal- und Transplantationschirurgie, Medizinische Hochschule Hannover, Konstanty-Gutschow-Straße 8, W-3000 Hannover 61

Bedeutung der simultanen arteriellen und portalen Reperfusion bei der Lebertransplantation

Impact of Simultaneous Declamping of Hepatic Artery and Portal Vein in Liver Transplantation

P. Palma[1], A.P. Gonzalez[1], M. Rentsch[1], M.D. Menger[1] und S. Post[2]

[1]Institut für Chirurgische Forschung, Ludwig-Maximilians-Universität, München
[2]Chirurgische Universitätsklinik, Heidelberg

Einleitung

Während der anhepatischen Phase kommt es bei klinischer Lebertransplantation, auch bei Verwendung eines Bypass, zum Blutstau im portalen Kreislauf und zur langsamen Erwärmung des Transplantats während Ischämie [1]. Zur Verkürzung der anhepatischen Phase wird daher von vielen Chirurgen die frühe portale Reperfusion mit nachfolgender arterieller Anastomosierung bevorzugt. Bisher ungeklärt ist die Frage, welche Auswirkungen diese initial fehlende arterielle Reperfusion für die frühe Funktion des Transplantats hat. In der vorliegenden Studie sollte der Einfluß simultaner (SA) im Vergleich zu verzögerter arterieller Reperfusion (VA) bei der Transplantation der Rattenleber auf verschiedene Indikatoren des Reperfusionsschadens, i.e. mikrovaskuläre Perfusion, Leukozyten-Akkumulation und hepatozelluläre Funktion *in vivo* quantitativ analysiert werden.

Material und Methoden

Nach Prämedikation mit Atropin (0,1 mg/kg s.c.) wurde bei 20 männlichen Lewis-Ratten (170–290 g) eine syngene orthotope Lebertransplantation in Äthernarkose durchgeführt. Die Leber des Spendertieres wurde "in situ" über die Aorta mit 10–15 ml kalter UW-Lösung (4°C) perfundiert (Perfusionsdruck von 100 cm Wassersäule) und 24 h bei 4°C in UW-Lösung gelagert. Bei der Empfänger-Operation wurde, um kardiale Komplikationen zu vermeiden, die Leber kurz vor Reperfusion mit 15 ml Ringer-Laktat (4°C) über die Portalvene ausgespült [2]. Die Reperfusion des Transplantats erfolgte durch Entfernen der Gefäßclips in folgender Reihenfolge: Suprahepatische Vena cava, infrahepatische Vena cava, Vena portae. Die arterielle Anastomosierung und Freigabe des Blutstroms erfolgte entweder simultan mit der portalen (SA-Gruppe, n = 8) oder verzögert 8 min nach portaler Reperfusion (VA-Gruppe, n = 12). Die Mikrozirkulation des linken Leberlappens des Transplantats wurde 30 bis 90 min nach portaler Reperfusion mittels intravitaler Fluoreszenzmikroskopie analysiert [2]. Azinäre Perfusion (Index: (Anzahl gut perfundierter + 0,5 × Anzahl irre-

Chirurgisches Forum 1993
f. experim. u. klinische Forschung
Becker/Beger/Hartel (Hrsg.)

gulär perfundierter)/(Gesamtzahl der untersuchten Azini) und sinusoidale Perfusion (in %) wurden nach i.v. Injektion von Na-Fluoreszein bestimmt. Die Akkumulation von Leukozyten in Sinusoiden und postsinusoidalen Venolen wurde nach in vivo Anfärbung der Leukozyten mit Rhodamin-G beurteilt. Die Quantifizierung der mikrozirkulatorischen Parameter erfolgte durch Bild-zu-Bild Videoanalyse. Die hepatozelluläre Funktion des Organs wurde durch Messung der Galleproduktion während 90 min Reperfusion bestimmt. Alle Ergebnisse sind als Mittelwert ± SEM (Standardfehler des Mittelwerts) angegeben. Zur statistischen Analyse wurde eine multifaktorielle Varianzanalyse durchgeführt.

Ergebnisse

Nach simultaner arterieller und portaler Reperfusion (SA) waren sowohl die azinäre als auch die sinusoidale Perfusion im Vergleich zu den arteriell verzögert reperfundierten Transplantaten (VA) signifikant ($p < 0{,}01$) verbessert (Tabelle 1). Die Zahl adhärierender Leukozyten war bei SA-Tieren sowohl in Sinusoiden als auch in postsinusoidalen Venolen deutlich niedriger als bei VA-Tieren. Zusätzlich fand sich nach simultaner Reperfusion im Vergleich zur VA-Gruppe während der ersten 90 min Reperfusion eine signifikant ($p < 0{,}05$) höhere Galleproduktion (Tabelle 1).

Tabelle 1. Mikrovaskuläre Perfusion, Leukozyten-Akkumulation und Organfunktion während 90 min Reperfusion nach Lebertransfusion bei der Ratte

	VA-Gruppe	SA-Gruppe	p-Wert
Mikrovaskuläre Perfusion			
Perfundierte Azini (Index)	0,64 ± 0,04	0,89 ± 0,03	p<0,01
Perfundierte Sinusoide (%)	78,9 ± 1,5	92,4 ± 1,1	p<0,001
Leukozytenadhärenz			
in Sinusoiden (pro mm^2 Leberoberfl.)	248 ± 12	205 ± 13	p<0,01
in postsinusoidalen Venolen (pro mm^2 Endothel)	650 ± 39	239 ± 29	p<0,01
Hepatozelluläre Funktion			
Gallefluß (ml/90 min/100 g Leber)	0,95 ± 0,4	2,24 ± 0,7	p<0,05

SA = simultane arterielle Reperfusion; VA = verzögerte arterielle Reperfusion. (Mittelwert ± Standardfehler des Mittelwerts; multifaktorielle Varianzanalyse)

Diskussion

Die Rekonstruktion der Arteria hepatica ist für die Reduktion des postischämischen Reperfusionsschadens auch im Modell der Rattenleber-Transplantation von entscheidender Bedeutung [3]. Zusätzlich berichteten Neuhaus und Mitarbeiter [4], daß sowohl bei experimenteller als auch bei klinischer Lebertransplantation durch simultane arterielle und portale Reperfusion die Freisetzung hepatozellulärer Enzyme (Indikator des hepatozellulären Schadens) im Vergleich zu verzögerter arterieller Reperfusion reduziert werden kann. Die vorliegende Studie zeigt, daß bei orthotoper Lebertransplantation in der Ratte nach 24 h kalter Ischämie durch simultane Freigabe von Vena portae und Arteria hepatica der mikrovaskuläre Perfusionsausfall, Leukozyten-Akkumulation und Transplantat-Dysfunktion signifikant vermindert sind. Sowohl das mikrovaskuläre Perfusionsversagen, als auch die Aktivierung, Akkumulation und Adhärenz von Leukozyten mit Freisetzung von Sauerstoff-Radikalen werden als spezifische Indikatoren des Reperfusionsschadens nach kalter Ischämie angesehen [5]. Verzögerte arterielle Reperfusion (VA) der transplantierten Lebern hatte eine deutliche Zunahme des Reperfusionsschadens zur Folge. Sowohl die Akkumulation von Leukozyten als auch das mikrovaskuläre Perfusionsversagen waren nach VA verstärkt. Weiterhin war bei verzögerter arterieller Reperfusion die initiale Galleproduktion signifikant niedriger, was eine Einschränkung der hepatozellulären Funktion des Transplantats widerspiegelt. Diese Ergebnisse legen nahe, bei klinischer Lebertransplantation zur Verminderung des Reperfusionsschadens die Reperfusion erst nach Fertigstellung der portalen und arteriellen Anastomose freizugeben.

Zusammenfassung

Mittels intravitaler Fluoreszenzmikroskopie (IVM) wurde der Einfluß der simultanen arteriellen Reperfusion auf die Mikrozirkulation und Primärfunktion bei der Lebertransplantation an der Ratte untersucht. Bei 20 männlichen Lewis-Ratten erfolgte in Äther-Anästhesie nach 24 h Konservierung in UW-Lösung eine syngene orthotope Lebertransplantation. Die arterielle Reperfusion erfolgte entweder simultan mit portaler (SA-Gruppe, n = 8) oder verzögert 8 min nach portaler Reperfusion (VA-Gruppe, n = 12). Die Mikrozirkulation wurde 60–90 min nach Reperfusion mittels IVM beurteilt. Die hepatozelluläre Funktion der Transplantate wurde anhand der Galleproduktion des Transplantats während der ersten 90 min Reperfusion bestimmt. Nach simultaner arterieller Reperfusion waren mikrovaskuläres Perfusionsversagen, Leukozyten-Akkumulation und -Adhärenz, sowie Transplantat-Dysfunktion signifikant geringer. Diese Ergebnisse legen nahe, zur Verminderung des Reperfusionsschadens bei klinischer Lebertransplantation die Reperfusion erst nach Fertigstellung der portalen und arteriellen Anastomose freizugeben.

Summary

The impact of simultaneous declamping of hepatic artery and portal vein on hepatic microcirculation and primary function of liver grafts was analyzed in vivo using intravital fluorescence microscopy (IVM). Under ether anesthesia orthotopic liver transplantation was performed in 20 male Lewis rats after cold storage of the liver in University of Wisconsin (UW) solution for 24 h. Arterial reperfusion was established either simultaneously with portal declamping (SA group, n = 8) or after a 8-min interval (VA group, n = 12). Quantitative analysis of the microcirculation was performed 60–90 min after onset of portal reperfusion by means of IVM. Hepatocellular function of the grafts was analyzed based on the bile flow during the first 90 min of reperfusion. SA resulted in significant reduction of leukocyte accumulation as well as improvement of microvascular perfusion and hepatocellular function. In view of these results, it would appear to be useful to complete both portal and arterial anastomoses before initiation of reperfusion in order to reduce microcirculatory deterioration and primary dysfunction in liver transplantation.

Literatur

1. Starzl TE, Demetris AJ (1990) Liver transplantation. A 31-year perspective. 1st ed. Year Book Medical Pibl., Chicago, pp 21–23
2. Post S, Rentsch M, Palma P, Gonzalez AP, Menger MD (1993) Assessment of microhemodynamics after liver transplantation by in vivo microscopy in the rat. Transplant Proc, im Druck
3. Post S, Menger MD, Rentsch M, Gonzalez AP, Herfarth C, Messmer K (1992) Impact of arterialization on hepatic microcirculation and leukocyte accumulation after liver transplantation in the rat. Transplantation 54:789–794
4. Neuhaus P, Brölsch CE, Ringe B, Pichlmayr R (1985) Experimental liver transplantation. In: Gips CH, Krom RAF (eds) Progress in liver transplantation. Nartinus Nijhoff, Boston, pp 13–22
5. Marzi I, Walcher F, Menger MD, Bühren V, Trentz O (1991) Microcirculatory disturbances and leukocyte adherence in transplanted livers after cold storage in Euro-Collins-, UW-, and HTK-solution. Transplant Int 4:45–50

Dr. med. P. Palma, Institut für Chirurgische Forschung, Klinikum Großhadern, Marchioninistraße 15, W-8000 München 70

Hepatocytentransplantation unter Einsatz dreidimensionaler, polymerer Stützgerüste und hepatotropher Stimulation

Hepatocyte Transplantation Using Three-Dimensional Polymer Scaffolds and Hepatotrophic Stimulation

P.M. Kaufmann[1,3], S. Uyama[1,2], T. Takeda[1], C.E. Brölsch[3] und J.P. Vacanti[1]

[1]Department of Surgery, Children's Hospital and Harvard Medical School, USA
[2]Second Department of Surgery, Kyoto University, Japan
[3]Department of General Surgery, University of Hamburg, Germany

Einleitung

Lebertransplantation ist die etablierte Therapie für Lebererkrankungen im Endstadium. Der Mangel an Spenderorganen nimmt jedoch weiterhin zu. Aus diesem Grund gibt es ein deutliches Interesse an Zelltransplantationsmethoden als Ersatztherapie für Enzymmangelerkrankungen und als supportive Therapie bei akutem und chronischem Leberversagen [1]. Unser Labor untersucht die Möglichkeiten zellbeladener, polymerer Matrizes als Mittel zur Schaffung neuen Ersatzgewebes [3]. Die erfolgreiche Hepatocytentransplantation in prävaskularisierte PVA Matrizes konnte bereits demonstriert werden.

Es ist bekannt, daß hepatotrophe Stimulation für die Erhaltung von Lebergewebe notwendig ist. Diese Stimulation wird durch komplette Hepatocytenmitogene wie EGF, TGFα und HGF-A sowie durch wachstumsfördernde Faktoren wie Insulin und Glukagon gewährleistet [4]. Die Mehrzahl dieser Faktoren stammt aus dem Ursprungsgebiet der Portalvene [5]. In dieser Studie soll nun geklärt werden, ob die Ansiedlung und Proliferation von transplantierten Hepatocyten durch den Einsatz einer portocavalen Shuntoperation in Kombination mit einer partiellen Hepatektomie verbessert werden kann.

Materialien und Methoden

Männliche LEW Ratten dienten als Spender bzw. Empfänger. Die Empfänger wurden in die Gruppen A, B und C aufgeteilt. Operationen wurden unter Methoxyfluranänästhesie durchgeführt. Vier PVA Schwämme (1,2 cm Durchmesser; 0,5 cm Höhe) wurden als Matrizes für die zu transplantierenden Hepatocyten in Mesenterialtaschen jedes Empfängers implantiert. Eine Woche zuvor wurde ein PCS (portocavaler Shunt) bei den Ratten der Gruppe B durchgeführt. Nach einer fünftägigen Prävaskularisationsphase für die PVA Matrizes folgte eine 70% HE in den Gruppen A und B sowie der Transplantation von 5×10^7 Hepatocyten in den Gruppen A,

Chirurgisches Forum 1993
f. experim. u. klinische Forschung
Becker/Beger/Hartel (Hrsg.)

B und C. Die Hepatocyten waren zuvor durch eine modifizierte Kollagenaseperfusionsmethode gewonnen worden [2]. Am Tag 0, 3 und 7 nach der Transplantation wurden aus jeder Gruppe 8 PVA Matrizes computergestützten morphometrischen Untersuchungen zur Quantifikation der Hepatocytenareale unterzogen. Hepatocytenareale wurden in $\mu m^2/60\ mm^2$ Schnittfläche (1,2 cm × 5 cm) angegeben. Zum Studium der DNA-Syntheserate wurden am 3. Tag nach der Hepatozytentransplantation (HCTx) BrdU-Färbungen in allen Gruppen durchgeführt. Der prozentuale Anteil der positiv gefärbten Hepatocyten an der Gesamtzahl wurde bestimmt.

Alle Ergebnisse wurden als Mittelwert und Standardfehler (SEM) angegeben. Zur Signifikanzanalyse wurde Student's t-Test angewandt und Werte $\leq 0{,}05$ als signifikant betrachtet.

Ergebnisse

Im Vergleich zum Hepatocytenareal am Tage der Transplantation ($139125 \pm 28439\ \mu m^2$) ist am 3. Tag ein Rückgang in allen drei Gruppen zu beobachten. Dieser Zellverlust ist am größten in Gruppe C verglichen mit den Gruppen A ($p = 0{,}005\ \mu m^2$) und B ($0{,}006\ \mu m^2$). Der Vergleich zwischen den Gruppen A ($60166 \pm 16148 \mu m^2$) und B ($107898 \pm 32396 \mu m^2$) zeigte höhere Werte für Gruppe B. Dieser Unterschied war jedoch nicht statistisch signifikant.

Sieben Tage nach HCTx war der Unterschied zwischen Gruppe C ($3217 \pm 2262 \mu m^2$) und Gruppe A ($11523 \pm 3076 \mu m^2$) nahezu signifikant ($p = 0{,}050$). Der Vergleich der Gruppen C und B ($84721 \pm 26841 \mu m^2$) ergab einen p Wert von 0,007. Ein signifikanter Unterschied fand sich auch zwischen den Gruppen A und B ($p = 0{,}013$) (Abb. 1).

Die Analyse der BrdU-Inkorporation am 3. Tag nach HCTx zeigte, daß in Gruppe C $1,20 \pm 0,66\%$ der Hepatocyten positiv bezüglich einer aktiven DNA Synthese waren. Der Wert für Gruppe A betrug $4,74 \pm 0,88\%$ und $4,46 \pm 0,67\%$ in Gruppe B. Die Unterschiede zwischen den Gruppen C und A ($p = 0{,}005$) sowie zwischen den Gruppen C und B ($p = 0{,}007$) waren signifikant (Abb. 2).

Diskussion

In den letzten Jahren hat unser Labor in Zusammenarbeit mit dem Massachusetts Institute of Technology Studien zur selektiven Zelltransplantation unter Einsatz künstlicher Polymere als Matrizes durchgeführt. PVA-Schwämme haben gegenüber natürlichen Implantationsregionen, wie z.B. der Milz, den Vorteil, größere Räume für die Zellansiedlung zu bieten. Um das Einwachsen und die Proliferation der Hepatocyten zu optimieren, wurde eine in-vivo Prävaskularisation der Matrizes etabliert. Dies gewährleistet außer der Versorgung mit nutritiven Substanzen einen verbesserten Zugang zu Faktoren, die die Viabilität und Proliferation der Hepatocyten beeinflussen. Die Ergebnisse dieser Studie deuten darauf hin, daß eine deutliche Erhöhung dieses Effektes durch eine 70%ige Hepatektomie des Empfängers erreicht wird.

Abgesehen von dem erhöhten absoluten Hepatocytenareal findet sich eine statistisch signifikante relative Steigerung der DNA Synthese am dritten Tag nach der HCTx im

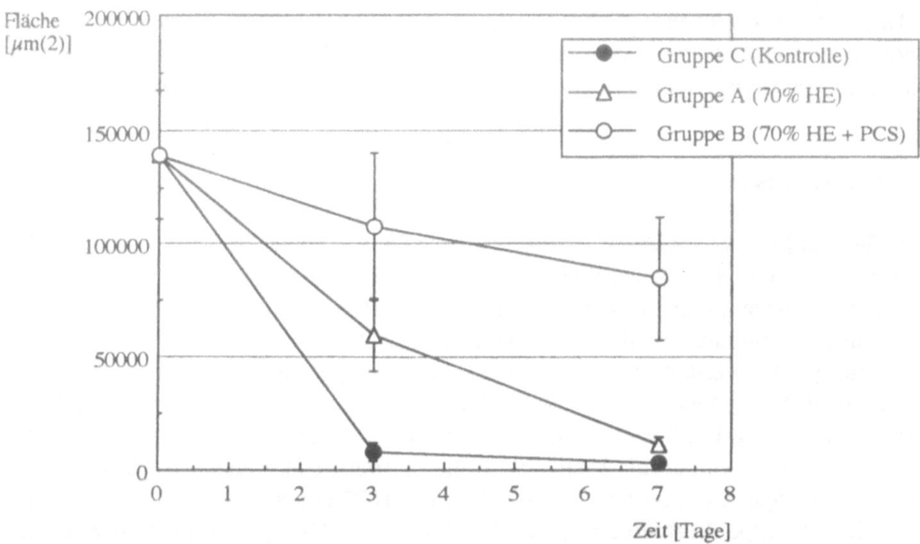

Abb. 1. Ergebnisse der morphometrischen Hepatocytenarealbestimmung in den PVA Matrizes am 3. und 7. Tag nach Transplantation sowie Ausgangswert am Tag der Transplantation. [μm^2 Hepatocyten pro 60 mm^2 Schnittfläche]

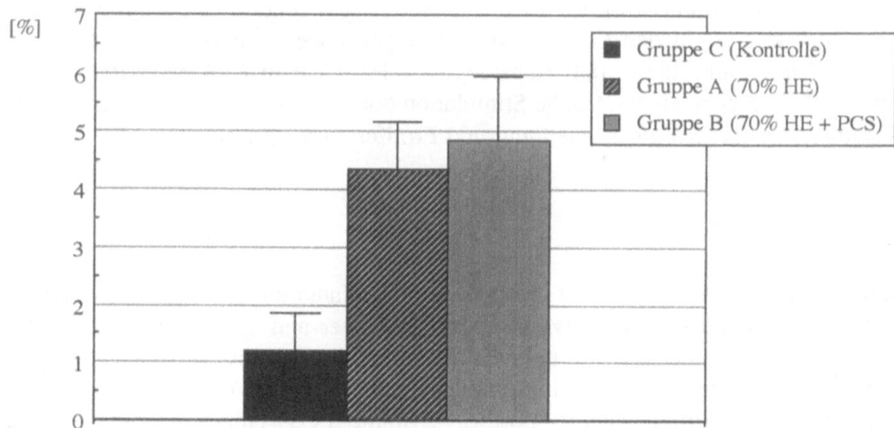

Abb. 2. Relativer Anteil der Hepatocyten mit aktiver DNA Synthese im BrdU-Test. Drei Tage nach HCTx. [% der Gesamthepatocytenfläche]

Vergleich zur nicht stimulierten Kontrollgruppe. Der Einfluß des PCS zeigt sich am 7. Tag nach der Transplantation in einem signifikant vergrößerten Zellareal, verglichen mit einer Stimulation durch partielle Hepatektomie alleine. Aber auch ohne PCS findet sich zu diesem Zeitpunkt ein signifikanter Unterschied zur nicht stimulierten Versuchsgruppe.

Diese Studie zeigt somit den erheblichen positiven Beitrag zur Optimierung der Ansiedlung und Proliferation von Hepatocyten durch die Kombination aus portocavalem Shunt und partieller Hepatektomie als Mittel der hepatotrophen Stimulation.

Zusammenfassung

Die Entwicklung von Methoden zur Transplantation großer Hepatozytenzahlen, bis hin zu einem Organäquivalent, stellt eine zukunftsträchtige Alternative zur etablierten Lebertransplantation bzw. Leberteiltransplantation dar. Bewährt hat sich hierbei der Einsatz dreidimensionaler, prävascularisierter Polyvinylalkohol-Matrizes (PVA). Es sollte geklärt werden, ob eine portocavale Shuntoperation (PCS) in Kombination mit einer 70% Hepatektomie die Ansiedlung und Proliferation transplantierter Hepatocyten verbessert. Dazu dienten männliche Lewisratten als Spender bzw. Empfänger. PVA-Schwämme wurden als Matrizes für die zu transplantierenden Hepatocyten implantiert. Gruppe A erhielt 5×10^7 Hepatocyten (HCTx) und eine 70% Hepatektomie (70% HE). Gruppe B erhielt PVS, 70% HE und HCTx. Gruppe C erhielt als Kontrolle nur HCTx. Morphometrische Untersuchungen zur Quantifikation der Hepatocytenareale fanden am Tag 0, 3 und 7 nach der Transplantation statt. Immunhistologie zum Studium der DNA Synthese wurde ebenfalls durchgeführt. Eine Woche nach HCTx zeigte die Gruppe B im Vergleich zu Gruppe A signifikant größere Hepatocytenareale ($p = 0{,}013$). Der Unterschied zwischen den Gruppen A und C war ebenfalls signifikant ($p = 0{,}005$). Immunhistologische Untersuchungen zeigten eine signifikant höhere DNA Syntheserate in den Gruppen A und B gegenüber Gruppe C ($p = 0{,}005$; $p = 0{,}007$). Wir schlußfolgern, daß Hepatocyten erfolgreich in PVA Matrizes transplantiert werden können. Hepatotrophe Stimulation durch portocavalen Shunt und partielle Hepatektomie fördern die Ansiedlung und Proliferation signifikant.

Summary

In the future the development of methods for transplantation of large hepatocyte numbers could provide an alternative to established liver and split liver transplantation. The use of three-dimensional prevascularized polyvinyl alcohol (PVA) scaffolds have allowed hepatocyte transplantation equivalent to a whole liver. The purpose of this study was to determine whether portocaval shunt (PCS) enhances engraftment and proliferation of transplanted hepatocytes if combined with a 70% hepatectomy (70% HE). Male Lewis rats served as donors and recipients, respectively. PVA sponges were implanted as matrices for the transplanted hepatocytes. Recipient animals were divided into three groups. Group A received 70% HE and transplantation of 5×10^7 hepatocytes. Group B received PCS, 70% HE, and hepatocyte transplantation (HCTx). Group C received only HCTx. Quantitative morphometric analysis of hepatocyte area was performed on day 0, 3, and 7 after transplantation. BrdU staining was performed to study DNA synthesis in the graft. We found that PCS and partial hepatectomy lead to significantly greater cell area 1 week after transplantation than 70% HE alone ($p = 0,013$). Seventy percent HE provided a significantly larger cell area than the controls ($P = 0,005$). BrdU staining revealed a significantly higher DNA synthesis rate in groups A and B compared with group C ($P = 0,005$; $P = 0,007$). In conclusion, hepatocytes can be successfully transplanted into PVA devices. Engraftment and proliferation can be significantly enhanced by using portocaval shunt and partial hepatectomy as hepatotrophic stimulation.

Literatur

1. Stein JE, Gilbert JC, Hansen LK, Schloo B, Ingber D, Vacanti JP (1991) Hepatocyte transplantation into prevascularized porous matrices. Abstract Book, 22nd Annual Meeting of the American Pediatric Surgical Association, Lake Buena Vista, Florida, May 15–18
2. Aiken J, Cima L, Schloo B, Mooney D, Johnson L, Langer R, Vacanti JP (1990) Studies in rat liver perfusion for optimal harvest of hepatocytes. J Pediatr Surg 25(1):140–145
3. Vacanti JP, Morse MA, Saltzman WM, Domb AJ, Perez-Atayde A, Langer R (1988) Selective cell transplantation using bioabsorbable artificial polymers as matrices. J Pediatr Surg 23(1):3–9
4. Michalopoulos GK (1990) Liver regeneration: molecular mechanisms of growth control. FASEB J 4:176–187
5. Fisher B, Szuch P, Levine M, Fisher ER (1971) A portal blood factor as the humoral agent in liver regeneration. Science 171:575–577

P.-M. Kaufmann, Department of Surgery, Children's Hospital and Harvard Medical School, USA

Die Rolle von präformierten natürlichen Antikörpern und Komplement bei der hyperakuten Abstoßung ex vivo xenogen perfundierter Herzen

The Role of Preformed Natural Antibodies and Complement for the Hyperacute Rejection of Ex Vivo Xenogeneic Perfused Hearts

M. Müdsam[1], M. Suckfüll[1], O. Pieske[1], G. Höbel[1], R. Babic[2] und C. Hammer[1]

[1]Institut für Chirurgische Forschung, Ludwig-Maximilians-Universität, München
[2]Institut für Pathologie, Ludwig-Maximilians-Universität, München

Einleitung

Die Transplantation von Organen einer Spezies auf eine andere führt innerhalb von Minuten oder wenigen Stunden zur hyperakuten Abstoßung. Die dafür verantwortlichen Vorgänge sind nicht geklärt. Präformierten natürlichen Antikörpern (PNAK) vom IgG und IgM Typ wird eine entscheidende Rolle bei der hyperakuten Abstoßung xenogener Organe zugeschrieben. Man ging bisher davon aus, daß PNAK das Komplementsystem klassisch aktivieren und so ein xenogenes Organ schädigen [1]. Kürzlich publizierte Ergebnisse von Johnston et al. 1991 [2] konnten zeigen, daß auch in Abwesenheit von PNAK xenogen transplantierte Organe hyperakut abgestoßen werden. Die Autoren nahmen daher an, daß das Komplementsystem auch über den alternativen Weg aktiviert werden kann. Ziel der vorliegenden Studie war es zu untersuchen, ob die hyperakute Abstoßung eines Xenografts in Anwesenheit von PNAK zur klassischen (Antikörper-vermittelt) oder zur alternativen Aktivierung des Komplementsystems führt. Diese Frage wurde an ex-vivo mit humanem Blut perfundierten und arbeitenden Schweineherzen überprüft [3].

Material und Methoden

Es wurden Halothan resistente Schweine (Deutsche Landrasse, 8 kg) als Organspender verwendet. Die Tiere wurden mit Azaperon, Ketaminhydrochlorid und Xylacin prämediziert, tracheostomiert und die Narkose mit Halothan und N_2O aufrechterhalten.

Nach medianer Sternotomie wurden V. azygos und hemiazygos ligiert. Vor der Kardioplegie mit Bretschneider Lösung wurden V. cava inferior und superior unterbunden und die Aorta abgeklemmt. Das Herz wurde mit 4°C kalter Ringerlösung gekühlt. Für die ex-vivo Perfusion wurden die Pulmonalvenen ligiert, das Herz aus dem Situs präpariert und Konnektoren in Aorta, linken Vorhof und Pulmonalarterie

Chirurgisches Forum 1993
f. experim. u. klinische Forschung
Becker/Beger/Hartel (Hrsg.)

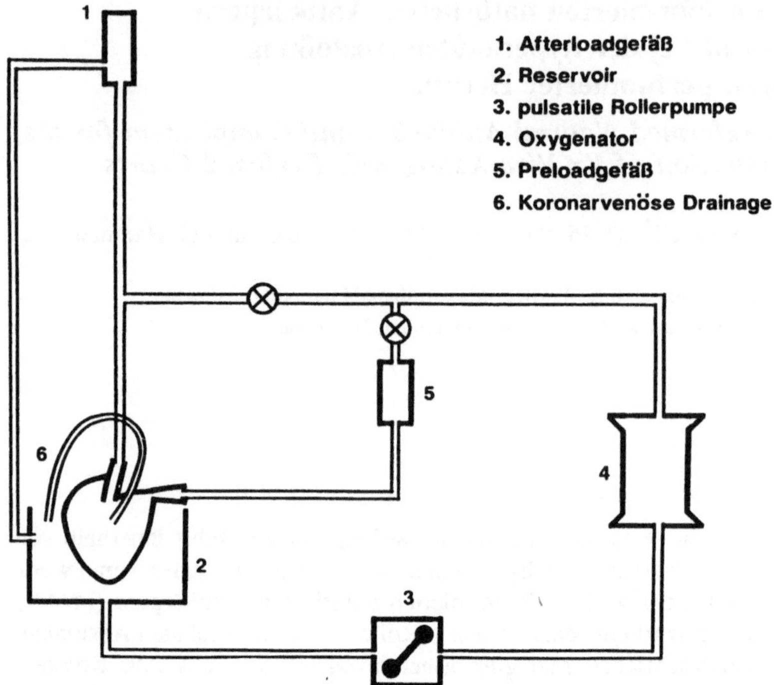

Abb. 1. Schematische Darstellung der Perfusionsanordnung eines "working heart model"

eingenäht. Nach 30 min Kardioplegiezeit wurde begonnen, das Herz im System zu perfundieren.

350 ml Blut wurden von einem Probanden unmittelbar vor Perfusionsbeginn gespendet, heparinisiert (50 I.U./ml) und mit Macrodex 6% (Knoll AG, Mannheim, Deutschland) auf einen Hämatokrit von 30% verdünnt.

Abbildung 1 zeigt das Perfusionssystem, das einer "working heart" Präparation entspricht. Blut gelangt über den linken Vorhof in den linken Ventrikel und wird gegen die Schwerkraft (entsprechend 55 mmHg) in ein Afterloadgefäß ausgeworfen. Von dort fließt es in ein Sammelgefäß und wird mittels einer pulsatilen Rollerpumpe über einen Oxygenator (DIDECO Masterflow; DIDECO s.p.a., P.O.Box 87, 41037 Mirandola, Italien) in ein Preloadgefäß geführt. Dieses ist 15 cm über dem linken Vorhof angeordnet, entsprechend einem definierten Preloaddruck von 11 mmHg. Die Versorgung des Myokards über die Koronarien wird durch die Pumparbeit des "working heart" wie in vivo gewährleistet. Das koronarvenöse Blut drainiert über das rechte Herz und die A. pulmonalis in das Sammelgefäß. Der Blut-pH wird durch Beimischung von CO_2 zu der für die Begasung des Oxygenators verwendeten Raumluft konstant gehalten. Calcium-Glukonat (500 mg/h; Braun Melsungen, Melsungen, Deutschland) und Glukose 20% (10 ml/h; Delta Pharma, 7417 Pfullingen, Deutschland) wurden über einen Perfusator appliziert.

Präformierte natürliche Antikörper-Titer wurden durch Hämagglutination von Schweineerythrozyten mit Plasma des Perfusats mit bzw. ohne Dithiothriol bestimmt.

Die komplement-lytische Aktivität des klassischen Weges wurde mittels mit Ambozeptor sensibilisierten Schaferythrozyten und Plasma des Perfusates bestimmt. Die durch Plasma verursachte Lyse wurde bei 578 nm spektrometrisch bestimmt und die Zeit bis zu einer Änderung der optischen Dichte von 500 Extinktionseinheiten gemessen (Behring Werke, Marburg, Deutschland).

Das Myokard wurde unmittelbar nach dem Versuch bei −75°C eingefroren. Für immunhistologische Färbungen wurden 4–6 μm dicke Schnitte angefertigt, luftgetrocknet und mit Aceton fixiert. Die endogene Peroxidase-Aktivität wurde mit H_2O_2 blockiert und unspezifische Bindungen durch Ziegenserum blockiert. Primärer und sekundärer Antikörper wurden hinzugefügt und Peroxidase mit Aminoethylcarbazol gefärbt. Polyklonale Antikörper vom Kaninchen gegen menschliches IgM, IgG, C1q, C4 und Faktor B wurden verwendet (DAKO Diagnostika GmbH, Hamburg, Deutschland). Polyklonale Peroxidase konjugierte Antikörper von der Ziege gegen Kaninchenimmunglobulin wurden als Zweitantikörper verwendet (DAKO Diagnostika GmbH, Hamburg, Deutschland).

Ergebnisse

Die mittleren PNAK-Titer vom IgM/IgG Typ sinken bereits innerhalb der ersten 5 min xenogener Perfusion von 1 : 128/1 : 8 auf 1 : 4/1 : 2 ab (Abb. 2). Die aus dem Serum absorbierten humanen Antikörper vom IgM und IgG-Typ lassen sich immunhistologisch vor allem auf dem Koronarendothel nachweisen. Die mittlere Komplementaktivität sinkt im Verlauf von 3-stündiger xenogener Perfusion von 70% auf 40% ab. Einen vergleichbaren Verlauf zeigt die mittlere Komplementaktivität auch bei autologer Perfusion (Abb. 3). Die immunhistologische Untersuchung des Komplementsystems weist den zentralen C3-Komplex im Myokard xenogen perfundierter Herzen nach. Allerdings können die ausschließlich bei klassischer Aktivierung des Komplementsystems auftretenden Fragmente C1q und C4 nicht nachgewiesen werden. Der als Marker für die Aktivierung des alternativen Weges gewählte Faktor B färbt sich immunhistologisch sowohl auf dem Koronarendothel als auch stellenweise auf der Oberfläche von Myozyten.

Zusammenfassung

Während xenogener ex-vivo Perfusion von Schweineherzen mit humanem Blut kommt es zur Absorption von PNAK vom IgM und vom IgG-Typ am Koronarendothel. Die im Hämoperfusat durch Aktivierung des klassischen Weges untersuchte Komplementaktivität nimmt im Verlauf von xenogener und autologer Perfusion in gleicher Weise ab. Dies ist durch die ex vivo Perfusionssituation bedingt; eine nennenswerte Aktivierung des klassischen Weges durch das Xenograft erfolgt nicht. Dies ist in Einklang mit den immunhistologischen Befunden. Zwar weist die Präsenz von C3d im Myokard auf eine Komplementaktivierung hin, diese erfolgt jedoch nicht über den klassischen

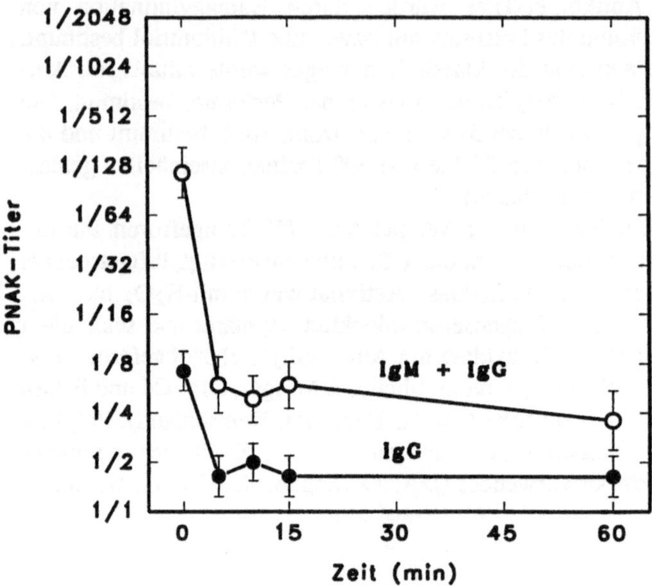

Abb. 2. Absorption präformierter natürlicher Antikörper während xenogener ex-vivo Perfusion von Schweineherzen mit humanem Blut. *Offene Kreise* entsprechen den mittleren Titern von IgG und IgM, *geschlossene Kreise* entsprechen den mittleren Titern von IgG (Spaltung mit DTT)

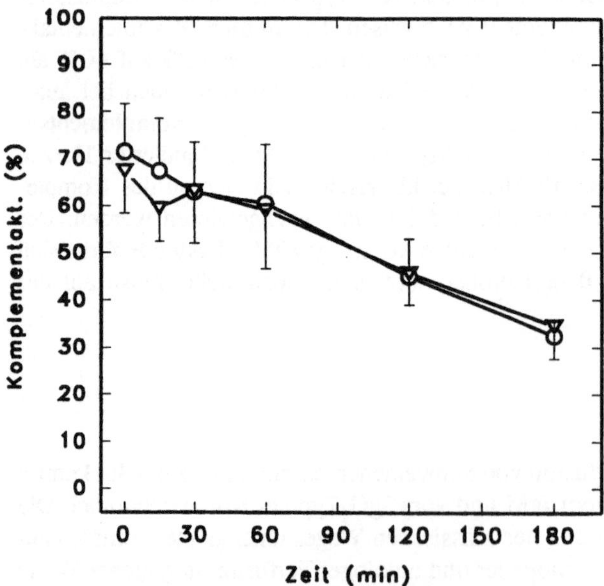

Abb. 3. Mittlere Komplementaktivitäten gemessen im Plasma während autologer (*Dreiecke*) und xenogener (*Kreise*) ex-vivo Perfusion von Schweineherzen mit humanem Blut

Weg; C1q und C4 konnten nicht nachgewiesen werden. Der Nachweis von Faktor B auf dem Koronarendothel ist indes als Marker für die Komplementaktivierung auf dem alternativen Weg zu werten. Wir gehen daher davon aus, daß die Komplement-vermittelte Schädigung eines Xenografts durch Aktivierung des alternativen Weges stattfindet und nicht durch Aktivierung des klassischen Weges.

Summary

Xenogeneic perfusion of porcine hearts with human blood leads to absorption of preformed natural antibodies (PNAB) at the coronary endothelium. Classically induced complement activity of the hemoperfusate decreases steadily during xenogeneic and autologous perfusion in a similar way. This is caused by the perfusion setting; xenogeneically perfused hearts induce no remarkable activation of the classical complement pathway. This is consistent with immunohistological findings. The presence of C3d in the myocardium proves complement activation. However, this is not induced by the classical pathway; C1q and C4 could not be demonstrated. Presence of staining for factor B on the coronary endothelium is a marker for complement activation via the alternative pathway. Therefore, we conclude, that complement-mediated damage during hyperacute rejection of a xenograft is induced by activation of the alternative pathway rather than the classical pathway.

Literatur

1. Platt JL, Fischel RJ, Matas AJ, Reif SA, Bolman RM, Bach FH (1991) Immunopathology of hyperacute xenograft rejection in a swine-to-primate model. Transpl 52:214–220
2. Johnston PS, Wang MWL, Wright L, White DJG (1991) Hyperacute rejection in the complete absence of antibody. Transpl Proc 23,1:877–879
3. Forty J, Metacalf M, White DJG, Wallwork J (1991) Development and use of an ex vivo heart model to study hyperacute xenograft rejection. Minerva Chir 46:123–127

Dr. M. Müdsam, Institut für Chirurgische Forschung, Ludwig-Maximilians-Universität, Marchioninistraße 15, W-8000 München 70

Signifikante Verlängerung des Transplantatüberlebens in einem stark inkompatiblen Rattensystem durch selektive Ausschaltung der α/β-TCR$^+$ T-Lymphozyten

Significant Prolongation of Graft Survival in a Strongly Incompatible Rat System by Selective Elimination of α/β-TCR$^+$ T-Lymphocytes

Ch. Dufter[1], J. Thies[1], S. Post[1], P. Terneß[2], S.C. Meuer[3] und G. Otto[1]

[1]Chirurgische Universitätsklinik, Heidelberg (Direktor: Prof. Dr. Ch. Herfarth)
[2]Institut für Transplantationsimmunologie, Heidelberg (Direktor: Prof. Dr. G. Opelz)
[3]Abteilung für Angewandte Immunologie, Deutsches Krebsforschungszentrum, Heidelberg (Direktor: Prof. Dr. S.C. Meuer)

Einleitung

Seitdem es Medawar erstmals gelungen ist, eine lebenslange Akzeptanz gegenüber fremdem Gewebe zu induzieren, steht die Frage nach den Mechanismen der Toleranzinduktion im Mittelpunkt immunologischer Forschung. Den Kliniker bewegen dabei hauptsächlich zwei Aspekte: die Funktionsfähigkeit eines transplantierten Organs zu verbessern und bedrohliche Abstoßungskrisen zu verhindern. Letztere sollten durch Vermeidung toxischer Immunsuppressiva, die die Gesundheit des Patienten gefährden, bewältigt werden [1]. Durch den Einsatz monoklonaler Antikörper, die modulierend in die T-Zellfunktion eingreifen, konnte ein verlängertes Transplantatüberleben induziert werden [2].

In den vorliegenden Untersuchungen im Rattensystem setzten wir den monoklonalen Antikörper R73 ein, der sich selektiv gegen den α/β-Rezeptor auf T-Lymphozyten richtet [3]. Die Präsenz von α/β-TCR$^+$ T-Lymphozyten wurde während des Behandlungszeitraumes mit durchflußzytometrischen Methoden ermittelt, und die Bildung von gegen R73 (= Mausimmunoglobulin) gerichteten Antikörpern im ELISA bestimmt.

Material und Methoden

Versuchstiere

Ingezüchtete, männliche Lewis-Ratten ($RT1^l$) als Organempfänger und DA-Ratten ($RT1^{avl}$) als Herztransplantatspender wurden vom Zentralinstitut für Versuchstierzucht in Hannover bezogen.

Operationsverfahren (Heterotope Herztransplantation)

Alle Operationsschritte wurden in Äther-Inhalationsnarkose ausgeführt. Nach der Explantation des Spenderherzens erfolgte der mikrochirurgische Wiederanschluß End-

Chirurgisches Forum 1993
f. experim. u. klinische Forschung
Becker/Beger/Hartel (Hrsg.)

zu-Seit in fortlaufender Nahttechnik mit 10/0 Polyamid heterotop an Aorta und V. cava inf. des Empfängertieres [4]. Die Transplantatfunktion wurde täglich im EKG überprüft. Zwischen Spender und Empfänger bestand eine starke Inkompatibilität hinsichtlich aller Klasse I- und II-Antigene des Haupthistokompatibilitätskomplexes.

Antikörper

Alkalische Phosphatase F(ab')$_2$-mouse anti-rat-IgG-F(ab')$_2$: zum Nachweis von Anti-R73-Antikörpern im ELISA; R73 mouse anti-rat-α/β-TCR-PE: Markierung des α/β-T-Zell-Rezeptors; OX19 mouse-anti-rat-CD5-FITC: pan-T-Zell-Marker; G4.18 mouse anti-rat-CD3-FITC: gerichtet gegen ein Oberflächenantigen, das mit dem T-Zell-Rezeptor assoziiert ist; Isotop-Kontrollantikörper als Negativkontrolle (alle von DIANOVA, Hamburg); X36 rat anti-mouse-κ-PE: Sekundärantikörper, zur Anfärbung des Maus-Antikörpers R73 (Becton-Dickinson, Heidelberg); R73 mouse anti-rat-α/β-TCR unkonjugiert (wurde freundlicherweise von Prof. Thomas Hünig, Institut für Immunologie und Virologie (Würzburg) zur Verfügung gestellt).

Durchflußzytometrie

Nach Auftrennung von 300 μl EDTA-Vollblut über Dichtegradientenzentrifugation, Erythrozytenlyse und Einstellen der Zellzahl auf 200 000 Zellen/100 μl wurden alle weiteren Inkubationsschritte mit sättigenden Antikörperkonzentrationen über jeweils 30 min bei 4° C durchgeführt: a) Inkubation mit 0,1 μg R73/100 μl; b) Zugabe von 10 μl eines rat anti-mouse-κ-PE Sekundärantikörpers, c) Abblocken freier Bindungsstellen mit 50 μl 5% Mausserum; d) Markierung der T-Zellen mit 0,6 μg anti-CD3-FITC bzw. 0,6 μg anti-Cd5-FITC. Die Ergebnisse wurden im FACScan (Becton Dickinson) ausgewertet.

ELISA (Nachweis von Anti-R73-Antikörpern)

Nach Beschichtung von 96-well-Mikrotiterplatten (Maxisorb, NUNC) mit 1,5 μg R73/Kavität wurden die Sera der Versuchstiere in einer Verdünnungsreihe aufgetragen. Die Extinktionswerte (Absorption bei 405 nm) wurden nach Inkubation mit einem F(ab')$_2$-mouse anti-rat-IgG-F(ab')$_2$-Antikörper und Substrat (PNP) mit den Positiv- und Negativkontrollen (Serum mit hohem Antikörpertiter bzw. ohne Antikörper) verglichen (Photometer SLT 340 ATC, SLT Instruments).

Ergebnisse

Transplantatüberlebenszeit

Gruppe I: junge Empfängertiere (6 Wochen)
Behandlungsschema: Tag −2 und −1 vor der Transplantation: je 1000 μg R73 ip, am Tag 0 (= Transplantation) und an den Tagen 3–18 Tagen jeden 3. Tag 100 μg R73 ip. Es lassen sich hinsichtlich der Transplantatüberlebenszeit zwei Untergruppen unterscheiden. Gruppe Ia: Bei 3 Tieren konnte eine langdauernde Verlängerung

der Transplantatüberlebenszeit (über 200 Tage) beobachtet werden. Gruppe Ib: Die Überlebenszeit bei 6 Tieren betrug 47 ± 22 Tage (Mittelwert ± SD).

Gruppe II: alte Empfängertiere (10 Wochen)
Gleiches Behandlungsschema.
Bei allen 14 Tieren dieser Gruppe wurde das Herztransplantat nach spätestens 33 Tagen abgestoßen, die mittlere Überlebenszeit betrug $19{,}6 \pm 5{,}2$ Tage.

Gruppe III (Kontrollgruppe): ohne Behandlung
Transplantatüberlebenszeit: $7 \pm 1{,}3$ Tage (s. Abb. 1)
Es zeigt sich sowohl eine signifikante Verlängerung der Transplantatüberlebenszeit bei den behandelten Tieren gegenüber der Kontrollgruppe, als auch innerhalb der behandelten Gruppe zwischen den jüngeren und älteren Tieren (p = 0,001; Wilcoxon-Test).

Prozentsatz der α/β-TCR$^+$ T-Lymphozyten

Zu Beginn der Behandlung nahm der Anteil der α/β-TCR$^+$ T-Lymphozyten im peripheren Blutbild ab. CD3-positive Zellen: Ausgangswert: 70%, Tag −1: 4%, Tag 0: 2%. Danach folgt ein stetiger Anstieg bis auf einen Wert von 64% am Tag 8. In der Einfachfärbung mit dem pan-T-Zell-Marker anti CD5 nahm die Zellzahl nach der Injektion von 72% auf 17% ab, erreichte aber bereits am Tag der Transplantation wieder einen Wert von 44%. Der Prozentsatz der T-Zellen in der Gruppe mit den älteren und jüngeren Tieren zeigte dabei einen ähnlichen Verlauf (s. Abb. 2).

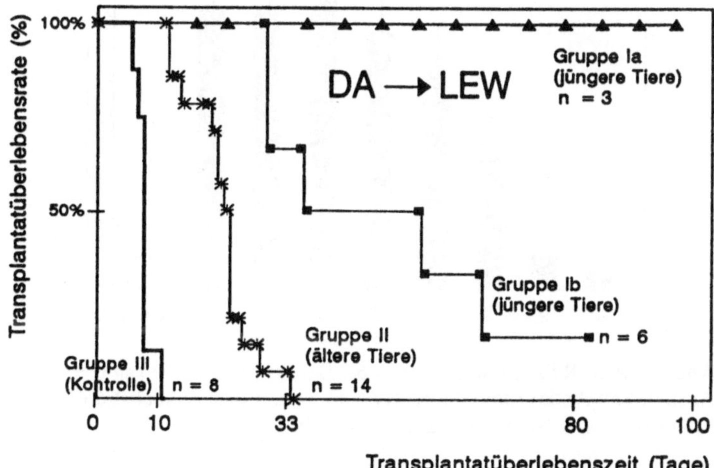

Abb. 1. Kaplan-Meier-Kurven der Herztransplantatüberlebenszeit bei Behandlung mit R73. Eine perioperative Behandlung mit dem monoklonalen anti-α/β-TCR-Antikörper R73 führt zu einer signifikanten Verlängerung der Überlebenszeit transplantierter Herzen. Bei 3 Tieren konnte sogar eine langdauernde Überlebenszeit (> 200 Tage) beobachtet werden

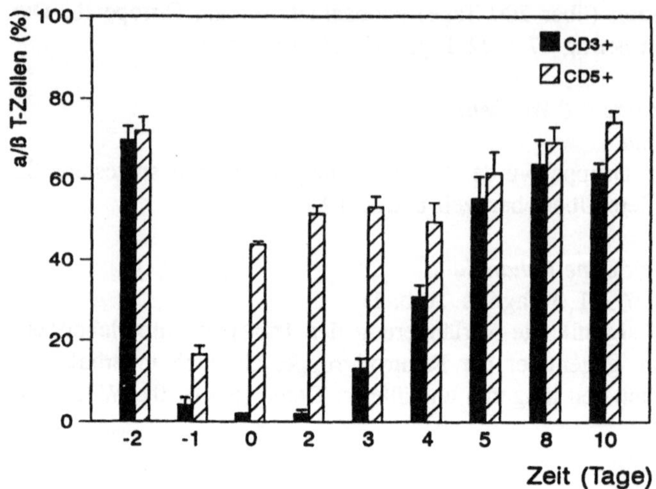

Abb. 2. Prozentsatz der α/β-Zellen während der Behandlung mit R73. Nach der ersten Gabe von R73 nimmt der Anteil CD3-positiver T-Zellen über einen Zeitraum von 5 Tagen von 70% auf 2% ab (Tag 0 = Transplantation). Danach erfolgt ein Anstieg auf Anfangswerte (n = 4). Der Anteil CD5-markierter T-Lymphozyten dagegen fällt nur kurzfristig auf 17% ab und erreicht bereits am Tag der Transplantation wieder einen Wert von 44%

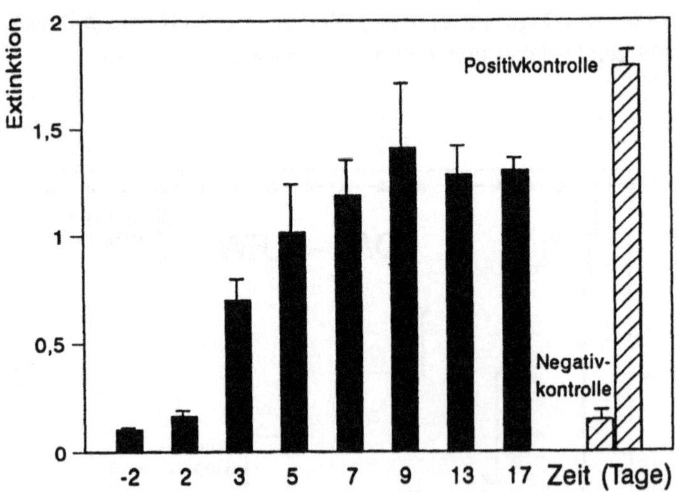

Abb. 3. Anti-R73-Antikörper (n = 6). Bereits am Tag 3 (Tag 0 = Transplantation) erfolgte ein Anstieg von Antikörpern gegen R73 im Serum der Versuchstiere. Vergleichend sind die Werte der Positiv- und Negativkontrolle angegeben

Anti-R73-Antikörper

Bereits drei Tage nach der Transplantation konnte im ELISA ein Anstieg von Antikörpern nachgewiesen werden, die sich gegen den monoklonalen Maus anti-α/β-TCR-Antikörper R73 richteten (s. Abb. 3).

Diskussion

Durch den Einsatz des monoklonalen α/β-Antikörpers R73 läßt sich eine signifikante Verlängerung der Überlebenszeit eines stark inkompatiblen Herztransplantates nachweisen, die in Einzelfällen sogar zu einem apparent endgültigen Einwachsen des fremden Organs führt. Dieser Effekt ist ausgeprägter in der Gruppe der jüngeren Tiere. Nach Behandlung mit R73 nimmt der Prozentsatz CD3-positiver T-Zellen über 5 Tage auf 2% ab. Dies ist am ehesten durch eine Modulation des α/β-T-Zell-CD3-Komplexes zu erklären. Gegen eine ausschließliche Depletion von T-Lymphozyten spricht der Befund, daß durch den unabhängigen pan-T-Zell-Marker CD5 bereits am Tag der Transplantation wieder ein Anteil von 44% gemessen werden konnte. Gleichzeitig mit der Zunahme der α/β-TCR$^+$ T-Lymphozyten am Tag 3 erfolgte ein Anstieg von Antikörpern gegen R73 im Serum der Versuchstiere, so daß bereits nach einer kurzzeitigen Behandlung die Wirkung von R73 durch die Bildung von Antikörpern blockiert wird. Der genaue Mechanismus der Toleranzinduktion (suppressive Zellen, Anergie, andere Faktoren) muß weiteren Versuchen vorbehalten bleiben.

Zusammenfassung

Die perioperative Gabe des selektiv gegen α/β-TCR$^+$ T-Lymphozyten gerichteten monoklonalen Antikörpers R73 führt bereits über einen kurzen Zeitraum zu einer signifikanten Verlängerung der Überlebenszeit eines heterotopen Herztransplantates. In Einzelfällen entwickelte sich sogar eine apparent definitive Transplantatakzeptanz (> 200 Tage). Während der Behandlung konnte eine kurzzeitige Abnahme des Anteils α/β-TCR$^+$ T-Lymphozyten über 5 Tage von 70% auf unter 2% gemessen werden. Anschließend folgte eine Rückkehr zu Anfangswerten. Gleichzeitig konnte die Bildung von Anti-R73 Antikörpern im Serum der Versuchstiere nachgewiesen werden.

Summary

Perioperative treatment with R73, a monoclonal antibody that is directed against the α/β T cell receptor, leads to a significant prolongation of a strongly incompatible heart allograft survival (Dague-Sprawley to Lewis rats). In some cases even long-lasting graft survival was achieved (> 200 days). In the course of the treatment, decrease of α/β T cell percentage from 70% to less than 2% was measured by fluorescence-activated cell sorter scanning over a period of 5 days, followed by return to normal values. After 5 days of treatment, anti-R73 antibodies were detected.

Literatur

1. Fabre JW (1992) Is tolerance a prospective for clinical research? Transplant Int 5 [Suppl 1]:571–577
2. Cobbold SP (1991) Monoclonal antibody therapy for the induction of transplantation tolerance. Immunol Letters 29:117–122
3. Hünig T, Wallny H-J, Hartley JK, Lawetzky A, Tiefenthaler G (1989) A monoclonal antibody to a constant determinant of the rat T-cell antigen receptor that induces T cell activation. J Exp Med 169:73–86
4. Ono K, Lindsey ES (1969) Improved technique of heart transplantation in rats. J Thorac Cardiovasc Surg 57:225

Diese Forschungsarbeit wurde unterstützt vom "Schwerpunkt Transplantation Heidelberg" des Landes Baden-Württemberg.

Herzlichen Dank für die freundliche Unterstützung an Martina Finger, Monika Jung, Christiane Hain und Tamer Koru.

Ch. Dufter, Chirurgische Universitätsklinik, Im Neuenheimer Feld 110,
W-6900 Heidelberg

Beeinflussung der Kalziumaufnahme und Antigenität biologischer Materialien durch Oberflächenbesiedlung mit homologen Zellen

Influence of Seeding with Homologous Cells on Calcium Uptake and Antigenicity of Biological Materials

M. Dahm[1], M. Husmann[2], O. Oster[3], W. Schmiedt[1], D. Prüfer[1] und H. Oelert[1]

[1]Klinik und Poliklinik für Herz-, Thorax- und Gefäßchirurgie, Universitätskliniken Mainz
[2]Institut für Mikrobiologie, Universitätskliniken Mainz
[3]Abteilung für Klinische Chemie, Universitätskliniken Mainz

Einleitung

Ein beträchtlicher Anteil biologischer Herzklappenprothesen muß innerhalb der ersten Dekade nach Implantation wegen Gewebedegeneration und Verkalkungen ausgetauscht werden [2]. Die Pathophysiologie der zugrundeliegenden Prozesse ist im Detail noch unklar [1]. Immunreaktionen als eine Ursache werden diskutiert: das histologische Bild mancher wegen Degeneration explantierter Bioprothese zeigt entzündliche Infiltrate mit Zerstörung der Kollagenstruktur. Eine wichtige Einflußgröße für die Progredienz dystropher Verkalkungen der Implantate ist der Einstrom von Plasmaproteinen in das avitale Fasergerüst mit Anlagerung von Kalzium.

Zielsetzung

In einer in-vitro und in-vivo Studie wurde getestet, ob die Besiedlung der Bioimplantate mit vitalen homologen Zellen deren Kalziumaufnahme und Antigenität reduzieren kann.

Methodik

Proben von in Glutaraldehyd konservierten Schweine- (GPV, n = 36) und Rinderperikardklappen (GBP, n = 40) sowie glycerinbehandeltem Rinderperikard (GlyBP, n = 33), die entweder nur gespült oder aber mit Fibrozyten aus den Herzen jugendlicher Ratten bewachsen waren, wurden mit Kulturmedium (RPMI 1640, 10% FCS, 1% Penicillin/Streptomycin) mit physiologischem Kalziumspiegel (2,3 mmol/l) inkubiert. Gleichermaßen vorbehandelte Proben wurden in die abdominellen Muskeln von Lewis-Ratten implantiert (GBP: n = 22, GPV: n = 24, GlyBP: n = 21). Nach 2 und 4 Wochen wurde atomabsorptionsspektroskopisch der Kalziumgehalt der Präparate bestimmt sowie ein ELISA und ein Lymphozytenproliferationstest durchgeführt, um die

Chirurgisches Forum 1993
f. experim. u. klinische Forschung
Becker/Beger/Hartel (Hrsg.)

B- und T-Zellreaktion gegen die Biomaterialien zu testen. Referenzpräparate wurden histologisch aufgearbeitet.

Ergebnisse

Alle unbesiedelten Biomaterialien verkalkten in-vitro mit der Zeit zunehmend. Die Oberflächenbesiedlung reduzierte die Kalziumaufnahme signifikant ($p < 0,01$). Die Ergebnisse der tierexperimentellen Untersuchungen untermauern die der in-vitro-Versuche: sie zeigen eine signifikante Reduktion des Kalzium-Gehalts der GBP und GlyBP-Implantate ($p < 0,05$), die vor Implantation mit Rattenfibrozyten besiedelt worden waren. Schweineklappen verkalkten in-vivo nur geringfügig.

Tabelle 1. Kalziumgehalt der unbesiedelten und besiedelten Biomaterialien nach in-vitro Inkubation mit kalziumhaltigem Medium bzw. nach Implantation bei der Ratte

		GBP	GPV	GlyBP
Zwei Wochen				
in-vitro	besiedelt	4,20 ± 1,70	4,21 ± 1,72	1,30 ± 0,41
	unbesiedelt	8,10 ± 1,73	11,16 ± 3,54	3,78 ± 0,72
in-vivo	besiedelt	0,28 ± 0,16	0,27 ± 0,05	0,19 ± 0,07
	unbesiedelt	0,86 ± 0,66	0,37 ± 0,10	0,39 ± 0,26
Vier Wochen				
in-vitro	besiedelt	7,06 ± 1,68	4,26 ± 1,07	3,39 ± 0,79
	unbesiedelt	17,41 ± 6,51	22,80 ± 6,16	16,30 ± 0,71
in-vivo	besiedelt	0,21 ± 0,07	0,33 ± 0,11	0,33 ± 0,24
	unbesiedelt	0,67 ± 0,37	0,39 ± 0,10	1,13 ± 0,44

Im Gegensatz zur Kontrollgruppe, wo alle Tiere spezifische Antikörper aufwiesen, konnten bei keinem der Tiere, deren GBP- oder GlyBP-Implantate an der Oberfläche mit homologen Rattenfibrozyten besiedelt waren, Antikörper gegen das Implantat nachgewiesen werden. GPV rief weder unbesiedelt noch besiedelt eine Antikörperantwort hervor.

Während in der Kontrollgruppe alle GBP-implantierten Tiere mit einer signifikanten T-Zell Proliferation reagierten, ließen sich nach Oberflächenbesiedlung nur bei einem Tier T-Zellaktivierungen nachweisen. Im Vergleich zu den Kontrollpräparaten fand sich bei den besiedelten Präparaten histologisch an der Grenzzone zwischen Implantat und Wirtsgewebe eine viel geringer ausgeprägte entzündliche Umgebungsreaktion.

Diskussion

Infolge des chemischen Fixationsprozesses mit Glutaraldehyd bestehen die heute eingesetzten Bioprothesen aus einem avitalen Fasergerüst aus Kollagen [3]. Die selektive Barrierefunktion vitaler Zellen für kospuskuläre und gelöste Blutbestandteile entfällt also völlig, so daß das Material vielen im Organismus abgelaufenen Diffusionsprozessen passiv unterworfen ist, insbesondere der Insudation von Plasmaproteinen und der Anlagerung von Kalzium an existente oder später exponierte Bindungsstellen. Die damit verbundene Verkalkung und die frühzeitige Gewebedegeneration der Implantate limitiert die Indikationen zur Implantation einer biologischen Herzklappenprothese.

Ein mögliches Konzept zur Verbesserung der unbefriedigenden Langzeitergebnisse erschien uns, das Material mit vitalen Zellen zu besiedeln. Die Oberflächenbesiedlung von Klappen mit homologen oder autologen Zellen könnte nämlich sowohl entzündliche Veränderungen verhindern, d.h. eine Modulation der Antigenität des Implantates bedingen, als auch als Barriere gegen Plasmaeinlagerungen dienen.

Die in-vitro-Studien zur Kalziumaufnahme von unbesiedelten Biomaterialien zeigen eindrucksvoll eine progressive Kalziumakkumulation in den verschiedenen Gewebeproben, wobei es sich in dem gezeigten Ausmaß um einen passiven Diffusionsprozeß handelt. Dieser ließ sich durch die Besiedlung der Gewebestücke mit Rattenfibrozyten signifikant reduzieren, nicht jedoch völlig eliminieren. Auch im Rattenmodell war die Oberflächenbesiedlung erfolgreich in der Reduktion der Mineralisation. Im Vergleich zur in-vitro Studie fallen sowohl das Ausmaß der Kalzifikation als auch das der Reduktion geringer aus. Ursache hierfür könnte sein, daß in der Umgebung des Implantates weniger Plasmaproteine und kalziumhaltiges Serum zur Verfügung stehen, während beides in-vitro im Überschuß vorhanden war. Hinzu kommt, daß alle Implantate mit zunehmender Versuchsdauer bindegewebig eingebaut werden und damit eine Diffusionsbarriere entsteht.

Neben dem Einfluß auf die Mineralisation wurde in den Kleintierstudien auch die Bedeutung der Oberflächenbesiedlung mit homologen Zellen für immunologische Reaktionen gegen die Implantate evaluiert. Es zeigt sich, daß durch die Besiedlung der GBP- und GlyBP-Implantate mit homologen Zellen die Antikörperproduktion und auch die T-Zellaktivierung signifikant reduziert werden. Ob die nachgewiesene Verzögerung der Mineralisation mit der Modulation der Immunreaktionen in Verbindung steht, erscheint allerdings sehr unwahrscheinlich.

Bereits publizierte tierexperimentelle Studien zur Reduktion der Mineralisation von Bioimplantaten setzten verschiedene Gruppen von Chemikalien ein, um die Biomaterialien chemisch zu modifizieren (Reduktion der Bindungsstellen für Kalzium, Ladungsänderung der Oberfläche, Surfactants). Während die klinische Anwendung dieser Konzepte aufgrund der Toxizität der Chemikalien bzw. der mangelnden technischen Praktikabilität bisher nicht möglich war, erscheint diese für das vorgestellte Konzept oberflächenbesiedelter Implantate aber sehr wohl realisierbar. Großtierversuche mit intrakardialen Implantaten müssen diese Ergebnisse allerdings noch weiter untermauern.

Zusammenfassung

Die Oberflächenbesiedlung biologischer Materialien mit Rattenfibrozyten erwies sich in-vitro und im Kleintierversuch als effizientes Verfahren sowohl zur Reduktion der Antigenität der Implantate als auch der passiven Kalziumaufnahme in die Präparate.

Summary

Surface seeding with homologous cells proves to be effective in reducing antigenicity of bioimplants and calcium accumulation in biological materials in-vitro and in the rat model.

Literatur

1. Barnhart GR, Jones M, Ishihara T, Chavez AM, Rose DM, Ferrans VJ (1982) Bioprosthetic valvular failure. J Thorac Cardiovasc Surg 83:618–31
2. Ferrans JV, Boyce SW, Billingham ME, Jones L, Ishihara T, Roberts WS (1980) Calcific deposits in porcine bioprostheses: structure and pathogenesis. Am J Card 46:721–34
3. Gallo I, Nistal F, Blasquez R, Arbe E, Artinano E (1988) Incidence of primary tissue failure in porcine bioprosthetic heart valves. Ann Thorac Surg 45:66–70

Dr. M. Dahm, Klinik und Poliklinik für Herz-, Thorax- und Gefäßchirurgie, Universitätskliniken Mainz, Langenbeckstraße 1, W-6500 Mainz

Das Schicksal der Knochentransplantate bei freier Patellarsehnenplastik

Micromorphological Investigations on the Bony Autografts in Bone-Patellar Tendon-Bone Transplants

M.A. Scherer[1], P. Böhm[2], R. Ascherl[3], M.-L. Schmeller[1], K. Herfeldt[1] und G. Blümel[1]

[1]Institut für Experimentelle Chirurgie, Technische Universität München (TUM)
[2]Orthopädische Universitätsklinik, Eberhard-Karls-Universität Tübingen
[3]Orthopädische Klinik und Poliklinik, TUM

Einleitung

Bereits 1943 vertrat Albee [1] die Meinung, daß nur die knöcherne Einheilung der transplantierten Knochenschuppen bei Patellarsehnentransplantaten die Rekonstruktion des vorhandenen Kreuzbandes definitiv sichern kann: "... the new ligament must maintain its tension and only bony anchorage will assure this when weightbearing and motion are allowed ...". Gerade im Rahmen des allgemeinen Trends zur Frühmobilisation sind Qualität und Quantität dieser knöchernen Inkorporation von Bedeutung. Unseres Wissens existiert zu diesem Problem keine zielgerichtete tierexperimentelle Untersuchung. Die Fragestellung bei diesem Versuchsvorhaben beschäftigt sich mit dem Schicksal der transplantierten Knochenschuppen bei freien Patellarsehnentransplantaten: Mit dem Einheilungs- und Resorptionsverhalten, sowie den Veränderungen der Übergangszone vom Band auf den Knochen.

Methodik

Nach Versuchsgenehmigung durch die Reg. v. Obb. wurde bei 34 weiblichen, erwachsenen Schafen (56–82 kg KG) in allgemeiner Intubationsnarkose eine freie Patellarsehnenplastik aus dem mittleren Drittel der Patellarsehne, modifiziert nach Wirth oder Brückner, durchgeführt: Mit der Schublehre wurde ein exakt 5 mm breiter, medianer Streifen mit einer anhängenden, dreieckigen Knochenschuppe von der Patella und einer trapezförmigen Schuppe von der Tibia gehoben, um 180° gedreht und durch isometrisch gelegte tibiale und femorale Bohrkanäle derart implantiert, daß die tibiale Knochenschuppe femoral verblockt wurde. Distale Fixation mit Zackenkranzunterlegscheibe und AO-Kortikalisschraube unter 40–60 N Vorspannung (Federwaage). Postoperativ erfolgte keine Analgesie. Den nicht immobilisierten Tieren wurden fluorochrome Farbstoffe verabreicht; nach 1, 3, 6 und 12 Monaten wurden sie getötet und die Präparate in 8 verschiedenen Schnittebenen u.a. für die Paraffinhistologie bzw. die unentkalkte Hartschnitthistologie aufgearbeitet. Parameter zur histologischen

Chirurgisches Forum 1993
f. experim. u. klinische Forschung
Becker/Beger/Hartel (Hrsg.)

Auswertung waren: Inkorporation der Knochenschuppe, Grad des Umbaues, Struktur des Knochen-Band-Überganges mit den Merkmalen normal/gestört/scholliger Zerfall/kein Zusammenhang, Ausbildung einer Neokortikalis mit den Merkmalen Defektbereiche/Formänderungen/geometrische Orientierung, Art und Umfang des Interface zwischen Transplantat und Lager sowohl hinsichtlich der Knochenschuppe als auch des Ligamentum patellae Transplantates.

Ergebnisse

Generalisierend läßt sich feststellen, daß die knöcherne Inkorporation der tibialen und patellaren Knochenschuppe durch die Morphologie des jeweiligen knöchernen Fragmentes, durch das Maß der Formschlüssigkeit zum knöchernen Lager und durch die biomechanische Belastung bestimmt wird. Neben dem unterschiedlichen Verhalten im tibialen vs. femoralen Transplantatlager, hat auch die geometrische Orientierung einen ganz entscheidenden Einfluß: Bei der Mehrzahl der Transplantate kommt es im ventralen und ventrolateralen Bereich zu einem besonders innigen Verbund zwischen dem Band und der Wand des Bohrkanals. Es kann jedoch nicht mit letzter Sicherheit ausgeschlossen werden, daß diese eindeutige geometrische Ausrichtung der Transplantatfunktion mit dem Versuchstier Schaf und der vorgegebenen Anatomie und Mechanik der Gelenksbewegung zusammenhängt.

Ganz sicher nicht speziesspezifisch ist die Tatsache, daß eine Aufarbeitung der Präparate in Serienschnitten eine beträchtliche Variabilität der Ergebnisse – auch innerhalb eines Versuchstieres – mit sich bringt. Diese Unterschiede erstrecken sich sogar bis auf die Ebene des Einzelschnittes: Sieht man den Bohrkanal im Lagerknochen als Zylinder an, dann ist bei keinem Transplantat eine homogene Ausprägung der Transplantatfixation bzw. des knöchernen Umbauvorganges über die gesamten 360° gegeben.

Im Rahmen dieser Arbeit steht das Verhalten der knöchernen Fragmente im Vordergrund. Im spongiösen Anteil des Transplantates kommt es innerhalb von 3 bis 6 Monaten zu einer kompletten und grenzschichtlosen Inkorporation. Die spongiösen Anteile sind stets vollständig eingeheilt, auch in den zentralen Osteonen sind Farbbanden der Markierung zu sehen. Das Transplantatvolumen, bzw. die beurteilbare Querschnittsfläche nimmt mit zunehmendem postoperativen Intervall ab. Ein Jahr postoperativ ist das Knochenfragment im ehemals spongiösen Anteil nur noch schwer von der Knochenneubildung des Lagers zu differenzieren. Im Gegensatz dazu steht das Verhalten der Kortikalis, die im ersten halben Jahr stets abgrenzbar ist und wenig Umbauaktivität zeigt. Die rein kortikalen Anteile weisen 6 Monate postoperativ noch vergleichsweise wenig fluorochrome Zeichnung auf, haben also einen geringen Knochenumbau und -anbau. Nach einem Jahr ist der Unterschied zwischen Transplantatkortikalis und Transplantatspongiosa leicht verwischt: Im Rahmen der ossären Integration kommt es zu einer zunehmenden Spongiosierung und Knochenneubildung. Als Sonderfall können Knochenschuppen mit überwiegenden oder gar ausschließlich kortikalen Anteilen zu einem beträchtlichen Oberflächenanteil durch ein Bindegewebs- oder Markgewebe-Interface vom Lagerknochen separiert sein. Der Umbauvorgang ist zwölf Monate postoperativ noch nicht abgeschlossen.

Der physiologische Ansatz der Patellarsehne am Knochen scheint in einem gewissen Rahmen erhalten zu bleiben. Früh postoperativ lassen sich histologisch weder bei der polychromen Sequenzmarkierung noch im Doppelkontrastbild gravierende Gefügestörungen nachweisen. Diese Aussage trifft allerdings nur für Sehnenanteile zu, die im Bohrkanal gestreckt verlaufen und augenscheinlich krafttragende Funktion hatten. Unbelastete Anteile zeigen schollige Veränderungen am Ansatz, eine Störung im Organisationsniveau des "crimping", eine quantitative und qualitative Reduktion der Pseudo-Sharpey-Fasern sowie letztendlich verschiedene Destruktionsformen im vierschichtigen Knochen-Band-Übergang. Die Umbauvorgänge in der Kompakta des Transplantats am Übergang zur transplantierten Sehne verlaufen sehr langsam. Der lokale Nachweis von Gefäßen ein Jahr postoperativ verläuft parallel mit einer Desintegration des Knochen-Band-Überganges und stellt somit kein positives Zeichen dar. Die Veränderungen an der Knochen-Band-Übergangszone kann man zwölf Monate postoperativ in vier Stadien einteilen: Stadium A entspricht der – sehr seltenen – subtotalen Resorption des Transplantates mit einer vollständigen Auflösung und Zerrüttung des Knochen-Band-Überganges. Begleitend kommt es dann auf diesem Schnittniveau zur Aufspleißung des transplantierten Bandes mit verstärkter Vaskularisation oder der Ausbildung von Fettzellen. Der Bohrkanal ist entrundet, die Bildung von Neokortikalis mit weiten Defektstrecken behaftet. Im Stadium B besteht der Knochen-Band-Übergang noch in einem begrenzten Areal, das Knochentransplantat ist großenteils umgebaut und zu einem beträchtlichen Volumenanteil resorbiert. Bei der Neokortikalis am Bohrkanal selber sind die Defektstrecken gegenüber Stadium A reduziert oder fehlen. Das Stadium C, prozentual am häufigsten zu finden, definiert sich als weitgehende Osteointegration der Knochenschuppe mit geringer Resorption und überwiegend erhaltenem Knochen-Band-Übergang. Der Bohrkanal ist zirkulär mit Neokortikalis nachgezeichnet, das Bandtransplantat mit Pseudo-Sharpey-Fasern an der Wand des Bohrkanals fixiert. Im Stadium D schließlich entspricht das histologische Bild einem "physiologischen" Knochen-Band-Übergang und einer vollständig knöchernen integrierten Knochenschuppe ohne signifikante Volumenreduktion. Dieses "Idealbild" ist nur selten anzutreffen.

Obwohl bei der Rekonstruktion der chronischen, eventuell auch der akuten Kreuzbandinsuffizienz die Forderung nach der kombinierten (Auto-)Transplantation von *Band und Knochen* seit langem erhoben wird [1], gehört dieses Thema nach Wroble und Brand [4] zu den "paradoxes in the history of the anterior cruciate ligament". Obwohl der Ansatz schlüssig ist, wird er nicht regelmäßig beachtet und nicht experimentell abgesichert. Die Verwendung von Bandtransplantaten mit ihrem knöchernen Ursprung und Ansatz erhöht die Chancen der Ausbildung einer funktionsfähigen Rekonstruktion. Die knöcherne Fixation reduziert die freie Länge des Transplantates und erhöht damit die im Vergleich zum gesunden Kreuzband materialspezifisch zu niedrige Steifigkeit eines Patellarsehnenstreifens. Aber auch im Hinblick auf die sekundäre Relaxation des Transplantats, also eine Elongation, eine Dehnung des unter Vorspannung fixierten Transplantats, verbürgt ein hoher Spongiosaanteil durch Impaktieren und hohe Haftreibung einen guten Primärsitz [3]. Der Umbau stellt ein Kontinuum dar [2]. In dieser Untersuchung ist es nicht möglich, einen Endpunkt anzugeben. In Übereinstimmung mit den arthroskopischen Befunden von Kohn am Patellarsehnentransplantat beim Menschen [2] wird das histologische Bild mit zunehmendem postoperativen Intervall "schlechter", d.h. es entfernt sich vom morphologischen Aspekt zum Zeitpunkt der Operation.

Aus dieser Untersuchung ergeben sich eindeutige *klinische Konsequenzen*: Für die Knochenschuppen bei freien Patellarsehnentransplantaten muß gefordert werden, daß sie 1. einen spongiösen Anteil tragen, daß 2. die Fixation im "press-fit" oder über Interferenzschrauben erfolgt, 3. auf die Orientierung der Knochenschuppe im Bohrkanal geachtet wird, 4. eine vollständige, zirkuläre knöcherne Fixation nicht erwartet werden kann und 5. auch 12 Monate postoperativ noch ein Umbauvorgang zu erwarten ist.

Zusammenfassung

Unter der Fragestellung nach dem Schicksal der transplantierten Knochenschuppen bei freien Patellarsehnentransplantaten wurde bei 34 Schafen eine freie Patellarsehnenplastik durchgeführt. Nach 1, 3, 6 und 12 Monaten wurden die Tiere getötet und in je 8 verschiedenen Schnittebenen (un-/entkalkt) beurteilt. Die knöcherne Inkorporation der Knochenschuppen wird durch die Morphologie des jeweiligen Fragmentes, durch das Maß der Formschlüssigkeit zum knöchernen Lager und durch die biomechanische Belastung bestimmt. Der Umbauvorgang ist zwölf Monate postoperativ noch nicht abgeschlossen. Die Ergebnisse werden in die Stadien A bis D klassifiziert, die vier verschiedenen Einheilungs- und Umbauzuständen entsprechen.

Als klinische Konsequenzen muß gefordert werden, daß die Knochenschuppen von Patellarsehnentransplantaten einen spongiösen Anteil tragen, daß die Fixation im "press-fit" oder über Interferenzschrauben erfolgt, auf die Orientierung der Knochenschuppe im Bohrkanal geachtet wird, und eine vollständige, zirkuläre knöcherne Fixation nicht erwartet werden kann und auch 12 Monate postoperativ der Umbauvorgang nicht abgeschlossen ist.

Summary

Objectives of the study were to investigate the fate of the bony fragments of free bone-patellar tendon-bone grafts for reconstruction of the anterior cruciate ligament. This type of reconstruction was performed in 34 sheep that were killed after a survival time of 1, 3, 6, and 12 months. Decalcified and undecalcified serial sections at eight different levels were performed on each specimen. The results were evaluated with the help of a semiquantitative verbal rating system. Osseous incorporation of the bony fragments predominantly depends on the morphology of the fragment itself, on the extent of geometrical congruity between transplant and host bone, and, finally, on the biomechanical load pattern. Incorporation is an ongoing process that is not terminated 12 months postoperatively. A classification system is proposed that accurately described four different levels of incorporation and morphological transplant integrity (stages A–D). Clinical consequences arising from this study are the following: bony fragments should include spongious bone; "press fit" or interference screws are a must; geometrical orientation of the transplant is an important factor, and transplant incorporation is a continuous process that takes longer than 12 months.

Literatur

1. Albee FH (1943) A new operation for the repair of the crucial ligaments of the knee. Am J Surg 60:349
2. Kohn D (1990) Arthroscopic evaluation of anterior cruciate ligament reconstruction using a free patellar tendon autograft. Clin Orthop Rel Res 254:220–224
3. Scherer MA, Ascherl R, Früh HJ, Mau H, Schmeller ML, Blümel G (1992) The impact of tension on the bone-ligament-interface in patellar tendon transplants for ACL-reconstruction. Transactions Soc Biomath 4th World Biomat Congr, 420 (abstract)
4. Wroble RR, Brand RA (1990) Paradoxes in the history of anterior cruciate ligament. Clin Orthop 259:183–191

Dr. med. Dr. med. habil. M.A. Scherer, Institut für Experimentelle Chirurgie, TUM, Rechts der Isar, Ismaninger Straße 22, W-8000 München 80

Optimierung des mikrobiologischen Keimnachweises bei der allogenen Knochentransplantation

An Optimized Screening Method of Bacterial Contamination in Allogeneic Bone Grafts

T. v. Garrel[1], J. Garbas[1], H. Knaepler[1] und R. Mutters[2]

[1]Klinik für Unfallchirurgie, Philipps-Universität, Marburg (Direktor: Prof. Dr. L. Gotzen)
[2]Institut für Mikrobiologie, Philipps-Universität, Marburg (Direktor: Prof. Dr. H.D. Klenk)

Einleitung

Das Risiko der Übertragung bakterieller Infektionserkrankungen mit dem kryokonservierten allogenen Knochentransplantat ist wesentlich höher als die virale Infektionsgefahr (HIV, Hepatitis B und C, CMV). Literaturangaben über die bakterielle Kontaminationsrate von unter "sterilen" Bedingungen entnommenen Knochentransplantaten schwanken zwischen 5%–65% [2, 3]. Diese Unterschiede lassen sich durch die unterschiedlichen mikrobiologischen Screening-Techniken erklären. Während die deutschen "Richtlinien zum Führen einer Knochenbank" aus dem Jahre 1990 nur eine einfache Abstrichuntersuchung der Transplantatoberfläche vorschreiben, werden an den Gewebebanken in den USA umfangreiche bakterielle Untersuchungen mit bis zu 200–300 mikrobiologischen Kulturen pro Organspender [3] vorgenommen. Als Keimnachweismethoden kommen das herkömmliche Abstrichverfahren mit einem Wattetupfer, die direkte Bebrütung einer Knochenprobe oder die Inkubation und Untersuchung der Spülflüssigkeit von allogenen Knochentransplantaten in Frage. Ziel dieser Untersuchung war es, die Sensitivität des Wattetupfer-Abstrichverfahrens zu testen und diese Methode mit anderen Verfahren zu vergleichen.

Material und Methode

Getestet wurden vier unterschiedliche Keimnachweismethoden:

1. das Abstrichverfahren mittels Wattetupfer (in Port-A-Cul Universal-Transportmedium) mit anschließender Inkubation in Thioglycolat-Medium bei 36°C für 72 h,
2. die Untersuchung einer Spülflüssigkeit der Knochenoberfläche (10minütige Spülung in 200 ml Ringer-Lösung) mit anschließender Ultrafiltration (bakteriendichter Membranfilter 0,2 μm) und Bebrütung des Filters in Thioglycolat-Nährmedium bei 36°C für 72 h,
3. die Untersuchung der Spülflüssigkeit durch 10 ml Probenentnahme und Inkubation in einem Blutkulturnährmedium (Bactec Plus, Becton und Dickinson),
4. der direkte Keimnachweis auf dem Knochen durch Inkubation der gesamten Knochenprobe in Thioglycolat-Medium bei 36°C für 72 h.

Chirurgisches Forum 1993
f. experim. u. klinische Forschung
Becker/Beger/Hartel (Hrsg.)

Als Knochenmaterial wurden entknorpelte, porcine Hüftköpfe verwendet (n = 20 je getestete Bakterienspezies), deren Oberflächenstruktur sehr ähnlich denen humaner Spongiosatransplantate ist. Durch eine Kurzzeitautoklavierung bei 134°C für 8 min wurden die Hüftköpfe primär sterilisiert. Anschließend wurden die Knochenproben durch eine Punktkontamination mittels einer Hamilton-Pipette mit jeweils 0,2 μl einer Bakteriensuspension (3×10^3 Keime/ml) durch einen unabhängigen Untersucher verkeimt. Getestet wurden klinikrelevante Problemkeime: Staphylococcus aureus, Enterococcus faecalis, E. coli, Proteus vulgaris und Bazillus pumilus. Die Kontamination erfolgte an unterschiedlichen Oberflächenlokalisationen auf dem Knochen.

Nach einer 10minütigen Antrocknungszeit wurden Oberflächenabstriche mit einem angefeuchteten sterilen Wattetupfer von einem zweiten Untersucher durchgeführt, wobei sorgfältig die gesamte Zirkumferenz der Hüftköpfe umfahren wurde. Zum weiteren Transport und zur Inkubation wurden Port-A-Cul Universal Transportmedien mit anschließender weiterer Differenzierung in Thioglycolat-Nährmedium verwendet. Nach diesem Untersuchungsschritt wurden die Hüftköpfe in 200 ml steriler Ringer-Lösung für 10 min intensiv gewaschen, so daß oberflächliche Zellen und Zellbestandteile der Spongiosa abgelöst wurden. Aus der daraus resultierenden Spülflüssigkeit wurde eine Probe von 10 ml steril entnommen und in eine Blutkulturmediumflasche injiziert (Bactec plus, Becton & Dickinson). Die restliche Spülflüssigkeit wurde mittels Vakuumfiltration durch einen bakteriendichten Membranfilter der Porengröße 0,2 μm filtriert und diese Filter anschließend in Thioglycolat-Nährmedium für 3 Tage bei 36°C inkubiert. Im vierten Untersuchungsschritt wurden die kontaminierten Hüftköpfe direkt in Thioglycolat-Nährmedium überführt.

Ergebnisse

Die qualitative und quantitative mikrobiologische Auswertung ergab folgende Resultate: Bei der Untersuchung der Knochenoberfläche durch Wattetupferabstriche konnte insgesamt nur an 65 der 100 getesteten Hüftköpfe eine bakterielle Besiedlung nachgewiesen werden. Dabei zeigte sich eine Abhängigkeit der Ergebnisse von der jeweils getesteten Keimspezies. So waren die Abstriche bei Proteus vulgaris mit 85% positiven Ergebnissen relativ zuverlässig, während die Resultate für Staphylococcus aureus mit ca. 45% als unpräzise zu betrachten waren. Bei der Oberflächenspülung waren keine Unterschiede zwischen der Technik der Probenentnahme in Blutkulturmedium und der Ultrafiltration zu finden. Beide Verfahren erwiesen sich mit 96% positiven Testergebnissen als zuverlässig. Noch präzisere Ergebnisse lieferte die direkte Inkubation der kontaminierten Knochenproben in Thioglycolat-Nährmedium. Hier konnte in allen 100 Proben ein positiver Keimnachweis geführt werden (Tabelle 1).

Diskussion

Ein Vorhandensein bakterieller Erreger auf allogenen Gewebetransplantaten konnte von unterschiedlichen Autoren durch intensive mikrobiologische Screeningverfah-

Tabelle 1. Bakteriologische Untersuchungsergebnisse bei Testung unterschiedlicher Keimnachweismethoden

	Keimnachweis: E. coli			
Proben	Blutkulturmedium	Tupfer	Tupfer Thioglycolat	Filter in Thioglycolat
K	+++	nd	nd	nd
1	+++	–	–	–
2	–	–	–	+++
3	+++	–	++	+++
4	+++	(+)	++	+++
5	+++	++	++	+++
6	+++	–	–	+++
7	+++	+	++	+++
8 Leerprobe	–	–	–	–
9	+++	–	–	+++
10	+++	–	–	+++
11	+++	–	–	+++
12	+++	–	++	+++
13	+++	+	++	+++
14	+++	–	–	+++
15	+++	++	++	+++
16	+++	–	++	+++
17	+++	–	–	+++
18 Leerprobe	–	–	–	–
19	+++	–	++	+++
20	+++	–	–	+++

+++: Reichlich Kolonien auf dem Agar (> 1000); ++: mäßig Kolonien auf dem Agar (> 50, < 1000); +: spärlich Kolonien auf dem Agar (bis zu 50); (+): weniger als 10 Kolonien auf dem Agar

ren in über 65% der untersuchten Proben nachgewiesen werden [3]. Dabei stellen koagulase-negative Staphylococcen (Staphylococcus epidermidis) und Proprionibakterien die häufigsten Erreger dar. Diese hohe Kontaminationsrate mit zumeist apathogenen bakteriellen Erregern läßt sich durch akzidentelle Besiedlung während der Transplantatentnahme und durch das häufige, transitorische Vorkommen apathogener Bakterien der normalen Hautflora im Blut auch von gesunden Patienten erklären.

Die in der Literatur zu findenden, stark divergierenden Angaben zur Kontaminationsrate allogener Knochentransplantate lassen sich nur durch die unterschiedlichen mikrobiologischen Untersuchungstechniken erklären. Dabei gibt es bislang wenige Arbeiten, die sich mit der Zuverlässigkeit und Sensitivität dieser Testmethoden beschäftigen. 1991 konnte die Marburger Arbeitsgruppe "Knochentransplantation" in einer vergleichenden Untersuchung zwischen Abstrich- und Spülflüssigkeitsverfahren zeigen, daß die Verwendung von Wattetupfern zum Nachweis einer möglichen bakteriellen Oberflächenkontamination von allogenen Knochentransplantaten eine äußerst unpräzise Methode darstellt (Sensitivität von 60%) [1]. 1992 fanden Veen [5] und Taylor [4] eine Sensitivität des Abstrichverfahrens von 44 bzw. 80%.

Die hier vorgelegten Ergebnisse zeigen, daß das herkömmliche Abstrichverfahren keine suffiziente Untersuchungstechnik zur Erfassung bakterieller Oberflächenkon-ta-minationen auf Knochentransplantaten darstellt. Die Oberflächenspülung mit anschließender mikrobiologischer Untersuchung sowie die direkte Inkubation von Transplantatproben führen zu weit aussagekräftigeren Ergebnissen und sollten daher beim Betreiben einer allogenen Gewebebank Verwendung finden.

Zusammenfassung

Bei der Transplantation allogener Gewebe stellt die Möglichkeit der Übertragung bakterieller Krankheitserreger ein großes Risiko dar. Dabei beträgt die Kontaminationsrate von unter "sterilen" Bedingungen gewonnenen Knochentransplantaten bis zu 65%. Das zum Keimnachweis bislang am häufigsten verwendete Abstrichverfahren mittels Wattetupfer bietet mit einer Sensitivität von 65% keine ausreichende Sicherheit zum Ausschluß einer bakteriellen Besiedlung. Die Spülung der Transplantatoberfläche in einer sterilen Lösung und anschließende mikrobiologische Untersuchung dieser Spülflüssigkeit oder die direkte Inkubation einer Knochenprobe stellen mit einer Sensitivität von über 95% wesentlich aussagekräftigere mikrobiologische Screeningverfahren dar.

Summary

There is a high risk of transmitting bacterial infectious diseases with the transplantation of human allogeneic tissue grafts. The contamination rates of bone grafts, gained under 'sterile' conditions, are found up to 65%. The commonly used swab culture technique with a cotton carrier has a sensitivity of 65% and is therefore insufficient to exclude bacterial contamination of the graft. Rinsing the transplant's surface or direct incubation of a probe of the transplant lead to a sensitivity of 95% and are much more accurate methods for bacterial screening.

Literatur

1. v. Garrel T, Knaepler H (1991) An optimized screening method of bacterial contamination of allogeneic bone grafts. 1st European Congress of Tissue Banks, 24.10.–26.10.91, Berlin
2. Kuner E, Keller H (1984) Knochenbank, Ausstattung, Gewebegewinnung, Kältekonservierung, Organisation, Sicherheit. Orthopäde 151:704–706
3. Malinin TI (1992) Acquisition and banking of bole allografts. In: Habal MB, Reddi AH (eds) Bone grafts and bone substitutes. Saunders, Philadelphia
4. Taylor A, Zanzi K, Burchardt H, Forsell J (1992) The reliability of utilizing a dry swab culturing method to validate tissue sterility post-lyophilization. 16th Annual Meeting – American Association of Tissue Banks 24.8.–26.8.92, San Diego
5. Veen MR, Bloem R, Petit P (1992) Bacteriology in bone banking. 1st Annual Meeting – European Association of Musculo-Skeletal Transplantation (EAMST), 4.4.–5.4.92, Brüssel

Dr. med. Th. von Garrel, Klinik für Unfallchirurgie, Philipps-Universität Marburg, Baldingerstraße, W-3550 Marburg

Die Störung der subchondralen Durchblutung und die histomorphologischen Veränderungen nach intraartikulären Fersenbeinfrakturen

Changes in Subchondral Perfusion and Histomorphological Alterations Following Intra-Articular Fractures of the Calcaneus

H.G. Braick[1], B. Krefft[2] und M. Hansis[1]

[1]Klinik und Poliklinik für Unfallchirurgie, Universität Bonn
[2]Radiologische Klinik, Universität Bonn

Einleitung

Die hohe Inzidenz einer posttraumatischen Arthroseentwicklung nach intraartikulären Trümmerfrakturen ist allgemein anerkannt. Ätiopathogenetisch wird sie überwiegend als Folge biomechanischer Störungen durch anatomische Inkongruenz, Instabilität oder Achsenfehlstellungen angesehen. Nutritive Beeinträchtigungen des hyalinen Gelenkknorpels, als Ort der Arthroseentstehung, können durch die veränderte Zusammensetzung der Synovialflüssigkeit aber auch möglicherweise durch die gestörte Perfusion des subchondralen Knochens bedingt sein.

Ziel der Untersuchung

Das Ziel der prospektiven Untersuchung an 20 intraartikulären, subtalaren Calcaneustrümmerfrakturen war die Evaluation einer Perfusionsveränderung im subchondralen Knochen und ihre Bedeutung für die Entwicklung degenerativer Veränderungen des hyalinen Gelenkknorpels im subtalaren Gelenk.

Material und Methode

Es wurden 15 intraartikuläre Fersenbeintrümmerfrakturen nach operativer Rekonstruktion und 5 nach konservativer Behandlung 8 bis 36 Monate nach der Verletzung in die Untersuchung einbezogen. Eingangsbedingung war der computertomographische Nachweis einer dislozierten subtalaren Fraktur. Das Untersuchungsprotokoll

Chirurgisches Forum 1993
f. experim. u. klinische Forschung
Becker/Beger/Hartel (Hrsg.)

umfaßte für alle Patienten die klinische Untersuchung, ergänzt durch das Beurteilungsschema nach *Merle d'Aubigne*; Röntgennativaufnahmen in 2 Ebenen, eine Computertomographie in sagittaler und cronaler Schichtung (Somatom Plus S, Siemens AG Erlangen), eine Magnetresonanztomographieuntersuchung mit T1-gewichteten SE-Sequenzen und T2-gewichteten FFE Sequenzen (Gyroscan T5, Philips AG Eindhoven). Nach der intravenösen Gabe von 0,1 mmol/kg Körpergewicht Gadolinium-DTPA wurden nochmals T1-gewichtete SE und TFE-Sequenzen zur Anfertigung der Kontrastmitteldynamik im Rückfußbereich durchgeführt.

Bei der Patientengruppe mit operativ rekonstruierten Fersenbeinfrakturen wurde zum Zeitpunkt der Osteosynthesematerialentfernung eine Videoarthroskopie des unteren Sprunggelenkes und eine Knorpel-Knochenbiopsie aus der Facies articularis post. des Calcaneus entnommen und histologisch aufgearbeitet.

Ergebnisse

Die 15 nach der von *Bezes* (1983) angegebenen Methode operativ behandelten Patienten (männlich 6, weiblich 4, Alter 22–58 Jahre, $\bar{x}$ 44) mit intraartikulären Fersenbeinfrakturen vom Typ B2–B4 nach *Essex-Lopresti* (1952) wurden 9 bis 36 Monate nach dem Trauma klinisch und radiologisch untersucht.

Nach den Kriterien von *Merle d'Aubigne* konnten 8 sehr gute, 6 gute und 1 mäßiges Ausheilungsergebnis festgestellt werden.

Die Röntgennativ- und die CT-Untersuchungen wurden hinsichtlich der Wiederherstellung der ursprünglichen Knochenform, der Rekonstruktion der Gelenkflächen und des knöchernen Durchbaues ausgewertet. Hier zeigte sich eine gute Übereinstimmung mit dem ermittelten klinischen Ergebnis. Nur bei dem Patienten mit mäßigem Ausheilungsergebnis konnte eine deutliche subtalare Gelenkstufe mit vermehrter Sklerosierung des betroffenen Gelenkabschnittes festgestellt werden.

Das MRT vermochte die ehemaligen Frakturzonen bis zu 36 Monate nach dem Trauma sicher abzugrenzen, abschnittsweise wurde der Verlust des subtalaren Gelenkknorpels dargestellt. In ehemals dislozierten großen Knorpel-Knochenfragmenten zeigte sich eine inhomogene Signalintensitätsverteilung, die bis zum Signalverlust in der T1-gewichteten Sequenz reichte.

Auch die kontrastmittelverstärkte T1-gewichtete Sequenz zeigte als Ausdruck der reduzierten Vaskularisation in einzelnen frakturangrenzenden Arealen eine deutlich verminderte bis fehlende Signalintensität. Die Kontrastmitteldynamik in der T1-gewichteten TFE-Sequenz stellte nach Subtraktion das Anreicherungsverhalten im Calcaneus dar. Es konnte hierbei eine verstärkte Anreicherung in den periläsionalen Bezirken mit deutlicher Abschwächung zum subtalaren Frakturbezirk nachgewiesen werden.

Das Signalverhalten in der T2 gewichteten FFE Sequenz zeigte mit zunehmendem zeitlichen Abstand zum Trauma zunächst eine hohe, nach mehr als 12 Monaten dann eine deutlich geringere Intensität im Frakturbezirk.

Zur Ermittlung der morphologischen Äquivalente konnte bei 7 Patienten zum Zeitpunkt der Osteosynthesematerialentfernung nach 8 bis 36 Monaten eine Knorpel-Knochenbiopsie nach arthroskopischer Inspektion aus der Facies art. post. entnommen werden. Es wurden in 6 von 7 Präparaten die Zeichen der degenerativen Chondropathie festgestellt. Der subchondrale Knochen zeigte in 4 von 7 Biopsiepräparaten partielle Knochennekrosen mit leeren Osteocytenhöhlen und in allen Proben regressive Veränderungen von kollagenem Bindegewebe mit chondroider Transformation.

Die Vergleichsgruppe der 5 konservativ behandelten intraarticulären Calcaneusfrakturen ergab bei der klinischen Prüfung 1 gutes, 1 mäßiges und 1 schlechtes Ergebnis 7 bis 36 Monate nach dem Trauma. Die Röntgennativ- und CT-Untersuchung bot alle Zeichen der in Fehlstellung verheilten Fersenbeinfrakturen. Neben der immer nachweisbaren Verwerfung des subtalaren Gelenkabschnittes mit Stufenbildung und Diastase zum Sustentaculum tali fand sich die ausgeprägte Abflachung des Tuber-Gelenkwinkels bei Impaktierung der hinteren Gelenkfacette. Nicht knöchern durchbaute Frakturzonen konnten bis 18 Monate nach dem Trauma beobachtet werden. Die MRT Untersuchung mit Kontrastmittelverstärkung in der T1-gewichteten SE Sequenz und der dynamischen Untersuchungstechnik zur Bestimmung der Kontrastmittelaufnahme zeigte ausgeprägte Destruktionen des Gelenkknorpels und eine deutliche Signalintensitätsminderung im subchondralen Frakturareal bei periläsionaler Intensitätssteigerung.

Diskussion

Die mögliche Entwicklung einer posttraumatischen Arthrose nach Gelenkfrakturen ist allgemein anerkannt. Ätiopathogenetisch wird sie überwiegend als Folge der biomechanischen Störung durch Inkongruenz, Instabilität und Achsfehlstellung angesehen [1]. Nutritive Störungen des hyalinen Gelenkknorpels – als Ort der Arthroseentstehung – können durch die veränderte Zusammensetzung der Synovialflüssigkeit, aber möglicherweise auch durch eine gestörte Vaskularisation [1, 4] des subchondralen Knochens bedingt sein.

Postoperative Untersuchungen an rekonstruierten intraartikulären Fersenbeinfrakturen wurden bisher überwiegend mit Röntgennativ- oder CT-Verfahren vorgenommen [2]. Der Vorteil der MRT liegt nicht zuletzt in der Fähigkeit, Gelenkknorpel und dessen pathologische Veränderungen, unter zusätzlicher Gabe von Gd-DTPA, mit hoher Genauigkeit darstellen zu können [5]. Durch unsere Untersuchungen an biomechanisch und anatomisch günstig rekonstruierten Fersenbeinfrakturen konnte im MRT der Nachweis subchondraler Vascularisationsstörungen mit partiellem Verlust des hyalinen Gelenkknorpels geführt werden. Die nichtinvasiv erhobenen Befunde konnten durch histomorphologische Untersuchungen mit dem Nachweis der degenerativen Chondropathie und partiellen Nekrose des subchondralen Knochen bestätigt werden.

Wesentlich ausgeprägter waren die pathologischen Veränderungen im MRT bei der Vergleichsgruppe konservativ behandelter intraartikulärer Fersenbeinfrakturen. Die im Vergleich auch klinisch wesentlich schlechteren Resultate dieser Gruppe lassen sich durch die Summation der ätiopathogenetischen Faktoren der posttraumatischen Arthrose erklären. Eine Analogie zu bekannten traumatisch entstandenen aseptischen Knorpel-Knochennekrosen, wie der Talusnekrose, der Scaphoidpseudarthrose oder der Femurkopfnekrose läßt sich hieraus ableiten [3].

Zusammensetzung

In einer prospektiven Studie wurden bei 15 operativ und 5 konservativ behandelten intraartikulären Fersenbeinfrakturen, 7 bis 36 Monate nach dem Trauma, kontrastmittelverstärkte MRT Untersuchungen zur Beurteilung der subtalaren Gelenkflächen vorgenommen. Bei 7 Patienten konnten Knorpel-Knochenbiopsien aus der hinteren subtalaren Gelenkfläche in Beziehung zu den MRT-Untersuchungsergebnissen gesetzt werden. Es ließ sich hierbei der Verlust oder die Degeneration des hyalinen Knorpels und die partielle subchondrale Knochennekrose bestätigen. Das Ausmaß der subtalaren Veränderungen zeigte eine direkte Beziehung zum klinischen Behandlungsergebnis.

Daher sind wir der Meinung, daß es sich bei der nachgewiesenen posttraumatischen Knorpeldegeneration nicht nur um eine unmittelbare Folge der Gelenkverletzung handelt, sondern daß die Vaskularisationsstörung des subchondralen Knochens ebenfalls einen Einfluß auf die Ätiologie der posttraumatischen Arthrose bei subtalaren Fersenbeinfrakturen hat. Die operative Rekonstruktion vermag den Einfluß dieses Faktors zu reduzieren und Reparationsvorgänge gegenüber der konservativen Behandlung zu beschleunigen, eine vollständige Verhinderung scheint jedoch nicht sicher möglich zu sein.

Summary

In 15 patients undergoing reconstructive surgery for intra-articular fractures of the calcaneus and five undergoing conservative therapy, magnetic resonance imaging (MRI) examinations including intravenous injection of Gd-DTPA were compared with the clinical outcome, results of computed tomography (CT) examination, plain radiographs, and biopsy specimen from the posterior subtalar joint. MRI was capable of depicting cartilage defects and reduction or loss of subchondral bone vascularity. There was a good correlation between clinical results, MRI, and histopathological findings showing partial aseptic necrosis. These findings recommend early reconstruction of intra-articular fractures of the calcaneus to prevent post-traumatic osteoarthritis.

Literatur

1. Friedebold G (1972) Die posttraumatische Arthrose. Hefte zur Unfallheilkd 110:127–140
2. Heuchmer T, Bargon G, Bauer G, Mutschler W (1992) Computertomographie nach intraarticulärer Kalkaneusfraktur. Unfallchirurg 95:31–36
3. Nägele M, Wilhelm K, Kuglstatter W, Bauer G, Schade G, Hahn D (1990) Ischämische Mondbeinnekrose. Unfallchirurg 93:562–564
4. Simank HG, Graf J, Fromm B, Niethard FU (1992) Welche Wirkung haben gelenknahe Frakturen auf den hyalinen Gelenkknorpel? Unfallchirurg 95:280–283
5. Reiser MF, Vahlensieck M, Schüller H (1992) Imaging of the knee joint with emphasis on magnetic resonance imaging. Radiol 2:87–94

Dr. H.G. Braick, Klinik und Poliklinik für Unfallchirurgie, Universität Bonn, Sigmund-Freud-Straße 25, W-5300 Bonn 1

Die 2-Kanal Laserdopplerflußmessung in der Verlaufsbeobachtung der offenen Fraktur – Eine experimentelle Untersuchung zur Revaskularisation von Knochengewebe

The Two-Channel Laser Doppler Flowmetry of Open Fractures – An Experimental Study of Cortical Bone Revascularization

J. Buchholz[1], W. Knopp[1], R. Schnabel[1], A. Ekkernkamp[1], K. Morgenroth[2] und G. Muhr[1]

[1]Chirurgische Klinik und Poliklinik, Berufsgenossenschaftliche Krankenanstalten Bergmannsheil, Bochum (Direktor: Prof. Dr. med. G. Muhr)
[2]Pathologisches Institut, Ruhr-Universität, Bochum (Direktor: Prof. Dr. med. K. Morgenroth)

Einleitung

Extremitätenverletzungen mit schwerer Weichteilschädigung stellen auch heute noch eine große Herausforderung für die Chirurgie dar. Nicht nur der Erhalt der so geschädigten Extremität, sondern auch die Wiedererlangung der Funktion bedingen sowohl für den Patienten als auch für den Chirurgen mannigfaltige Probleme.

Erkrankungszeiträume von mehr als 18 bis 24 Monate nach solchen Verletzungen sind keine Seltenheit. Die sozioökonomischen Folgekosten belaufen sich oft, unabhängig von etwaigen Rentenzahlungen, auf mehr als 250 000 DM.

Der Hauptbezug bei offenen und geschlossenen Frakturen mit Weichteilschaden liegt im klinischen Alltag in der Versorgung von Unterschenkelfrakturen. Diese Frakturen und deren Komplikationen sind es, die maßgeblich Einfluß nehmen auf die Dauer der Rekonvaleszenz, die Wiederherstellung der Mobilität und die Möglichkeit der beruflichen wie sozialen Wiedereingliederung. Ursächlich sind dafür zwei Gründe miteinander verknüpft: 1. Die gestiegene Mobilität in unserer Gesellschaft führt immer mehr zu einer Zunahme von Verletzungen in diesem Bereich. 2. Der Unterschenkel ist nicht wie andere Regionen des Körpers von einem zirkulären polsternden Muskelmantel umgeben. Dadurch ergibt sich, daß die einwirkenden Kräfte zum einen einen direkteren schädigenderen Einfluß auf die Knochen des Unterschenkels ausüben und zum anderen, daß der ohnehin schon schwach ausgeprägte Weichteilmantel durch das Trauma in Mitleidenschaft gezogen wird. Der natürliche Schutz des Knochens vor Mikroorganismen wird zerstört und gleichzeitig die Vaskularisation zur Aufrechterhaltung der regenerativen Prozesse unterbrochen. Daher ist die Gefahr groß, daß zum einen langstreckige Knochenanteile nekrotisch werden und verloren gehen und/oder zum anderen eine Osteomyelitis entsteht. Die Beurteilung, ob freiliegendes Knochengewebe noch ausreichend durchblutet ist, unterliegt bis dato allein der subjektiven Beurteilung durch den Chirurgen im Rahmen der operativen Versorgung oder der Dekortication durch das Auftreten von Blutpunkten aus der Kortikalis.

Chirurgisches Forum 1993
f. experim. u. klinische Forschung
Becker/Beger/Hartel (Hrsg.)

Fragestellung

Im Rahmen einer experimentellen Untersuchung sollte daher der Frage nachgegangen werden, ob ein Meßverfahren wie die 2-Kanal Laserdopplerflußmessung in der Lage ist, den Zustand der Durchblutung des kortikalen Knochens als reproduzierbare Maßeinheit wiederzugeben, und ob diese Maßzahlen mit der parallel durchgeführten histologischen Beurteilung dieses Knochengewebes bzgl. seiner Vitalität korrelieren.

Material und Methode

Als Versuchsmodell zur Erzeugung einer offenen Fraktur wurden, unterteilt in zwei Gruppen zu je 40 Tieren, Kaninchen der Rasse "Weiße Neuseeländer" verwendet. Standardisiert wurde bei allen Tieren in Narkose eine Tibiafraktur durch Heraussägen eines Kortikalisdeckels aus dem linken Hinterlauf erzeugt. Der Frakturbereich wurde zudem deperiostiert und der Markraum ausgeräumt. Ohne Verschluß der Haut oder Weichteile blieb dann der Frakturbereich für 3 Tage (Gruppe I) oder 7 Tage (Gruppe II) offen und wurde dann durch einen lokalen Muskellappen des M. gastrocnemius nach Debridement gedeckt. Die Frakturstabilisierung erfolgte durch eine Schraubenosteosynthese mittels zweier Kortikalisschrauben. Im Intervall von 1 bis 16 Wochen nach der plastischen Deckung der Fraktur wurden die Tiere eingeschläfert und der Frakturbereich klinisch, histomorphologisch (Färbung: Elastica van Giesson und Hämatoxillin-Eosin) wie auch rasterelektronenmikroskopisch untersucht.

Sowohl im Rahmen der Frakturerzeugung als auch bei der Muskellappendeckung wurde die Mikrozirkulation des geschaffenen Kortikalisdeckels, der Kortikalis im Gewebeverband und des Periostes mittels der Laserdopplerflußmessung bestimmt. Zudem wurde ebenfalls in Narkose die gleiche Messung vor Sakrifizierung der Tiere durch nochmalige Freilegung des Kortikalisdeckels durchgeführt.

Zur Anwendung kam dabei das Laserdopplerflußmeßgerät MBF 3D der Firma Moor mit zwei Lasern der Typenklasse BS 4803 Typ 3B mit elektronischer Laserdiodenstabilisierung und Thermostabilität durch Peltierelemente. Mit einer Eindringtiere von 1,5 mm wird das ausgesandte Laserlicht durch die sich bewegenden Erythrozyten abgelenkt und reflektiert. Dabei unterliegt es einer Frequenzverschiebung entsprechend dem Dopplereffekt. Durch Verwendung spezieller Prozessoralgorithmen besteht eine direkte Proportionalität zwischen der Anzahl der Erythrozyten im vom Laserlicht durchströmten Gewebe und dem Mittelwert ihrer Geschwindigkeit. Als Maßzahl dient dabei das Produkt der sich bewegenden Erythrozyten (CONC) und ihrer Geschwindigkeit (SPEED), welches als Blutfluß (FLUX) bezeichnet wird.

Ergebnisse

Die Auswertung der histologischen Befunde zeigte, daß die Veränderungen nach Ausmaß und Form gleichförmig in den zeitlich differierenden beiden Gruppen ausgebildet waren. Sowohl in der Frühphase der ersten vier Wochen nach Muskellappenplastik als auch in der Spätphase nach 8 bis 16 Wochen war in der Gruppe II mit der

Weichteildeckung nach 7 Tagen der Umfang der Knochennekrose und das Ausmaß der Osteomyelitis so groß, daß sich nur in Ansätzen überhaupt ein Hinweis auf das Einheilen des Kortikalisdeckels ergaben. In der Gruppe I hingegen entwickelte sich aus der Kontaktzone zwischen Muskellappen und Knochen ein Granulationsgewebe, dessen Kapillarisierungsgrad sukzessive bis zur vierten Woche anstieg. Parallel dazu bildeten sich aus der Muskulatur Gefäße, die mit der Kortikalis in Kontakt traten. Gleichzeitig bildeten sich unter der Oberfläche des an den Kortikalisdeckels angrenzenden Knochengewebes Kapillarsprossen aus. Osteoklasten bauen parallel dazu den Knochen an der Grenzfläche ab. Durch Proliferation von Fibroblasten aus dem periostalen Weichgewebe wurde anschließend Faserknochen neu gebildet.

Bei immer weiter zunehmendem Kapillarisierungsgrad nach der vierten Woche nach Muskellappenplastik wurde dann bis zur achten Woche der Frakturspalt durch Faserknochen überbrückt und der Kortikalisdeckel reintegriert. Im weiteren Verlauf folgte dann der Ersatz des Faserknochens durch lamilläres Knochengewebe. Die bindegewebige Grenzschicht zwischen Muskulatur und Kortikalisdeckel hatte sich dann wie ein Neoperiost auf den Kortikalisdeckel gelegt und entsandte Kapillaren in die trabekulären Zwischenräume des Knochens.

Zur Festlegung der Referenzbereiche der einzelnen Gewebearten Kortikalisdeckel (D), Kortikalis (C), Periost (D) und Muskulatur (M) wurde zunächst im links/rechts Seitenvergleich bei 20 Tieren die LDF mit beiden Lasersonden vorgenommen. Unter Festlegung eines Signifikanzniveaus von 80% fand sich dabei ein arithmetisches Mittel für den Kortikalisdeckel nach völliger Entfernung aus dem Knochenverbund von 2,685 FLUX und für die Kortikalis von 22,23 FLUX (Tabelle 1).

Tabelle 1. Berechnung des Stichprobenumfanges für die Gewebearten D = Kortikalisdeckel, K = Kortikalis, P = Periost und M = Muskulatur

	D	K	P	M
Gesamteinheit (N)	20	20	20	20
Arithmetisches Mittel	2,685	22,24	39,24	94,19
Varianz	0,48555	22,2394	21,4784	639,813
Signifikanzniveau	80%	80%	80%	80%
Notwendiger Stichprobenumfang der LDF-Messung	9,75809	9,8953	9,9293	9,8622

Die in Form arbitraischer Units ermittelten Zahlenwerte der Laserdopplerflußmessung (LDF) zeigten dann im Verlauf von 1–16 Wochen nach durchgeführter Muskellappenplastik einen strengen signifikanten Verlauf mit guter Korrelation zu den histomorphologischen Ergebnissen. Ausgehend von einem durchschnittlichen Wert für Kortikalisgewebe im Knochenverbund von 22 FLUX sank dieser Wert nach vollständiger Herausnahme aus dem Knochenverbund auf Werte zwischen 1–5 FLUX mit einem Mittelwert von 2,6 FLUX ab. Bei den Tieren der Gruppe I mit einer frühen Muskellappenplastik und damit klinischer und histologischer Einheilung dieses Knochendeckels stiegen dann parallel zur Reintegration die Meßwerte der LDF auf die normalen Werte von kortikalem Knochengewebe im Verlauf bis zur 16. Woche an. Bei den Tieren der

Gruppe II mit plastischer Deckung der offenen Fraktur nach 7 Tagen hingegen kam es im zeitlichen Verlauf bis zur achten Woche nur zu einem geringen Anstieg der Werte auf maximal 15 FLUX. Bei keinem einzigen Tier dieser Gruppe wurde der Wert der normalen Kortikalisdurchblutung erreicht. Im Zeitraum bis zur 16. Woche fielen dann die Werte parallel zum klinischen und histomorphologischen Befund mit den Zeichen der Knochennekrose und Osteomyelitis wieder auf Werte zwischen 5 und 10 FLUX ab.

Schlußfolgerungen

Im Rahmen einer tierexperimentellen Untersuchung über die Versorgung einer offenen Fraktur mit Weichteilschaden konnte histomorphologisch gezeigt werden, daß im Tiermodell eine Revaskularisation von kortikalem Knochengewebe über die Weichteildeckung mittels Muskellappen bis zu einem Zeitintervall von 3 Tagen nach Eintritt des Traumas sinnvoll ist. Eine zeitlich spätere Versorgung hingegen kann den Eintritt der Knochennekrose und die Entstehung einer Osteomyelitis nicht mehr verhindern. Übertragen auf die von Östrup 1982 nachgewiesene maximale Überlebenszeit der menschlichen Knochenzelle von 5 Tagen bedeutet dies, daß in diesem Zeitraum die Versorgung der offenen Fraktur mit Weichteilschaden einschließlich einer evtl. notwendigen Muskellappenplastik abgeschlossen sein muß [3]. Trotz der von Ketterl et al. [2] nachgewiesenen Fähigkeit, die vitales Muskelgewebe bei der Therapie der chronischen Osteomyelitis erbringt, ist eine spätere Deckung der offenen Fraktur nicht als sinnvoll anzusehen. Die Bestimmung der Mikrozirkulation von Knochengewebe mittels Laserdopplerflußmessung [4, 5] erfährt durch die Anwendung des neuen Lasergerätes MBF 3D mit zwei Meßsonden eine deutliche Bereicherung [1], da sie durch den Vergleich beider Sonden untereinander sichere und genauere Ergebnisse über die Mikrozirkulation liefert. In unserer Untersuchung deckten sich diese zudem voll und ganz mit den histomorphologischen und auch klinischen Ergebnissen im Rahmen der Weichteildeckung von offenen Frakturen. Im Tierexperiment war die LDF in der Lage, eine definierte Grenze zwischen vitalem und avitalem kortikalen Knochengewebe aufzuzeigen, die gleichzeitig dem klinischen Bild der Einheilung bzw. der Nekrose entsprach. Hierdurch ist unseres Erachtens die Möglichkeit gegeben, im klinischen Einsatz erstmalig bei der Behandlung offener Frakturen, wie auch im Rahmen der Osteomyelitisbehandlung, durch den Einsatz der Laserdopplerflußmessung eine definitive Grenze zwischen durchblutetem und damit überlebensfähigem und nicht mehr durchblutetem Knochengewebe zu ziehen. Eine Minimierung von Knochenverlust bei gleichzeitiger Vermeidung des Belassens von nekrotischem Knochengewebe in situ wäre damit zu erreichen.

Zusammenfassung

In einer experimentellen Studie mit Kaninchen konnten wir nachweisen, daß nur bis zum dritten Tag nach Setzen des Traumas eine plastische Versorgung mit einem Muskellappen die Gewähr für eine Revaskularisation von kortikalem Knochengewebe bot. Bei einer späteren Weichteilsanierung nach 7 Tagen konnte das Entstehen einer kompletten Knochennekrose nicht mehr verhindert werden. Die Durchführung der Laserdopplerflußmessung und deren Meßergebnisse mittels der 2-Kanal Sondentechnik zeigte klar abgrenzbare Grenzwerte zwischen vitalem und avitalem Knochen und spiegelte mit der Höhe der Meßwerte auch den klinischen und histomorphologischen Zustand bzgl. der Revaskularisation oder Nekrose des Knochens eindeutig wieder.

Summary

In an experimental study using adult rabbits, we found that only in the first 3 days after trauma a reconstruction of soft tissue damage with a muscle flap will be successful in revascularizing cortical bone. Later reconstruction will lead to necrosis of the bone. The use of the two-channel laser Doppler flowmetry in this study showed a clear difference between vascularized and nonrevascularized cortical bone, reflecting the clinical and histological outcome of revascularization or necrosis of cortical bone.

Literatur

1. Barnett NJ, Dougherty G, Pettinger SJ (1990) Comparative study of two laser Doppler blood flowmeters. J Med Engineering Technology 14 (6):243–249
2. Ketterl R, Ascherl R, Feller AM, Stzeinau HU, Stübinger B, Blümel G (1991) Revaskularisation durch Muskellappen bei avaskulärem und infiziertem Knochen. Langenbecks Arch Chir [Suppl] Chir Forum, pp 1–7
3. Östrup LT (1982) Free bone transfer. Scand J Plast Reconstr Surg 14 [Suppl]:103
4. Swiontkowski MF, Schlehr F, Collins JC, Sanders R, Pou A (1988) Comparison of two laser-Doppler flowmetry systems for bone blood flow analysis. Calcif Tissue Int 43:103–107
5. Swiontkowski MF, Senft D (1992) Cortical bone microperfusion: Responde to ischemia and changes in major arterial blood flow. J Orthop Res 10:337–343

Dr. J. Buchholz, Chirurgische Klinik und Poliklinik, Krankenanstalten Bergmannsheil, Universitätsklinik, Gilsingstraße 14, W-4630 Bochum 1

Endotoxin im Blutplasma von Patienten nach Trauma
Endotoxin in Blood Plasma of Trauma Patients

W. Strecker[1], O. Gonschorek[1], L. Kinzl[1], D. Berger[2] und H.G. Beger[2]

[1]Abteilung für Unfallchirurgie (Direktor: Prof. Dr. L. Kinzl), Universität Ulm
[2]Abteilung für Allgemeinchirurgie (Direktor: Prof. Dr. H.G. Beger), Universität Ulm

Zielsetzung

Die Spätletalität nach Trauma wird in erster Linie durch Organversagen (OV) und Sepsis verursacht. Dabei kommt dem Darm als Schockorgan eine zentrale Bedeutung zu. Das hämorrhagisch-traumatische Schockgeschehen bewirkt eine Minderperfusion der Darmmukosa. Darüberhinaus bewirken Schädigungen der Lunge eine intestinale Hypoxie. Weitere Schädigungsmechanismen, wie der Reperfusionsschaden, führen zum Zusammenbruch der Darmbarriere, zur Translokation von Endotoxin (ET) und schließlich von Bakterien aus dem Darmlumen in das portalvenöse Blut. Die konsekutiv freigesetzten Mediatoren, wie Interleukin 1 und Tumor-Nekrose-Faktor, triggern Folgereaktionen, die zum OV und zur Sepsis führen [3].

Der klinische Nachweis einer zentralen Rolle des ET in dem postulierten pathophysiologischen Geschehen nach Trauma steht bislang aus. Ziel unserer Untersuchung war die Bestimmung der Endotoxin-Plasmaspiegel bei schwerverletzten Patienten mit unterschiedlichem Verletzungsmuster.

Methodik

Im Zeitraum Juli 1991 bis Juni 1992 wurden an der Chirurgischen Universitätsklinik Ulm 97 polytraumatisierte Patienten aufgenommen. 40 Patienten aus diesem Kollektiv entsprachen den strengen nachfolgenden Aufnahmekriterien (Tabelle 1). Insbesondere sollte eine bakterielle Kontamination von äußeren Wunden ebenso ausgeschlossen sein wie traumatische Eröffnungen des Gastrointestinaltraktes und des bronchopulmonalen Systems.

Bei allen 40 Patienten wurde nach Abschluß der Diagnostik der jeweilige Injury Severity Score (ISS) ermittelt (Tabelle 2), sowie im weiteren Verlauf der Goris-Score als Parameter des OV [2]. Entsprechend der im Vordergrund stehenden Verletzungen wurden die Patienten einer der folgenden 4 Verletzungsgruppen zugeordnet: I Lungenkontusion; II Schädel-Hirn-Trauma II°/III°; III Extremitätenfrakturen; IV Schwere Kombinationsverletzungen.

Arterielle Blutproben wurden in einem festgelegten zeitlichen Raster nach Trauma abgenommen: direkt nach Aufnahme im Schockraum, nach weiteren 30 und 60 min; nach 2, 4, 6, 8, 10 und 12 h; nach 1, 2, 3, 4, 5, 8 und 10 Tagen.

Chirurgisches Forum 1993
f. experim. u. klinische Forschung
Becker/Beger/Hartel (Hrsg.)

Tabelle 1. Aufnahmekriterien der untersuchten Patienten

Einschlußkriterien

1. Stumpfes Thoraxtrauma
2. Schädel-Hirn-Trauma mit pos. CT-Befund
3. Frakturen von mindestens 2 großen Röhrenknochen
4. Jede Kombination von 1.–3.

Ausschlußkriterien

1. Alter < 16 und > 80 Jahre
2. Gravidität
3. Immundefizienz
4. Kontaminierte offene Frakturen
5. Perforierende Traumen von Thorax oder Abdomen
6. Therapiefreies Intervall > 30 Minuten
7. Rettungszeiten > 2 Stunden

Endotoxin (ET): Die ET-Konzentration im Blutplasma wurde mittels Limulus-Amöbozyten-Lysat-Test nachgewiesen [1]. Die Sensitivität des Tests liegt bei 0,02 EU/ml, entsprechend 1,7 pg ET/ml Plasma.

Statistik: Die bei den Vergleichen zwischen den einzelnen Verletzungsgruppen angegebenen Daten stellen Mittelwerte $\bar{x} \pm$ SEM dar. Die Signifikanzen wurden mit dem t-Test nach Student für ungepaarte Stichproben berechnet. Das Signifikanzniveau wurde mit $p < 0{,}01$ festgelegt.

Ergebnisse

Von den 40 Patienten, die die Aufnahmekriterien erfüllten, waren 34 Männer und 6 Frauen. Ihr Alter lag zwischen 16 und 78 Jahren ($\bar{x}$ = 43,7 Jahre). Die Verletzungsschwere zeigte eine Streuung zwischen 11 und 54 Punkten ISS ($\bar{x}$ = 23). Der Goris-Score war am niedrigsten in der Patientengruppe II (Extremitätenfrakturen) mit 0,8 Punkten und am höchsten in der Patientengruppe I (Lungenkontusion) mit 4 Punkten (Tabelle 2). 7 der 40 Patienten erlagen ihren Verletzungen. Grund war in 6 Fällen ein verletzungsbedingter Hirntod, in 1 Fall ein hämorrhagischer Schock.

Im zeitlichen Verlauf nach Trauma (Abb. 1) sind in den ersten 5 Tagen anhaltend hohe ET-Spiegel in der Patientengruppe mit Thoraxtrauma nachweisbar. Mäßig erhöhte ET-Spiegel persistieren bei den Verletzten mit Kombinationsverletzungen. Bei den Patienten der Gruppen II und III hingegen ist bereits 24 h nach dem Unfallereignis eine weitgehende Normalisierung der ET-Spiegel eingetreten.

Die Unterschiede der ET-Spiegel am Aufnahmetag zwischen den einzelnen Verletzungsgruppen sind zum Teil hochsignifikant ($p < 0{,}005$), insbesondere zwischen den Gruppen I und II sowie zwischen II und IV. Keinerlei Korrelation besteht zwischen dem jeweiligen mittleren ET-Spiegel der einzelnen Verletzungsgruppen und der jeweiligen Verletzungsschwere, ausgedrückt durch den ISS.

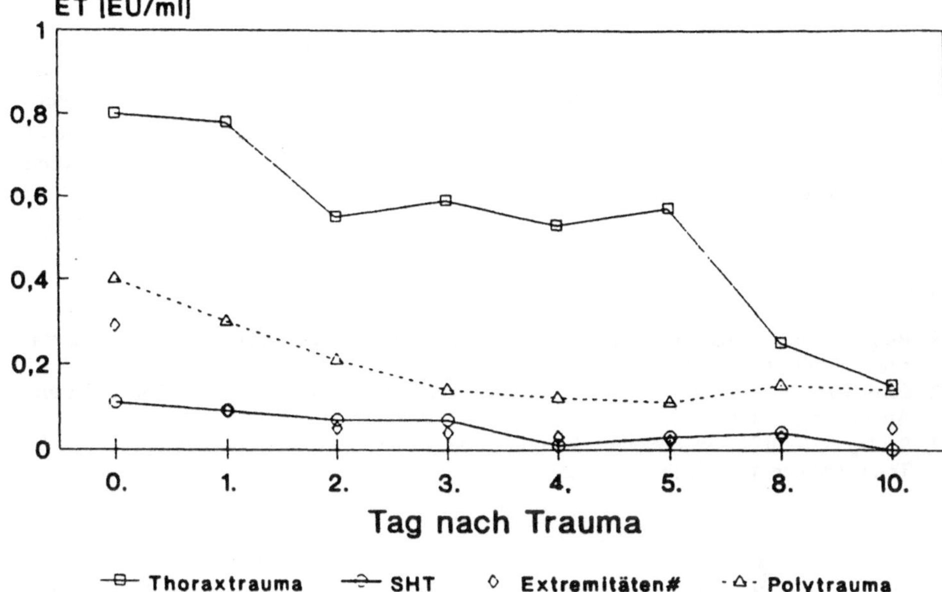

Abb. 1. Endotoxinkonzentrationen im Blutplasma von unfallverletzten Patienten im zeitlichen Verlauf nach Trauma

Tabelle 2. Patientendaten, Injury Severity Score und Goris-Score in den einzelnen Verletzungsgruppen

Verletzungs-gruppe	n	m/w	Alter	ISS	OV (Goris-Score)
I	6	5/1	46,8	17	4
II	12	9/3	48,5	20	1,4
III	8	7/1	40,8	12	0,8
IV	14	13/1	40,3	35	2,9
Gesamt	40	34/6	43,7	23	2,2

Zusammenfassung

1. Bei entsprechender Verletzungsschwere (ISS) finden sich hohe Endotoxinspiegel bei Traumapatienten mit Lungenkontusion, während die Endotoxinspiegel bei Patienten nach Schädelhirntrauma nur mäßiggradig erhöht sind. Dieser Unterschied ist hochsignifikant.
2. Unfallverletzte mit Extremitätenfrakturen als Hauptdiagnose sowie solche mit schweren Kombinationsverletzungen zeigen mittelgradige Anstiege der Endotoxinspiegel am Aufnahmetag.
3. Es besteht keine Beziehung zwischen Verletzungsschwere (ISS) und posttraumatischer Endotoxinämie.

Summary

Mean endotoxin (ET) concentrations are significantly higher in patients suffering from thoracic trauma than in patients with brain injury in the acute phase after severe trauma. Patients with limb fractures and combined injuries had moderate increases of ET concentrations during the first day after trauma. There is no correlation between the Injury Severity Score and ET levels.

Literatur

1. Berger D, Beger HG (1990) Endotoxin binding proteins of human serum: Are there therapeutic implications? Clin Chir Acta 162:289
2. Goris RJA, te Boekhorst TPA, Nuytinck JKS, Gimbrère JSF (1985) Multiple-organ failure. Arch Surg 120:1109
3. Schlag G, Redl H (1988) Neue Erkenntnisse der Pathogenese des Schockgeschehens in der Traumatologie. Unfallchirurgie 14:3

Dr. W. Strecker, Abteilung für Unfallchirurgie, Chirurgische Universitätsklinik Ulm, Steinhövelstraße 9, W-7900 Ulm

Xanthinoxidase: Mediator der Aktivierung polymorphkerniger Granulozyten nach Trauma?

Xanthine Oxidase: Mediator of Polymorphonuclear Leukocyte (PMNL) Activation During Ischemia/Reperfusion in Humans?

S. Rose, J. Dike, M. Fiebrich, P. Weber und V. Bühren

Chirurgische Universitätsklinik, Homburg/Saar

Einleitung

Wesentliches Merkmal des posttraumatischen Ischämie/Reperfusionssyndromes (z.B. nach hypovolämischem Schock, Großreplantation) ist eine fulminante vaskuläre Permeabilitätsstörung, die in vielen Fällen zum beatmungspflichtigen respiratorischen Versagen führt. Entscheidender Faktor in der Entwicklung des Organversagens sind endotheliale Membranschäden, welche nach derzeitigen Vorstellungen vorwiegend durch die Wirkung toxischer Sauerstoffradikale aus der Xanthinoxidase-Reaktion oder dem "respiratory burst" aktivierter polymorphkerniger Granulozyten induziert werden [1]. Friedl zeigte nach Tourniquet-Ischämie am Menschen bereits Minuten nach Öffnen der Blutsperre ein deutliches Ansteigen der Xanthinoxidase-Aktivität im Plasma [2].

Ziel der vorliegenden Studie war es, den zeitlichen Verlauf der Granulozyten-Aktivierung nach Skelettmuskel-Reperfusion zu untersuchen. Über die potentielle Blockade der Xanthinoxidase-Aktivierung durch den kompetitiven Xanthinoxidase-Inhibitor Allopurinol [3] sollte die Bedeutung dieses Enzymsystems für die PMNL-Aktivierung im Ischämie/Reperfusionssyndrom abgeschätzt werden. Daneben wurde die Wirkung des nicht-steroidalen Antiphlogistikums und Cyclooxygenase-Hemmers Indomethazin auf die PMNL-Aktivierung überprüft.

Material und Methode

Patientenkollektiv

Bei 23 Patienten (18–60 Jahre) mit Tourniquet-Ischämie der oberen Extremität nach handchirurgischen Eingriffen wurde aus der oberflächlichen Cubitalvene sowohl der ischämischen (ipsilateral) als auch der nicht-ischämischen Kontrollextremität (kontralateral) vor Ischämie und bis 90 min nach Eröffnung des Tourniquet (Reperfusion) heparinisiertes Vollblut entnommen. Polymorphkernige Granulozyten (PMNL) wurden mittels Percoll-Gradient isoliert. Als Leukozyten-Funktionsparameter wurden PMNL-Myeloperoxidase (MPO), PMNL-Sauerstoffradikal-Produktion (SRP), PMNL-Elastase und Luminol-verstärkte Chemilumineszenz (LCL) quantifiziert.

Chirurgisches Forum 1993
f. experim. u. klinische Forschung
Becker/Beger/Hartel (Hrsg.)

Gruppe A: unbehandelt, n = 9, durchschnittliche Ischämiezeit (IZ) 67±15 min; *Gruppe B:* Allopurinol (300 mg p.o.) 12 h und 2 h vor Ischämiebeginn, n = 6, IZ: 72 ± 15 min; *Gruppe C:* Indomethazin (50 mg p.o.) 2 h vor Ischämiebeginn, n = 6, IZ: 69±29 min.

Meßmethoden

PMNL-Myeloperoxidase: Guaiacol-Assay mit Quantifizierung des Tetraguaiacol-Komplex nach PMNL-Lyse mit Triton-X100 (0,1%) bei 470 nm.

PMNL-Sauerstoffradikalproduktion: Ferricytochrom C-Reduktionsassay mit Quantifizierung der Sauerstoffradikalproduktion bei 550 nm. "Discontinuous Assay" mit und ohne Inhibition durch Superoxid Dismutase. PMNL-Stimulation mit Phorbol-Myristat-Acetat unter Plasma-Einfluß.

PMNL-Elastase: Immun-Assay (Fa. Boehringer, Ingelheim, Deutschland)

PMNL-Chemilumineszenz: Quantifizierung der Luminol-verstärkten Lichtemission nach Aktivierung gesunder Spender-PMNL mit Phorbol-Myristat-Acetat unter Plasma-Einfluß (Integral, Peak).

Harnsäure: Uricase-PAP-Methode (Fa. Boehringer, Ingelheim, Deutschland)

Statistik

Varianzanalyse (ANOVA) und abhängiger t-Test (Systat, Evanston, IL). Testergebnisse mit $p < 0,05$ wurden als statistisch relevant betrachtet. Die Versuchsergebnisse sind als Mittelwerte ± Standardabweichung des Mittelwertes dargestellt.

Ergebnisse

PMNL, isoliert aus dem Venenblut der Kontrollarme aller drei Versuchsgruppen, zeigten über den gesamten Versuchszeitraum keine signifikanten Änderungen von PMNL-MPO, PMNL-SRP, Plasma-Elastase oder -Harnsäure. Im Gegensatz dazu stiegen in den Ischämiearmen inbehandelter Patienten *60 min nach Reperfusion* PMNL-MPO. PMNL-SRP und Plasma-Elastase signifikant ($p < 0,05$) im Vergleich zum Kontrollarm oder zum Zeitpunkt vor Ischämie an (Tabelle 1). Vor und nach diesem Zeitpunkt waren keine signifikanten Veränderungen dieser Parameter an der reperfundierten Extremität nachweisbar.

Der signifikante MPO-Anstieg nach Reperfusion wurde sowohl in der Allopurinol- als auch Indomethazin-behandelten Gruppe nicht beobachtet. PMNL, isoliert 60 min nach Reperfusion ischämischer Extremitäten von Allopurinol- und Indomethazin-behandelten Patienten, zeigten eine signifikant verringerte ($p < 0,05$) Phorbolester-stimulierte Sauerstoffradikalproduktion in Gegenwart des eigenen Plasmas.

Tabelle 1. PMNL-Funktionsparameter sowie Harnsäure- und Elastase-Plasmaspiegel 60 min nach Eröffnung des Tourniquet im kontralateralen Kontrollarm (C) und ipsilateralen reperfundierten Arm (I)

		MPO (mU)	SRP (nmol/min/ 10^6 cells)	Elastase (g/ml)	Harnsäure (mg/dl)
A.	C	547 ± 57	51 ± 4	22 ± 2	$5,7 \pm 0,2$
	I	976 ± 83^a	68 ± 4^a	60 ± 3^a	$6,2 \pm 0,2$
B.	C	498 ± 30	50 ± 30	28 ± 2	$3,9 \pm 0,2^b$
	I	463 ± 24^b	22 ± 3^b	71 ± 8^a	$3,9 \pm 0,2^b$
C.	C	412 ± 33	31 ± 1	30 ± 2	$3,9 \pm 0,3^b$
	I	400 ± 28^b	43 ± 4^b	80 ± 13^a	$3,7 \pm 0,1^b$

[a] $p < 0,05$ vs. Kontrollarm
[b] $p < 0,05$ vs. Ischämiearm der Gruppe A

Wurden diese Plasmen mit PMNL gesunder Spender inkubiert, so zeigten sich weder für die unbehandelte noch für die beiden behandelten Gruppen signifikante Effekte auf die PMNL-Sauerstoffradikal-Produktion oder Luminol-verstärkte Chemilumineszenz.

Während der signifikante Anstieg der PMNL-Elastase im Plasma zum Zeitpunkt 60 min nach Reperfusion durch Allopurinol- und Indomethazin unbeeinflußt blieb, wurde in diesen beiden Gruppen eine signifikant niedrigere Plasma-Harnsäure-Konzentration im Vergleich zur unbehandelten Gruppe beobachtet.

Schlußfolgerungen und Diskussion

1. Der Nachweis aktivierter polymorphkerniger Granulozyten ("respiratory burst") 60 min nach Reperfusion ischämischer Skelettmuskulatur korreliert mit einem signifikanten Anstieg von Fluoreszenz-Produkten und Hinweisen auf einen Radikal-induzierten Membranschaden [2]. Gesteigerte Aktivität des Myeloperoxidase-Systems impliziert eine potentielle Schädigung der Mikrozirkulation nachfolgender Organsysteme, insbesondere der Lunge als direkt nachgeschaltetem Filter.

2. Unter Berücksichtigung der im gleichen Modell gezeigten frühen Xanthinoxidase-Aktivierung zeigt die deutliche Hemmung der PMNL-Aktivierung durch Allopurinol eine mögliche "Trigger"-Rolle des Xanthinoxidase-Systems für die Induktion des sekundären, Granulozyten-bedingten Reperfusionsschadens. Diese Hypothese wird durch die deutliche Verminderung der Plasma-Harnsäurekonzentration unter Allopurinol-Behandlung gestützt.

3. Eine dem Allopurinol vergleichbare Beeinflussung der PMNL-Funktion durch Indomethazin läßt auf eine Beteiligung Cyclooxygenase-abhängiger Arachidonsäure-Derivate oder auch Prostaglandin-induzierter Sauerstoffradikal-Produktion schließen.

Vorläufige Messungen der Phospholipase A_2-Aktivität zeigen auch, daß sowohl Indomethazin- als auch Allopurinol-Behandlung die Aktivität dieses Schlüsselenzyms beeinflussen. Allerdings lassen sich aufgrund der vorliegenden Daten noch keine gesicherten Rückschlüsse auf die spezifische Rolle von Arachidonsäure-Derivaten in Bezug auf das Xanthinoxidase-System, die PMNL-Aktivierung oder auch umgekehrt ziehen.

4. Der fehlende Einfluß von Allopurinol und Indomethazin auf den PMNL-Elastase Anstieg im Plasma zeigt einen differenzierten Aktivierungs- und Kontrollmechanismus für die verschiedenen PMNL-Enzymsysteme.

5. Die Beobachtung, daß in allen Versuchsgruppen die spezifischen Plasmaeffekte auf die PMNL-SRP nicht an gesunden Spender-PMNL reproduziert werden konnten, läßt vermuten, daß der PMNL-"respiratory burst" nicht nur durch die Freisetzung spezifischer inhibierender und supprimierender Mediatoren, sondern auch während der Passage des PMNL durch das reperfundierte Gefäßgebiet kontrolliert und moduliert wird. In diesem Zusammenhang spielt die PMNL-Endothel-Interaktion eine entscheidende Rolle und könnte zum spezifischen "priming" der granulozytären Signal- und Rezeptorsysteme führen [4, 5].

Zusammenfassung

An Patienten mit Tourniquet-Ischämie der oberen Extremität konnte am reperfundierten Arm 60 min nach Eröffnung der Blutsperre ein signifikantes Ansteigen der PMNL-Sauerstoffradikalproduktion (SRP), PMNL-Myeloperoxidase-Aktivität wie auch der PMNL-Elastase im Plasma gezeigt werden. Der PMNL-"respiratory burst" wurde durch Vorbehandlung der Patienten sowohl mit dem kompetitiven Xanthinoxidase-Hemmer Allopurinol (300 mg p.o., 12 und 2 h vor Ischämie) als auch mit dem Cyclooxygenase-Hemmer Indomethazin (50 mg p.o., 2 h vor Ischämie) in Gegenwart des Plasmas signifikant gehemmt. Dieses Plasma zeigte allerdings keinen Effekt auf die SRP oder Luminol-verstärkte Chemilumineszenz gesunder Spender-PMNL. Die deutliche Senkung der Plasma-Harnsäure-Konzentration durch beide Therapeutika ist als indirekter Hinweis auf eine verminderte Xanthinoxidase-Aktivität zu werten. Diese Beobachtungen lassen eine potentielle Mediatorrolle der frühen Xanthinoxidase-Aktivierung für den sekundären PMNL-"respiratory burst" nach Ischämie/Reperfusion vermuten. Inwieweit Arachidonsäurederivate diese Mechanismen verstärken und kontrollieren ist Ziel weiterer Untersuchungen. Neben dem Einfluß humoraler Mediatoren scheint ein spezifisches Priming der PMNL durch Interaktion mit dem Gefäßendothel wesentlich.

Summary

Polymorphonuclear leukocytes (PMNL) were isolated from the cubital vein blood of patients undergoing tourniquet ischemia of the upper extremity. At 60 min after release of the tourniquet, PMNL demonstrated a significant "respiratory burst" in the presence of plasma and an increase in plasma elastase activity. Pretreatment with allopurinol (300 mg p.o., 12 and 2 h before ischemia) and indomethacin (50 mg p.o., 2 h before ischemia) significantly inhibited PMNL-oxygen free radical production and PMNL-myeloperoxidase activity, but did not affect plasma elastase concentrations. Xanthine oxidase activation might be a "trigger" mechanism to induce PMNL "respiratory burst" during ischemia/reperfusion events. Specific plasma effects were not reproducible in healthy donor PMNL, suggesting that in addition to soluble plasma mediators (e.g., cytokines, complement), PMNL endothelial cell interactions might contribute to a specific "priming" of leukocytes during reperfusion. Whether arachidonic acid derivatives are involved in these mechanisms has to be studied by further analyses of prostaglandin and leukotriene profiles.

Literatur

1. Granger DN (1988) Role of xanthine oxidase and granulocytes in ischemia-reperfusion injury. Am J Physiol 255 (Heart Circ Physiol 24):H1269–H1275
2. Friedl HP, Smith DJ, Till GO, Thomson PD, Louis DS, Ward PA (1990) Ischemia-reperfusion in humans. Appearance of xanthine oxidase activity. Am J Physiol 136:491–495
3. Hille R, Massey V (1982) Tight binding inhibitors of xanthine oxidase. Pharmacol Ther 14:249–263
4. Marzi I, Knee K, Bühren V, Menger M, Trentz O (1992) Reduction by superoxide dismutase of leukocyte-endothelial adherence after liver transplantation. Surgery 111:90–97
5. Jutila MA (1992) Leukocyte traffic to sites of inflammation. APMIS 100:287–293

Dr. med. S. Rose, Abteilung für Unfallchirurgie, Chirurgische Universitätsklinik, W-6650 Homburg/Saar

Korrelation von D-Dimeren zu Verletzungsschwere und Thromboserisiko bei unfallchirurgischen Patienten

d-Dimer Levels Correlate with Injury Severity and Pathologic Thrombosis in Trauma Patients

U. Schmidt[1], B.L. Enderson[2], J.P. Chen[2], M. Nerlich[1] und H. Tscherne[1]

[1]Unfallchirurgische Klinik, Medizinische Hochschule Hannover
[2]University of Tennessee Graduate School of Medicine, Knoxville, USA

Einleitung

D-Dimere werden bei der Spaltung von Faktor XIII-quervernetztem Fibrin gebildet. Der Anstieg der Dimere gilt als Indikator eines hyperkoagulabilen Zustandes in der Initialphase nach akutem Trauma, prolongierte Verläufe dieses Zustandes können das Auftreten einer "pathologischen" Thrombose beeinflussen.

Das Ziel dieser prospektiven Studie war es, Veränderungen der D-Dimer Spiegel spezifischen Organsystemveränderungen zuzuordnen und diese mit dem Auftreten von Thrombosen und Lungenembolien zu korrelieren.

Methodik

41 erwachsene Patienten (32 männlich, 9 weiblich, mittleres Alter 33 Jahre, 18–81 Jahre) wurden während eines 5monatigen Zeitraumes in die Studie aufgenommen. Die prospektive Auswahl der Patienten erfolgte bezüglich spezifischer isolierter Verletzungen. Patienten, die eine Heparinisierung erhalten hatten, wurden von der Studie ausgeschlossen.

Die Blutentnahme erfolgte bei Klinikaufnahme, dann 1, 2, 4, 6 Tage nach Aufnahme und weiter im wöchentlichen Rhythmus via Punktion peripherer Venen.

Die Bestimmung der D-Dimere erfolgte mit zwei Methoden, dem D-Dimer Latex Agglutinationstest (American Dade, Miami, Florida, USA) und dem D-Dimer ELISA Verfahren (American Diagnostica, New York, New York, USA). Die statistische Analyse erfolgte mit dem Spearman Rank Sum Test mit Signifikanzen von $p < 0{,}05$.

Ergebnisse

Die D-Dimer Spiegel, die nach beiden Methoden bestimmt wurden, wurden mit dem Injury Severity Score (ISS) der Patienten korreliert. Tabelle 1 zeigt die Korrelation der D-Dimer Spiegel zur Verletzungsschwere nach dem ISS aufgeteilt nach spezifischen

Chirurgisches Forum 1993
f. experim. u. klinische Forschung
Becker/Beger/Hartel (Hrsg.)

Tabelle 1. Korrelation der D-Dimere (Latex-Test) mit der Verletzungsschwere nach dem ISS bei Klinikaufnahme

	n	Korrelation	p
insgesamt	41	0,580	0,0001
Schädel/Hirn	8	0,860	0,006
Wirbelsäule mit Neurologie	8	0,832	0,010
Untere Extremität	10	0,232	0,548
Polytrauma	11	0,454	0,187
andere	4	–	–

Verletzungen. Auffallend ist eine signifikante Korrelation bei Patienten mit isoliertem Schädel/Hirn Trauma und isolierten Wirbelsäulenverletzungen mit Neurologie.

Beide Messungen zeigten bei Klinikaufnahme die höchsten Werte, mit einem allmählichen Rückgang zu Normalwerten an den folgenden Tagen.

2 der 41 Patienten entwickelten klinisch Symptome einer Lungenembolie (LE), die durch eine Ventilations-/Perfusionsszintigraphie bestätigt wurde. Ein Patient mit einem kompletten Querschnitt nach Wirbelsäulenverletzung entwickelte an beiden Unterschenkeln eine tiefe Beinvenenthrombose. Bei allen 3 Patienten folgte nach initialem Rückgang der D-Dimer Werte (Latex und ELISA) ein Wiederanstieg (Abb. 1) bereits mehrere Tage, bevor klinisch die Diagnose der Thrombose bzw. Lungenembolie gestellt werden konnte. 3 andere Patienten entwickelten klinisch eine LE-Symptomatik, jedoch konnte per Pulmonalisangiographie diese ausgeschlossen werden. Keiner dieser Patienten entwickelte einen Wiederanstieg der D-Dimere bis 4–8 μg/ml.

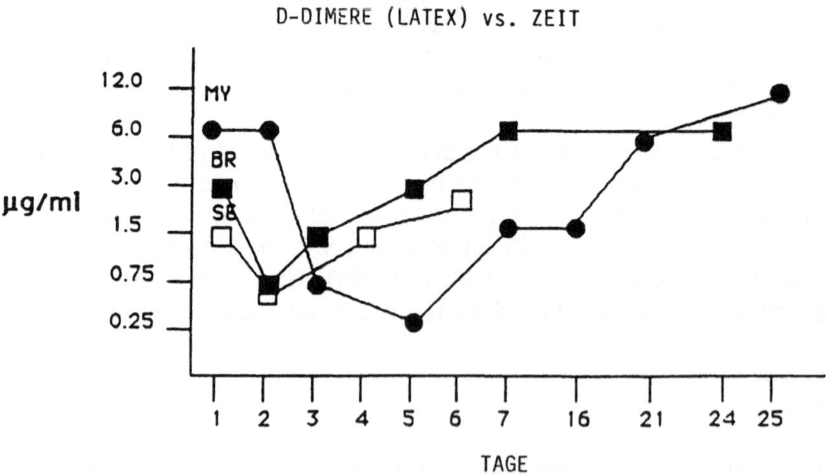

Abb. 1. Zeitverlauf der D-Dimere (Latex) bei 3 Patienten (MY, BR, SE) mit Thrombose bzw. Lungenembolie

Diskussion

Unfallchirurgische Patienten erfahren in der Initialphase nach Trauma eine Periode der Hyperkoagulabilität und Hyperfibrinolyse, gefolgt von einem Abfall der fibrinolytischen Aktivität [1, 2].

Patienten mit Verletzungen des zentralen Nervensystems zeigen eine Korrelation zwischen Verletzungsschwere und D-Dimer Spiegel, also der Höhe der Hyperkoagulabilität. Diese Ergebnisse stehen in Übereinstimmung mit Studien, die eine erhöhte Inzidenz der Thrombose und Lungenembolie bei diesen Patienten zeigen.

Lichey et al. [3] beschrieben den Nutzen der D-Dimer Messung (ELISA) in der Diagnostik der Lungenembolie.

Charakteristisch für Patienten mit pathologischer Thrombose ist ein allmählicher Wiederanstieg der D-Dimer Spiegel, mehrere Tage vor Auftreten klinischer Symptome. Dieser Wiederanstieg ist jedoch nicht ausschließlich spezifisch hinsichtlich des Auftretens einer Thrombose bzw. Lungenembolie. Die Bestimmung der D-Dimer Werte ermöglicht jedoch die Erfassung von Patienten mit erhöhtem Risiko der Thrombose. Ein Wiederanstieg der D-Dimere nach initialem Rückgang scheint bei Patienten ohne Sepsis und ARDS ein Risikofaktor zu sein. Maßnahmen wie prophylaktische Heparinisierung bzw. das Setzen eines Vena cava Schirmes können getroffen werden, um die Möglichkeit einer tödlichen Lungenembolie zu minimieren. Weiterhin unterstützt die Messung der D-Dimer Spiegel die Diagnostik bei klinischem Verdacht auf Thrombose oder Lungenembolie.

Zusammenfassung

Diese prospektive Studie untersucht die Messung von D-Dimer Spiegeln nach akutem Trauma als Indikator der Hyperkoagulabilität, welche diese Patienten einem erhöhten Risiko hinsichtlich der Entwicklung einer pathologischen Thrombose zuordnet. 41 Patienten wurden untersucht, um die Anwendung der D-Dimer Bestimmung hinsichtlich des Thromboserisikos zu definieren. Ein Wiederanstieg der D-Dimere war charakteristisch bei Patienten, die eine Lungenembolie entwickelten, jedoch verursachte ebenfalls Sepsis oder ein ARDS ähnliche Verläufe. Patienten mit Verletzungen des zentralen Nervensystems zeigten eine signifikante Korrelation der D-Dimer Spiegel mit der Verletzungsschwere nach dem Injury Severity Score, jedoch nicht polytraumatisierte Patienten oder Patienten mit Verletzung der unteren Extremität. D-Dimer Bestimmungen stellen somit eine einfache, schnelle und relativ kostengünstige Methode dar, um Patienten mit erhöhtem Thromboserisiko zu erfassen.

Summary

This prospective study examines the measurement of d-Dimer cross-linked fibrin degradation products (d-Dimer XDPs) as an indicator of hypercoagulability, which places a trauma patient at risk of developing pathologic thrombosis. Forty-one trauma patients were studied to evaluate the potential use of d-Dimer XDP levels in evaluating the risk of pathologic thrombosis. A secondary increase in d-Dimer XDP levels was found to occur in patients with pulmonary embolism, although sepsis and acute respiratory distress syndrome (ARDS) can also cause a late increase. d-Dimer XDP levels in patients with central nervous system injuries demonstrated significant correlations with the injury severity, but not in patients with multiple system or single lower extremity injuries. However, determining d-Dimer levels appears to provide an easy, relatively inexpensive means of evaluating trauma patients for the risk of pathologic thrombosis.

Literatur

1. Bennett B, Towler HMA (1985) Hemostatic response to trauma. Br Med Bull 41:274–280
2. Enderson BL, Chen JP, et al. (1991) Fibrinolysis in multisystem trauma patients. J Trauma 31:1240
3. Lichey J, Reschowski I et al. (1990) D-Dimer is a highly specific and sensitive parameter in the diagnosis of lung embolism. Fibrinogen 4: Current Basis and Clinical Aspects. Elsevier, Amsterdam, pp 209–212

Dr. med. U. Schmidt, Medizinische Hochschule Hannover, Unfallchirurgische Klinik, Postfach 610180, W-3000 Hannover 61

Tierexperimentelle Untersuchungen zur Einheilung einer augmentierten Hydroxylapatitkeramik in einem Tibiasegmentdefekt beim Schaf

The Healing of a Segmental Defect in the Sheep Tibia Filled with an Augmented Hydroxylapatite Ceramic

B. Wippermann, P. Junge, H. Zwipp und H. Tscherne

Unfallchirurgische Klinik, Medizinische Hochschule Hannover

Einleitung

Die Auffüllung von Knochendefekten insbesondere im diaphysären Bereich stellt in der Unfallchirurgie nach wie vor ein aktuelles Problem dar. Die autologe Knochenverpflanzung gilt weiterhin als das Standardverfahren der ersten Wahl, an ihren Ergebnissen müssen sich alls Konkurrenzverfahren messen. Nachteilig bei diesem Verfahren ist einerseits die Notwendigkeit des zusätzlichen Eingriffs und andererseits die limitierte Verfügbarkeit. Der allogene Knochenersatz hat neben seiner geringeren osteoinduktiven Potenz noch den Nachteil der primären Infektionsgefahr durch Aids [4] und Hepatitis sowie der häufigen Spätinfekte. Durch diese Entwicklungen wurde das Interesse an Knochenersatzstoffen neu belebt. Diese sollten einerseits unbegrenzt und ohne Morbidität für den Patienten verfügbar sein und andererseits den osteogenen Eigenschaften der autologen Knochenverpflanzung nahe kommen. Es gibt Hinweise in der Literatur, daß der Zusatz von Knochenmark die Einheilung von Keramiken verbessern kann [2]. In dieser Studie sollten 2 Fragen geklärt werden: 1. Kann eine Hydroxylapatitkeramik aus boviner Spongiosa (Fa. Merck, Darmstadt, Deutschland) einen Tibiasegmentdefekt zuverlässig überbrücken? 2. Kann die Einheilung der Keramik durch Beladung mit 0,2 g basic Fibroblast Growth Factor (bFGF) (Fa. Merck, Darmstadt, Deutschland), mit autologem Knochenmark oder mit einer Kombination dieser Substanzen verbessert werden?

Methoden

Als Versuchsmodell diente ein einseitiger 2 cm langer (entspricht 10% der Knochenlänge) Tibiasegmentdefekt beim mindestens 2 Jahre alten weiblichen Schwarzkopfmutterschaf. Insgesamt wurden für diesen Versuch 48 Tiere mit einem Durchschnittsgewicht von 70,3 kg operiert. In Intubationsnarkose mit Halothan – Lachgas wurde der Tibiasegmentdefekt mit einer sonderangefertigten schmalen DC-Platte versorgt. Die Platte hatte die Dimensionen einer 8-Lochplatte, bei der die beiden zentralen Schraubenlöcher nicht angelegt waren. Insgesamt 7 Tiere konnten wegen

Chirurgisches Forum 1993
f. experim. u. klinische Forschung
Becker/Beger/Hartel (Hrsg.)

Komplikationen (proximale Tibiafraktur früh postoperativ n = 5, Pneumonie n = 1, Narkosezwischenfall n = 1) nicht ausgewertet werden. Es wurden 6 Versuchsgruppen gebildet, in denen der Defekt bei den auswertbaren Tieren wie folgt aufgefüllt wurde: 1. Keramik allein (n = 7), 2. Keramik + bFGF (n = 6), 3. Keramik + autologes Knochenmark (n = 8), 4. Keramik + bFGF + autologes Knochenmark (n = 7), 5. autologe Spongiosaplastik vom hinteren Beckenkamm (n = 7), 6. keine Auffüllung (n = 6). Zusätzlich wurde eine Achillotendotomie durchgeführt, da nur so eine vorübergehende Entlastung sichergestellt werden konnte. Postoperativ wurde ein Morphinderivat zur Schmerzbekämpfung verabreicht.

Der Keramikzylinder hatte einen Durchmesser von 20 mm und eine Höhe von ebenfalls 20 mm. Nach Herstellerangaben betrug die Gesamtporosität 30 bis 80 Vol.% bei einer Porenweite von ca. 100–1500 μm. Das Porensystem war interkonnektierend, der Mittelwert aller Porendurchmesser lag bei 450 μm.

Es wurde ein rekombinanter, humaner, basischer Fibroblastenwachstumsfaktor verwandt. Das Protein hat ein Molekulargewicht von ca. 17–18 k Dalton und einen isoelektrischen Punkt von 9,8. Das monomere bFGF-Konzentrat wird mit Puffer und einem Stabilisator versetzt und anschließend lyophilisiert.

Das Knochenmark (10 ml) wurde unmittelbar präoperativ mittels Jamshidi-Punktion vom hinteren Beckenkamm gewonnen, mit 50 I.E. Heparin versetzt und der Keramikzylinder darin getränkt. Die Zylinder nahmen durchschnittlich 4,7 ml des Markes auf. Vorversuche hatten gezeigt, daß mit diesem Verfahren der Keramikkörper vollständig durchtränkt ist.

Nach 6–8 Wochen belasteten alle Tiere die operierte Extremität voll und wiesen ein normales Gangbild auf. Am Ende der 3monatigen Beobachtungszeit wurden die Tiere mit i.v. Injektion von T61 getötet. Beide Tibiae wurden explantiert, von anhängendem Weichgewebe befreit und die Implantate entfernt. Die beiden Knochenenden wurden in Modellgips eingegossen, so daß der Defektbereich und proximal sowie distal davon 1 cm frei blieb. Damit waren auch sämtliche Schraubenlöcher eingegossen. Es erfolgte die Torsionsprüfung der Tibia in einer Materialprüfmaschine im Seitenvergleich mit der nicht operierten Gegenseite bis zum Versagen mit einer Winkelgeschwindigkeit von 20°/min. Es wurde mit einem X/Y Schreiber eine Drehmoment/Winkel-Kurve aufgezeichnet und ausgewertet. Der Frakturtyp wurde nach White und Panjabi [5] in vier Gruppen eingeteilt. Typ I: Bindegewebiges Versagen im Defektbereich, Typ II: Knöchernes Versagen im Defektbereich, Typ III: Knöchernes Versagen durch Defekt und angrenzenden Knochen, Typ IV: Knöchernes Versagen außerhalb des Defektbereiches.

Ergebnisse

Bei der manuellen Prüfung des Defektes zeigte sich von den 41 Präparaten eine bindegewebige Heilung in insgesamt 14 Fällen. Davon entfielen auf die einzelnen Gruppen: Keramik 3/7, Keramik + FGF 2/6, Keramik + Mark 1/8, Keramik + Mark + FGF 3/7, Spongiosa 0/7, Leerdefekt 5/6. In der Mehrzahl der Präparate mit bindegewebiger Heilung war es zu einer Lockerung der Platte gekommen, so daß wir davon ausgehen, daß eine Ausheilung nicht mehr eingetreten wäre. Bei der biomechanischen

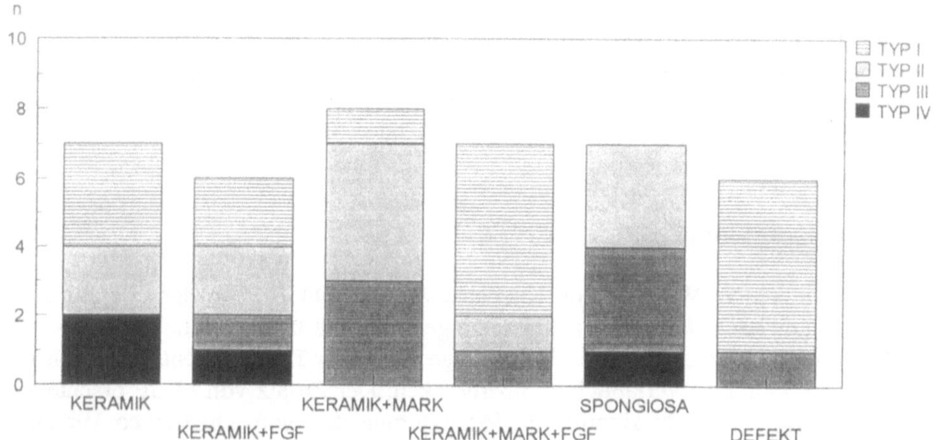

Abb. 1. Verteilung der Frakturtypen bei der Torsionsprüfung nach White und Panjabi. *Typ I*, bindegewebiges Versagen im Defektbereich; *Typ II*, knöchernes Versagen im Defektbereich; *Typ III*, knöchernes Versagen durch Defekt und angrenzendem Knochen; *Typ IV*, knöchernes Versagen außerhalb des Defektbereiches

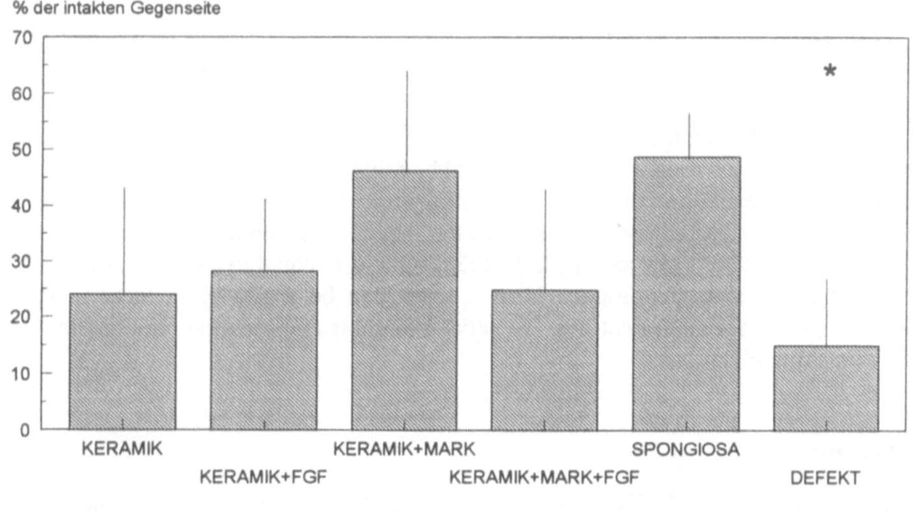

Abb. 2. Maximales Drehmoment (Mittelwert und Standardabweichungen) bei der Rotationsprüfung in den einzelnen Versuchsgruppen

Prüfung wiesen diese Präparate eine sehr geringe Steifigkeit und niedrige Drehmomentwerte auf (entsprechend Typ I). Die Verteilung der Frakturmechanismen ist in Abb. 1 zusammengefaßt. Die Mittelwerte und Standardabweichungen des maximal erreichten Drehmomentes, ausgedrückt in % der intakten Gegenseite, sind in Abb. 2

zusammengefaßt. Die statistische Analyse mittels Kruskal-Wallis-Test ergab einen signifikanten Unterschied zwischen den Versuchsgruppen. Im Newman-Keuls-Test fand sich jeweils kein Unterschied zwischen den Gruppen Keramik + Mark und Spongiosa einerseits sowie zwischen den übrigen Keramik-Gruppen andererseits. Alle Gruppen unterschieden sich signifikant von dem Leerdefekt.

Zusammenfassung

Die osteoinduktive Wirkung von Knochenmark und bFGF ist in der Literatur mehrfach nachgewiesen. Unsere Ergebnisse zeigen, daß die hier geprüfte Keramik in der 3-Monats-Kontrolle allein nicht in der Lage ist, einen Tibiasegmentdefekt von etwa 10% der Schaftlänge verläßlich zu überbrücken. Der Zusatz von bFGF brachte zwar eine geringe, aber nicht signifikante Verbesserung des biomechanischen Verhaltens. Die mit autologem Knochenmarksaspirat getränkte Keramik ergab mit der autologen Spongiosaplastik vergleichbare Werte. Da autologes Knochenmark durch Beckenkammpunktion leicht und in großer Menge bei geringem Komplikationsrisiko zu gewinnen ist, scheint uns diese Kombination auch für den klinischen Einsatz sehr vielversprechend.

Summary

The osteoinductive properties of bone marrow and basic fibroblast growth factor (bFGF) are well documented in the literature. Our results show that porous hydroxylapatite ceramic by itself is unable to reliably bridge a 2-cm segmental defect in the sheep tibia. The addition of bFGF moderately improved the biomechanical results, but these changes were statistically insignificant. When the ceramic block was penetrated with autologous bone marrow aspirate, the results were equal to autologous cancellous bone grafting. Since autologous bone marrow can be aspirated in large quantities without significant complications, we believe that this combination may be promising for clinical applications.

Literatur

1. Connolly JF, Guse R, Tiedemann J, Dehne R (1991) Autologous marrow injection as a substitute for operative grafting of tibial nonunions. Clin Ortho 266:259–270
2. Grundel RE, Chapman MW, Yee T, Moore DC (1991) Autogenic bone marrow and porous biphasic calcium phosphate ceramic for segmental bone defects in the canine ulna. Clin Ortho 266:244–258
3. Jingushi S, Heydermann A, Kana SK, Macey IR, Bolander M (1990) Acidic fibroblast growth factor injection stimulates cartilage enlargement and inhibits cartilage gene expression in rat fracture healing. J Orthop Res 8:364–371
4. Simonds RJ, Holmberg SD, Hurwitz RL, Coleman TR, Bottenfield S, Conley LJ, Kohlenberg SH, Castro KG, Dahan BA, Schable CA, Rayfield MA (1992) Transmission of human immunodeficiency virus type I from a seronegative organ and tissue donor. New Engl J Med 326 (11):726–732

5. White III AA, Panjabi MM, Southwick WO (1977) The four biomechanical stages of fracture repair. J Bone Joint Surg 59-A:188–192

Dr. med. B.W. Wippermann, Unfallchirurgische Klinik, Medizinische Hochschule Hannover, Konstanty-Gutschow-Straße 8, W-3000 Hannover 61

Das nerval gestielte vordere Kreuzbandtransplantat*

Anterior Cruciate Ligament Transplants

J. Grüber[1], W. Lierse[2], Ch. Bertram[1], Ch. Eggers[1] und A. Friedrich[1]

[1]Abteilung für Unfall-, Wiederherstellungs- und Handchirurgie, Allgemeines Krankenhaus St. Georg (Leiter: Priv. Doz. Dr. Ch. Eggers), Hamburg
[2]Abteilung für Neuroanatomie (Direktor Prof. Dr. W. Lierse), Anatomisches Institut, Universitätsklinik Eppendorf, Hamburg

Einleitung

Die Rekonstruktion des vorderen Kreuzbandes ist heute immer noch vom Stabilitätsgedanken geprägt. Das erweiterte mechanische Verständnis von Knieinnenverletzungen und konsequentes therapeutisches Vorgehen haben zu einer wesentlichen Verbesserung der mechanischen Komponenten geführt. Die neuromuskuläre Stabilität bleibt weiterhin unberücksichtigt. Auch nach aufwendigen Rekonstruktionen erreichen viele Patienten die einstige sportliche Leistungsstufe nicht wieder. Mögliche Ursachen für die schlechten Ergebnisse ist die vollständige Desintegration von Stabilität, Durchblutung und neuromuskulärer Steuerung. Nur eine vollständige Wiederherstellung aller 3 Systeme kann zu einer restitutio ad integrum führen.

Der Nachweis eines muskulären Reflexes (vorderer Kreuzbandreflex) nach mechanischer Reizung von Kreuzbändern gelang 1986 [1]. In der ischiocruralen Muskulatur fanden sich bei axialer Dehnung des vorderen Kreuzbandes reguläre muskuläre Reizantworten nach 25–32 mS. Die Bandstrukturen haben neben der rein mechanischen Haltefunktion auch die Funktion von Stellgliedern in einem Regelkreis, dessen Einzelheiten noch ungeklärt sind. Wenn durch die Einbeziehung von nervalen Strukturen als Augmentat der Schutzreflex erhalten wird, kann so ein erweitertes Therapiekonzept zur Verbesserung der Ergebnisse nach Bandplastiken nicht nur am Knie beitragen.

Ziel der Untersuchung war es, den partiellen Erhalt des vorderen Kreuzbandreflexes beim Kreuzbandersatz durch Augmentation des Transplantates mit Faszienstreifen aus der synergistischen Muskulatur zu zeigen.

Methodik

In einem ersten Eingriff wurde an Schafen nach vollständiger Entfernung des vorderen Kreuzbandes eine Bandplastik mit dem mittleren Drittel des Lig. patellae durchgeführt.

* Das Projekt wurde unterstützt durch die Deutsche Forschungsgemeinschaft (Gr 921/3).

Chirurgisches Forum 1993
f. experim. u. klinische Forschung
Becker/Beger/Hartel (Hrsg.)

1. Nervalgestieltes Transplantat (10 Tiere): Verwendet wurde ein freies Transplantat, das transossär in den Insertionen an Ansatz und Ursprung durch zwei Bohrkanäle geführt und mit einer Kleinfragmentschraube fixiert wurde. Zusätzlich wurde ein Faszienstreifen des M. gluteobiceps durch die Fossa poplitea in das Kniegelenk gebracht und auf das Transplantat aufgesteppt.

2. Kontrollgruppe (6 Tiere): Verwendet wurde ein freies Transplantat wie oben beschrieben. Auf die Augmentation wird verzichtet.

3. Referenzgruppe: Die Gelenke der nicht versorgten Gegenseite wurden als Referenz für die diversen Untersuchungen genutzt (Anatomie, Histologie und EMG). Ein zweiter Eingriff erfolgte vor Tötung der Tiere nach 1,5 Jahren zum Nachweis der vorderen Kreuzbandreflexes bei 7 Tieren mit nerval gestieltem Transplantat, bei 2 Tieren der Kontrollgruppe und bei 4 Gelenken der Referenzgruppe. Für diesen Eingriff wurde das Kniegelenk unter Operationsbedingungen über den bei der ersten Operation verwendeten Zugang eröffnet. Das Kreuzband wird am Ansatz (tibial) desinseriert. Geschont wurden der Ursprung (femoral) und die Gefäßnervenstiele:
1. Die A. genus media und der MAN (Medial Articular Nerve) treten aus der Fossa poplitea an das Band heran.
2. Das nervalgestielte Augmentat, das nach der "over the top" Methode durch die Fossa poplitea an das Transplantat geführt wurde.

Nach Durchflechtung des Kreuzbandes/Transplantates mit einem Dexonfaden und Verspannung durch Zug erfolgte die axiale Dehnung. Zum Nachweis von Reizantworten wurden im EMG Ableitungen über dem M. gluteobiceps, M. semimembranosus und der Vastusgruppe mittels Nadelelektroden vorgenommen.

Ergebnisse

Bei vier Gelenken, die primär nicht operiert wurden, konnte während der Kontrolloperation der vordere Kreuzbandreflex nach axialer Dehnung des desinserierten Bandes nachgewiesen werden (Abb. 1a). Das Ergebnis entspricht den aus der Literatur bekannten Ergebnissen und reproduziert den beim Menschen beschriebenen LCA-Reflex beim Schaf [1].

Bei den mit einem nerval gestielten Transplantat operierten Tieren fand sich eine Reizantwort im M. gluteobiceps (Abb. 1b). Diese Reizantwort ist im EMG ähnlich der nach Dehnung des intakten vorderen Kreuzbandes. In den anderen Muskelgruppen der Beuge- und Streckmuskulatur fanden sich keine Antworten (Abb. 1c).

Das Patellarsehnentransplantat war bei 14 von 16 Tieren eingeheilt. Bei zwei nervalgestielten Transplantaten fand sich kein intakter Kreuzbandersatz, sondern lediglich ein leerer synovialer Schlauch. Die Membrana synovialis wurde analog dem o.b. Vorgehen axial gedehnt, ohne daß eine Reizantwort aufgezeichnet werden konnte (Abb. 1d).

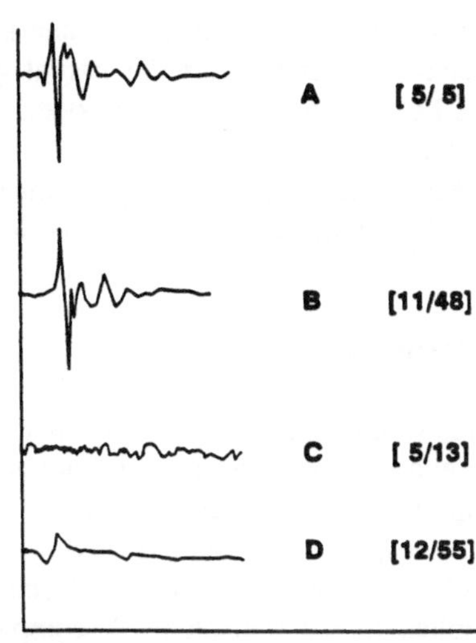

Abb. 1a–d. EMG nach:
a axialer Dehnung des intakten vorderen Kreuzbandes Ableitung M. gluteobiceps,
b axialer Dehnung des intakten nervalgestielten Patellarsehnentransplantates Ableitung M. gluteobiceps,
c axialer Dehnung des intakten nervalgestielten Patellarsehnentransplantates Ableitung Vastus-Gruppe,
d axialer Dehnung des leeren synovialen Schlauches Ableitung M. gluteobiceps

Diskussion

Mit dieser Untersuchung kann gezeigt werden, daß ein nerval gestieltes Transplantat des vorderen Kreuzbandes, bestehend aus Patellarsehne und Faszienstreifen der synergistischen Muskulatur, unter axialer mechanischer Belastung ein ähnliches Reflexverhalten zeigt wie das intakte vordere Kreuzband. Inwieweit ein neuromuskulärer Regelkreis durch dieses Verfahren wiederhergestellt wird, bleibt weiteren Untersuchungen vorbehalten.

Die auf das Postulat von Denti beruhende Hypothese, daß die im Patellarsehnentransplantat gefundenen Mechanorezeptoren einen neuromuskulären Regelkreis ermöglichen, konnte in der Kontrollgruppe widerlegt werden, da hier eine Reflexantwort nicht nachgewiesen werden konnte. Die Mechanorezeptoren, die nach Einheilung eines freien Patellarsehnentransplantates histologisch gefunden werden, können einen physiologischen Regelkreis nicht aufrecht erhalten, da nach der Entnahme des freien Transplantates jeglicher nervaler Anschluß fehlt.

Zusammenfassung

In dieser tierexperimentellen Studie konnte gezeigt werden, daß eine Bandplastik zum Ersatz des vorderen Kreuzbandes beim Schaf, welche mit einem nerval gestielten Faszienstreifen des M. gluteobiceps augmentiert wurde, nach Dehnung des Transplantates zu einer Reizantwort im M. gluteobiceps führt. In einer Kontrollgruppe, ohne nerval gestielten Fascienstreifen, konnten keine EMG-Potentiale abgeleitet werden. Ein Vergleich der Reizantwort der nerval gestielten Kreuzbandplastik mit dem Reizmuster des LCA-Reflexes des nicht ooperierten Kniegelenkes zeigte eine ähnliche Potentialverteilung.

Mit dieser neuartigen Operationsmethode konnte tierexperimentell neben der mechanischen auch eine neuromuskuläre Funktion wiederhergestellt werden.

Summary

This study demonstrates that replacing the anterior cruciate ligament of sheep with a patellar tendon transplant and augmenting this with part of the fascia of the gluteobiceps muscle led to a contraction of this muscle after traction is applied to the transplant. This response was documented with an electromyogram (EMG). In a control group without augmentation with a fascial strip, no response was seen after traction was applied to the transplant. A comparison of the electromyographic response of the transplant with the fascial strip and the normal LCA reflex of a knee that has not been operated on shows almost identical potentials.

This study shows that in sheep the mechanical as well as the neuromuscular function could be replaced by a patella tendon transplant augmented with a strip of the fascia from the gluteobiceps muscle.

Literatur

1. Grüber J, Wolter D, Lierse W (1986) Der vordere Kreuzbandreflex (LCA-Reflex). Unfallchirurg 89:551–554

Dr. med. J. Grüber, Allgemeines Krankenhaus St. Georg, Abteilung für Unfall-, Wiederherstellungs- und Handchirurgie, Lohmühlenstraße 5, W-2000 Hamburg 1

Morphometrische Untersuchungen zur Veränderung des Kollagenfibrillendurchmessers in einem Patellarsehnentransplantat nach Kreuzbandersatz

Morphometric Analysis of Changes in Collagen Fibril Diameter in the Patellar Tendon Autograft After Cruciate Ligament Reconstruction

U. Bosch[1], H. Möller[1], T. Iburg[1], B. Decker[2], W.J. Kasperczyk[1] und H.J. Oestern[3]

[1]Unfallchirurgische Klinik, Medizinische Hochschule Hannover
[2]Abteilung für Zellbiologie und Elektronenmikroskopie, Medizinische Hochschule Hannover
[3]Unfallchirurgische Klinik, Allgemeines Krankenhaus, Celle

Einleitung

In Sehnen und Ligamenten beeinflussen die koaxiale Anordnung der fibrillären Strukturen, vornehmlich von Kollagenfasern, entlang der Belastungsachse sowie der Verteilungsmodus der Kollagenfibrillendurchmesser (KFD) die mechanischen Eigenschaften dieser Gewebe [3]. Das autogene Patellarsehnentransplantat (PST) erfährt als Kreuzbandersatz eine merkliche Schwächung seiner mechanischen Eigenschaften [1]. Ziel dieser Studie war die morphometrische Analyse der Kollagenfibrillen hinsichtlich ihres Durchmessers in einem autogenen PST bis zu 2 Jahren nach Ersatz des hinteren Kreuzbandes (LCP).

Material und Methodik

Bei 30 zweijährigen, reinrassigen Schafen (Deutsches Schwarzkopfschaf) wurde in Intubationsnarkose das LCP des linken Hinterlaufes standardisiert mit einem freien, autogenen PST ersetzt. Postoperativ erfolgte keine Protektion des operierten Beines. Nach Abschluß der Wundheilung hatten die Tiere freien Auslauf in der Herde.

Nach 2, 6, 16, 26, 52 und 104 Wochen wurden bei jeweils 5 Tieren nach Gabe von T 61 standardisiert Gewebeproben aus dem PST entnommen. Nach Immersionsfixierung erfolgte die Einbettung der Proben in Epon. Ultradünnschnitte (quer, 50–60 nm) wurden nach Kontrastierung mit Bleizitrat und Uranylazetat an einem Philips Elektronenmikroskop EM 201 bei 30 000facher Vergrößerung fotodokumentiert. Die morphometrische Auswertung erfolgte interaktiv mit einem Bildanalysegerät (IBAS-AT). Pro PST wurden bei 20 repräsentativen Filmnegativen in einem Meßfenster, das einem 1 μm^2 großen Gewebeareal entsprach, die KFD interaktiv unter Berücksichtigung der Prinzipien für Messungen von punktförmigen Objekten in einem definierten Meßfenster erfaßt. Die Meßwerte wurden einer von sechs empirisch ermittelten Größenklassen zugeordnet. Der mittlere KFD pro Gruppe und der

Chirurgisches Forum 1993
f. experim. u. klinische Forschung
Becker/Beger/Hartel (Hrsg.)

prozentuale Flächenanteil der Kollagenfibrillen pro μm^2 wurden errechnet. Die Patellarsehne (PS) und das LCP aus fünf Kniegelenken von nicht operierten, 2jährigen Schafen dienten als Kontrolle. Signifikante Unterschiede zwischen den Gruppen wurden mit Hilfe des Kruskal-Wallis-Test ermittelt. Als Signifikanzniveau wurde $p < 0{,}05$ gewählt.

Ergebnisse

Der Verteilungsmodus der relativen Häufigkeit der KFD ließ bei der PS und beim LCP (Kontrolle) sowohl dicke als auch dünne Kollagenfibrillen erkennen (Abb. 1).

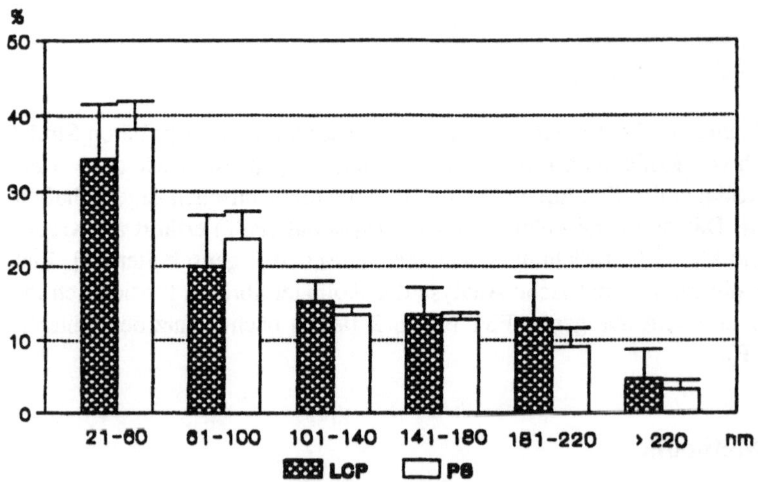

Abb. 1. Prozentuale Häufigkeitsverteilung der Kollagenfibrillendurchmesser in 6 Größenklassen beim hinteren Kreuzband (*LCP*) und bei der Patellarsehne (*PS*) der Kontrolltiere

Beim PST zeigte sich im Vergleich zu den Kontrollen eine zunehmende Linksverschiebung im Verteilungsmodus mit einer eindeutigen Zunahme der relativen Häufigkeiten von dünnen Kollagenfibrillen (Abb. 2a und b). Der mittlere KFD nahm im Verlauf signifikant ab ($H = 26{,}4$; $p < 0{,}05$). Bis zur 16. Woche post OP kam es zwischen den einzelnen Meßzeitpunkten jeweils zu einer signifikanten Abnahme von 100,7 nm (PS) auf 49,5 nm (PST). Bis zum Versuchsende zeigte sich eine nicht signifikante Zunahme auf 55,8 nm (Abb. 3).

Im PST war der prozentuale Flächenanteil der Kollagenfibrillen pro μm^2 zu jedem post OP Zeitpunkt signifikant geringer als in der PS und im LCP der Kontrollen ($H = 25$; $p < 0{,}05$; Abb. 4).

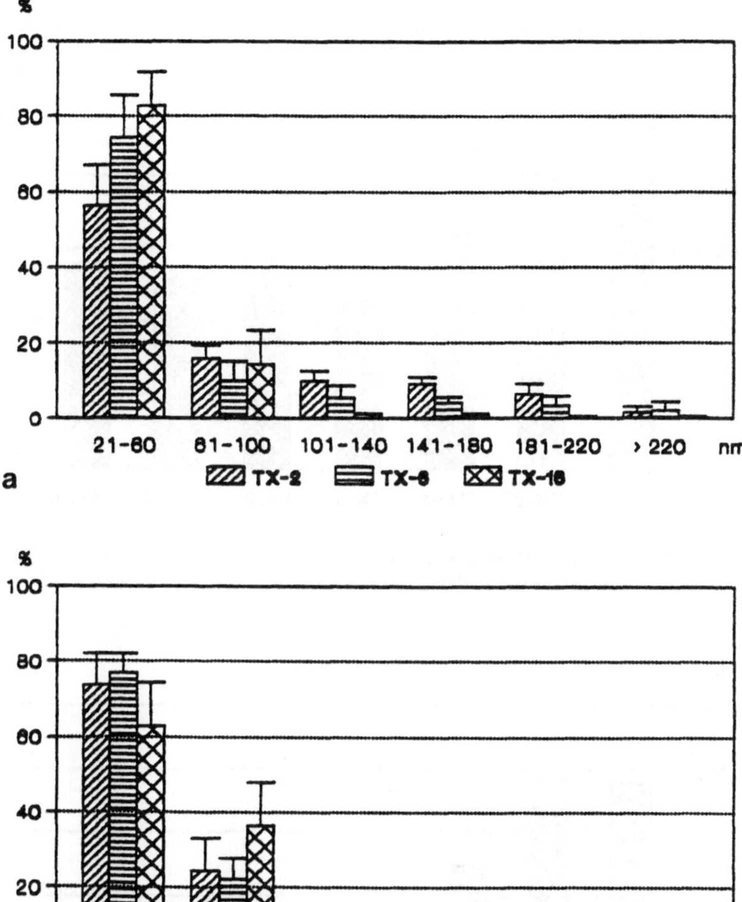

Abb. 2. Prozentuale Häufigkeitsverteilung der Kollagenfibrillendurchmesser in 6 Größenklassen. **a** Patellarsehnentransplantat (*TX*) 2, 6 und 16 Wochen postoperativ. **b** Patellarsehnentransplantat 26, 52 und 104 Wochen postoperativ

Diskussion

Das auffälligste Ergebnis ist die Linksverschiebung des Verteilungsmodus der KFD im PST zugunsten dünner Kollagenfibrillen. Bereits innerhalb der ersten 16 Wochen post OP nahm die relative Häufigkeit der Kollagenfibrillen mit einem Durchmesser bis 100 nm um rund 60% von 61,7% (PS) auf 97,1% zu und änderte sich mit 98,8% bis zur 104. Woche post OP nicht mehr wesentlich. Dies steht in Einklang mit dem erheblichen Abfall der mechanischen Eigenschaften des PST [1]. Für dickere Kolla-

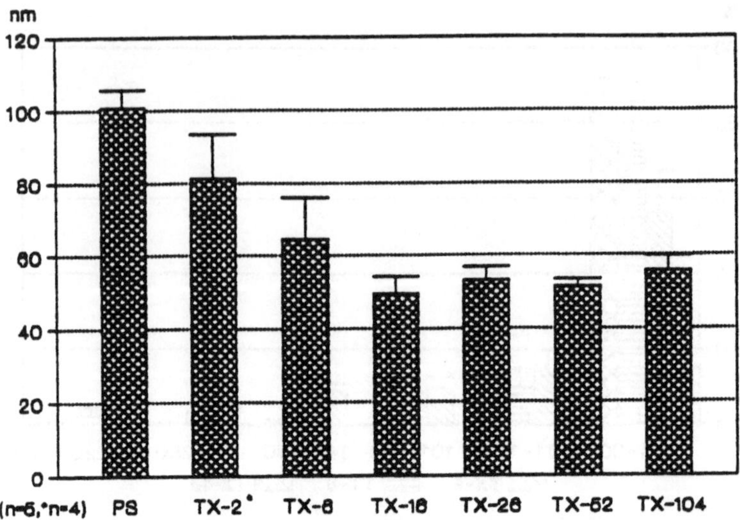

Abb. 3. Mittlerer Kollagenfibrillendurchmesser (Mittelwert ± SD) bei der Patellarsehne (*PS*) der Kontrolltiere sowie beim Patellarsehnentransplantat (*TX*) zu unterschiedlichen Zeitpunkten postoperativ

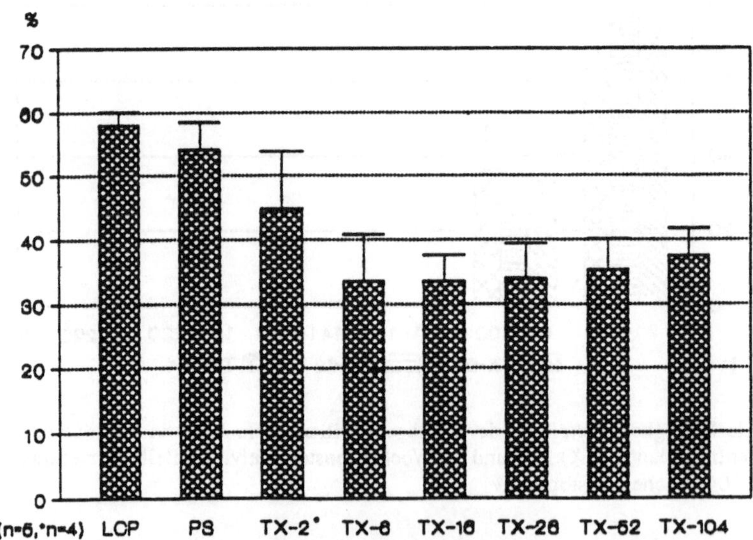

Abb. 4. Prozentualer Flächenanteil der Kollagenfibrillen pro μm^2 beim hinteren Kreuzband (*LCP*), bei der Patellarsehne (*PS*) und beim Patellarsehnentransplantat (*TX*) zu unterschiedlichen Zeitpunkten postoperativ

genfibrillen wird eine größere Dichte an intrafibrillären, stabilen kovalenten Bindungen postuliert und damit eine größere Zugfestigkeit als für dünnere Kollagenfibrillen angenommen [3]. Zwischen der 16. und 104. Woche post OP kam es zu einer gewissen

Verschiebung innerhalb der zwei kleinsten Größenklassen. Die relative Häufigkeit in der Größenklasse 21–60 nm nahm von 82,8% auf 62,2% ab zugunsten einer Zunahme der relativen Häufigkeit in der Größenklasse 61–100 nm. Dies läßt ein gewissen radiales Wachstum von Kollagenfibrillen durch Anlagerung von Kollagenmonomeren vermuten [3]. Entsprechend der Veränderung des Verteilungsmodus nahm der mittlere KFD bereits in den ersten 16 Wochen post OP um 50% ab. Trotz der Zunahme der Kollagenfibrillenanzahl pro μm^2 nahm die von Kollagen bedeckte Fläche pro μm^2 signifikant ab, da die Zunahme auf einer Vermehrung von nur dünnen Kollagenfibrillen beruhte. Ähnliche Beobachtungen wurden bei der Heilung von Sehnengewebe nach Ruptur oder Tenotomie gemacht [2, 4].

Demnach können reparative Prozesse im Bindegewebe originäre Strukturen nicht wieder herstellen. Die Ergebnisse sind für die Beurteilung der Belastbarkeit einer Kreuzbandersatzplastik von klinischer Relevanz und können eine Ursache für Spätinsuffizienzen von biologischen Transplantaten darstellen.

Zusammenfassung

Die Kollagenfibrillendurchmesser wurden in einem autogenen Patellarsehnentransplantat nach Ersatz des hinteren Kreuzbandes in einem Schafsmodell über 2 Jahre postoperativ mittels einer morphometrischen Untersuchung analysiert. Bereits in der Frühphase post OP kam es zu einer deutlichen Zunahme der relativen Häufigkeit von dünnen Kollagenfibrillen, verbunden mit einem signifikanten Abfall des mittleren Kollagenfibrillendurchmessers und der von Kollagen bedeckten Fläche pro μm^2. Auch nach 2 Jahren kam es hinsichtlich der Kollagenfibrillen zu keiner Angleichung an eine Sehne oder Ligament.

Summary

After posterior cruciate ligament reconstruction by a patellar tendon autograft, the alterations in collagen fibril diameter distribution, mean fibril diameter, and the area covered by collagen were estimated up to 2 years postoperatively. In the autograft, there was a considerable increase of small fibrils and a significant decrease of the mean fibril diameter and of the area covered by collagen up to week 16. As far as the collagen fibril diameters were concerned, normal values were not reestablished within 2 years of the operation.

Literatur

1. Bosch U, Kasperczyk WJ (1992) Healing of the patellar tendon autograft after posterior cruciate ligament reconstruction – a process of ligamentization? Am J Sports Med 20:558–566
2. Matthew CA, Moore MJ (1991) Regeneration of rat extensor digitorum longus tendon: the effect of a sequential partial tenotomy on collagen fibril formation. Matrix 11:259–268

3. Parry DAD, Barnes GRP, Craig AS (1978) A comparison of the size distribution of collagen fibrils in connective tissues as a function of age and a possible relation between fibril size distribution and mechanical properties. Proc R Soc Lond (Biol) 203:305–321
4. Williams IE, Craig AS, Parry DAD, Goodship AE, Shah J, Silver IA (1985) Development of collagen fibril organization and collagen crimp patterns during tendon healing. Int J Biol Macromol 7:275–282

Gefördert durch AO-Stiftung, B. Braun-Stiftung und Hauptverband der gewerblichen Berufsgenossenschaften.

Dr. U. Bosch, Unfallchirurgische Klinik, Medizinische Hochschule Hannover, Konstanty-Gutschow-Straße 8, W-3000 Hannover 61

Kräfteverteilung zwischen Patellarsehnenersatz des vorderen Kreuzbandes und parallel geschaltetem Augmentationsband als Funktion unterschiedlicher Vorspannungen

Load Sharing Between Patellar Tendon Replacement of the Anterior Cruciate Ligament and a Parallel-Running Augmentation Cord as a Function of Different Preloads

U. Becker[1], H. Kiefer[1], L. Dürselen[2] und G. Haas[1]

[1]Abteilung für Unfallchirurgie, Hand-, Plastische und Wiederherstellungschirurgie (Ärztl. Dir.: Prof. Dr. L. Kinzl), Universitätsklinik Ulm
[2]Abteilung für Biomechanik und Unfallchirurgische Forschung (Dir.: Prof. Dr. L. Claes), Universität Ulm

Für die Wiederherstellung der Kniegelenksstabilität nach Ruptur des vorderen Kreuzbandes ist derzeit die Kombination eines autologen Patellarsehnentransplantates (BTB) mit einem synthetischen Augmentationsband weit verbreiteter Standard [4]. Sie soll eine frühfunktionelle Aktivität erlauben und klinisch eine gute Langzeitstabilität versprechen [3]. Beweise für eine tatsächliche Streßreduktion des BTB durch das Augmentationsband stehen jedoch noch aus. In dieser Arbeit wird die Kräfteverteilung zwischen einem BTB und einer neuen, synthetischen, verzögert resorbierbaren Kordel aus Polydioxanon (PDS) als Funktion unterschiedlicher Vorspannungen untersucht.

Material und Methoden

An 9 intakten Leichenknien (männlich, Durchschnittsalter 29 J.) wurde das vordere Kreuzband reseziert und mit Hilfe eines Isometriemeßzielgerätes (Kinemetric, Fa. Richards) durch ein 10 mm breites BTB-Transplantat aus dem zentralen Drittel des Lig. patellae ersetzt, wobei das femorale Knochenblöckchen im Bohrloch mit einer Interferenz-Schraube fixiert wurde. Eine 2 mm dicke, u-förmig gedoppelte, ventral des Transplantates parallel anliegende Kordel aus PDS (Fa. Ethicon) wurde femoral mit 2 Staples (Fa. Richards) in Gürtelschnallentechnik verankert. Die tibialen Enden beider Komponenten (BTB und Kordel) wurden mit flexiblen Stahldrähten in Ringkraftaufnehmern befestigt und konnten reibungsfrei im 12 mm Bohrkanal der Tibia gleiten. In einem Kniebelastungssimulator, der die zwangfreie Bewegung zwischen 0 und 110° erlaubte [2], wurden beide Bandersatzkomponenten zwischen 0 und 100 N in Streckstellung vorgespannt. Während dreier Bewegungszyklen mit einer Winkelgeschwindigkeit von 10°/sec wurden die in BTB und Kordel auftretenden Kräfte getrennt gemessen. Anschließend erfolgte ein vorderer Schubladentest (Lachman-Test) mit 130 N bei 20° Beugung, entsprechend der klinisch üblichen Arthrometrie mit dem KT-1000 Arthrometer. Nach Versuchsende wurden die BTB-Transplantate entnommen

Chirurgisches Forum 1993
f. experim. u. klinische Forschung
Becker/Beger/Hartel (Hrsg.)

und zur Erstellung von Kraftdehnungsdiagrammen in einer Materialprüfmaschine bis zur Reißgrenze gedehnt. Distales Femur und Tibiakopf wurden mit Hilfe von Hilfslinien anthropometrisch zur Beurteilung der Lage der Bohrlöcher vermessen.

Ergebnisse

1. Kräfteverteilung zwischen BTB und Kordel bei passivem Bewegungszyklus: Die im BTB bei passiver Beugung auftretenden Kräfte zeigen bei allen Präparaten, unabhängig von der Vorspannung, ein qualitativ einheitliches Muster mit einem Maximum in Streckung, einem starken Abfall um bis zu 50% bis 20° Beugung, einer Plateauphase und schließlich einem weiteren Abfall bei maximaler Beugung. Eine Erhöhung der Vorspannung der Kordel von 10 auf 100 N führt bei 4 Kniegelenken zu einer Reduktion der im BTB auftretenden Kräfte um ca 20% (Abb. 1). Bei den übrigen 5 Präparaten kann durch Erhöhung der Vorspannung der PDS-Kordel keine oder nur eine geringfügige Reduktion der Kraft im BTB erzielt werden.

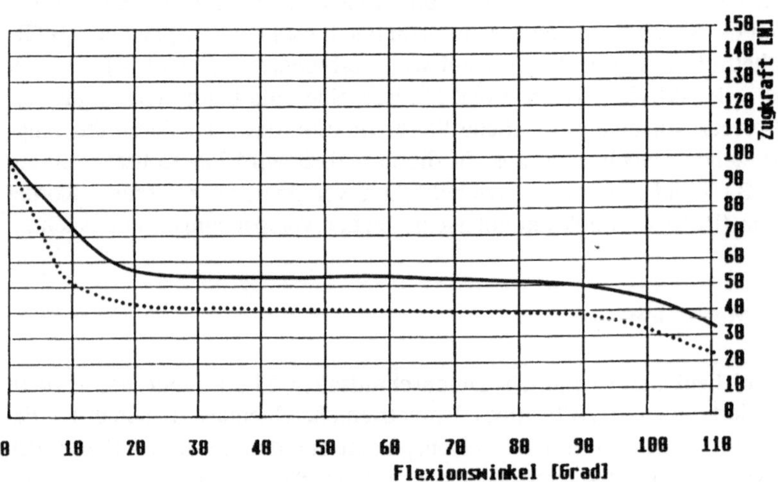

Abb. 1. Gemessene Bandkräfte im BTB bei passivem Bewegungszyklus. Vorspannung im BTB 100 N. Eine Erhöhung der Vorspannung der PDS-Kordel von 10 N (*durchgezogene Linie*) auf 100 N (*gepunktete Linie*) führt zu einer Reduktion der im BTB gemessenen Kräfte

2. Kräfteverteilung zwischen BTB und Kordel beim Lachman-Test: Die bei einer vorderen Schubladenbelastung von 130 N im BTB auftretenden Kräfte werden durch die Vorspannung der Kordel einheitlich im Sinne einer Reduktion beeinflußt (Abb. 2). Bei geringerer Vorspannung des BTB sind die Unterschiede weniger ausgeprägt.

3. Dehnungen und Ausrißkräfte: Bei einer Zugkraft von 100 N und einer Zuggeschwindigkeit von 10 mm/sec treten Dehnungen zwischen 2,3 und 4,7% auf. Die Reißkräfte der isolierten Transplantate betragen im Mittelwert 1172 N.

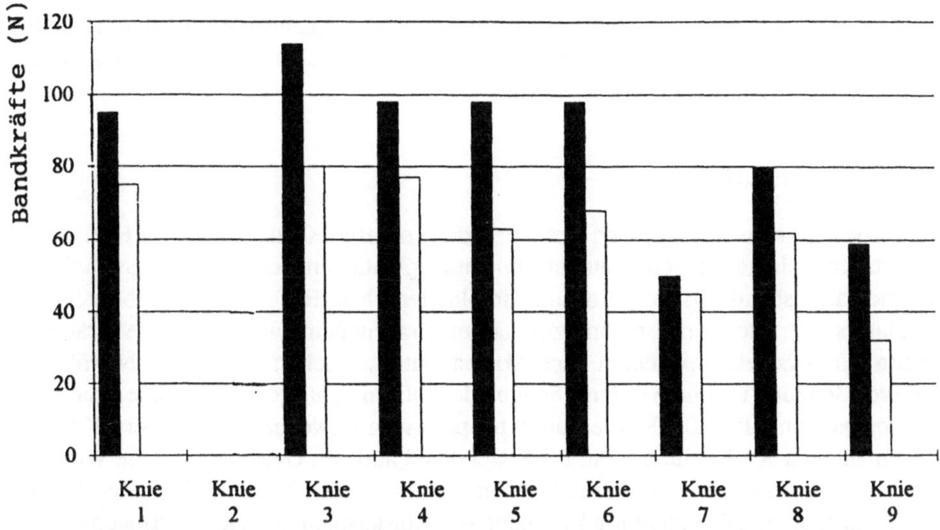

Abb. 2. Gemessene Bandkräfte im BTB beim Lachman-Test. Vorspannung im BTB 100 N. Der Effekt höherer Vorspannung der PDS-Kordel (*weiße Säule*: 100 N, *schwarze Säule*: 10 N) ist bei allen Knien deutlich (Knie 2 wegen präparatorischer Mängel nicht verwertbar)

4. Anthropometrische Messungen: Die Lage der femoralen Bohrkanäle variiert trotz präoperativer Isometriemessung stark. Bei 4 Kniegelenken liegt der intraartikuläre Bohrkanaleingang (gewünscht) dorsal. Bei den 5 anderen Präparaten, die, wie unter Abschnitt 1 erwähnt, eine geringere Kräftereduktion im BTB durch Vorspannungserhöhung der Kordel zeigten, liegen die Bohrlocheingänge teilweise bis zu 12 mm weiter ventral.

Diskussion

Der Nutzen eines synthetischen Augmentationsbandes zum Schutz des Transplantates wird kontrovers diskutiert [1, 3, 4]. In unserem Experiment können die im Transplantat auftretenden Kräfte durch eine parallel geschaltete Augmentationskordel reduziert werden. Voraussetzung hierfür ist jedoch eine korrekte isometrische Implantation beider Bandersatz-Komponenten. Sie wurde bei uns trotz Isometriemessung nicht in allen Fällen erreicht, was jeweils prompt zu einer geringeren Kraftreduktion im BTB durch die Kordel führte. In der Literatur finden sich unterschiedliche Angaben über die Höhen der Vorspannung [1, 3]. Unter den beschriebenen experimentellen Bedingungen läßt sich die Notwendigkeit einer Vorspannung der Augmentationskordel nachweisen, um eine Minderbelastung des Transplantates zu bewirken. Mit der höchsten Vorspannung von 100 N ließ sich dabei der ausgeprägteste Effekt erzielen.

Ungeklärt bleiben jedoch die folgenden Fragen:

1. Wieviel bleibt in vivo im zeitlichen Verlauf von der initialen Vorspannung erhalten?
2. Welche Vorspannung beeinflußt die Einheilung und "Ligamentisation" des Transplantates am günstigsten?

Zusammenfassung

An 9 Leichenknien wurden nach Resektion des vorderen Kreuzbandes mit Hilfe eines Isometriemeßzielgerätes ein Patellarsehnentransplantat und ein parallel geschaltetes Augmentationsband aus Polydioxanon implantiert. Mit Hilfe eines Kniebelastungssimulators mit integrierter rechnergesteuerter Kraftmeßeinheit wurden die Kräfte in beiden Bandersatzkomponenten nach Vorspannung zwischen 0 und 100 N während passiver Beugung und bei vorderer Schubladenbelastung aufgezeichnet. Die Erhöhung der Vorspannung der PDS-Kordel führte bei passivem Bewegungszyklus bei 4 Kniegelenken zu einer Kraftreduktion im BTB. Bei den 5 anderen Gelenken war die Wirkung aus implantationstechnischen Gründen weniger ausgeprägt. In allen Fällen der Schubladenbelastungen läßt sich durch Erhöhung der Kordelspannung eine Verringerung der im Transplantat auftretenden Kräfte nachweisen.

Summary

BTB ligament replacement was performed in nine cadaveric knee joints after resection of the anterior cruciate ligament (ACL). Grafts were augmented with a parallel-running polydioxanon (PDS) cord. Using a computer-directed pneumatic load apparatus, both components were prestressed with loads between 0 and 100 N. Forces in the BTB and the PDS cord were measured during passive flexion and anteriorly directed load (Lachman's test). In four knees increased prestress of the PDS caused reduction of forces in the BTB during the passive motion cycle. Due to the implantation technique this effect could not be demonstrated in the other five knees. In all joints undergoing Lachman's test, increased prestress of the PDS reduced the forces in the BTB.

Literatur

1. Holzmüller W, Rehm KE, Perren SM (1992) Mechanische Eigenschaften PDS-augmentierter Patellarsehnentransplantate zur Rekonstruktion des vorderen Kreuzbandes. Unfallchirurg 95:306–310
2. Kiefer H, Dürselen L, Claes L (1992) Experimentelle Untersuchungen zur Biomechanik des Kniebandapparats. Hefte Unfallheilkunde 221. Springer, Berlin Heidelberg New York
3. Noyes FR, Barber SD (1992) The effect of ligament-augmentation device on allograft reconstruction for chronic ruptures of the anterior cruciate ligament. J Bone Joint Surg 74A:960–972
4. Schabus R (1988) Die Bedeutung der Augmentation für die Rekonstruktion des vorderen Kreuzbandes. Acta Chir Austr [Suppl] 76

Dr. U. Becker, Abteilung für Unfallchirurgie, Hand-, Plastische und Wiederherstellungschirurgie, Universität Ulm, Steinhövelstraße 9, W-7900 Ulm

Effekt medikamentös bedingter Darmmotilitätsstörungen auf bakterielle Translokation*

Effect of Drug-Induced Changes in Small-Intestinal Motility on Bacterial Translocation

P.M. Kueppers[1], T.A. Miller[2], C.Y. Chen[2], C. Herfarth[1] und F.G. Moody[2]

[1]Chirurgische Klinik, Universität Heidelberg
[2]Department of Surgery, University of Texas Health Science Center, Houston, Texas, USA

Einleitung

Die Translokation teilungsfähiger enteraler Bakterien aus dem Darmlumen in Lymphstrombahn, Blut und ferne Organe wird als Auslöser von Sepsis bei traumatisierten Patienten diskutiert [1]. Als verantwortliche Mechanismen gelten bakterieller Überwuchs, eingeschränkte Barrierefunktion der Mukosa, sowie eingeschränkte Immunfunktion, die jeweils allein oder in Kombination den bisher beschriebenen Tiermodellen mit bakterieller Translokation zugrunde liegen [2, 3, 4]. Herabgesetzte Darmmotilität wiederum ist eine Ursache für bakteriellen Überwuchs. Untersucht wurde anhand zweier Modelle medikamentöser Suppression der Darmmotilität in der Ratte, ob dies zu bakteriellem Überwuchs im Darmlumen und zu bakterieller Translokation führt. Wir unterschieden dabei Translokation von Bakterien in MLN vom Auftreten von Bakterien im Blut und fernen Organen. In zwei getrennten Versuchsserien wurde durch zwei Substanzen mit unterschiedlichem Wirkungsmechanismus eine vergleichbar ausgeprägte Störung der Darmmotilität herbeigeführt. Die Folgen bezüglich Besiedelung des Darmlumens und bakterieller Translokation in Lymphknoten, Blut und ferne Organe wurden gegenübergestellt.

Methodik

Gruppen männlicher Sprague-Dawley Ratten (Harlan Lab, Houston, TX, USA) wurden 4 Tage mit Morphin bzw. Clonidin behandelt. Beide Substanzen wurden subcutan verabreicht. Wegen der schnellen Toleranzentwicklung wurde Morphin kontinuierlich und in steigender Dosierung von 4 mg/kg an Tag 1, bis 7,8 mg/kg an Tag 4 infun-

* Unterstützt durch NIH GM38529 und DFG KU782/1-1.

Chirurgisches Forum 1993
f. experim. u. klinische Forschung
Becker/Beger/Hartel (Hrsg.)

diert. Clonidin wurde zweimal täglich injiziert, in einer Dosierung von 0,5 mg/kg am Morgen und 1,0 mg/kg am Abend. Es wurde jeweils eine Kontrollgruppe mit Injektionen von Kochsalzlösung gegenübergestellt. Im Morphinexperiment wurde parenteral ernährt, um der Malnutrition entgegenzuwirken (Parenteral Nutrition Kit, Baxter, Deerfield, IL, USA, plus MVI-12, Rorer, Fort Washington, PA, USA). Alle Tiere wurden bei geregelter Raumtemperatur und Tag-/Nachtzyklus in metabolischen Käfigen mit mindestens fünftägiger Akklimatisationszeit gehalten. Therapie- und Kontrolltiere im Clonidinexperiment hatten freien Zugang zu Futter (Ralston Purina, St. Louis, MO, USA) und Wasser. Alle Tiere im Morphinexperiment wurden fünf Tage vor Beginn der Behandlung mit einem zentralen Venenkatheter und einem Subkutankatheter ausgestattet. Diese waren über einen Drehmechanismus mit Infusionssystemen verbunden, der den Tieren freie Bewegung im Käfig erlaubte. Der Versuchsgruppe, mit subcutanem Morphin und totaler parenteraler Ernährung, wurden hierbei zwei Kontrollen zugeordnet. Eine Gruppe erhielt nur Kochsalzlösung und hatte freien Zugang zu Futter, die andere wurde parenteral ernährt und erhielt Kochsalzlösung subcutan. In beiden Versuchsreihen wurde bei 6 Tieren je Gruppe die intestinale Transitzeit im Dünndarm gemessen. Alle diese Tiere wurden fünf Tage vor dem Experiment mit einem Duodenalkatheter ausgestattet. Am Ende wurde darüber 0,1 ml einer 5 mmolaren Lösung fluoreszenzmarkierter Dextrane (durchschnittliches Molekulargewicht 10000 Dalton) appliziert. Nach 25 min wurde der Dünndarm entnommen, in 10 gleiche Teile geteilt und der Gehalt an Marker pro Segment bestimmt. Bei allen anderen Tieren wurde steril der MLN-Komplex, Blut, Leber, Milz und ein Mesenterialabstrich entnommen. Mit Hilfe mikrobiologischer Standardmethoden wurde darin Keimzahl und -Art bestimmt. In mindestens 6 Tieren aus jeder Gruppe wurde außerdem eine quantitative Bestimmung aller nachweisbaren Keime in einem 5 cm langen Segment aus Duodenum, Jejunum, Ileum und Coecum durchgeführt.

Ergebnisse

Morphin- und Clonidinbehandlung führten zu einer gleichermaßen ausgeprägten Reduktion des intestinalen Transports. Das Zentrum der Markerverteilung lag mit 36 ± 2 bzw. 40 ± 3 % der Dünndarmlänge signifikant ($p < 0{,}01$) proximaler als in den zugehörigen Kontrollgruppen (60 ± 3 und 59 ± 5%). Parenterale Ernährung alleine hatte keinen Einfluß auf die intestinale Transitgeschwindigkeit (58 ± 3%). Beide Behandlungen führten auch zur bakteriellen Überwucherung in Dünn- und Dickdarm. Die Gesamtzahl an CFU war im Duodenum, Ileum und Coecum erhöht (Tabelle 1). Die Inzidenz des Nachweises von lebenden Bakterien in den MLN betrug bei beiden Behandlungen 100% (Tabelle 2). Die Gruppe mit alleiniger parenteraler Ernährung wies in 50% Bakterien in den MLN auf. Über 100 CFU/MLN lag die Zahl der Bakterien allerdings nur in 6%, während 100% der morphinbehandelten und 92% der clonidinbehandelten Tiere diesen häufig angegebenen Schwellenwert überschritten. Die durchschnittliche Zahl von CFU/MLN war unter Morphin gegenüber zugehöriger Kontrolle und alleiniger parenteraler Ernährung erhöht. Das gleiche trifft auch für die Clonidinbehandlung zu (Tabelle 2). Außerhalb von Lymphknoten konnte in 93% der morphinbehandelten Tiere an einem oder mehreren Orten Keime nachgewiesen werden; im Einzelnen zu 67% in der Leber, 53% im Blut und jeweils 47% in Milz und Peritonealabstrich. Demgegenüber konnte aus keinem clonidinbehandelten oder parenteral ernährten Tier in einem dieser Organe ein einziger Keim angezüchtet werden (Tabelle 2).

Tabelle 1. Gesamtzahl aller nachweisbaren Bakterien in verschiedenen Darmabschnitten als log 10 colony forming units pro Gramm Gewebe

Behandlung	Duodenum	Jejunum	Ileum	Coecum
Morphin	5,28 ± 0,88[a]	6,25 ± 0,75	9,14 ± 0,25[a]	10,86 ± 0,11[a]
Kontrolle	3,33 ± 0,37	5,59 ± 0,29	7,05 ± 0,48	9,65 ± 0,37
Parenterale Ernährung	2,77 ± 0,44	5,68 ± 0,81	7,99 ± 0,13[a]	10,20 ± 0,42
Clonidin	5,90 ± 0,31[a]	6,35 ± 0,49	8,14 ± 0,36[a]	10,44 ± 0,23[a]
Kontrolle	2,78 ± 0,55	5,24 ± 0,43	7,00 ± 0,32	0,31 ± 0,18

[a] $p < 0,05$ versus Kontrolle

Tabelle 2. Bakterielle Translokation zu mesenterialen Lymphknoten (MLN) sowie Blut, Leber, Milz und Peritoneum (ferne Organe)

Behandlung	Inzidenz MLN	CFU/MLN mean ± SEM	Inzidenz ferne Organe
Morphin	15/15[a]	2079 ± 811[a]	14/15[a]
Kontrolle	2/14	13 ± 9	0/14
Parenterale Ernährung	8/16	33 ± 14	0/16
Clonidin	15/15[a]	757 ± 193[a]	0/15
Kontrolle	2/8	73 ± 48	0/8

[a] $p < 0,05$ versus Kontrolle. CFU: colony forming units

Zusammenfassung

Morphin und Clonidin führen zu einer vergleichbaren Suppression des intestinalen Transits. Dies führt in unserer Studie zu bakteriellem Überwuchs und dem Auftreten hoher Zahlen teilungsfähiger Keime in den mesenterialen Lymphknoten. Bakterielle Translokation in die Blutbahn oder ferne Organe trat jedoch nur nach Morphin, nicht aber in Zusammenhang mit Clonidinbehandlung auf. Wir folgern, daß bakterieller Überwuchs und vermehrtes Auftreten von Darmkeimen in den lokalen Lymphknoten allein nicht zur Auslösung von Sepsis ausreicht. Dazu ist ein weiterer Faktor notwendig, den Morphin, nicht jedoch Clonidin, aufweist. Dies könnte der immunsuppressive Effekt des Morphins sein, was angesichts der häufigen Anwendung von Opiaten weitere Untersuchungen erfordert.

Summary

Morphine and clonidine administration results in comparable suppression of intestinal transit. In our study this effect leads to bacterial overgrowth and high numbers of viable bacteria in the mucocutaneous lymph node (MNL), but bacterial translocation to blood or distant organs was seen only after morphine was administered. We conclude that bacterial overgrowth and increasing numbers of enteric bacteria in local lymph nodes is not sufficient to cause sepsis. An additional factor is necessary which is supplied by morphine, but not clonidine. This might be the immunosuppressive effect of morphine. Considering the regular use of opioids, further investigation is needed.

Literatur

1. Wilmore DW, Smith RJ, O'Dwyer ST, Jacobs DO, Ziegler TR, Wang X (1988) The gut: A central organ after surgical stress. Surgery 104:917–923
2. Deitch EA (1990) Bacterial translocation of the gut flora. J Trauma 30:184–189
3. Steffen EK, Berg RD (1983) Relationship between cecal population levels of indigenous bacteria and translocation to the mesenteric lymph nodes. Infect Immun 39:1252–1259
4. Barber AE, Jones WG, Minei JP, Fahey TJ, Lowry SF, Shires GT (1991) Bacterial overgrowth and intestinal atrophy in the etiology of gut barrier failure in the rat. Am J Surg 161:300–304
5. Berg RD, Wommack E, Deitch EA (1988) Immunosuppression and intestinal bacterial overgrowth synergistically promote bacterial translocation. Arch Surg 123:1359–1364

Dr. P.M. Kueppers, Chirurgische Klinik der Universität Heidelberg, Im Neuenheimer Feld 110, W-6900 Heidelberg

Monoklonaler Antikörper gegen das Leukozytenadhäsionsmolekül MAC-1 (CD11b) verhindert die postischämische Leukozytenadhärenz in vivo

Monoclonal Antibody Against the Leukocyte Adhesion Molecule MAC-1 (CD11b) Prevents Postischemic Leukocyte Adherence In Vivo

R. Hecht, D. Nolte, A. Botzlar, M.D. Menger und K. Meßmer

Institut für Chirurgische Forschung, Klinikum Großhadern, Universität München

Einleitung

Ischämie und Reperfusion bewirken eine Aktivierung von Leukozyten; diese können über spezifische Adhäsionsmoleküle am Endothel postkapillärer Venolen adhärieren, ins umliegende Gewebe emigrieren und durch Bildung von Sauerstoffradikalen sowie Freisetzung von Entzündungsmediatoren zur Manifestation des postischämischen Reperfusionsschadens beitragen [1, 2]. Der Vorgang der Adhäsion und Emigration wird durch β_2-Integrine (CD11/CD18) mediiert. Durch Blockade dieser leukozytären Adhärenzmoleküle könnte das Ausmaß des postischämischen Reperfusionsschadens mittels spezifischer Antikörper signifikant vermindert werden [3, 4].

Quantitative intravitalmikroskopische Untersuchungen zum Nachweis der Effekte monoklonaler Antikörper auf die postischämische Leukozytenadhärenz sind bisher in der Mikrozirkulation des quergestreiften Muskels nicht durchgeführt worden. Es war daher das Ziel dieser Studie, die Effekte des monoklonalen Antikörpers anti-MAC-1, der gegen die CD11b-Untereinheit des CD11/CD18-Rezeptorkomplexes gerichtet ist, im quergestreiften Rückenhautmuskel der Balb/C-Maus zu untersuchen.

Methodik

Tiermodell: Die Versuche wurden an 20–23 g schweren Balb/C-Mäusen durchgeführt, denen in Allgemeinanästhesie (100 mg Ketanest + 30 mg Rompun $\times$ kg^{-1} KG s.c.) ultraleichte Titankammern in die Rückenhaut sowie venöse Verweilkatheter in die Vena jugularis implantiert wurden. Dieses Modell erlaubt in Anlehnung an das Rückenhautkammermodell beim syrischen Goldhamster [2] die intravitalmikroskopische Untersuchung der Mikrozirkulation eines feinen quergestreiften Hautmuskels. Darüberhinaus ermöglicht dieses neue Tiermodell die Analyse der biologischen Bedeutung von Adhäsionsmolekülen auf der Oberfläche von Leukozyten und mikrovaskulärem Endothel, da für die Spezies Maus spezifische Antikörper gegen die verschiedenen Adhäsionsmoleküle zur Verfügung stehen.

Chirurgisches Forum 1993
f. experim. u. klinische Forschung
Becker/Beger/Hartel (Hrsg.)

Intravitalmikroskopie: In jedem Versuchstier wurden 4–6 postkapilläre Venolen (20–60 μm Ø) vor Induktion einer 3 h Ischämie definiert. Die identischen Gefäßsegmente wurden im weiteren Ablauf des Versuchs mehrfach analysiert. Die Leukozyten wurden mit dem Floureszenzfarbstoff Rhodamin 6G (10 $\mu g\ kg^{-1}\ min^{-1}$ i.v.) intravital angefärbt, die mikroskopischen Bilder auf Videoband aufgezeichnet und off-line mit Hilfe eines computergestützten Mikrozirkulationsanalysesystems [5] bezüglich Änderungen des Gefäßdurchmessers und der Leukozyten/Endothel-Interaktion ausgewertet. Adhärente Leukozyten wurden angegeben als Anzahl der Zellen pro mm^2 Gefäßoberfläche, die sich innerhalb einer Beobachtungsdauer von 30 sec nicht vom Endothel lösten. Die Erythrozytenfließgeschwindigkeit wurde off-line mit Hilfe des Software-Systems "Capi-Flow" bestimmt.

Versuchsprotokoll: Die Versuchstiere wurden randomisiert der Kontrollgruppe (n = 5) bzw. der Testgruppe (n = 5) zugeteilt. 48–72 h nach Implantation der Rückenhautkammern und venösen Verweilkatheter wurden Ausgangswerte für die Leukozyten/Endothel-Interaktion, Gefäßdurchmesser und Erythrozytenfließgeschwindigkeit bestimmt. Anschließend wurde das Gewebe in der Kammer einer dreistündigen Ischämie ausgesetzt; die Messungen wurden 0,5 h und 2 h nach Reperfusion in den identischen Gefäßabschnitten wiederholt. 10 Minuten vor Reperfusion erhielten die Tiere einen Bolus von anti-MAC-1 (1 mg kg^{-1} KG i.v., Boehringer Mannheim) gefolgt von einer kontinuierlichen Infusion (22 $\mu g\ kg^{-1}\ min^{-1}$ i.v.) während der ersten 0,5 h Reperfusion. Kontrolltiere erhielten äquivalente Volumina eines nicht-bindenden Isoantikörpers ($Fc_{\gamma 2a}$).

Ergebnisse

Bei den mit $Fc_{\gamma 2a}$-behandelten Kontrolltieren erfolgte nach 3 h Ischämie und nachfolgender Reperfusion ein dramatischer Anstieg der postischämischen Leukozytenadhärenz, die ihr Maximum zwei Stunden später erreichte. Ein nahezu ähnlicher Verlauf konnte bei mit 0,9% NaCl behandelten Tieren beobachtet werden, weshalb auf eine Darstellung der Ergebnisse dieser Kontrollgruppe verzichtet wurde. Nach Behandlung mit dem monoklonalen Antikörper anti-MAC-1 war die postischämische Leukozytenadhärenz signifikant vermindert (Abb. 1).

Diskussion

Das Modell der Rückenhautkammer bei der Balb/C-Maus erlaubt erstmals, die biologische Bedeutung der für die Leukozyten/Endothel-Interaktion verantwortlichen Adhäsionsmoleküle bei Ischämie und Reperfusion intravitalmikroskopisch am nichtanästhesierten Versuchstier quantitativ zu erfassen. Durch selektive Blockade dieser Rezeptoren wird es möglich, die funktionelle Rolle der verschiedenen leukozytären und endothelialen Adhäsionsmoleküle *in vivo* zu untersuchen.

In dieser Studie konnte durch selektive Blockade des Adhärenzrezeptors MAC-1 (CD11b), der vor allem auf neutrophilen Granulozyten, nicht jedoch auf Lympho-

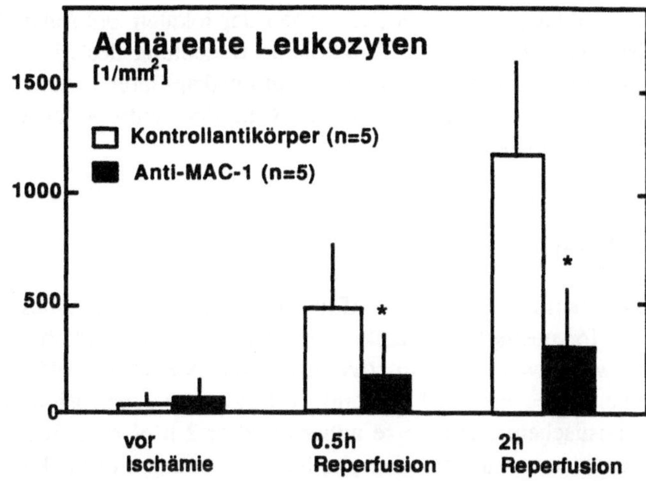

Abb. 1. Leukozytenadhärenz in postkapillären Venolen vor Induktion einer dreistündigen Ischämie auf den Rückenhautmuskel der Balb/C Maus und 0,5 h und 2 h nach Reperfusion. 10 Minuten vor Reperfusion wurde den Tieren entweder anti-MAC-1 (anti-CD11b, 1 mg kg^{-1} KG) oder der nicht-bindende Kontrollantikörper $Fc_{\gamma 2a}$ (1 mg kg^{-1} KG) intravenös infundiert. Adhärente Leukozyten sind angegeben als Zahl pro mm^2 Endotheloberfläche. Mittelwerte ± SD, * $p < 0,05$ vs. Kontrollantikörper, Wilcoxon Test

zyten exprimiert wird, die postischämische Leukozytenadhärenz nahezu vollständig blockiert werden. Die Infusion des Antikörpers führte dabei im Vergleich zur Kontrolle zu keiner Veränderung des prozentualen Anteils langsam rollender Leukozyten. Die Tatsache, daß die Parameter Blutfließgeschwindigkeit und Gefäßdurchmesser in beiden Versuchsgruppen die gleichen Veränderungen erfuhren, erlaubt, die Veränderungen der Mikrohämodynamik als Ursache der postischämisch gesteigerten Leukozyten/Endothel-Interaktion auszuschließen.

Unsere Beobachtungen belegen die zentrale Bedeutung neutrophiler Granulozyten in der frühen Reperfusionsphase und legen die selektive Blockade von Leukozytenadhäsionsmolekülen als gezielte Therapie bei Krankheitszuständen, wie Schock, Sepsis und Polytrauma, nahe, bei denen eine temporäre Hemmung der Leukozytenadhärenz erwünscht sein kann.

Zusammenfassung

Die funktionelle Bedeutung der Blockade des Leukozytenadhäsionsmoleküls MAC-1 (CD11b) für die postischämische Leukozytenadhärenz am Endothel postkapillärer Venolen wurde im Modell der Rückenhautkammer der Balb/C-Maus erstmals *in vivo* untersucht. Dreistündige Ischämie und nachfolgende Reperfusion führten bei Kontrolltieren nach 2 h Reperfusion zu einem dramatischen Anstieg der postischämischen Leukozytenadhärenz. Dieser Effekt konnte durch Infusion des spezifischen Antikörpers anti-MAC-1 effektiv vermindert werden ($p < 0,05$). Die beobachteten Effekte waren unabhängig von Veränderungen der lokalen Mikrohämodynamik. Unsere Ergebnisse unterstreichen die funktionelle Bedeutung des MAC-1 Rezeptors für die postischämische Leukozytenadhärenz in postkapillären Venolen des quergestreiften Muskels und weisen auf die zentrale Rolle der neutrophilen Granulozyten in der frühen Reperfusionsphase hin.

Summary

The functional importance of blocking the leukocyte adhesion molecule MAC-1 (CD-11b) for postischemic leukocyte adhesion to the endothelium of postcapillary venules was investigated in vivo using the dorsal skinfold chamber model in Balb/C mice. Three hours of ischemia followed by reperfusion induced a drastic increase of postischemic leukocyte adhesion after 2 h of reperfusion in control animals. This phenomenon was effectively reduced by infusion of the blocking antibody anti-MAC-1 ($p < 0.05$). The observed effects were independent of local microhemodynamic changes. Our results underline the functional importance of the MAC-1 receptor in postischemic leukocyte adhesion in postcapillary venules of the striated muscle and point to the central role of neutrophils in the early reperfusion period.

Literatur

1. Granger DN, Benoit JN, Suzuki M, Grisham MB (1989) Leukocyte adherence to venular endothelium during ischemia-reperfusion. Am J Physiol 257:G683
2. Nolte D, Bayer M, Lehr HA, Becker M, Krombach F, Kreimeier U, Messmer K (1992) Attenuation of postischemic microvascular disturbances in striated muscle by hyperosmolar saline dextran. Am J Physiol 263:H1411–H1416
3. Simpson PJ, Todd RF, Mickelson JK, Fantone JC, Gallagher KP, Lee KA, Tamura Y, Cronin M, Lucchesi BR (1990): Sustained limitation of myocardial reperfusion injury by a monoclonal antibody that alters leukocyte function. Circulation 81:226
4. Vedder NB, Winn RK, Rice CL, Chi EY, Arfors KE, Harlan JM (1988) A monoclonal antibody to the adherence-promoting leukocyte glycoprotein, CD18, reduces organ injury and improves survival from hemorrhagic shock and resuscitation in rabbits. J Clin Invest 81:939
5. Zeintl H, Sack F-U, Intaglietta M, Messmer K (1989) Computer assisted leukocyte velocity measurement in intravital microscopy. Int J Microcirc Clin Exp 8:293

Dr. R. Hecht, Institut für Chirurgische Forschung, Klinikum Großhadern, Marchioninistraße 15, W-8000 München 70

α/β TCR gerichtete monoklonale Antikörper-Therapie in der Ratte: Vorbehandlung mit mAb R73 induziert immunologische Anergie mit langfristigem Transplantatüberleben und Verhinderung von Sensibilisierung*

α/β-T cell Receptor Targeted Monoclonal Antibody Therapy in the Rat: Pretreatment with mAb R73 Induces Immunological Anergy Associated with Long-Term Allograft Survival and Abrogation of Host Sensitization

F. Jakobs[1], S. Westerholt[1], T. Sewczik[1], N. Zantl[1], W.W. Hancock[2] und C.D. Heidecke[1]

[1]Chirurgische Klinik der TU München
[2]Department of Pathology and Immunology, Monash Medical School, Prahran, Australia

Einleitung

Monoklonale Antikörper (mAb) mit Spezifitäten gegen T-Lymphozyten und deren Subpopulationen sind zunehmend Bestandteil immunsuppressiver Therapiestrategien. mAbs werden zur Prophylaxe und Therapie von Abstoßungsreaktionen im Konzert mit anderen Immunsuppressiva eingesetzt. Darüberhinaus werden mAbs zur Induktion von Toleranz im Tierexperiment verwendet. Der Mechanismus der zugrundeliegenden Areaktivität ist noch weitgehend unverstanden. In dieser Studie wurde der Einfluß eines mAb gegen α/β T-Zell-Rezeptor (TCR) tragende Lymphozyten (mAb R73 [1]) auf das Transplantatüberleben von Rattenherztransplantaten und die in situ T-Zell-Aktivierung in einem akut zellulären und einem gemischt vaskulär/zellulären Abstoßungsmodell untersucht.

Methodik

mAb-Therapie: R73 ist ein Maus-anti-Ratte IgG_1 mAb mit Spezifität gegen Ratten-α/β TCR [1]. R73 wurde in verschiedenen Konzentrationen (0,01–5 mg/kg) über 3 und 7 Tage i.v. vor oder nach der Organtransplantation appliziert. Cyclosporin A (CsA) wurde in therapeutischer Dosierung (15 mg/kg i.m.) nach der Organentnahme über 7 Tage injiziert.

Organtransplantation: Heterotope Herztransplantate wurden an ingezüchteten Ratten (BN($RT1^n$) auf LEW($RT1^l$)) in Äthernarkose an die infrarenalen großen Gefäße End-zu-Seit anastomosiert. Das Transplantatüberleben wurde täglich durch Palpation in

* mit Unterstützung der DFG (He 1248/2-3 + 1248/2-4).

Chirurgisches Forum 1993
f. experim. u. klinische Forschung
Becker/Beger/Hartel (Hrsg.)

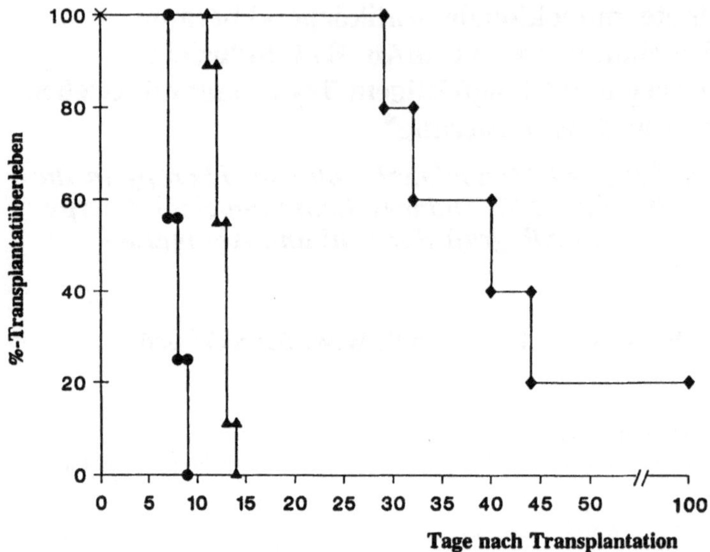

Abb. 1. Effekt von α/β TCR gerichteter Therapie mit mAb R73 auf das Transplantatüberleben von Rattenherzallotransplantaten in Abhängigkeit vom Therapiezeitpunkt (akutes Abstoßungsmodell). ● Kontrollen (n = 13), ▲ 0,1 mg/kg R73 post transplantationem (Tag 0 bis 6) (n = 9), ♦ 0,1 mg/kg R73 prä transplantationem (Tag −7 bis −1) (n = 5)

der Flanke überprüft. Zur Sensibilisierung (akzeleriertes Abstoßungsmodell) wurden 7 Tage vor der Herztransplantation (d −7) orthotope BN Hautallotransplantationen (2 Transplantate von 2,5 cm Durchmesser auf dem Rücken) durchgeführt.

Immunhistologie: Serielle Cryostatschnitte (4 μm) wurden zur Lokalisation von Zytokinen in Aceton fixiert und nach Inkubation mit einem Panel von Antikörpern (Ab) einer Peroxidase-Antiperoxidase-Färbung unterzogen (Spezifität und Quelle der Abs [2]). Zytokin- und Endothel-Färbung wurden semiquantitativ anhand der Anfärbung intra- und extrazellulärer (Zytokine in und um mononukleäre Zellen) bzw. kontinuierlicher (Endothelium) Strukturen ausgewertet.

Ergebnisse

Transplantatüberleben akutes Abstoßungsmodell: Unbehandelte LEW-Ratten stießen heterotope BN-Herztransplantate in $7,8 \pm 0,8$ Tagen ab. Die Applikation von mAb R73 beginnend unmittelbar postoperativ über 3 bzw. 7 Tage führte zu einer dosisabhängigen Verlängerung des Herztransplantatüberlebens. Die Verlängerung des Transplantatüberlebens war ab 0,1 mg/kg signifikant (Abb. 1) und unabhängig davon, ob über 3 oder 7 Tage therapiert wurde (Ergebnisse nicht gezeigt). Im Gegensatz hierzu führte die präoperative Therapie (Tag −7 bis −1) bei einer Dosierung von 0,1 mg/kg zu einem langfristigen Transplantatüberleben (Median > 40 Tage, $p < 0,0007$, Abb. 1), während 0,01 mg/kg ineffektiv waren ($8,4 \pm 0,9$ Tage, n.s.).

Transplantatüberleben akzeleriertes Abstoßungsmodell: BN-Herzallotransplantate wurden nach vorheriger Sensibilisierung durch BN-Hauttransplantate von LEW-Ratten binnen 36 h abgestoßen ($1,4 \pm 0,5$ Tage). Therapie mit mAb R73 nach der Herztransplantation verlängerte das Transplantatüberleben dosisabhängig [$2,7 \pm 0,7$ Tage bei 0,01 mg/kg mit nachfolgendem Plateau zwischen 0,1 und 5 mg/kg ($7,0 \pm 1,4$ Tage bei 5 mg/kg, $p < 0,07$)]. Therapie während der Sensibilisierungsphase (Tag -7 bis -1) ergab ebenfalls eine dosisabhängige Verlängerung des Transplantatüberlebens (0,01 mg/kg $1,5 \pm 0,6$ Tage, n.s. und 0,1 mg/kg $12,7 \pm 0,6$ Tage, $p < 0,002$). Um zu überprüfen, ob die α/β TCR gerichtete Therapie mit R73 in der Lage war, die durch Hauttransplantation induzierte Sensibilisierung zu verhindern, wurde R73 (0,1 mg/kg) vor oder während der Sensibilisierungsphase gegeben gefolgt von einer postoperativen CsA Therapie (15 mg/kg über 7 Tage nach der Herztransplantation). Dieses Regime erzeugte ein langfristiges Transplantatüberleben (> 100 Tage, $p < 0,001$), während die alleinige CsA-Therapie im akzelerierten Abstoßungsmodell das Transplantatüberleben nur auf $15,2 \pm 1,6$ Tage verlängerte.

Immunhistologie: In Kontrolltieren zeigte sich zum Zeitpunkt der maximalen Zellinfiltration der Transplantate im akuten Abstoßungsmodell (Tag 5) eine Zytokinproteinproduktion von TNF-α, IL-2 und IFN-γ, welche an infiltrierenden mononukleären Zellen sowie an Endothelzellen nachweisbar war (Tabelle 1). Therapie mit effektiven Dosen R73 (0,1 mg/kg) supprimierte diese in-situ Zytokinexpression (Tabelle 1). Die Suppression der Zytokinexpression war bei postoperativ therapierten Tieren nur temporär. Bei präoperativer Therapie wurde zusätzlich eine starke Markierung für IL-4 an mononukleären und Endothelzellen beobachtet. Im akzelerierten Abstoßungsmodell wurden vergleichbare Zytokinexpressionsmuster wie im akuten Modell ohne und mit R73 Therapie gefunden.

Tabelle 1. Immunhistologie von Herzallotransplantaten unter und nach α/β TCR gerichteter Therapie mit mAb R73 im akuten Abstoßungsmodell[1,2]

Marker	Kontrollen	0,1 mg/kg prä-Tx	0,1 mg/kg post-Tx
IL-2	10–20% MNC	< 1% MNC	< 1% MNC
IFN-γ	10–20% MNC < 5% endo	< 1% MNC	< 1% MNC
TNF-α	10–20% MNC > 50% endo 10–20% Myozyten	5–10% MNC 25–50% endo glatte Muskulatur	< 1% MNC

[1] n = 2–4 Organe/Gruppe von Ratten, die am Tag 5–6 nach Herztransplantation entnommen wurden

[2] Abkürzungen: endo Endothelium; MNC mononukleäre Zellen

Kontrollen = untherapierte Ratten; 0,1 mg/kg prä-Tx = Ratten mit präoperativer R73-Applikation (Tag -7 bis -1); 0,1 mg/kg post-Tx = Ratten mit postoperativer R73-Applikation (Tag 0 bis 6)

Diskussion

α/β TCR gerichtete Therapie mit mAb R73 wurde erstmals parallel bei akuter zellulärer und gemischt humoraler/zellulärer (akzelerierter) Transplantatabstoßung durchgeführt. Die Ergebnisse zeigen, daß relativ niedrige Dosen von R73 nur dann das Transplantatüberleben verlängern, wenn diese vor dem Kontakt mit Alloantigen appliziert wurden, und daß das gleiche Therapieregime effektiv die akzelerierte Transplantatabstoßung verhindert. Die Tatsache, daß die postoperative Therapie der akuten Abstoßung über einen weiten Dosisbereich nur eine mäßige Verlängerung des Transplantatüberlebens erbrachte, war unerwartet, da in Autoimmunmodellen der mAb R73 die spezifischen Läsionen erfolgreich verhinderte bzw. therapierte [3].

Die α/β TCR gerichtete Therapie vor der Antigenpräsentation in Form des Transplantats war in beiden untersuchten Modellen effektiv: Im akuten Abstoßungsmodell verlängerte sie langfristig das Transplantatüberleben. Dies wurde auch unter CD4 gerichteter Therapie beobachtet [4]. In sensibilisierten Transplantatempfängern konnte die akzelerierte Abstoßung ähnlich wie unter CD4 gerichteter Therapie [4] verhindert werden. Die sich nachfolgend entwickelnde akute Abstoßung wurde durch CsA kupiert.

Die Mechanismen, die zu dem Status der verminderten Reaktivität gegenüber Allotransplantaten führen, sind bislang nicht geklärt. Wenngleich sowohl unter laufender wie nach beendeter α/β TCR gerichteter Therapie die in situ T-Zell-Aktivierung anhand der fehlenden Zytokinexpression abgeschaltet erscheint, unterscheiden sich jedoch beide Therapie-Modalitäten dahingehend, daß bei fehlendem Alloantigen in Form des Transplantats ein Status der temporären Anergie erzeugt wird, währenddessen das nachfolgend transplantierte Organ langfristig überleben kann. Möglicherweise induziert die Injektion von anti-α/β TCR mAbs über eine unvollständige T-Zell-Aktivierung eine immunologische Anergie bei fehlendem zweiten Signal durch Antigen präsentierende Zellen [5]. Unsere Daten könnten eine Rationale für neue Therapiestrategien darstellen, die das Armamentarium der gegenwärtig durchgeführten postoperativen Immunsuppression erweitern.

Zusammenfassung

Therapie mit mAb R73 führte zu einer dosisabhängigen Verlängerung des Transplantatüberlebens von Rattenherztransplantaten in einem akuten und akzelerierten Abstoßungsmodell. Langfristiges Transplantatüberleben und Verhinderung von Sensibilisierung waren nur bei präoperativer Applikation des mAb zu erzielen. Die in-situ Zytokinexpression war unter der Therapie dramatisch reduziert.

Summary

mAb therapy using R73 produced a dose-dependent prolongation of rat cardiac allograft survival in both acute and accelerated rejection models. Pre- but not posttransplant mAb therapy was required to achieve long-term graft survival and abrogation of sensitization. In-situ cytokine expression was dramatically inhibited during mAb therapy.

Literatur

1. Hünig T, Wallny HJ, Hartley JK, Lawetzky A, Tiefenthaler G (1989) A monoclonal antibody to a constant determinant of the rat T cell antigen receptor that induces T cell activation: Differential reactivity with subsets of immature and mature T lymphocytes. J exp Med 169:73–86
2. Hancock WW, Sayegh MH, Sablinski T, Kut JP, Kupiec-Weglinski J, Milford EL (1992) Blocking of mononuclear cell accumulation, cytokine production and endothelial activation within rat cardiac allografts by CD4 monoclonal antibody therapy. Transplantation 53:1276–1280
3. Jung S, Krämer S, Schluesener HJ, Hünig T, Toyka K, Hartung HP (1992) Prevention and therapy of experimental neuritis by antibody against T cell receptors α/β. J Immunol 148:3768–3775
4. Sablinski T, Sayegh MH, Hut JP, Tilney NL, Milford EL, Kupiec-Weglinski JW (1992) The importance of targeting the Cd4+ T cell subset at the time of antigenic challenge for induction of prolonged vascularized allograft survival. Transplantation 53:219–221
5. Schwarz RH (1990) A cell culture model for T lymphocyte clonal anergy. Science 248:1349–1356

Dr. C.D. Heidecke, Chirurgische Klinik, TU München, Ismaninger Straße 22, W-8000 München 80

Experimentelle Analyse der Antikörpersättigung in humanen Kolonkarzinomen

Experimental Analysis of Antibody Saturation in Human Colon Carcinoma

E. Löhde[1], M. Lück[1], H. Schlicker[1], G. Barzen[2] und E. Kraas[1]

[1]Chirurgische Abteilung und Abteilung für Nuklearmedizin, Krankenhaus Moabit, Berlin
[2]Abteilung für Nuklearmedizin, Rudolf-Virchow Universität, Berlin

Einleitung

In der interdisziplinären Therapie und Diagnostik des kolorektalen Karzinoms hat das Konzept des immunologischen "tumor targeting" wichtige Bedeutung. Trotz verbesserter Detektionsverfahren bleiben die Ergebnisse der Radioimmunszintigraphie jedoch kontrovers. Sehr gute Ergebnisse im Tiermodell stehen einer zu geringen Antikörperanreicherung in Tumoren beim Menschen gegenüber.

Grundlagen der Antikörperbindung in *humanen* Kolontumoren sind nach wie vor weitgehend ungeklärt. Es fehlen quantifizierende Basisdaten über die mAk Anreicherung und mögliche Sättigungsgrenzen im Tumorgewebe.

Ziel der Untersuchung war: 1. nach *in vivo* Applikation den mAk-Gehalt im Tumorgewebe zu bestimmen; 2. mit Hilfe eines extrakorporalen Perfusionssystems für humane Kolonkarzinome zu untersuchen, inwieweit die mAk Anreicherung durch *ex vivo* Perfusion des Tumors noch erhöht werden kann und 3. die Sättigungsgrenze von Tumoren für mAk zu bestimmen.

Vorgestellt werden die Ergebnisse für den klinisch zugelassenen mAk BW431/26 IgG1 anti human CEA.

Methode

In vivo Applikation: Bei Patienten mit bekanntem Primärkarzinom des Kolons (n = 10) wurden prä op. 2 mg mAk BW431/26 m Tc99 i.v. appliziert. Die szintigraphische TM-Lokalisation erfolgte 24 h p.i. und die Operation 48 h p.i.. Post op. wurden unterschiedliche Gewebeproben entnommen, die angereicherte Aktivität im Bohrloch bestimmt und die mAk Menge nach Halbwertszeitkorrektur errechnet.

Ex vivo Applikation: Entnahme des Kolonresektates (n = 41) und arterielle Kanülierung. Einbringen in ein oxygeniertes extrakorporales Perfusionssystem mit pulsativer Durchströmung bei 37°C. Fluß, Druck, pH, Temperatur wurden laufend überwacht. Als Perfusionsmedium wurden Erythrozytenkonzentrat in HSA und heparinisierter Ringerlösung eingesetzt. In den Perfusionskreislauf wurde der Tc99 gekoppelte mAk

Chirurgisches Forum 1993
f. experim. u. klinische Forschung
Becker/Beger/Hartel (Hrsg.)

BW431/26 eingegeben und die Anreicherung im Tumor kontinuierlich szintigraphisch analysiert. Es wurden unterschiedliche mAk Konzentrationen von 0,05–12 μg/ml eingesetzt. Nach 45 min erfolgte die Auswaschphase über weitere 45 min mit Antikörperfreiem Medium. Die szintigraphische Analyse und Parameterkontrolle wurde kontinuierlich fortgesetzt. Es folgten Gewebeprobenanalysen.

Ferner wurden zuvor *in vivo* mit dem mAk BW431/26 (Tc99 gekoppelt) markierte Tumore (n = 6) zusätzlich extrakorporal mit dem mAk BW431/26 (J131 gekoppelt) perfundiert. Die spezifische Aufnahme der jeweiligen Radionuklide wurde quantitativ analysiert.

Ergebnisse

In vivo Anreicherung: Bei allen Patienten verblieb der mAk in der Zirkulation 48 h ± 4 h bis zur Operation. Die Lokalisation des Primärtumors *in vivo* gelang 4x sicher, 1x fraglich und 3x nicht. Die Szintigraphie des Resektates post op. zeigte stets eine gute Anreicherung der mAk im Tumor. Zusätzlich kamen Lymphknoten direkt zur Darstellung.

Zentraler Meßpunkt war die mAk Menge, die im Tumor akkumulierte. Bei einer mittleren mAk Konzentration im Kreislauf von 0,4 μg/ml initial wurden vom Tumorgewebe im Mittel nur 0,26 μg/g aufgenommen. Dabei zeigte sich eine heterogene mAk Verteilung mit Bindungsprävalenz auf luminalem Tumorgewebe.

Extrakorporale Anreicherung: Nach Applikation des mAk im extrakorporalen Perfusionssystem ergab sich im Vergleich zur *in vivo* Bindung ein hochgradig übereinstimmendes Muster. Bei einer vergleichbaren mAk Konzentration im Perfusat von 0,6–1

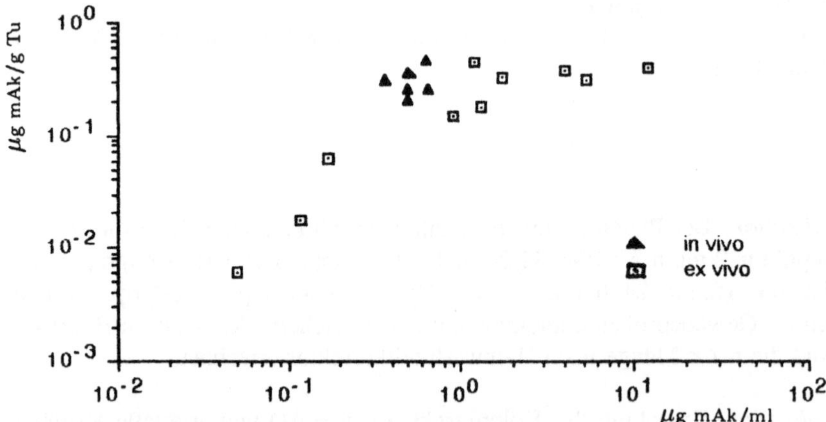

Abb. 1. Vergleich der Antikörperanreicherung in humanen Kolonkarzinomen in vivo und ex vivo. Bei Erhöhung der mAk-Konzentration im Perfusat wird ein Sättigungsplateau für die mAk in einem Bereich von etwa 0,3 μg/g erreicht. Die *in vivo* bei Patienten eingesetzte mAk Menge von 0,4 μg/ml reicht offensichtlich für das Erreichen der maximalen mAk Aufnahme im Tumor aus

μg/ml nahmen die Tumore 0,29 μg/g Gewebe im Mittel auf. Die Aufschlüsselung der mAk Verteilung im Gewebe ergab ebenfalls die Prävalenz der Bindung auf luminalen Tumoranteilen (x = 0,33 μg/g).

Zur Ermittlung von Sättigungsgrenzen wurde das 0,12–30fache der *in vivo* verwendeten mAk Konzentration eingesetzt. Es zeigte sich, daß Kolonkarzinome nicht mehr als etwa 0,3 μg mAk/g fest gebunden aufnehmen können (Abb. 1). Eine Erhöhung des mAk Angebotes führte nicht mehr zur Erhöhung der mAk Aufnahme.

In vivo und ex vivo Anreicherung: Die Frage der Tumorsättigung nach *in vivo* Applikation wurde zusätzlich geprüft durch additive Perfusion der *in vivo* markierten Tumore im extrakorporalen System. Unter Verwendung unterschiedlicher Radioisotope (mAk BW431/26 Tc99 *in vivo* und mAk BW431/26 J131 *ex vivo*) zeigte sich, daß 48 h nach *in vivo* Applikation noch über 90% der Antigene im Tumor abgesättigt sind und keine erneute Bindung des mAk BW431/26 J131 möglich ist.

Diskussion

Die entscheidende und in der Literatur kontrovers diskutierte Frage in der Radioimmunodetektion ist, wieviele Antikörper können im Tumor aufgenommen werden und gibt es eine Sättigung?

In der vorliegenden Arbeit wurden diese Fragen erstmalig experimentell für humane Tumore beantwortet. Zunächst wurde die Menge Antikörper bestimmt, welche bei definierter Antikörperapplikation im Tumor anreichert. Ausgegangen wurde von den in der klinischen Diagnostik eingesetzten 2 mg pro Patient. Sowohl in der *in vivo* und *ex vivo* Analyse wurde eine mittlere Antikörperanreicherung im Bereich um 0,3 μg Antikörper pro Gramm Tumor ermittelt. Dies liegt in dem in der Literatur berichteten Aufnahme von 0,002%–0,03% der applizierten Antikörpermenge im Tumor [3].

Mit Hilfe der extrakorporalen Perfusion wurde erstmalig das Sättigungsplateau für humane Kolonkarzinome definiert. In einer Versuchsreihe mit unterschiedlichen Antikörperkonzentrationen konnte gezeigt werden, daß ab einem Bereich von etwa 0,4 μg Antikörper pro ml Perfusat die maximale Aufnahmekapazität der Tumore für den mAk erreicht wird. Eine weitere Erhöhung der Antikörperkonzentration führt nicht zur Erhöhung der Antikörperbindung im Tumor (Abb. 1).

Dieses experimentell erhobene Ergebnis wurde zusätzlich gestützt durch die kombinierte *in vivo* und *ex vivo* Untersuchungen. Es konnte gezeigt werden, daß – in Übereinstimmung mit der experimentellen Sättigungskurve – bei Patienten nach Applikation von 2 mg Antikörper (= etwa 0,4 μg/ml Blut) tatsächlich die vollständige Absättigung erreichbarer Antigene im Tumor erreicht wird. Mehr als 90% der Bindungsstellen waren nach 48 h noch besetzt. Diese Aussagen sind grundlegend für künftige Konzepte der Radioimmuntherapie und -Diagnostik von Kolonkarzinomen.

Zusammenfassung

Ziel war es, im Rahmen des immunologischen "tumor targeting" Basisdaten für die Antikörperanreicherung in humanen Kolonkarzinomen zu erarbeiten. Untersuchungen nach *in vivo* Applikation des mAk BW431/26 anti human CEA wurden mit experimentellen Daten der mAk Anreicherung in einem extrakorporalen oxygenierten Perfusiossystem für humane Kolonkarzinome korreliert. In enger Übereinstimmung ergab sich, daß humane Kolontumore nur die limitierte Menge etwa 0,3 μg mAk/g Gewebe aufnehmen können. Dieses Sättigungsplateau wird ab einer Antikörperkonzentration von etwa 0,4 μg/ml im Perfusat erreicht. Eine höhere Antikörperdichte führt nicht zur erhöhten Anreicherung im Tumor.

Summary

The aim of the study was to analyze basic data of antibody accumulation in human colon carcinoma, this being a prerequisite for immunotargeting. The antibody mAk BW431/26 anti-human CEA was administered in vivo as well as in an experimental extracorporal oxygenized perfusion system for human colon carcinoma. In close correlation the data show a saturation limit for mAb in tumors of 0.3 μg/g. This can be reached by a concentration of circulating mAb of 0.4 μg/ml. Further increase of mAb will not intensify mAb uptake in tumor tissue.

Literatur

1. Epenetos AA, Snook D, Durbin H, Johnson PM, Taylor Papadimitriou J (1986) Limitations of radiolabeled monoclonal antibodies for localization of human neoplasms. Cancer Res 46:3183–91
2. Löhde E, Schwarzendahl P, Schlicker H, Abri O, Kalthoff H, Matzku S, Epenetos AA, Kraas E (1990) Accumulation characteristics of human colon carcinomas after monoclonal antibody ex vivo perfusion. Br J Cancer [Suppl]X:12–14
3. Sedlacek HH, Schulz G, Steinstraesser A, Kuhlmann L, Schwarz A, Seidel L, Seemann G, Kraemer H-P, Bosslet K (1988) Monoclonal antibodies in tumor therapy. In: Eckhardt S, Hozner JH, Nagel GA (eds) Contributions to oncology, vol 32

Dr. E. Löhde, Chirurgische Abteilung und Abteilung für Nuklearmedizin, Krankenhaus Moabit, 1000 Berlin

Impact of Endothelial Cell-Seeding with Omentally Derived Microvascular Cells on the Long-Term Patency and Neointimal Hyperplasia in Small-Diameter Dacron Grafts

Autotransplantation von mikrovaskulären Endothelzellen des Omentums mit kleinlumigen Dacronprothesen: Langzeitdurchgängigkeit und Neointimabildung

M. Pasic[1], W. Müller-Glauser[1], M. Lachat[1], P. Bittermann[2], L. von Segesser[1], and M. Turina[1]

[1]Clinic for Cardiovascular Surgery, University Hospital Zurich, Switzerland
[2]Sulzer Medical Technology, Ltd., Winterthur, Switzerland

Introduction

Although it has been shown that endothelial cell-seeding may reduce anastomotic intimal hyperplasia in animals with good early and midterm results [1], no long-term data are available. Anastomotic hyperplasia is characteristic of the normal healing process, but its precise control and the influence of complete endothelialization of a seeded prosthetic graft have still not been completely understood [2]. Microvascular cells derived from omental tissue allow immediate high-density seeding; however, the isolates contain not only endothelial cells, but also a variety of other cell types [3]. Despite approximately 95% endothelialization at 4 weeks, an inner capsule continues to accumulate beneath the endothelial monolayer [4], remaining a potential hazard for late occlusion during the long-term period [5].

In this study we reported the impact of seeding with microvascular cells derived from omental tissue on long-term patency and proliferation of a subendothelial layer in small-diameter Dacron grafts.

Material and Methods

Studies were performed in 13 mongrel dogs initially weighing 20–30 kg. Dogs were cared for according to the European Convention on Animal Care. The experiments were reviewed and approved by the Ethical Committee of the University Hospital Zurich.

Four-mm-internal diameter and 6-cm-length uncrimped Dacron grafts of a water porosity of 700 ml/cm^2/min were seeded during the preclotting with autologous plasma, and implanted end-to-end into the carotid arteries after excision of a 6-cm-long arterial segment. Microvascular endothelial cells were harvested from omental tissue according to the method of Schmidt et al. [4] with some modifications. Seeding

Chirurgisches Forum 1993
f. experim. u. klinische Forschung
Becker/Beger/Hartel (Hrsg.)

density of $1.75 \pm 0,44 \times 10^6$ endothelial cells/cm^2 of graft surface. All dogs received dipyridamole (75 mg/day) and acetylsalicylic acid (325 mg/day) orally for 4 weeks, beginning 1 and 4 days prior to surgery, respectively.

Approximately 0.5 ml aliquot of the cells was removed for a cell count, cell identification, and tissue culture. The number of cells was calculated from fluorometric DNA measurements. Endothelial cells were identified by their typical cobblestone morphology at confluence by biochemical testing for the specific rapid receptor-mediated uptake of acetylated low-density lipoprotein labeled with a fluorescent probe and examined with phase contrast and epifluorescence. Smooth muscle cells were identified by marking with α-smooth muscle actin γ-globulin asm-1 and visualization by a fluorescent labeled secondary antibody.

Graft patency was determined by arteriography immediately after the operation, followed by angiography after 1, 4, 26, and 52 weeks. The prostheses were explanted 6 months (n = seven dogs) and 1 year (n = six dogs) after surgery. After macroscopic examination the grafts were studied by light and scanning electron microscopy. The mean thickness of the neointima within 10 mm of the suture lines, as well as of the central part of the graft, was measured on hematoxylin-eosin stained cross section using a computer-assisted image-analyzing system.

Data are presented as mean value $\pm$ standard deviation. Statistical comparison of neointimal thickenings were made with an unpaired t test. A P value less than 0.05 was considered to be significant.

Results

All grafts were patent throughout the study period of 12 months (patency rate of 100%). Angiograms of the grafts showed smooth intimal surfaces. Macroscopically, the luminal surfaces of the grafts were smooth and shiny without atheromatous plaques or anastomotic thickening (Fig. 1).

Histological studies revealed a cellular lining of the grafts with highly organized subendothelial layers (Fig. 2). Transmural vasa vasorum were only occasionally noted. Scanning electron microscopy showed a cellular lining of a complete monolayer of cells with endothelial-like morphology in all examined areas (Fig. 3).

Light microscopic evaluation showed that the mean neointimal tissue thickness of the seeded Dacron grafts was greater at 26 weeks than at 52 weeks (Table 1). However, no statistically significant difference was found. The central graft areas were thicker than proximal or distal anastomotic regions, showing no anastomotic hyperplasia.

Table 1. Thickness (mm) of the proximal, central, and distal regions at 26 and 52 weeks after implantation of the Dacron grafts seeded with omentally derived microvascular cells in dogs ($\pm$ SD)

	26 weeks	52 weeks
Proximal	0.325 ± 0.095	0.267 ± 0.122
Central	0.386 ± 0.154	0.313 ± 0.101
Distal	0.319 ± 0.077	0.250 ± 0.078

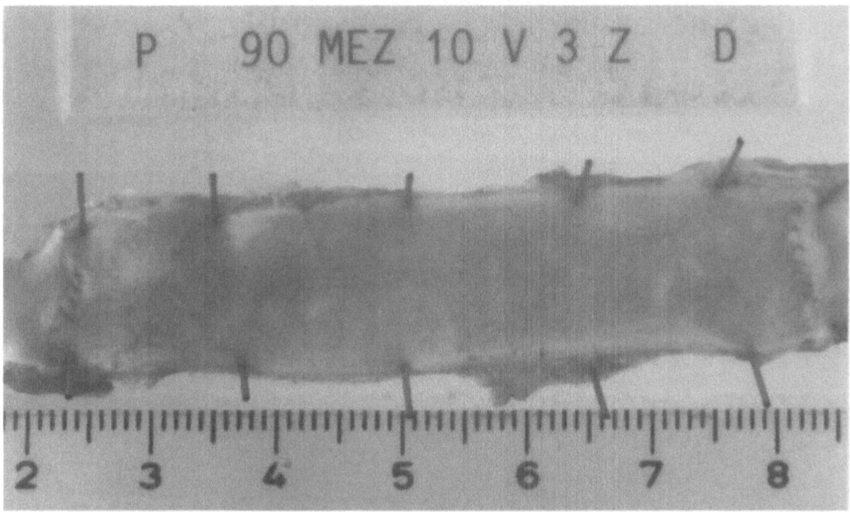

Fig. 1. Macroscopic appearance of the luminal surface of the seeded graft explanted 12 months after insertion

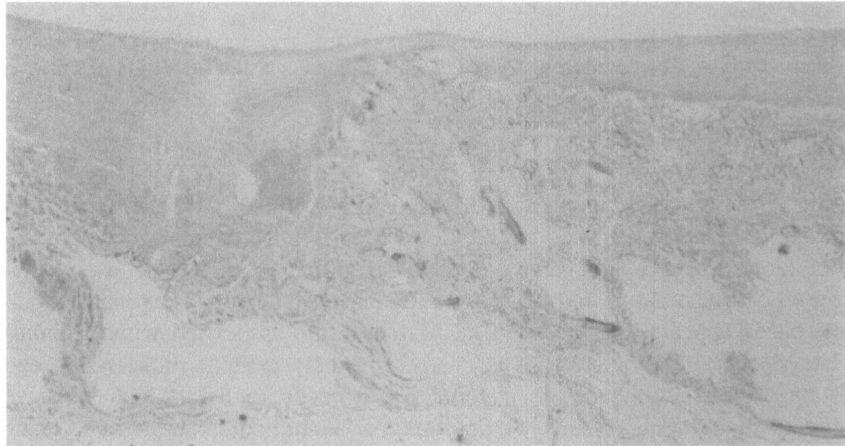

Fig. 2. Light microscopy (hematoxylin-eosin): photomicrographs of cross section of the anastomosis showed anastomotic neointimal tissue without extensive subendothelial thickness

Discussion

Our study supports the hypothesis that endothelial cell seeding improved late patency rate and reduces neointimal hyperplasia in endothelial-like lining above the highly organized subendothelial multilayers, without development of late anastomotic hyperplasia.

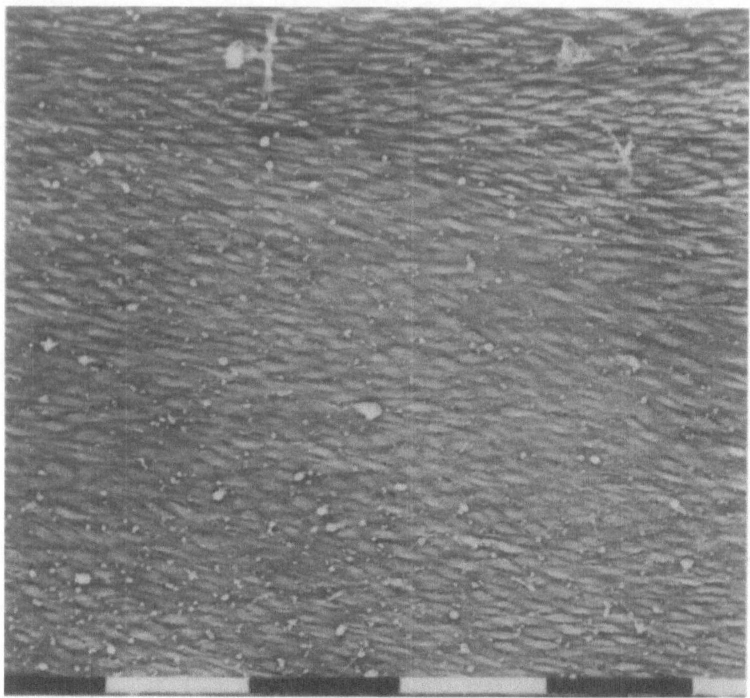

Fig. 3. Scanning electron micrograph of Dacron graft seeded with omentally derived microvascular cells; a confluent of endothelial-like cells with minimal platelet or cellular deposition (*white bar*: 0.1 mm)

Intimal hyperplasia is a characteristic fibromuscular cellular response to vascular injury during vascular reconstruction [2]. It leads to intimal or neointimal proliferation after reconstruction with vein or prosthetic grafts, or in a host artery after endarterectomy, atherectomy, and coronary angioplasty. On gross examinations, intimal hyperplasia appears as a white, firm, fibrous lesion associated with thrombus only at late stages. Histologically, it is characterized by cellular proliferation and accumulation of extracellular matrix material which occurs as a result of excessive proliferation of smooth muscle cells [1]. Formation of neointimal hyperplasia occuring after implantation of prosthetic vascular grafts is not identical to intimal proliferation after endarterectomy or angioplasty, especially due to chronic inflammatory responses associated with implanted synthetic grafts.

Neointimal hyperplasia in the area of the distal anastomoses accounts for more than 20% of late failure of infrainguinal prosthetic graft revascularization [6]. After prosthetic graft reconstruction, the migration of smooth muscle cells from the anastomosis is always preceded by endothelial cells [2]. In contrast to occlusions after angioplasty or atherectomy which tend to appear in the first 6 months, the stenosing intimal lesions of autogenous or prosthetic grafts usually appear later after surgery [6].

The potential for endothelial cell seeding and antiplatelet agents to promote patency and to reduce anastomotic intimal hyperplasia has been shown in animals [1, 7]. Anastomotic intimal hyperplasia after a 16-week study period is inversely related to the extent of luminal endothelial cell coverage of small-diameter Dacron prostheses seeded with enzymatically derived autologous venous endothelial cells [7]. High density endothelial cell seeding without antiplatelet agents inhibits neointimal hyperplasia up to 6 weeks after carotid endarterectomy in dogs [8].

In this study we showed that endothelial cell seeding with omentally derived microvascular cells improved long-term patency and did not cause late neointimal hyperplasia of small-diameter Dacron grafts in dogs.

Summary

In this study we examined influences on long-term patency and neointimal hyperplasia of small-diameter Dacron grafts seeded with enzymatically derived microvascular cells from omental tissue in a canine model. In 13 mongrel dogs microvascular cells were enzymatically harvested from omentum and seeded prior to the graft implantation onto 6-cm-long uncrimped Dacron prostheses with an internal diameter of 4 mm with seeding density of $1.75 \pm 0.44 \times 10^6$ cells/cm^2 of graft surface. All dogs received dipyridamole (75 mg/day) and acetylsalicylic acid (325 mg/day) orally for 4 weeks. The prostheses were explanted 6 months ($n = 7$ dogs) and 1 year ($n = 6$ dogs) after surgery. All grafts were patent throughout the study. Microscopic examination showed a confluent luminal coverage with endothelial-like cells and highly organized subendothelial tissue layers, but without anastomotic neointimal hyperplasia. We conclude that one-stage endothelial cell seeding with omentally derived microvascular cells improved long-term patency of small-diameter Dacron grafts, without development of late neointimal hyperplasia.

Acknowledgements

The authors thank M.-C. Mensel, C. Probst, R. Werschler, and Mr. F. Rieser for technical assistance with the cell culture, seeding procedure, the scanning electron microscopy, and the morphometric evaluations of the histologic sections; A. Gartenmann and B. Ajro for histological specimens; A. Huber for engineering assistance; B. Leskosek, S. Egger-Rühle, Y. Amacher, and A. Avdyli for excellent operative assistance; and O. Reinhard for preparing the illustrations. Scanning electron microscopy was done at the Institute of Anatomy, University of Zürich, Zürich, Switzerland. Operations were performed at the Veterinary Faculty, University of Zürich, Zürich, Switzerland.

The study was supported by the Kommission zur Förderung der wissenschaftlichen Forschung, Bern, Switzerland, Projekt No. 1576, 1724.1, and 2178-1, and by Sulzer Medical Technology, Ltd., Winterthur, Switzerland.

References

1. Graham LM, Vincent CK, Brothers TE, Harrell KA, Darvishian D, Sell R, Burkel WE, Stanley JC (1988) Efficacy of antiplatelet agents in promoting patency and reducing anastomotic hyperplasia of endothelial cell seeded and unseeded ePTFE grafts. Surg Forum 39:348–350
2. Chervu A, Moore WS (1990) An overview of intimal hyperplasia. Surg Gynecol Obstet 171:433–447
3. Sterpetti AV, Hunter WJ, Schultz RD, Sugimoto JT, Blair EA, Hacker K, Chasan P, Valentine J (1988) Seeding with endothelial cells derived from the microvessels of the omentum and from the jugular vein: a comparative study. J Vasc Surg 7:677–684
4. Schmidt SP, Monajjem N, Evancho MM, Pippert TR, Sharp WV (1988) Microvascular endothelial cell seeding of small-diameter Dacron vascular grafts. J Invest Surg 1:35–44
5. Herring M, Baughman S, Glover J, Kesler K, Jesseph J, Campbell J, Dilley R, Evan A, Gardner A (1984) Endothelial seeding of Dacron and polytetrafluoroethylene grafts: the cellular events of healing. Surgery 96:745–754
6. Quiñones-Baldrich WJ, Alfredo AP, Ahn SS, Baker JD, Machleder HI, Moore WS (1992) Long-term results of infrainguinal revascularization with polytetrafluoroethylene: a ten-year experience. J Vasc Surg 16:209–217
7. Graham LM, Brothers TE, Vincent CK, Burkel WE, Stanley JC (1991) The role of an endothelial cell lining in limiting distal anastomotic intimal hyperplasia of 4-mm-I.D. Dacron grafts in a canine model. J Biomed Mat Res 25:525–533
8. Bush HL, Jakubowski JA, Sentissi JM, Curl GR, Hayes JA, Deykin D (1987) Neointimal hyperplasia occurring after carotid endarterectomy in a canine model: effect of endothelial cell seeding vs. perioperative aspirin. J Vas Surg 5:118–125

M. Pasic, M.D., Sc.D., Clinic for Cardiovascular Surgery, University Hospital Zürich, Rämistraße 100, CH-8091 Zürich, Switzerland

Primäre exokrine Insuffizienz der Bauchspeicheldrüse nach Gastrektomie

Primary Exocrine Insufficiency of the Pancreas After Total Gastrectomy

J. Böhm[1], M. Büchler[1], H. Friess[1], P. Malfertheiner[2] und H.G. Beger[1]

[1]Allgemeinchirurgie, Chirurgische Klinik I, Universität Ulm
[2]Abteilung für Gastroenterologie, Universität Ulm

Einleitung

Das Auftreten einer Maldigestion wird nach Magenresektion häufig beobachtet. Es werden verschiedene Ursachen für diese Maldigestion verantwortlich gemacht, so der Verlust der peptischen Vorverdauung, die Ausschaltung des Duodenums, die Störung der gastrointestinalen Motorik und das Auftreten einer sekundären Pankreasinsuffizienz als Folge einer pankreatikocibalen Asynchronie. Das Auftreten einer primären Insuffizienz der Bauchspeicheldrüse nach totaler Gastrektomie wird bisher nur von einem Autor beschrieben [1]. Ziel unserer Arbeit war es, beim selben Patientenkollektiv, vor und 3 Monate nach Gastrektomie, mittels Sekretin-Zärulein-Test, einem standardisierten direkten Pankreasfunktionstest, die exokrine Pankreasfunktion zu untersuchen.

Patienten und Methoden

Bei 15 Patienten mit Magenkarzinom (12 Männer, 3 Frauen, mittleres Alter 64,5 Jahre) wurde 14 Tage vor geplanter totaler Gastrektomie ein Sekretin-Zärulein-Test durchgeführt. Die Patienten erhielten eine Nakayama-Rekonstruktion mit Pouch (10 cm) und Erhalt der Duodenalpassage, so daß dieselben Patienten 3 Monate nach Gastrektomie nochmals demselben Pankreasfunktionstest zugeführt werden konnten. Postoperativ war die Durchführung des Sekretin-Zärulein-Testes bei 7 Patienten möglich. Bei den übrigen Patienten war die Operation palliativ oder es bestand postoperativ der klinische oder radiologische Verdacht auf eine Progredienz des Tumorleidens. Zur Durchführung des Sekretin-Zärulein-Testes wurde nach 12stündiger Nahrungskarenz eine doppellumige Gastroduodenalsonde gelegt, deren korrekte Lage mittels Durchleuchtung überprüft wurde. Über eine halbe Stunde wurde dann die Basalsekretion abgesaugt. Eine Stunde lang wurde das durch Stimulation mit Sekretin, in der Dosierung 1 U/kg/h, sezernierte Sekret abgesaugt. Für eine weitere Stunde wurde das Sekret abgesaugt, das durch Stimulation mit Sekretin, in der Dosierung 1 U/kg/h, und zusätzlich mit Zärulein, in der Dosierung 120 ng/kg/h, sezerniert wird. Ermittelt

Chirurgisches Forum 1993
f. experim. u. klinische Forschung
Becker/Beger/Hartel (Hrsg.)

wurde die Menge des sezernierten Duodenalsekretes, dessen pH, sowie der Gehalt an Trypsin, Chymotrypsin, Amylase und Bicarbonat im Duodenalsekret. Zur Statistik wurde ein Wilcoxon-Test für unverbundene Stichproben angewandt. Die Ergebnisse sind als Mediane wiedergegeben.

Resultate

Der Vergleich der Sekretionsleistung unter maximaler Stimulation mit Sekretin (1 U/kg/h) und Zärulein (120 ng/kg/h) zeigte eine deutliche Einschränkung der Sekretionskapazität des exokrinen Pankreas 3 Monate nach erfolgter Magenresektion. So reduzierte sich das Volumen des Duodenalsekrets von präoperativ 410 ml/h auf postoperativ 95 ml/h um 77%. Ebenfalls verringerte sich der Gehalt an Enzymen, welche unter maximaler Stimulation gewonnen wurden. Die Trypsinsekretion ging von präoperativ 10 942 U/h auf postoperativ 1 159 U/h zurück, was einer Reduktion um 89% entspricht (Abb. 1). Die Ausschüttung an Chymotrypsin war von präoperativ 5 707 U/h auf postoperativ 496 U/h, also um 91% reduziert (Abb. 2). Die Sekretion von Amylase erniedrigte sich von präoperativ 58 165 U/h auf postoperativ 14 986 U/h um 74% (Abb. 3). Auch der im Duodenalsekret bestimmte Gehalt an Bicarbonat war von präoperativ 25 mVal/h auf 2 mVal/h im postoperativ durchgeführten Sekretin-Zärulein-Test um 92% reduziert (Abb. 4).

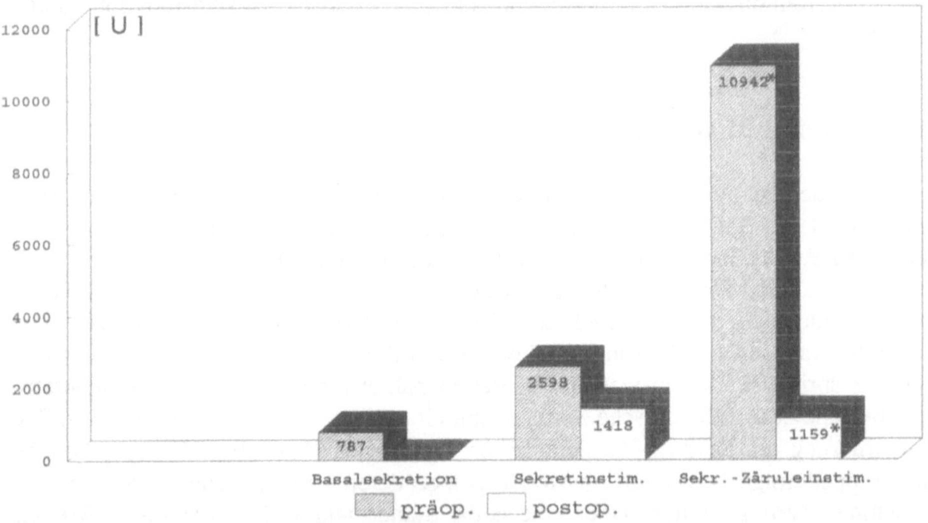

Abb. 1. Trypsingehalt des Duodenalsekrets im Sekretin-Zärulein-Test; präoperativ 15 Pat.; postoperativ 7 Pat.; Werte als Mediane; * $p < 0,009$

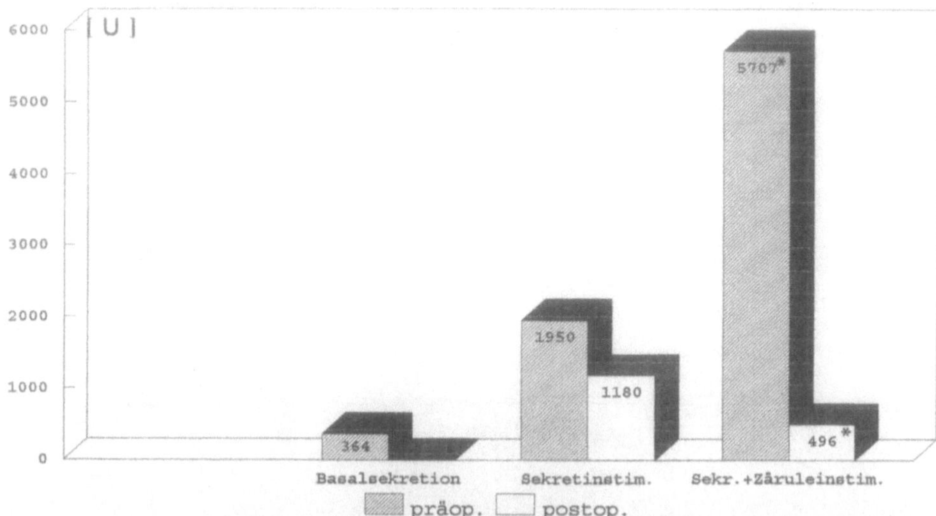

Abb. 2. Chymotrypsingehalt des Duodenalsekrets im Sekretin-Zärulein-Test; präoperativ 15 Pat.; postoperativ 7 Pat.; Werte als Mediane; * $p < 0{,}021$

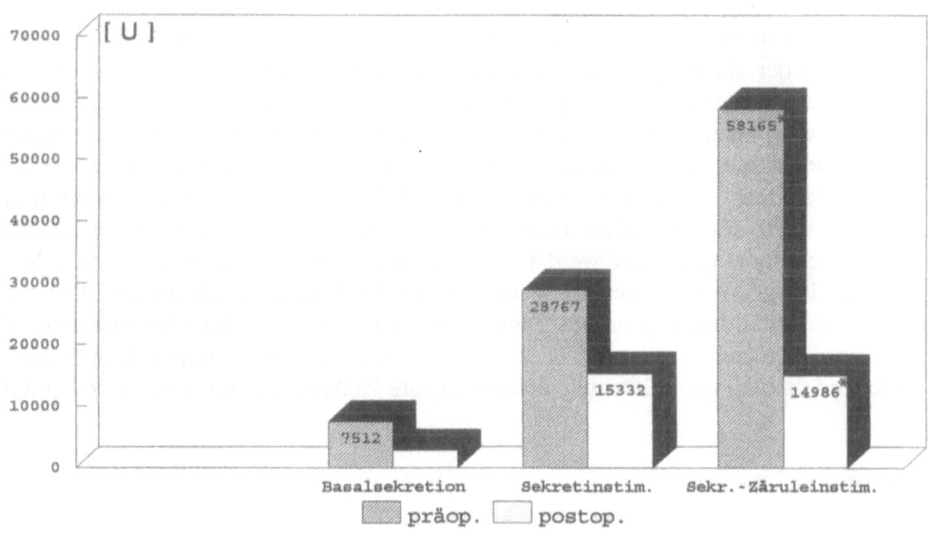

Abb. 3. Amylasegehalt des Duodenalsekrets im Sekretin-Zärulein-Test; präoperativ 15 Pat.; postoperativ 7 Pat.; Werte als Mediane; * $p < 0{,}009$

Diskussion

Unsere Daten zeigen eine deutliche Einschränkung der Sekretionskapazität des exokrinen Pankreas 3 Monate nach Gastrektomie und sprechen somit im Falle der untersuchten Patienten für das Auftreten einer primären exokrinen Insuffizienz der Bauch-

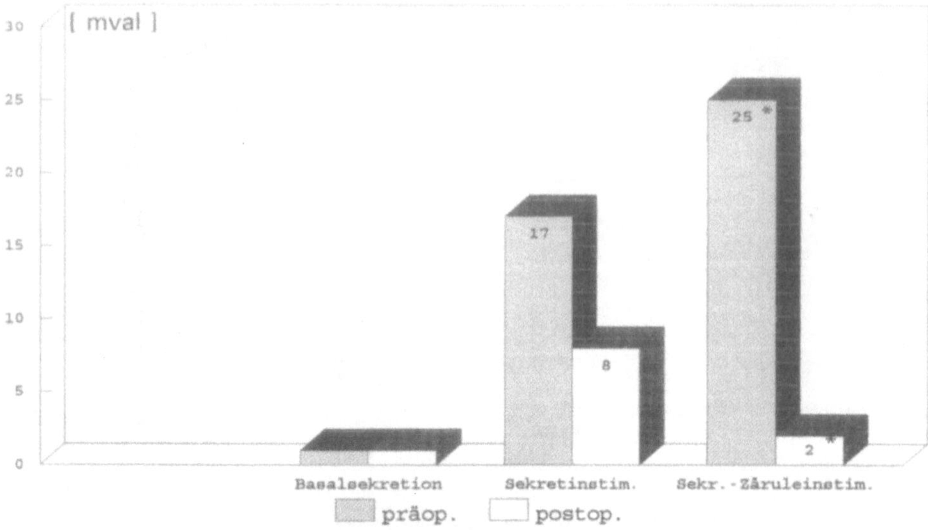

Abb. 4. Bicarbonatgehalt im Duodenalsekrets unter Sekretin-Zärulein-Stimulation; präoperativ 15 Pat.; postoperativ 7 Pat.; Werte als Mediane; * $p < 0{,}009$

speicheldrüse nach Magenresektion. Die mögliche Ursache dieser primären exokrinen Insuffizienz der Bauchspeicheldrüse sehen wir in der Gastrektomie mit Lymphknotendissektion. Durch diesen Eingriff kommt es zu einer Denervation des Pankreas. Eine tierexperimentelle Studie konnte zeigen, daß es bei extrinsischer Denervation des Hundepankreas nach Nahrungsstimulation zu einer Reduktion der Proteinsekretion des Pankreas um annähernd 88% kommt [2]. Auch beim Menschen kann nach Denervation im Rahmen einer Pankreastransplantation ein Sistieren der exokrinen Pankreassekretion beobachtet werden [3]. In Übereinstimmung hierzu besteht die Vorstellung, daß beim Menschen die Pankreassekretion hauptsächlich abhängig ist von einer cholinergen Innervation des Organs, und der hormonale Stimulus mittels CCK als Neuromodulator fungiert [4]. Dies wäre auch eine Erklärung dafür, daß trotz hochdosierter Stimulation mit Zärulein keine adäquate Pankreassekretion zustande kommt.

Zusammenfassung

Die Untersuchung der exokrinen Funktion der Bauchspeicheldrüse mittels Sekretin-Zärulein-Test vor und 3 Monate nach totaler Gastrektomie zeigte, unter maximaler Stimulation mit Sekretin (1 U/kg/h) und Zärulein (120 ng/kh/h), eine signifikante Reduktion der Sekretionskapazität des exokrinen Pankreas. Das Volumen des Duodenalsekretes war um 77%, der Gehalt an Bicarbonat um 92%, die Ausschüttung von Trypsin um 89%, sowie der Gehalt an Chymotrypsin bzw. Amylase um 91% bzw. 74% reduziert. Diese Daten dokumentieren zum erstenmal eine primäre exokrine Insuffizienz der Bauchspeicheldrüse nach Gastrektomie. Die Ursache sehen wir in der verfahrensbedingten Denervation des Pankreas mit Zerstörung enteropankreatischer und gastropankreatischer Reflexbahnen im Rahmen der Gastrektomie mit Lymphknotendissektion.

Summary

Pancreatic exocrine function was investigated using exogenous stimulation with secretin (1 U/kg h^{-1}) and cerulein (120 ng/kg h^{-1} before and 3 months after total gastrectomy. In response to exogenous stimulation we found a significant reduction of the pancreatic secretory capacity 3 months after total gastrectomy compared with the secretory capacity before. The reduction in output was 77%, 89%, 91%, 74%, and 92%, respectively, for volume, trypsin, chymotrypsin, amylase, and bicarbonate. For the first time the results of the present study prove the occurrence of a primary exocrine insufficiency of the pancreas following total gastrectomy. We conclude that denervation of the pancreas and loss of extrinsic reflexes due to gastrectomy with lymphadenectomy lead to primary exocrine pancreatic insufficiency.

Literatur

1. Gullo L, Costa PL, Ventrucci M, Mattioli S, Viti G, Labo G (1979) Exocrine pancreatic function after total gastrectomy. Scand J Gastroent 14:401–407
2. Köhler H, Nustede R, Barthel M, Schafmayer A (1992) Einfluß der extrinsischen Denervation des Pankreas auf die nahrungsstimulierte Pankreassekretion und die Freisetzung von Cholezystokinin und Neurotensin beim Hund. Z Gastroenterol 30:125–129
3. Hopt UT, Büsing M, Schareck WD, Becker HD (1991) The bladder drainage technique in pancreas transplantation – the Tübingen experience. Diabetologia 34:24–27
4. Adler G, Beglinger C, Braun U, Reinshagen M, Koop L, Schafmayer A, Rovati L, Arnold L (1991) Interaction of the cholinergic system and cholecystokinin in the regulation of the endogenous and exogenous stimulation of pancreatic secretion in humans. Gastroenterology 100:537–543

J. Böhm, Abteilung für Allgemeine Chirurgie, Universitätsklinik Ulm,
Steinhövelstraße 9, W-7900 Ulm

Positiver Einfluß von Cholecystokinin (CCK)-Rezeptorantagonisten auf die Nahrungsaufnahme und das Körpergewicht nach Gastrektomie bei der Ratte

Cholecystokinin Receptor Antagonists Increase Food Intake and Body Weight After Gastrectomy in the Rat

T.T. Zittel*, B. v.Elm, R.K. Teichmann und H.D. Becker

Abteilung für Abdominalchirurgie, Chirurgische Universitätsklinik Tübingen
(Direktor: Prof. Dr. H.D. Becker)

Einleitung

Gewichtsverlust nach Gastrektomie ist ein bekanntes klinisches Problem. Erst in den letzten Jahren wurde eine verminderte kalorische Nahrungsaufnahme nach Gastrektomie festgestellt und als Teilursache des Gewichtsverlustes vermutet [1]. Gastrektomie führt bei Ratten ebenfalls zu Gewichtsverlust und zu einer Zunahme der postprandialen CCK-Ausschüttung [2, 3]. Da CCK die Nahrungsaufnahme hemmt [4], könnte CCK Mitursache des Gewichtsverlustes nach Gastrektomie sein. Ziel unserer Studie war es, den Effekt von spezifischen CCK-A (MK329) bzw. CCK-B (L365,260) Rezeptorantagonisten auf den Gewichtsverlust und die Nahrungsaufnahme nach Gastrektomie bei der Ratte zu untersuchen.

Methodik

Erwachsene männliche Lewis-Ratten (300-350 g) wurden in Einzelkäfigen unter kontrollierten Bedingungen gehalten (20°C, 12 h/12 h hell-dunkel Rhythmus). Die tägliche Nahrungsaufnahme wurde bei unoperierten und gastrektomierten Ratten (Rekonstruktion nach Roux-en-Y) zwischen dem 30. und 40. postoperativen Tag gemessen. In einer separaten Studie wurden gastrektomierte Ratten vom 20. bis zum 100. postoperativen Tag auf eine zwölfstündige Fütterungsperiode während der Dunkelphase beschränkt. Unmittelbar vor und 6 h nach Beginn der Fütterungsperiode wurde täglich entweder Vehikel, MK329 oder L365,260 (jeweils 0,01 und 0,1 mg/kg) intraperitoneal injiziert. Am Ende der Fütterungsperiode wurde die jeweilige Nahrungsaufnahme (Altromin Rattentrockenfutter) gemessen und in Relation zum präoperativen Körpergewicht (KG) gesetzt.

* Gefördert durch DFG-Stipendium Zi 415/1-1.

Chirurgisches Forum 1993
f. experim. u. klinische Forschung
Becker/Beger/Hartel (Hrsg.)

Statistik

Alle Daten sind als Mittelwert ± Standardabweichung des Mittelwertes angegeben. Differenzen zwischen den verschiedenen Gruppen wurden mittels ANOVA (Varianzanalyse), gefolgt von Fisher's LSD (least significant difference) Test, analysiert. Eine Wahrscheinlichkeit von $p < 0{,}05$ wurde als signifikante Differenz bewertet.

Ergebnisse

Gastrektomie reduzierte die tägliche Nahrungsaufnahme um 19% im Vergleich zu unoperierten Ratten (s. Abb. 1). Mit Vehikel behandelte gastrektomierte Ratten verloren bis zum 100. postoperativen Tag signifikant mehr Gewicht als mit MK329 oder L365,260 behandelte gastrektomierte Ratten (s. Abb. 2). Mit Vehikel behandelte gastrektomierte Ratten nahmen zwischen dem 20. und 100. postoperativen Tag signifikant weniger Trockenfutter/100 g präoperatives KG auf als mit MK329 oder L365,260 behandelte gastrektomierte Ratten (s. Tabelle 1).

Tabelle 1. Nahrungsaufnahme vom 20. bis zum 100. postoperativen Tag nach Gastrektomie

Postop. Tag	Vehikel (n=12)	MK329 0,01mg/kg (n=5)	MK329 0,1mg/kg (n=5)	L365,260 0,01mg/kg (n=6)	L365,260 0,1mg/kg (n=6)
20–39	108 ± 5g	107 ± 8g	123 ± 8g[a]	129 ± 7g[a]	114 ± 7g
40–59	104 ± 3g	111 ± 4g	120 ± 4g[b]	118 ± 4g[b]	115 ± 4g[a]
60–79	99 ± 4g	104 ± 6g	108 ± 6g	104 ± 5g	115 ± 3g[a]
80–99	93 ± 4g	103 ± 6g	106 ± 6g	104 ± 5g	104 ± 5g
20–99	404 ± 10g	426 ± 16g	457 ± 16g[b]	457 ± 14g[b]	449 ± 14g[a]

Nahrungsaufnahme in Relation zum präoperativen Körpergewicht (g Nahrungsaufnahme/100 g präoperatives Körpergewicht)
[a] $p < 0{,}05$ vs Vehikel
[b] $p < 0{,}01$ vs Vehikel

Diskussion

Als Ursache des Gewichtsverlustes nach Gastrektomie wurde bisher vor allem eine Malabsorption aufgrund mangelnder Stimulation des Pankreas und beschleunigter Dünndarmpassage diskutiert [5]. Häufig handelt es sich aber lediglich um eine marginale Malabsorption, und insbesondere die Resultate hinsichtlich der Geschwindigkeit der Dünndarmpassage nach Gastrektomie sind widersprüchlich. Eine veränderte CCK-Ausschüttung als mögliche Teilursache des Gewichtsverlustes nach Gastrektomie stellt einen neuen Ansatzpunkt dar. In unserer Studie reduzierten CCK-A bzw. CCK-B Rezeptorenantagonisten den postoperativen Gewichtsverlust bis zum 100. postoperativen

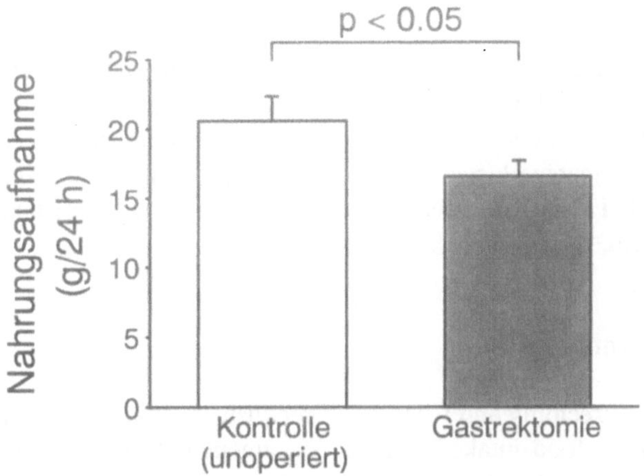

Abb. 1. Nahrungsaufnahme pro 24 h nach Gastrektomie. Gastrektomierte Ratten (▩, n = 4) konsumieren signifikant weniger Futter pro 24 h als unoperierte Ratten (□, n = 4) bei gleichem Körpergewicht (347 ± 7 vs 377 ± 10 g)

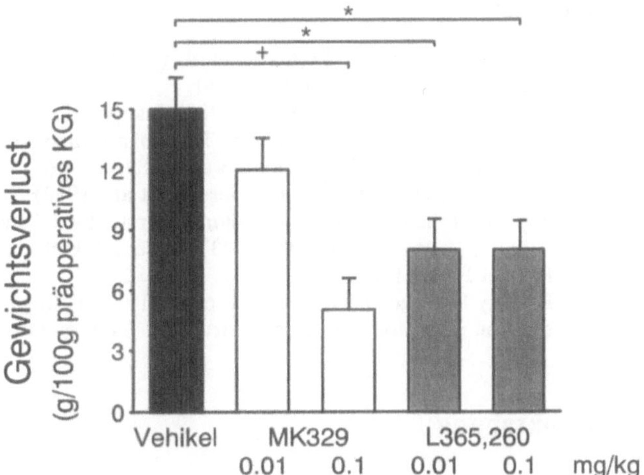

Abb. 2. Effekt von CCK-Rezeptorantagonisten auf den Gewichtsverlust nach Gastrektomie. MK 329 (□) bzw. L365,260 (▩) reduzieren den postoperativen Gewichtsverlust signifikant. Angaben in g/100 g präoperatives Körpergewicht. * p < 0,05, + p < 0,01

Tag um 66 bzw. 46%. Dies korrelierte mit einer Zunahme der postoperativen Nahrungsaufnahme um 11–13%. Unsere Ergebnisse deuten auf eine Beteiligung von CCK als Teilursache des Gewichtsverlustes und der verminderten Nahrungsaufnahme nach Gastrektomie hin.

Zusammenfassung

Gastrektomie mit Rekonstruktion nach Roux-en-Y bei Ratten reduzierte das Körpergewicht und die tägliche Nahrungsaufnahme um 15 bzw. 19%. Behandlung mit CCK-A oder CCK-B Rezeptorantagonisten führte zu einer Reduktion des postoperativen Gewichtsverlustes um 46–66% und zu einer Zunahme der Nahrungsaufnahme um 11–13%. CCK könnte somit Teilursache des Gewichtsverlustes nach Gastrektomie sein.

Summary

Gastrectomy and Roux-en-Y reconstruction in rats decreased body weight by 15% and daily food intake by 19%. Treatment with cholecystokinin (CCK) A or B receptor antagonists after gastrectomy reversed body weight loss by 46%–66% and improved food intake by 11%–13%. Thus, CCK could be partly responsible for body weight loss after gastrectomy.

Literatur

1. Braga M, Zuliani W, Foppa L, et al. (1988) Food intake and nutritional status after total gastrectomy. Br J Surg 75:477–480
2. Zittel T, Niebel G, Thiede A (1989) Interposition oder Roux-en-Y Rekonstruktion nach totaler Gastrektomie bei Ratten: Ergebnisse einer kontrollierten experimentellen Studie. Langenbecks Arch Chir, Chir Forum 1989:163–167
3. Büchler M, Malfertheiner P, Friess H, et al. (1989) Cholecystokinin influences pancreatic trophism following total gastrectomy in rats. Int J Pancreatol 4:261–271
4. Gibbs J, Young R, Smith G (1973) Cholecystokinin decreases food intake in rats. J Comp Physiol Psychol 84:488–495
5. Bradley E, Isaacs J, Del Mazo J, et al. (1977) Pathophysiology and significance of malabsorption after Roux-en-Y reconstruction. Surgery 81:684–690

Danksagung

Wir danken R.M. Freidinger von Merck, Sharp & Dohme für die Überlassung der CCK-Rezeptorantagonisten.

Dr. med. T.T. Zittel, CURE/VA Wadsworth, Building 115, Room 115, Los Angeles, CA 90073, USA

Experimentelle vaskularisierte Kniegelenkstransplantation an einem Hundemodell: Frühergebnisse nach Allotransplantation und Replantation

Vascularized Knee Joint Transplantation in a Canine Model: Early Results After Allografting and Autografting

R. Rosso[1], D. Schäfer[1], R. Fricker[1], R. Schläpfer[1], J. Brennwald[2] und M. Heberer[1]

[1]Allgemeinchirurgische Klinik (Vorsteher: Prof. Dr. med. F. Harder) und Orthopädische Klinik (Vorsteher: Prof. Dr. E. Morscher), Universität Basel, Schweiz
[2]AO Forschungsinstitut (Vorsteher: Prof. Dr. S. Perren), Davos, Schweiz

Einleitung

Schwere Gelenkdestruktionen können durch Knochentumore, Gelenkinfekte oder Trauma entstehen. Amputation und Arthrodese sind die klassischen Behandlungsformen. Heute werden hingegen rekonstruktive Verfahren angestrebt [1, 2]. Dies wurde durch Verbesserungen der adjuvanten onkologischen Therapie, der antibiotischen Behandlung und vor allem der Endoprothetik möglich. Allerdings bleibt die dauerhafte Prothesenverankerung aufgrund langer Hebelarme, insbesondere bei jungen, körperlich aktiven Patienten, schwierig. Zudem besteht ein nicht unerhebliches Infektrisiko. Es wurde deshalb auch versucht, Gelenkflächen durch osteochondrale Transplantate, die zur Herabsetzung der Antigenität tiefgefroren wurden, wiederherzustellen. Komplikationen, insbesondere Infekte und Instabilität, sind aber auch bei diesen Verfahren häufig [2]. Eine weitere Alternative stellt die vaskularisierte Gelenktransplantation dar, für die experimentelle Techniken beschrieben wurden [3, 4, 5]. Die vorliegende Untersuchung soll funktionelle und morphologische Resultate nach primär vaskularisierter Allotransplantation und vaskularisierter Replantation vergleichen. Wir berichten hier über funktionelle Resultate drei Monate nach der Operation.

Material und Methoden

Als Versuchstiere wurden einjährige, skelettreife Hunde (16 bis 24 kg) verwendet. Bei vier Tieren wurde eine vaskularisierte Replantation durchgeführt. Vier Hunde dienten als Gelenkspender für vier weitere Tiere, bei denen eine vaskularisierte Allotransplantation unter Immunsuppression durchgeführt wurde. Die Zuordnung von Gelenkspendern zu Empfängern erfolgte aufgrund der Ergebnisse von gemischten Lymphozytenkulturen (one way MLC). Präformierte Antikörper wurden ausgeschlossen (negatives Crossmatch). Die Immunsuppression mit Cyclosporin A als Monotherapie wurde beim Empfänger eine Woche vor der Transplantation begonnen. Das Unter-

Chirurgisches Forum 1993
f. experim. u. klinische Forschung
Becker/Beger/Hartel (Hrsg.)

suchungsprotokoll war von der Ethischen Kommission des Veterinäramts Basel-Stadt genehmigt.

Operationstechnik: Operiert wurde jeweils das linke Kniegelenk. Die am Kniegelenk inserierenden Muskeln wurden 1 bis 2 cm distal der Insertion durchtrennt. Mit Hilfe einer Schablone wurden Femur und Tibia schräg osteotomiert. Die Durchtrennung der A. und V. poplitea erfolgte distal des Abgangs der A. caudalis femoris distalis. Nach Spülung des Explantates mit Eurocollins-Lösung erfolgte die Osteosynthese mit 3,5 AO-LCDCP-Platten (Stratec Medical, CH-4437 Waldenburg, Schweiz). Die End-zu-End-Anastomose von A. und V. poplitea wurden unter dem Operationsmikroskop durchgeführt. Die beim Hund vorhandene A. saphena sichert bei dieser Technik die Durchblutung des Unterschenkels distal des Kniegelenks. Die Muskelreadaptation erfolgte mit resorbierbarem Nahtmaterial. Bei den Transplantationen erfolgte die synchrone Entnahme bei Spender und Empfänger, die Implantation entsprach der Replantation. Die Ischämiezeit bei der Replantationsgruppe betrug im Durchschnitt 130, bei der Transplantationsgruppe 169 min. Der Eingriff erfolgte unter antibiotischer Prophylaxe mit Imipenem-Cilastin (MSD, CH-8152 Glattbrugg, Schweiz). Postoperativ wurde für drei Wochen eine Gipshülse angelegt.

Untersuchungsverfahren: Nach der unmittelbar postoperativen Phase (2 Wochen) wurden rotes und weißes Blutbild, Elektrolyte und Kreatinin monatlich bestimmt. Die Cyclosporin-A-Vollblutkonzentration der transplantierten Hunde wurde 14tägig dokumentiert. Die statische Belastung der Hinterbeine wurde präoperativ und 4wöchentlich postoperativ bei jedem Hund mit einem Doppelwägesystem gemessen (Mettler Instrumente Schweiz AG). Jeder Untersuchung wurden fünf Messungen zu je 30 sec Dauer zugrundegelegt. Eine bildgebende Gefäßuntersuchung erfolgte präoperativ, unmittelbar postoperativ sowie nach einem und nach drei Monaten: Sowohl die arterielle, als auch die venöse Anastomose wurden mittels Duplexsonografie untersucht, wobei der arterielle Blutfluß gemessen wurde. Zur Beurteilung der Osteotomieheilung wurden Röntgenbilder des operierten Kniegelenks in zwei Ebenen sechs und zwölf Wochen postoperativ angefertigt.

Ergebnisse

Drei Monate postoperativ waren alle Operationswunden verheilt. Klinisch waren alle operierten Gelenke stabil. Kein Gelenk zeigte einen klinisch faßbaren Erguß. Mittels Duplexsonografie wurde nachgewiesen, daß arterielle und venöse Anastomosen während der gesamten Beobachtungszeit offen waren. Es gab keine Hinweise auf relevante Stenosen. Radiologisch fand sich in allen Osteotomiebereichen an Tibia und Femur eine deutliche Kallusbildung nach sechs Wochen. Bei den transplantierten Tieren war die Kallusbildung nach sechs und zwölf Wochen deutlich ausgeprägter als nach Replantation. Dies betraf Tibia und Femur gleichermaßen. Nach drei Monaten waren alle Osteotomien geheilt, und es fanden sich keine Hinweise auf Implantatlockerung. Der Gelenkspalt war radiologisch bei allen Kniegelenken sechs und zwölf Wochen postoperativ erhalten. Die Cyclosporinspiegel zeigten einen konstanten Verlauf im therapeutischen Bereich mit Ausnahme von zwei Tieren, bei denen je einmal ein Cyclosporin-A-Spiegel unterhalb des therapeutischen Minimums von 150 ng/l gemessen wurde (77 und 93 ng/l). Diese Konzentrationen wurden gleichentags durch Erhöhung der Dosis korrigiert. Klinisch entwickelte kein Tier eine Abstoßungsreaktion.

In der Replantationsgruppe wurde eine statische Belastung nach einem Monat bei drei, nach zwei Monaten bei allen Tieren festgestellt. In der Transplantationsgruppe belasteten nach einem Monat nur ein Hund und nach drei Monaten drei Tiere die operierte Extremität (Abb. 1). Ein Hund entlastete permanent.

Komplikationen: Bei einem Hund kam es aufgrund eines intraoperativen Hämoglobinabfalls von 16,1 auf 3,3 g/dl postoperativ zu einer passageren Amaurose. Das gleiche Tier entwickelte einen Monat postoperativ eine papillomatöse Hautveränderung, die zu dauerhafter Entlastung und eingeschränkter passiver Gelenkbeweglichkeit führte.

Diskussion

Experimentelle Untersuchungen zur vaskularisierten Gelenktransplantation beim Hund wurden bereits 1968 von Judet und Padovani vorgestellt [3]. 1980 publizierten Goldberg et al. und 1989 Doi et al. experimentelle Untersuchungen [4, 5], deren Design mit der vorliegenden Studie vergleichbar war. Die erneute Durchführung eines so aufwendigen Versuchs muß vor dem Hintergrund der Ergebnisse dieser früheren Untersuchungen begründet werden. Judet und Padovani führten 28 Replantationen und

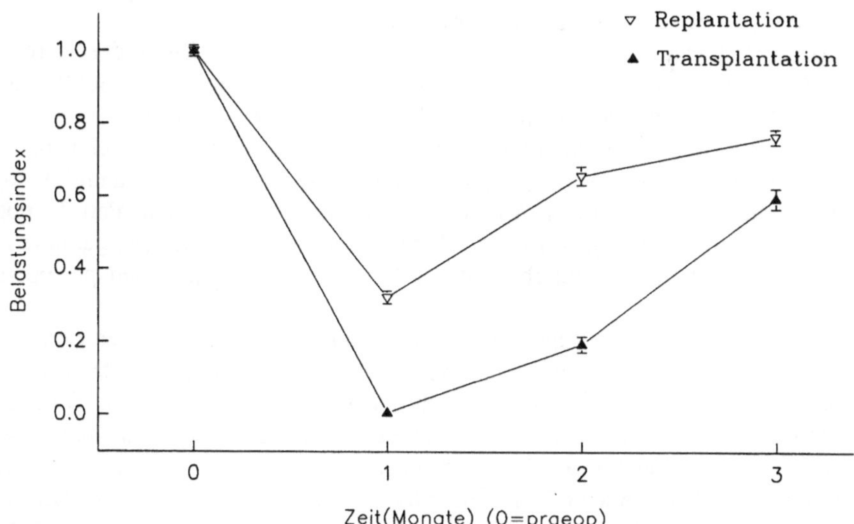

Abb. 1. Belastungsindex. Relative statische Belastung des operierten linken Hinterbeins bezogen auf die Summenbelastung beider Hinterbeine und den Wert des präoperativen Belastungsindex (Mittelwert ± Standardfehler)

21 Transplantationen durch. Nur vier replantierte Tiere konnten über ein Jahr verfolgt werden und zeigten offene Anastomosen und geheilte Osteotomien; histologisch wurden vitale Chondro- und Osteozyten nachgewiesen. Die übrigen Tiere konnten wegen Anastomosenproblemen, Komplikationen der Osteosynthese, Muskelnekrosen und Infekten nicht ausgewertet werden. Bei den transplantierten Tieren konnte der Verlauf bei keinem länger als drei Wochen verfolgt werden. Hier spielte vermutlich die damals inadäquate Immunsuppression mit Antilymphozytenserum und Korticosteroiden eine Rolle. Goldberg et al. untersuchten drei Gruppen: Replantation (n = 38), Transplantation unter Immunsuppression mit Azathioprin und Prednison (n = 8) sowie Transplantation unter Immunsuppression mit Azathioprin, Prednison und Antilymphozytenserum (n = 24). Nur sechs replantierte Tiere konnten über neun Monate evaluiert werden. Die restlichen Tiere mußten wegen Anastomosenproblemen, instabiler Osteosynthesen und Infekten von der Nachuntersuchung ausgeschlossen werden. Bei allen acht ohne Antilymphozytenserum immunsupprimierten Tieren kam es zur Transplantatabstoßung. Von den 24 mit Antilymphozytenserum behandelten Hunden überlebten zwölf Tiere neun bis zwölf Monate, die übrigen wurden wegen Infekten oder Anastomosenproblemen euthanasiert. Die evaluierten sechs Tiere der Replantationsgruppe wiesen ein gut funktionierendes Knie ohne Knorpeldegeneration, die fünf transplantierten ein mäßig funktionsfähiges Gelenk mit degenerativen Knorpelveränderungen auf. Detaillierte funktionelle Daten wurden nicht mitgeteilt. – In einer neueren Untersuchung konnten Doi et al. einige Probleme dieser Untersuchungen lösen, insbesondere durch die Kombination von Cyclosporin-A und Azathioprin. Nach vaskularisierter Replantation ohne Immunsuppression überlebten vier von sechs Tieren mit guten klinischen und histologischen Ergebnissen. Nach vaskularisierter Transplantation unter Immunsuppression konnten drei von fünf Tieren evaluiert werden (eine Abstoßung, ein Anastomosenproblem). Das klinische Ergebnis war gut, jedoch fehlten auch in dieser Arbeit funktionelle Verlaufskontrollen.

Insgesamt bietet das Hundemodell folgende Vorteile: Die Größe der Tiere erlaubt gebräuchliche Osteosyntheseverfahren, nicht invasive Prüfungen der Gefäßanastomosen und Untersuchungen des Gangbilds. Das Kniegelenk ist sehr gut zugänglich, eine En bloc-Resektion ist möglich und es handelt sich um ein belastetes Gelenk. Infolge der doppelten arteriellen Versorgung des Hinterlaufs durch A. poplitea und A. saphena genügt eine einzige arterielle Anastomose im Bereich der proximalen A. poplitea, wobei die Blutversorgung des Unterschenkels durch die A. saphena garantiert wird. Zudem erleichtert die Trainierbarkeit der Versuchstiere die prä- und postoperativen Untersuchungen.

Wir haben bei einer Gruppe vaskularisierte autologe Replantationen durchgeführt. Diese Gruppe ist wichtig, da keine Abstoßungsvorgänge das Resultat beeinflussen können. Die Gelenke sind ausschließlich den Folgen von operativem Trauma, temporärer Ischämie und Gelenkdenervation unterworfen. Die Ergebnisse dienten als Referenz für die allogene Transplantation unter Immunsuppression mit Cyclosporin A. Die Tatsache, daß alle acht Tiere drei Monate mit offener Anastomose bei konsolidierter Osteotomie überlebten, führen wir im wesentlichen auf die Technik (stabile Osteosynthese, mikrochirurgisch durchgeführte Anastomose) sowie die sorgfältige Betreuung der Tiere mit täglicher Kontrolle zurück. Die Kooperationsfähigkeit der Tiere wurde ferner konsequent für postoperative funktionelle Untersuchungen genutzt. Die günstigen Ergebnisse nach drei Monaten legen eine weitere Evaluation der Gelenktransplantation am Großtiermodell nahe. Falls auch die klinischen Resultate nach sechs Monaten überzeugen und durch die histologische Auswertung bestätigt werden, sollte die vaskularisierte Gelenktransplantation im Hinblick auf eine potentielle klinische Anwendung weiter exploriert werden. Allerdings wird eine klinische Transplantation bei nicht-vitaler Indikation nur dann Realität werden, wenn die Probleme der lebenslangen Immunsuppression gelöst werden können.

Zusammenfassung

An einem Hundemodell wurden die dreimonatigen Ergebnisse von vier vaskularisiert replantierten und vier vaskularisiert transplantierten Kniegelenken unter Immunsuppression mit Cyclosporin A verglichen. Nach drei Monaten waren alle Osteotomien geheilt und die Gefäßanastomosen durchgängig. Alle vier replantierten Hunde belasteten die operierte Extremität, bei den transplantierten hingegen nur drei von vier Tieren. Die Cyclosporinspiegel lagen im therapeutischen Bereich. Diese Ergebnisse rechtfertigen die weitere Evaluation der Kniegelenktransplantation im Großtiermodell.

Summary

Four vascularized knee joint replants were compared to four vascularized allotransplants (immunosuppressive medication using cyclosporin A) over a 3-month period. After this time, all osteotomies had healed, all anastomoses were patent, and the levels of cyclosporin A in the blood were within the therapeutic range throughout the period of investigation. In the replant group, all four dogs were fully weightbearing, in contrast to three out of four in the transplant group. These results encourage further long-term evaluation of vascularized joint transplantation in a canine model.

Literatur

1. Simon MA, Aschliman MA, Thomas N, Mankin HJ (1986) Limb-salvage treatment versus amputation for osteosarcoma of the distal end of the femur. JBJS 68A:1331–1337
2. Mankin HJ, Doppelt SH, Sullivan TR, Tomford WW (1982) Osteoarticular and intercalary allograft transplantation in the management of malignant tumors of bone. Cancer 50:613–630
3. Judet H, Padovani JP (1968) Transplantation d'articulation complète avec rétablissement circulatoire immédiat par anastomoses arterielles et veneuses. Mem Acad Chir (Paris) 94:520–526
4. Goldberg VM, Porter BB, Lance EM (1980) Transplantation of the canine knee joint on a vascular pedicle. JBJS 62A:414–424
5. Doi K, DeSantis G, Singer DI, Hurley JV, O'Brien B, McKay SM, Hickey MJ, Murphy BF (1989) The effect of immunosuppression on vascularized allografts. A preliminary report. JBJS 71A:576–582

Dr. med. R. Rosso, Department Chirurgie, Kantonsspital Basel, CH-4031 Basel, Schweiz

Beurteilung eines Schwerverletztenkollektivs nach Kriterien der Major Trauma Outcome Study (MTOS): Minimierung des "preventable trauma death" und Optimierung der Versorgungsqualität durch ein traumatologisch besetztes Rettungssystem

Evaluation of Severely Injured Patients According to the Major Trauma Outcome Study (MTOS): Decrease of "Preventable Trauma Deaths" and Optimized Trauma Care by a Trained Surgical Staff in an Emergency Unit

M. Holch[1], M. Muggia[2], D. Otte[1], M.L. Nerlich[3] und H. Tscherne[1]

[1]Unfallchirurgische Klinik, Medizinische Hochschule Hannover
(Direktor: Prof. Dr. H. Tscherne)
[2]Department of Surgery, University Hospital, Hadassah University, Jerusalem, Israel
[3]Abteilung Unfallchirurgie, Chirurgische Universitätsklinik, Regensburg
(Leiter: Prof. Dr. M.L. Nerlich)

Einleitung

Zur Effizienzbeurteilung präklinischer Versorgungsstrategien muß ein Zusammenhang zwischen der quantifizierbaren zugrundeliegenden Schädigung des Verletzten und dem Enderfolg der durchgeführten Maßnahmen hergestellt werden. Nach Scoring des zu beurteilenden Patientenguts, u.a. mittels Injury Severity Score (ISS) [2] und Glasgow Coma Scala [4], ermöglicht die Major Trauma Outcome Study (MTOS) [5] anhand des Verletzungsschweregrads die Ermittlung von verstorbenen Patienten mit einer zumindest theoretischen Überlebenschance aufgrund eines nicht zwangsläufig tödlichen Verletzungsmusters. Dargestellt werden soll der Einfluß der integrierten Unfallversorgung durch das "Trauma System" (TS: Rettungshubschrauber plus Notaufnahme) einer Unfallchirurgischen Klinik der Maximalversorgung auf das Überleben polytraumatisierter Patienten durch

1) Definition einer Gruppe von Fällen eines "preventable death" nach MTOS-Kriterien und Bewertung der Relevanz der durchgeführten präklinischen Maßnahmen,
2) Bewertung der präklinischen Versorgungsqualität und der Entscheidung zur primären Traumazentrum-Zuführung hinsichtlich des definitiven "outcome" und der Durchführungsrate bei verschieden strukturierten Rettungssystemen.

Methode

Von 1973 bis 1989 liegen die konsekutiv dokumentierten Verletzungsmuster und Versorgungsmaßnahmen von 8894 Unfallopfern vor. Sie wurden aus einem epidemio-

Chirurgisches Forum 1993
f. experim. u. klinische Forschung
Becker/Beger/Hartel (Hrsg.)

logisch repräsentativen regionalen Unfallforschungsprojekt mit Stichprobencharakter rekrutiert [3]. Diese Gesamtpopulation beinhaltet 661 tödlich Schwerverletzte sowie die korrespondierenden 110 schwerstverletzten Überlebenden mit einem mittleren ISS von $37,8 \pm 9,1$ Punkten (Auswahlkriterium: ISS > 20). Aus der Gruppe der 661 Verstorbenen erfolgte die Auswahl von 192 Fällen mit möglicher Überlebenschance nach GCS- und ISS-Einstufung (basierend auf AIS 1985) [1] durch erfahrene Unfallchirurgen. Der allein durch die Verletzungsschwere begründbare Tod nach Trauma wird definiert durch Vorliegen eines der Kriterien [1, 2, 4]:

1) primärer, traumabedingter Herz-Atemstillstand,
2) ISS = 75 Punkte, MAIS = 6 Punkte,
3) ISS > 45 Punkte bei einem Alter > 50 Jahre.

Als sicher nachvollziehbare Kriterien der notärztlichen Versorgung wurden gewählt und Erhebungsprotokollen und Krankenakten überprüft:

1) die Intubation und Beatmung vor Ort,
2) Einleitung einer Volumentherapie über mindestens zwei periphere Zugänge und Infusion von mindestens 1000 ml Flüssigkeit bis Klinikeinlieferung,
3) die Notarzt-Entscheidung zur primären Einlieferung in ein Traumazentrum.

Ergebnisse

Zur Auswertung gelangen 102 Verstorbene mit einer theoretischen Überlebenschance, d.h. 29% der Grundpatienten (n = 661) weisen kein zwangsläufig tödliches Verletzungsmuster auf. Diese 192 plus 110 überlebende Personen mit einem mittleren ISS von $37,8 \pm 9,1$ Punkten verteilen sich auf drei Beobachtungszeiträume: 1973 bis 1978, 1979 bis 1984 und 1985 bis 1989.

Tabelle 1 zeigt den Rückgang des Anteils von Verstorbenen mit nicht zwangsläufig tödlichem Verletzungsmuster und die Abnahme des Anteils solcher tödlichen Verletzungsfolgen, welche durch frühe präklinische Oxygenierung und eine suffiziente Volumentherapie vermieden werden können.

Tabelle 2 zeigt die Zunahme der relevanten Notarztmaßnahmen Intubation und Volumentherapie sowie die signifikant häufigere primäre Traumazentrumzuführung, welche in Kombination mit den vorgenannten Maßnahmen eine nachweisbare Optimierung des präklinischen Vorgehens darstellt. Sie wurde im Vorgehen des Rettungssystems des Traumazentrums öfter nachvollziehbar als in jenem anderer Rettungssysteme der Erhebungsregion.

Der Überlebensanteil (n = 110 mit mittlerem ISS = 37,8) an der Gesamtpopulation (n = 661 + 110) zeigt in Abhängigkeit von der Entscheidung "primäre Traumazentrum-Zuführung" einen signifikanten Unterschied im outcome:

primäre Traumazentrum-Zuführung – nein: 22,3% Überlebende,
primäre Traumazentrum-Zuführung – ja: 31,7% Überlebende.

Tabelle 1. Rückgang des Anteils von Verstorbenen mit nicht zwangsläufig tödlichem Verletzungsmuster und Abnahme des Anteils solcher tödlicher Verletzungsfolgen (hämorrhagischer Schock und Schockfolgeerkrankungen), welche durch frühe präklinische Oxygenierung und eine suffiziente Volumentherapie vermieden werden können

	1973–1978	1979–1984	1985–1989	
Anteil theoretisch Überlebender am Gesamtkollektiv:	39%	26%	19%	χ^2 $p < 0,05$; Mantel-Hänszel $p > 0,001$
Abnahme der Todesursache:				
Schweres SHT	11,8%	12,0%	9,5%	Ø Signifikanz
hämorrhag. Schock	8,3%	4,4%	2,5%	χ^2 $\alpha => 0,95$
Schockfolgeerkrankungen	10,6%	6,0%	4,4%	χ^2 $\alpha => 0,95$

Tabelle 2. Zunahme der relevanten Notarztmaßnahmen Intubation und Volumentherapie sowie signifikant häufigere primäre Traumazentrumzuführung im Zeitverlauf. Diese werden im Vorgehen des Rettungssystems des Traumazentrums öfter beobachtet als in jenem anderer Rettungssysteme der Erhebungsregion

	1973–1978	1979–1984	1985–1989		1973–1989	
Optimierte Versorgung:				durch:	AR	TS
primäre Intubation	57%	61%	88%	χ^2 $p < 0,05$	59%	66%
ausreich. Vol.-Therapie	60%	69%	88%	χ^2 $p < 0,05$	41%	56%
Max. Therapie + Traumazentrum	30%	39%	71%	χ^2 $p < 0,05$	24%	47%

Diskussion

Ein Zusammenhang zwischen der verbesserten präklinischen Beatmungstherapie und Volumenersatztherapie mit dem Rückgang von Todesfällen infolge Volumenmangelschock und Hypoxygenierung bei prinzipiell therapierbaren Verletzungsmustern ist ersichtlich. Erwartungsgemäß profitiert die schwere Organläsion des höhergradigen SHT nicht signifikant von dieser Effizienzsteigerung, auch wenn ein tendenziell positiver Einfluß von Intubation und Frühbeatmung auf outcome des SHT bekannt ist [4]. Ursächlich ist die nachweisbare, signifikante Optimierung invasiver präklinischer Maßnahmen, deren Effizienz durch die primäre Transportentscheidung ins Zentrum gesteigert wird.

Die unterschiedliche Behandlung gleichschwerverletzter Patientenkollektive durch verschiedene Erstversorgungssysteme weist hin auf die Bedeutung der frühestmöglichen Erfassung und realistischen Ersteinschätzung des Verletzungsmusters als Basis der Entscheidung zur optimierten Primärversorgung. Diese wird vom Traumazentrum-gestützten Rettungsmittel mit unfallchirurgisch geschulter Arztbesetzung nachweisbar öfter und mit höherem Überlebenserfolg bei gleichschwer verletzten Patienten durchgeführt.

Zusammenfassung

Anhand eines Kollektivs schwerverletzter Unfallopfer wird gezeigt, wie über den Beobachtungszeitraum im Zusammenhang mit Verbesserung der präklinischen Versorgung die Häufigkeit vermeidbarer Todesfälle zurückgeht. Die unterschiedliche Durchführung der konsequenten Erstversorgung durch verschiedene Notarztsysteme weist auf die Bedeutung der frühen chirurgischen Befunderhebung und Verletzungsmusterklassifizierung als Entscheidungsgrundlage hin.

Summary

A decrease in preventable deaths due to hypoxia or hemorrhagic shock in a population of severely injured patients was demonstrated during a 15-year period. Improved preclinical trauma care results in an increased survival rate following severe trauma. Appropriate preclinical trauma treatment is more often practiced by a trauma unit than by other emergency units staffed by emergency doctors without surgical training.

Literatur

1. American Association for Automotive Medicine (1985) The Abbreviated Injury Scale. American Association for Automotive Medicine, Morton Grove, Illinois (USA)
2. Copes WS, Champion HR, Sacco WJ, Lawnick MM, Keast SL, Bain LW (1988) The Injury Severity Score revisited. J Trauma 29:69–77
3. Dilling J, Otto D (1986) Die Bedeutung örtlicher Unfallerhebungen im Rahmen der Unfallforschung. Unfall- und Sicherheitsforschung im Straßenverkehr, Heft 56:59, Bundesanstalt für Straßenwesen
4. Nerlich ML, Holch M, Kant CJ, Muggia-Sullam M, Stange W, Otte D, Tscherne H (im Druck) Die Wertigkeit der Glasgow Coma Scale (GCS) in der primären Beurteilung Mehrfachverletzter mit schwerem Schädel-Hirn-Trauma. Hefte Unfallheilkd
5. Champion HR, Copes WS, Sacco WJ, Lawnick MM, Keast SL, Bain LW (1990) The Major Trauma Outcome Study: Establishing national norms for trauma care. J Trauma 30:1356–1365

Dr. med. M. Holch, Unfallchirurgische Klinik, Medizinische Hochschule, Konstanty-Gutschow-Straße 8, W-3000 Hannover 61

Die minimal invasive Lungenresektion im Tierversuch: Technik und erste Ergebnisse der thorakoskopischen Pneumonektomie

Minimally Invasive Pulmonary Resection in Animal Experiments: Techniques and Preliminary Results of Thoracoscopic Pneumonectomy

H.A. Gaissert, Hon-Chi Suen, B.F. Meyers und J.C. Wain

General Thoracic Surgical Unit, Massachusetts General Hospital, Boston, USA

Einleitung

Minimal invasive Methoden in der Lungenresektion versprechen postoperative Vorteile durch eine geringere Beeinträchtigung der Atemmechanik, erträglichere Schmerzen und raschere Genesung. Vor allem die Vermeidung der Aufdehnung von Rippen trägt zur postoperativen Erhaltung der physiologischen Brustwandfunktion bei. Der Einsatz der Thorakoskopie ist gerechtfertigt, wenn Mortalitäts- und Morbiditätsrisiken mit herkömmlichen Methoden vergleichbar sind und die Radikalität onkologischer Eingriffe nicht beeinträchtigt wird. Zurückhaltung besteht gegenwärtig gegenüber thorakoskopischen Resektionen, die eine Kontrolle der Hilusstrukturen voraussetzen. Gründe für diese Vorsicht sind die geringe klinische Erfahrung, das unbekannte Risiko von Blutungen und das Fehlen eines manuellen Zugangs und üblicher Nahttechnik. Wir untersuchten deshalb in einem Tiermodell die Anwendbarkeit thorakoskopischer Methoden auf die Pneumonektomie mit dem Ziel, eine Operation mit reproduzierbarer Kontrolle der Hilusgefäße zu entwickeln und Aussagen über den postoperativen Heilungsverlauf zu machen.

Methodik

Die video-assistierte thorakoskopische linksseitige Pneumonektomie wurde im erwachsenen Schaf (40–60 kg) in 6 Akut- und 18 Langzeitversuchen vorgenommen. Eingriffe wurden in Intubationsnarkose mit selektiver Okklusion des linken Hauptstammbronchus und in rechter Seitenlage durchgeführt. Die Länge der Trachea erforderte in größeren Tieren eine Tracheostomie, um die Position des Okklusionskatheters bronchoskopisch zu kontrollieren. Üblicherweise wurden 6 Interkostalzugänge für Kamera, Retraktion und Instrumente angelegt. Aufgrund des ovalen Querschnitts des Lungenhilus ermöglichten zwei zwerchfellnahe Zugänge für das Thorakoskop, ventral und dorsal, eine übersichtliche Bildgebung der Hilusstrukturen. Zunächst wurde die hintere Hilusregion dargestellt, die Pleura eröffnet und die untere Pulmonalvene frei-

Chirurgisches Forum 1993
f. experim. u. klinische Forschung
Becker/Beger/Hartel (Hrsg.)

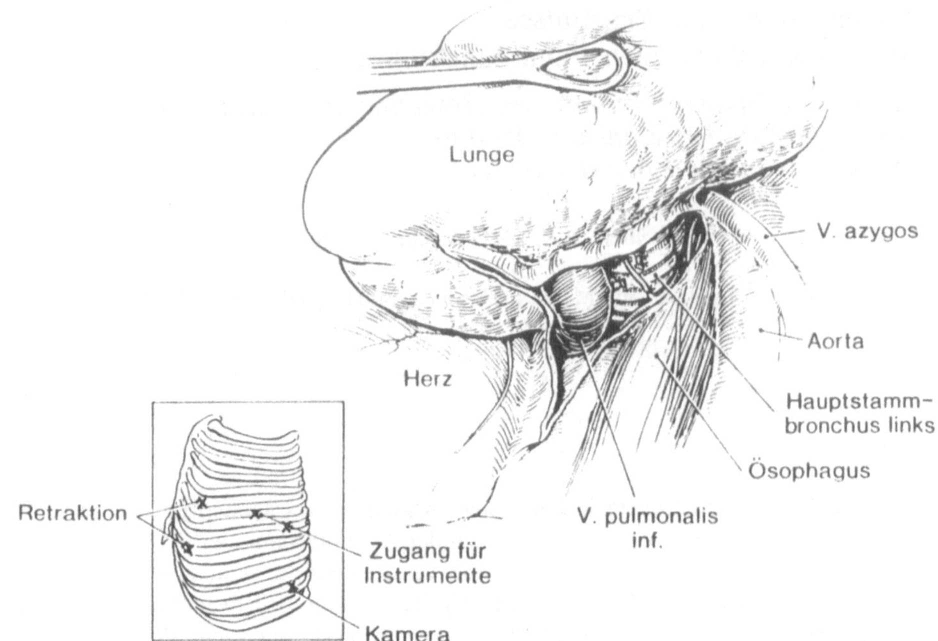

Abb. 1. Infero-dorsale Ansicht des Lungenhilus durch das Thorakoskop. Die Lunge ist nach vorn retrahiert, die Pleura ist eröffnet und ein dorsaler Ast der V. pulm. inf. ist durchtrennt. Eckeinsatz zeigt die Position der Instrumente in der linken Thoraxseite

gelegt (Abb. 1). Daraufhin wurden in der vorderen Hilusregion die Gefäßstrukturen unter direkter videoskopischer Kontrolle freigelegt (Abb. 2). Die obere und untere Pulmonalvene und die Pulmonalarterie wurden doppelt unterbunden mit Fixationsligatur und durchtrennt. Der Hauptstammbronchus wurde abgesetzt und der Stumpf mit Einzelknopfnähten (4-0 Vicryl) geschlossen. Bronchus und Gefäße wurden manuell mit einem endoskopischen Nadelhalter und regulärem atraumatischen Nahtmaterial genäht. Ventilation mit positivem Druck bestätigte den luftdichten Bronchusverschluß. Die resezierte Lunge wurde intakt durch eine etwa 10 cm lange Interkostalinzision entfernt. Der Pleuralkraum wurde mit Cephalosporin-haltiger Lösung ausgewaschen, und Wunden wurden schichtweise verschlossen.

In 6 Akutbeobachtungen wurde der Versuch nach Operation beendet. In 18 Langzeitversuchen schloß sich eine postoperative Beobachtung über 21 Tage an. Die Tracheostomie wurde nach Operation durch Naht verschlossen. Am Ende des Beobachtungszeitraumes wurde unter Narkose linksseitig thorakotomiert und die linke Hilusregion einschließlich Bronchusstumpf und Gefäßstümpfen entnommen und untersucht. Jede Separation der Bronchusnaht bezeichneten wir als Stumpfinsuffizienz und die Anwesenheit von Eiter oder übelriechendem Wundsekret in der Pleurahöhle als Empyem.

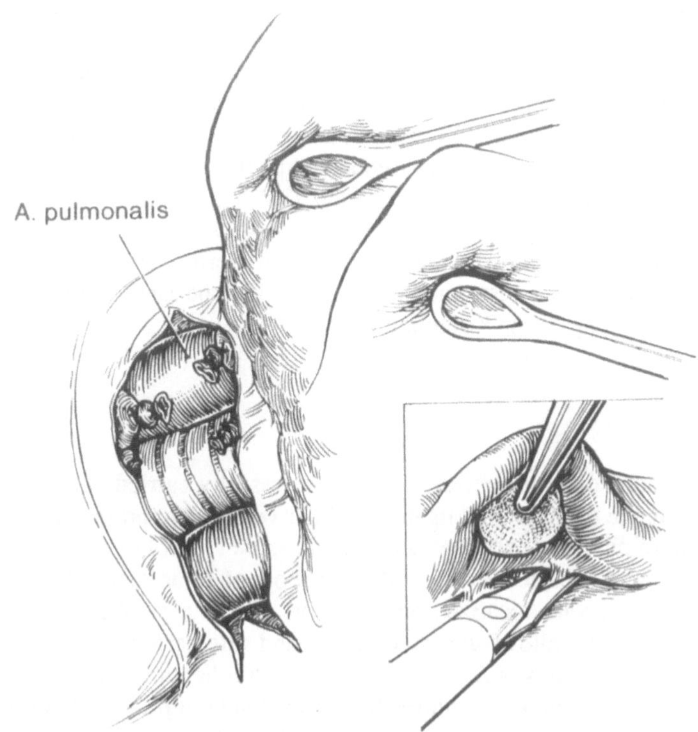

Abb. 2. Infero-ventrale Ansicht der Lungenhilus durch das Thorakoskop. Mit dorsaler Retraktion der Lunge sind die centralen Hilusstrukturen durch die eröffnete Pleura sichtbar. Die obere Pulmonalvene ist ligiert und durchtrennt. Der Eckeinsatz zeigt die Freilegung der Pulmonalarterie

Ergebnisse

Die Bilddarstellung der Pleurahöhle aus zwei Kamerapositionen erlaubte eine ungehinderte Beobachtung der gesamten Hilusregion. Die manuelle Technik ermöglichte die präzise Isolation von Gefäßen und Anlegung der Ligaturen. Blutungen traten selten auf, waren stets beherrschbar und führten in keinem Fall zum Verlust des Tieres.

Die Resektion der Lunge wurde in allen Tieren erfolgreich beendet. In der Akutgruppe führte die Dislokation eines Bronchialblockers zu Atemwegsverlegung und Tod eines Tieres. In 18 Spätbeobachtungen fand sich in 3 Tieren eine Bronchusstumpfinsuffizienz, in einem von diesen mit lokalisiertem Empyem. Der Defekt war jeweils begrenzt und mit Lockerung oder Abwesenheit von Einzelnähten verbunden. Intraoperativer Blutverlust in diesen Tieren war gering (< 100 ml). In 15 gab es keine Komplikationen des Bronchusverschlusses. Gefäßligaturen waren intakt in allen Tieren, und Nachblutungen traten nicht auf.

Zusammenfassung

Eine experimentelle Methode der thorakoskopischen Pneumonektomie wird beschrieben mit individueller Gefäßligatur und Nahtverschluß des Bronchus. Diese Operation ermöglicht eine exakte Freilegung und Unterbindung der Pulmonalgefäße. In 3 von 18 Schafen trat nach 21tägiger Beobachtung eine Insuffizienz des Bronchusstumpfes auf, mit lokalisiertem Empyem bei einem Tier. Video-assistierte Thorakoskopie erlaubt die reproduzierbare und sichere Durchführung der Pneumonektomie. Die hohe Inzidenz der Bronchusstumpfinsuffizienz in diesem Tiermodell erfordert eine Verbesserung von Nahttechnik und Instrumenten, oder zusätzliche Deckung mit lebendem Gewebe zur Reduzierung dieser Komplikation.

Summary

Thoracoscopic pneumonectomy is successfully carried out in an ovine model using a technique of individual ligation of hilar vessels and bronchial suture closure. This procedure provided excellent access and secure control of pulmonary vascular structures. Bronchial dehiscence occurred in three out of 18 animals observed for 21 days and was associated with localized empyema in one animal. We conclude that video-assisted thoracoscopy allows the reproducible and safe performance of pneumonectomy. Most bronchial stumps will heal without any complications; however, the high incidence of bronchial stump leak requires further technical improvement of instruments and suture technique or coverage of the stump with viable tissue to reduce this complication.

Literatur

1. Kalso E, Perttunen K, Kaasinen S (1992) Pain after thoracic surgery. Acta Anaesthesiol Scand 36:96–100
2. McKneally MF (1992) Lobectomy without a rib spreader [editorial]. Ann Thorac Surg 54:2
3. Lewis RJ, Sisler GE, Caccavale RJ (1992) Imaged thoracic lobectomy: Should it be done? Ann Thorac Surg 54:80–83
4. Mathisen DJ (1992) Don't get run over by the bandwagon [editorial]. Chest 102:4–5

Dr. H.A. Gaissert, General Thoracic Surgical Unit, Massachusetts General Hospital, Boston, MA., USA

Die Freisetzung inflammatorischer Mediatoren aus Monozyten (MØ) bei posttraumatischem Sepsissyndrom – Einfluß von Cyclooxygenase-Metaboliten

Release of Inflammatory Mediators by Monocytes (MØ) from Patients with Septic Shock Syndrome – Influence of Cyclooxygenase Metabolites

D. Jarrar[1], W. Ertel[1], V. Thiele[1], J. Kenney[2], E. Faist[1] und F.W. Schildberg[1]

[1]Chirurgische Klinik und Poliklinik, Klinikum Großhadern, Ludwigs-Maximilians-Universität München
[2]Syntex Research, Inc., Palo Alto, CA, USA

Einleitung

Die überschießende Freisetzung endogener inflammatorischer Mediatoren (Tumor-Nekrose-Faktor-α, Interleukin-1β) aus Makrophagen/Monozyten (MØ) wird für das septische Multiorganversagen (MOF) verantwortlich gemacht [1]. Der Arachidonsäuremetabolit Prostaglandin E_2 (PGE_2) reguliert über einen negativen Feedback-Mechanismus die Transkription, Translation und Sekretion von TNF-α und auf Translationsebene die IL-1β Aktivität [2]. Obwohl PGE_2 in Zellkulturen die TNF-α und IL-1β Freisetzung aus LPS-stimulierten Monozyten hemmte, ist der Einfluß von Arachidonsäuremetaboliten auf die Freisetzung von Zytokinen aus MØ von septischen Patienten ungeklärt. Es war das Ziel dieser Studie, die Sekretion von TNF-α und IL-1β sowie deren Regulation durch Arachidonsäuremetabolite bei manifestem Sepsissyndrom zu untersuchen.

Material und Methoden

Fünfzehn Patienten mit manifestem Sepsissyndrom wurden in die Studie aufgenommen, nachdem sie mindestens 5 der folgenden Einschlußkriterien erfüllten [1]: 1. Temperatur $> 38,3°C$ oder Hypothermie ($< 35,5°C$); 2. Tachykardie mit einer Herzfrequenz > 90 Schlägen/min; 3. Hypotension mit einem systolischen Druck < 90 mmHg oder Katecholaminpflichtigkeit > 5 μg/kg KG·min; 4. Leukozytose > 15000 Zellen/ml oder Leukopenie < 3000 Zellen/ml; 5. Verbrauchskoagulopathie mit einer PTT $>$

Chirurgisches Forum 1993
f. experim. u. klinische Forschung
Becker/Beger/Hartel (Hrsg.)

und/oder einem Thrombozytenabfall um mindestens 50% des Ausgangswertes; 6. Hypoxie, definiert als $paO_2 < 75$ mmHg oder einem Horowitz-Quotienten (paO_2/FiO_2) ≤ 250. In der Kontrollgruppe wurden 15 gesunde, altersentsprechende Probanden untersucht. Nach Erfüllung der Einschlußkriterien und Aufnahme in die Studie wurde den Patienten heparinisiertes Vollblut entnommen und *ex vivo* mit Lipopolysaccharid (LPS: 1,0 μg/ml; Difco, Detroit, MI, USA) mit oder ohne dem Cyclooxygenasehemmer Ibuprofen (0,1 mg/ml; Sigma, St. Louis, MO, USA) stimuliert. Das stimulierte Vollblut wurde in einnem Brutschrank bei 37°C und 5% CO_2-Atmosphäre auf einem Rotor gedreht, um eine Adhärenz der Monozyten zu vermeiden. Nach einer Inkubation von 8 h wurden die mononukleären Zellen mittels eines Dichtegradienten (Ficoll, d = 1,077, Seromed, Biochrom KG, Berlin, FRG) von Erythrozyten und Granulozyten getrennt. Die Überstände wurden gesammelt und bis zur Messung der Zytokine bei –70°C eingefroren. Die TNF-α und IL-1β-Spiegel in den Vollblutüberständen wurden mittels Bioassay (WEHI 164 Zytotoxizitätsassay [3]) und Elisa (IL-1β [4]) gemessen. Die Werte der Zytokinsekretion wurden auf 1×10^6 Monozyten/ml Vollblut korrigiert.

Ergebnisse

Die Freisetzung von TNF-α und IL-1β in humanem Vollblut von Patienten mit manifestem Sepsissyndrom war im Vergleich mit dem gesunden Kontrollkollektiv um 95% bzw. um 75% signifikant ($p \leq 0,05$) reduziert. Die Hemmung der Cyclooxygenase mit Ibuprofen führte in der Kontrollgruppe zu einer deutlich gesteigerten TNF-α-Freisetzung (+ 61%), während die IL-1β-Sekretion unbeeinflußt blieb. In der Gruppe mit Sepsissyndrom führte die Hemmung der Cyclooxygenase ebenfalls zu einer signifikanten Erhöhung der TNF-α-Freisetzung. Trotz einer deutlich höheren Steigerung der TNF-Sekretion (+ 40%) in der Sepsisgruppe blieb die signifikante Suppression der TNF-α-Sekretion aus MØ septischer Patienten bestehen. Ibuprofen hatte in der Sepsisgruppe keinen Einfluß auf die IL-1β-Sekretion.

Tabelle 1. Freisetzung von TNF-α und IL-1β in humanem Vollblut nach Stimulation mit LPS (1 μg/ml) über 8 h

	TNF-α [U/ml]		IL-1β [ng/ml]	
	LPS	LPS+Ibuprofen	LPS	LPS+Ibuprofen
Kontrollgruppe	341 ± 52	557 ± 83	43330 ± 3090	49415 ± 2910
Sepsisgruppe	20 ± 10[a]	104 ± 51[a]	10955 ± 4940[a]	16591 ± 5106[a]

X ± SEM; ANOVA: [a] $p \leq 0,05$ Kontrolle versus Sepsis
Sekretionswerte auf 1×10^6 Monozyten korrigiert

Diskussion

Das Sepsissyndrom führte zu einer signifikanten Hemmung der TNF-α- und IL-1β-Sekretion. Die Hemmung der Zytokinausschüttung steht im Widerspruch zu bisher publizierten Daten, die erhöhte TNF-α und IL-1β-Plasmaspiegel bei Patienten mit Sepsissyndrom beschrieben. Aus unseren Daten läßt sich schließen, daß die Freisetzung von inflammatorischen Mediatoren durch negativ regulatorische Mechanismen gehemmt wird. Diese Hypothese deckt sich mit Daten von Schmid et al. [5], daß sich nach mehrmaligen Infusionen von Endotoxin beim Menschen eine Endotoxintoleranz einstellt und die reaktive Mediatorausschüttung ausbleibt [5]. Wir überprüften in dieser Studie die Möglichkeit eines inhibitorischen Einflusses von Cyclooxygenaseprodukten (z.B. PGE_2), wie es von Kunkel et al. in *in vitro* Versuchen beschrieben wurde. Unsere Daten lassen die Schlußfolgerung zu, daß PGE_2 teilweise für die erniedrigte Sekretion von TNF-α verantwortlich sein könnte, da die Hemmung der Cyclooxygenase zu einer verbesserten TNF-α-Freisetzung vor allem bei septischen Patienten führte. Unsere Ergebnisse lassen im Vergleich zu früheren Studien nicht den Schluß zu, daß Arachidonsäuremetabolite im Vollblut die IL-1β-Sekretion negativ beeinflussen. Weitere Studien müssen die Bedeutung einer reduzierten CD14 Expression und/oder eines erniedrigten "LPS-binding protein" für die Synthesehemmung der TNF-α und IL-1β-Sekretion zeigen.

Zusammenfassung

Das manifeste Sepsissyndrom führte zu einer signifikanten Suppression der TNF-α- und IL-1β-Sekretion aus Monozyten septischer Patienten. Die Hemmung der Cyclooxygenase im Vollblut resultierte in einer partiellen Wiederherstellung der TNF-α-Freisetzung, während die IL-1β-Sekretion unbeeinflußt blieb. Die Suppression der Zytokinfreisetzung aus Monozyten septischer Patienten läßt sich somit nur teilweise durch den inhibitorischen Einfluß von Arachidonsäuremetaboliten erklären.

Summary

Septic shock results in a significant suppression of tumor necrosis factor (TNF) α and interleukin 1β (IL-1β) secretion by monocytes from septic patients. After the inhibition of the cyclooxygenase we observed a partial restitution of the TNF-α secretion, while the IL-1β release remained unaltered. These results indicate that the decreased release of TNF-α and IL-1β by monocytes from patients suffering from systemic infection is only partially due to metabolites of the cyclooxygenase pathway.

Literatur

1. Bone RC (1991) The pathogenesis of sepsis. Ann Int Med 115:457–469
2. Scales WE, Chensue SW, Otterness I, Kunkel SL (1989) Regulation of monokine gene expression: Prostaglandin E_2 suppresses tumor necrosis factor but not interleukin-1α or β-mRNA and cell-associated bioactivity. J Leukoc Biol 45:416-421
3. Eskandari MK, Nguyen DT, Kunkel SL, Remick DG (1990) WEHI 164 subclone 13 assay for TNF: Sensitivity, specificity and reliability. Immun Invest 19:69–79
4. Kenney JS, Masada MP, Eugui EM, Delustro BM, Mulkins MA, Allison AC (1987) Monoclonal antibodies to human recombinant interleukin 1 (IL-1)β: Quantitation of IL-1β and inhibition of biological activity. J Immunol 138:4236
5. Schmid P, Mackensen A, Galanos C, Engelhardt R (1992) Induction of hyporesponsiveness to LPS in cancer patients by daily application in escalating doses. 2nd Conference of the International Endotoxin Society (Vienna), 1992

D. Jarrar, c/o Dr. W. Ertel, Chirurgische Klinik und Poliklinik, Klinikum Großhadern, Ludwig-Maximilians-Universität München, Marchioninistraße 15, W-8000 München 70

Tumornekrosefaktor-α (TNF-α) induziert indirekt über die Freisetzung von Cyclooxygenasemetaboliten die Hemmung zellulärer Immunfunktionen

Tumor Necrosis Factor α Indirectly Induces the Inhibition of Cellular Immune Functions by Metabolites of the Cyclooxygenase Pathway

W. Ertel[1], I.H. Chaudry[2] und F.W. Schildberg[1]

[1]Chirurgische Klinik und Poliklinik, Klinikum Großhadern, Ludwig-Maximilians-Universität München
[2]Shock and Trauma Research Laboratories, Department of Surgery, Michigan State University, East Lansing, USA

Einleitung

Schock, Trauma, Verbrennungen und ausgedehnte chirurgische Eingriffe führen über eine Aktivierung von Makrophagen zu einer erhöhten Synthese und Sekretion von Tumornekrosefaktor-α (TNF-α) [1, 2]. Zahlreiche *in vitro* Studien [3] belegen, daß TNF-α zu einer signifikanten Steigerung der Prostaglandinsynthese und im besonderen von PGE_2 führt. Die erhöhte Freisetzung von PGE_2 aus Makrophagen könnte für die nach Trauma und Verbrennung auftretende Immunsuppression eine entscheidende Rolle spielen, da PGE_2 zu einer massiven Hemmung des zellulären und humoralen Immunsystems führt. Aus diesen Ergebnissen läßt sich die Hypothese ableiten, daß TNF-α *indirekt* über die erhöhte Freisetzung von PGE_2 für die posttraumatische Immunsuppression verantwortlich sein könnte. Es war das Ziel dieser Studie, den Einfluß von rekombinantem TNF-α (rTNF-α) auf Funktionen des zellulären Immunsystems zu untersuchen. Um Effekte von TNF-α auf kardiopulmonale und metabolische Funktionen auszuschließen, wurde eine niedrige Dosierung von rTNF-α verwendet.

Methoden

Als Versuchstiere wurden 6 Wochen alte männliche C3H/HeN-Mäuse verwendet. Die Injektion von rTNF-α (0,1 μg/g Körpergewicht; spezifische Aktivität $1,2 \times 10^7$ U/mg rTNF-α; Endotoxinkontamination 0,12 ng/mg rTNF-α) und von Ibuprofen (2 μg/g Körpergewicht) erfolgte über die Schwanzvene entsprechend dem Protokoll in Tabelle 1. Die Tiere wurden nach 1, 12 und 24 h eingeschläfert. Peritonealmakrophagen wurden mit Hilfe der Peritoneallavage gewonnen und über einen Adhärenzschritt gereinigt. Nach Stimulation mit LPS (1 μg/ml) wurden die Zellüberstände abzentrifugiert und bei −70°C eingefroren. Die Messung der PGE_2-Spiegel erfolgte mit RIA. Splenozytenkulturen wurden entsprechend früherer Protokolle [4] präpariert. Nach Stimu-

Chirurgisches Forum 1993
f. experim. u. klinische Forschung
Becker/Beger/Hartel (Hrsg.)

lation mit Con A (2,5 μg/ml) über 24 h wurde die Splenozytenproliferation über den Einbau von ^{3}H-Thymidin gemessen [4]. Die Interleukin-2 (IL-2)-Freisetzung aus Splenozyten wurde nach Stimulation mit Con A über 48 h aus den Splenozytenüberständen mit dem CTLL-20-Bioassay gemessen [4].

Tabelle 1. Studienprotokoll für die Injektion von rTNF-α, Ibuprofen und Placebo. Es wurden 4 Versuche pro Gruppe durchgeführt. Alle Substanzen wurden i.v. in die Schwanzvene verabreicht

Gruppe	Vorbehandlung		rTNF	NaCl
	Ibuprofen	NaCl		
1	–	+	+	–
2	+	–	+	–
3 (Kontrolle I)	+	–	–	+
4 (Kontrolle II)	–	+	–	+

Ergebnisse

Die Injektion einer niedrigen Dosierung von rTNF-α führte weder zu signifikanten Veränderungen der Pulsfrequenz und des Blutdrucks, noch zu metabolischen Veränderungen. Es wurde keine Letalität beobachtet. Die Injektion von NaCl mit oder ohne Ibuprofen (Gruppe III und IV) verursachte weder eine erhöhte Sekretion von

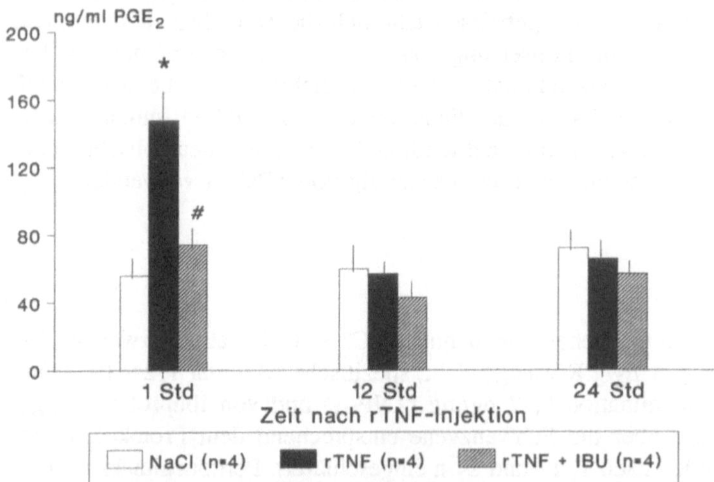

Abb. 1. Freisetzung von PGE$_2$ [ng/ml] aus Peritonealmakrophagen (PMØ) nach Stimulation mit LPS (1 μg/ml) über 24 h. Die PMØ-Kulturen wurden 1, 12 und 24 h nach Injektion von Placebo, rTNF-α oder rTNF-α plus Ibuprofen präpariert. Die Messung von PGR$_2$ aus PMØ erfolgte mit RIA. X $\pm$ SEM; * $p < 0{,}05$ rTNF-α versus NaCl; # $p < 0{,}05$ rTNF-α versus rTNF-α + Ibuprofen; ANOVA

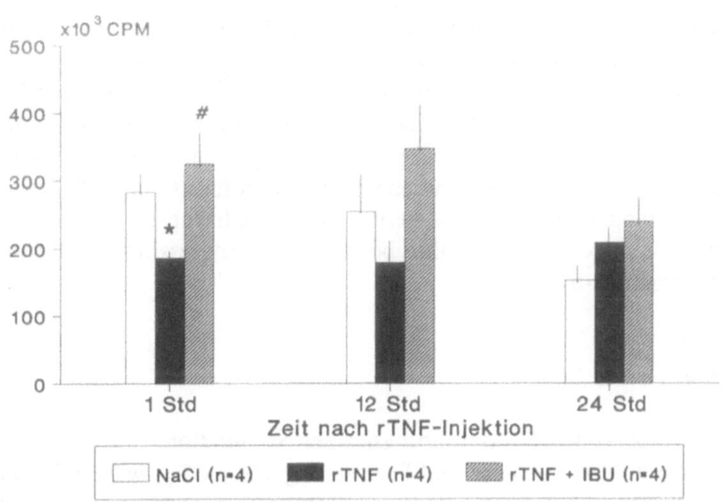

Abb. 2. Splenozytenproliferation [$\times 10^3$ CPM] nach Stimulation mit Con A (2,5 μg/ml) über 24 h. Die Splenozytenkulturen wurden 1, 12 und 24 h nach Injektion von Placebo, rTNF-α oder rTNF-α plus Ibuprofen präpariert. Die Messung der Proliferationskapazität erfolgte über den Einbau von ^{3}H-Thymidin. X ± SEM; * $p < 0{,}05$ rTNF-α versus NaCl; # $p < 0{,}05$ rTNF-α versus rTNF-α + Ibuprofen; ANOVA

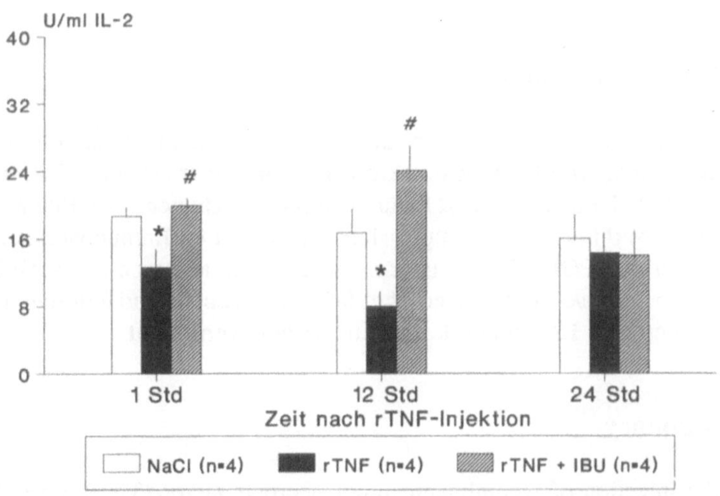

Abb. 3. Freisetzung von IL-2 [U/ml] aus Splenozyten nach Stimulation mit Con A (2,5 μg/ml) über 48 h. Die Splenozytenkulturen wurden 1, 12 und 24 h nach Injektion von Placebo, rTNF-α oder rTNF-α plus Ibuprofen präpariert. Die Messung von IL-2 aus Splenozyten erfolgte mit dem CTLL 20-Proliferationsassay. X ± SEM; * $p < 0{,}05$ rTNF-α versus NaCl; # $p < 0{,}05$ rTNF-α versus rTNF-α + Ibuprofen; ANOVA

PGE_2 aùs Peritonealmakrophagen, noch eine Hemmung bzw. Stimulation von Splenozytenfunktionen. Die Injektion einer niedrigen Dosierung von rTNF-α (Gruppe I) führte nach 1 h zu einer erhöhten Freisetzung von PGE_2 aus Peritonealmakrophagen. Gleichzeitig fand sich nach Injektion von rTNF-α eine signifikante Hemmung der IL-2-Synthese und eine Suppression der Splenozytenproliferation. Die Vorbehandlung mit dem Cyclooxygenasehemmer Ibuprofen (Gruppe II) verhinderte die erhöhte Freisetzung von PGE_2 aus Peritonealmakrophagen und verhinderte ($p < 0{,}05$) die nach alleiniger TNF-Injektion beobachtete Suppression der Splenozytenblastogenese und der IL-2-Synthese.

Diskussion

Die Gabe von rTNF-α führte zu einer Stimulation von Peritonealmakrophagen mit einer erhöhten Synthese und Freisetzung von PGE_2, während wichtige Splenozytenfunktionen gehemmt wurden. Im Gegensatz hierzu verhinderte die Vorbehandlung mit Cyclooxygenasehemmern die Suppression der Splenozytenfunktionen und senkte signifikant die Freisetzung von PGE_2. Diese Ergebnisse lassen die Schlußfolgerung zu, daß TNF-α *indirekt* über eine erhöhte Sekretion von immunsuppressiven Prostaglandinen (z.B. PGE_2) eine Hemmung zellulärer Immunfunktionen verursacht. Somit könnte die erhöhte Sekretion von Tumornekrosefaktor-α nach Schock, Trauma, Verbrennungen oder ausgedehnten chirurgischen Eingriffen für die posttraumatische Immunsuppression eine entscheidende Rolle spielen.

Zusammenfassung

Die Injektion einer niedrigen Dosierung von rekombinantem TNF-α führte zu einer Aktivierung von Peritonealmakrophagen mit einer erhöhten Sekretion von PGE_2 und zu einer Hemmung von zellulären Immunfunktionen. Die Hemmung der Cyclooxygenase verhinderte die Suppression von zellulären Immunparametern bei gleichzeitig erniedrigter PGE_2-Freisetzung. Diese Ergebnisse lassen die Schlußfolgerung zu, daß TNF-α *indirekt* über eine erhöhte Sekretion von sekundären immunsuppressiven Mediatoren eine Hemmung des Immunsystems verursacht.

Summary

The injection of recombinant tumor necrosis factor (TNF)-α results in an activation of peritoneal macrophages with an increased release of PGE_2 and a significant suppression of the cellular immune system. Pretreatment with cyclooxygenase inhibitors before injection of rTNF-α, however, attenuated rTNF-α induced inhibition of cellular immune functions. These data lead us to conclude that TNF-α causes suppression of the immune system *indirectly* via activation of macrophages with an increased release of immunosuppressive arachidonic acid metabolites.

Literatur

1. Takayama TK, Miller C, Szabo G (1990) Elevated tumor necrosis factor-α production is concomitant to elevated prostaglandin E_2 production by trauma patients' monocytes. Arch Surg 125:29–35
2. Ertel W, Morrison MH, Ayala A, Chaudry IH (1991) Chloroquine attentuates hemorrhagic shock-induced suppression of Kupffer cell antigen presentation and major histocompatibility complex class II antigen expression through blockade of tumor necrosis factor and prostaglandin release. Blood 78:1781–1788
3. Bachwich PR, Chensue SW, Larrick JW, Kunkel SL (1986) Tumor necrosis factor stimulates interleukin-1 and prostaglandin E_2 production in resting macrophages. Biochem Biophys Res Comm 136:94–101
4. Ertel W, Morrison MH, Ayala A, Dean RE, Chaudry IH (1992) Interferon-γ attenuates hemorrhage-induced suppression of macrophage and splenocyte functions and decreases susceptibility to sepsis. Surgery 111:177–187

Dr. W. Ertel, Chirurgische Klinik und Poliklinik, Klinikum Großhadern, Ludwig-Maximilians-Universität München, Marchioninistraße 15, W-8000 München 70

Trauma- und sepsisbedingte Inhibition der Interleukin-2 (IL-2) Synthese und IL-2 mRNA Expression ist reversibel durch direkte Phosphokinase C (PKC) Aktivierung

Trauma and Sepsis-Induced Inhibition of Interleukin-2 (IL-2) Synthesis and IL-2 mRNA Expression is Reversible via Direct Phosphokinase C (PKC) Activation

S. Zimmer[1], C. Schinkel[1], J.-P. Kremer[2], E. Faist[1] und F.W. Schildberg[1]

[1]Chirurgische Klinik und Poliklinik, LMU München
[2]GSF, Institut für experimentelle Hämatologie, München

Einleitung

Die traumainduzierte Suppression des T-Zellwachstumsfaktors IL-2 ist eine der folgenschwersten Funktionsstörungen der spezifischen Immunantwort, da aufgrund der daraus resultierenden mangelnden klonalen T-Zellexpansion die Entstehung opportunistischer Infektionen bei Schwerstverletzten begünstigt, respektive die anerge Reaktionslage des kritisch kranken Patienten nicht durchbrochen werden kann.

Die Inhibition der IL-2 Biosynthese erfolgt sofort mit dem Trauma, ist innerhalb der ersten Stunden nachweisbar und persistiert abhängig von Traumaqualität und Verletzungsausmaß über Wochen und Monate [1]. Nach Ausschluß anderer ätiologischer Faktoren wurde postuliert, daß dieses Phänomen letztlich auf eine mechanistische Beeinflussung des T-Zellaktivierungsprozesses zurückzuführen sein muß [2]. Neben einer dominierenden Suppressorrolle innerhalb der Niederregulierung der T-Zellaktivierung durch den Monozyten (MØ)-Mediator Prostaglandin E_2 (PGE_2) wurde als weiterer Mechanismus der T-Zelldysfunktion eine fehlerhafte transmembranöse Signalübertragung, die zur Induktion einer adäquaten IL-2 Synthese notwendig ist, postuliert. Ziel der hier dargestellten Untersuchungen war 1.) die Lokalisation des IL-2 Synthesedefekts durch die parallele Analyse der IL-2 mRNA Expression und der IL-2 Proteinsynthese und 2.) der Nachweis eines möglichen transmembranösen Signalübermittlungsdefektes durch die Verwendung von Phorbolester, einem Substrat, welches unter Umgehung der Second Messenger Kaskade direkt die Proteinkinase C (PKC) der T-Zelle aktivieren kann.

Patienten und Methoden

In die Studie wurden 14 Traumapatienten (9 Mehrfachverletzungen, 5 Schwerbrandverletzungen, 11 Männer, 3 Frauen, 38 ± 5 Jahre, Injury Severity Score (ISS) 34 ± 2 Punkte) sowie 8 Patienten mit einem post-traumatischen Sepsissyndrom (7 Männer,

Chirurgisches Forum 1993
f. experim. u. klinische Forschung
Becker/Beger/Hartel (Hrsg.)

1 Frau, 56 ± 5 Jahre, Elebute Sepsis Score 22 ± 7 Punkte) aufgenommen. Mononukleäre Blutleukozyten (PBMC) wurden an den konsekutiven Tagen (D) 1, 3, 5, 7 und 10 nach Trauma, respektive nach Erstmanifestation des Sepsissyndroms über einen Separationsgradienten isoliert und als Zellsuspension aufbereitet. Diese PBMC Kulturen wurden dann mit dem Mitogen Phythämagglutinin (PHA) allein (48 h Inkubation) oder in Kokultur mit Phorbol Myristate Acetate (PMA) (Inkubationszeit 4 h respektive 20 h) stimuliert. Nach Terminierung der Zellkulturen wurde die IL-2 Eiweißsynthese mittels Bioassay (humane ConA Blasten) aus den Kulturüberständen bestimmt, während aus den verbliebenen PBMC's ein Zellysat präpariert wurde. Aus diesem Lysat wurde dann die IL-2 nach Northern Blotting durch radioaktive Hybridisierung mit der spezifischen cDNA autoradiographisch dargestellt und quantifiziert.

Die statistische Analyse der Ergebnisse erfolgte mittels Student's t-Test, wobei als Signifikanzniveau $p \leq 0{,}05$ gewählt wurde. Alle Werte sind als Mittelwerte ± S.E.M. ausgedrückt.

Ergebnisse

Die PHA induzierte IL-2 Synthese war an allen Untersuchungstagen verglichen mit den Normalwerten ($0{,}62 \pm 0{,}04$ U/ml) in beiden Patientenkollektiven deutlich supprimiert (Tabelle 1). In den PHA/PMA stimulierten PBMC Kulturen (Normalwert $1{,}25 \pm 0{,}12$ U/ml bei einer Inkubationszeit von 20 h) war die IL-2 Synthese an konsekutiven Tagen nach Trauma respektive nach Manifestation des Sepsissyndromes nicht vermindert und lag immer im Normbereich.

Tabelle 1. IL-2 Protein Konzentrationen (U/ml) der PBMC Überstände nach Stimulation mit PHA allein (48 h) oder unter Zusatz von Phorbolester (PMA) als Kostimulus (20 h) an konsekutiven Tagen nach Trauma und im Verlauf eines Sepsissyndroms

IL-2 (U/ml)	Trauma					
	D1	D3	D5	D7	D10	
PHA	0,27	0,40	0,41	0,29	0,27	
± S.E.M.	0,06[a]	0,05[a]	0,09[a]	0,08[a]	0,09[a]	
PHA/PMA	1,29	1,26	1,26	1,18	1,16	
± S.E.M.	0,14	0,12	0,12	0,06	0,04	
IL-2 (U/ml)	Sepsis					Kontrolle
	D1	D3	D5	D7	D10	
PHA	0,31	0,27	0,20	0,26	0,26	0,62
± S.E.M.	0,10[a]	0,08[a]	0,09[a]	0,08[a]	0,10[a]	0,04
PHA/PMA	1,24	1,25	1,27	1,19	1,16	1,25
± S.E.M.	0,06	0,05	0,06	0,02	0,07	0,12

[a] $p < 0{,}05$ der Patientenkollektive gegenüber der Kontrollgruppe. X ± S.E.M.

Das IL-2 mRNA Signal in PHA-stimulierten Kulturen war in den Zellen gesunder Kontrollen immer präsent, wenn auch deutlich schwächer als die Transkriptionsintensität nach PHA/PMA Kostimulation. In beiden Patientenkollektiven dagegen war nach PHA Stimulation nie ein IL-2 mRNA Signal sichtbar, während nach PHA/PMA Kostimulation bei 10 von 11 evaluierbaren Autoradiographien ein deutliches IL-2 mRNA-Signal, identisch mit der Intensität der Kontrollzellkulturen, nachweisbar war (Abb. 1b). Die Signalintensität in den PHA/PMA stimulierten PBMC Kulturen war bezeichnenderweise bei 3 Patienten mit einem komplizierten septischen posttraumatischen Verlauf deutlich beeinträchtigt oder nicht nachweisbar. In Abb. 1a und 1b ist die IL-2 Proteinsynthese in PHA und PHA/PMA stimulierten PBMC Kulturen von einem Patienten mit ausgedehntem Verbrennungstrauma (38% der Gesamtkörperoberfläche), sowie die dazu korrespondierende Autoradiographie dargestellt. Eine beeindruckende Übereinstimmung zwischen IL-2 mRNA Expression und IL-2 Proteinsynthese konnte in diesem Fall dokumentiert werden.

Diskussion

Durch die hier dargestellten Untersuchungsdaten konnte nachgewiesen werden, daß die Verwendung von Phorbolester, einem Substrat, das die Aktionskaskade essentieller Second Messenger Substanzen innerhalb des Ablaufes der Signaltransmission nach Antigenstimulus imitieren und die PKC direkt aktivieren kann, eine Restitution der IL-2 mRNA Expression und der IL-2 Proteinsynthese bewirkt. Daraus ist zu folgern, daß die Veränderung der Expression der IL-2 mRNA und der IL-2 Proteinausschüttung nach Trauma nicht durch einen konstitutionellen Defekt bedingt ist, sondern im wesentlichen auf einer alterierten Signalübermittlung zwischen Zellmembran und Zellkern beruht. Die Analyse der korrespondierenden Profile der mRNA Expression und der Proteinsynthese für IL-2 zeigte eine sehr gute Übereinstimmung zwischen Genexpression und Lymphokinproduktion und legte die weitere Schlußfolgerung nahe, daß die streßinduzierte Veränderung der IL-2 Synthese im wesentlichen auf der Transkriptionsebene reguliert wird.

Eine weitere funktionelle Komponente, welche für die Störung der frühen T-Zellaktivierung und der daraus folgenden Unterdrückung der IL-2 Synthese verantwortlich ist, ist die PGE_2-mediierte Erhöhung des intrazellulären zyklischen Adenosinmonophosphates (cAMP), ein Phänomen, welches insbesondere unter dem modulierenden Einfluß von Endotoxin gesehen wird und auf der massiven Stimulierung von Adenylatcyclase, dem verantwortlichen Enzym für die cAMP Bildung, beruht. Gestützt auf unsere neuesten klinischen in-vivo Ergebnisse über den Einfluß immunmodulierender Substanzen, wie Cyclooxygenasehemmer und cGMP Induktoren [3], vermuten wir, daß die IL-2 mRNA Expression und die IL-2 Eiweißproduktion gerade unter Streßbedingungen über die postulierte Interaktion zweier Regulationswege [4] erfolgt: Über den vorwärtsregulierenden Polyphosphoinositit – PKC – Calzium – Calmodulinweg und den Adenylatcyclase – cAMP – Proteinkinase A mediierten Inaktivierungsweg. Abhängig jeweils von den individuellen in-vivo Serumbedingungen dominieren die einzelnen Regulationssysteme das Nettoergebnis der Lymphokinsynthese.

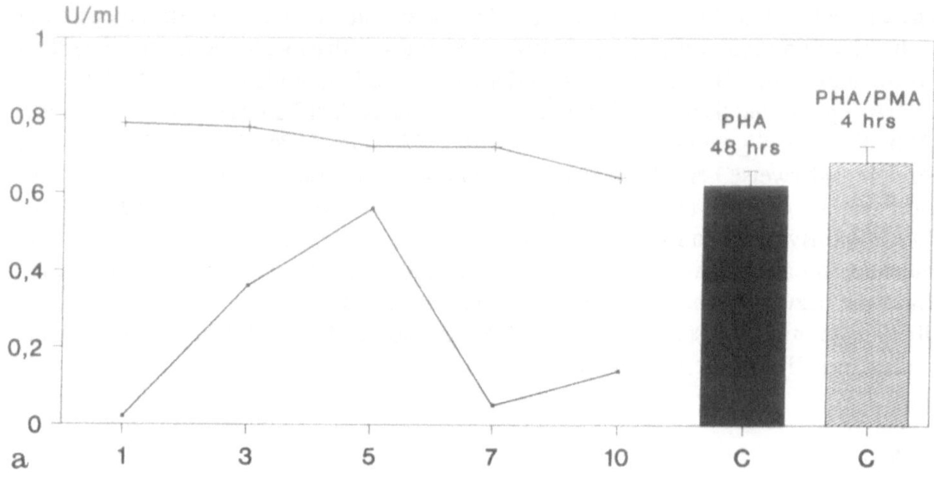

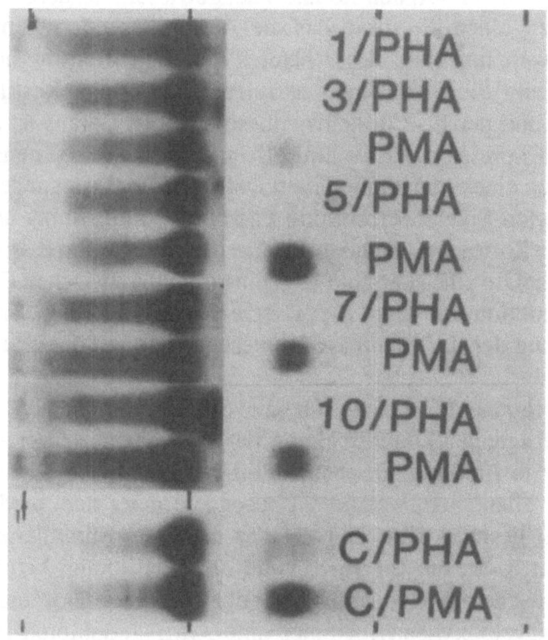

Abb. 1a,b. **a** PHA 48 h Stimulation (—•—) und PHA/PMA 4 h Stimulation (—+—) induzierte IL-2 Konzentration in den PBMC Kulturen eines Verbrennungspatienten (m, 54 Jahre, ISS 25 Punkte) während des posttraumatischen Verlaufes im Vergleich mit dem jeweiligen Kontrollkollektiv (*C*). **b** Zur Il-2 Proteinsynthese in a korrespondierende Darstellung der IL-2 mRNA Expression von PHA und PHA/PMA stimulierten PBMC Kulturen an konsekutiven Tagen nach Trauma. Die zelluläre Gesamt-RNA wurde aus den in Kultur genommenen Zellen isoliert und für die weitere Untersuchung wurden jeweils 10μg RNA verwendet. Nach Northern Blotting wurde die RNA mit ^{32}P markierten IL-2 cDNA Proben hybridisiert. Gleiche RNA-Mengen wurden mit muriner 28S rRNA nachgewiesen. *C*: mRNA Expression für IL-2 der T-Zellen einer gesunden Kontrollperson

Zusammenfassung

Das Ziel dieser Studie war es, detaillierte Erkenntnisse über die gestörten Mechanismen der T-Zellaktivierung unter Streßbedingungen nach Trauma und in der Sepsis zu gewinnen. Durch den Vergleich von IL-2 mRNA Expression und der entsprechenden IL-2 Proteinsynthese in Mitogen stimulierten mononukleären Leukozytenkulturen an konsekutiven Tagen nach Trauma, respektive nach Erstmanifestation eines Sepsissyndroms, wurde die Hauptregulationsebene der IL-2 Synthese bestimmt. Durch die Verwendung von Phorbolester (PMA) als Kostimulus zu dem Mitogen (PHA) sollte nachgewiesen werden, ob die inadäquate IL-2 Synthese möglicherweise durch eine fehlerhafte Aktivierung der Second Messenger Kaskade in der T-Zelle bedingt ist. Unsere Ergebnisse zeigen, daß die beeinträchtigte IL-2 Synthese in diesen Patientengruppen weitestgehend durch Störungen auf der Transkriptionsebene verursacht ist. Durch den zusätzlichen Einsatz von PMA konnte die IL-2 Produktion sowohl auf mRNA-Ebene als auch auf Ebene der Proteinfreisetzung vollständig normalisiert werden. Daraus ist zu folgern, daß die gestörte IL-2 Synthese nach Trauma und bei Sepsis nicht konstitutionell defekt ist, sondern vielmehr durch eine fehlerhafte Signalübermittlung von der T-Zellmembran zum Zellkern bedingt wird.

Summary

The current study was undertaken to further elucidate the mechanisms of dysfunctional T-cell activation under stressful traumatic and septic conditions. The major regulatory level of interleukin-2 (IL-2) release was determined by parallel analysis of IL-2 mRNA expression and IL-2 protein synthesis in mitogen-stimulated mononuclear leukocyte cultures on consecutive days postinjury and postsepsis. By using phorbol myristate acetate (PMA) as a costimulus together with phytohaemagglutin (PHA) we wanted to examine whether inadequate IL-2 synthesis is possibly due to defective signal transduction on the level of second messengers. Our data indicate that defective IL-2 synthesis under stressful conditions is largely regulated on the level of transcription. The administration of PMA could well restitute IL-2 mRNA expression and IL-2 protein synthesis. Thus, it was concluded that IL-2 synthesis following major trauma and during sepsis syndrome is not constitutionally defective, but most likely attributable to alterations in the transmission of signals from the cell membrane to the nucleus.

Literatur

1. Faist E, Mewes A, Baker CC, Strasser T, Alkan SS, Rieber P, Heberer G (1987) Prostaglandin E_2 (PGE_2) dependent suppression of interleukin-2 (IL-2) production in patients with major trauma. J Trauma 27:837–848
2. Hoyt DB, Pinney E, Ozkan AN (1989) Trauma peptide T-cell suppression: Mechanisms of action. In: Faist E, Ninnemann J, Green D (eds) Immune consequences of trauma, shock and sepsis. Springer, Berlin Heidelberg, pp 293–296

3. Faist E, Markewitz A, Fuchs D, Lang S, Schildberg FW (1991) Immunomedulatory therapy with thymopentin and indomethacin: Successful restoration of interleukin-2 synthesis in patients undergoing major surgery. Ann Surg 214:264–275
4. Kammer GM (1988) The adenylate cyclase – cAMP – protein kinase A pathway and regulation of the immune response. Immunol Today 9:222–229

S. Zimmer, Chirurgische Klinik und Poliklinik, Klinikum Großhadern, Ludwig-Maximilians-Universität, Marchioninistraße 15, W-8000 München 70

Der Einfluß von Sauerstoffradikalen auf die Granulation von PMN-Leukozyten

The Influence of Oxygen Radicals on the Granulation of Polymorphonuclear Leukocytes

B. Poch, M.H. Schoenberg, F. Gansauge, S. Gansauge und H.G. Beger

Abteilung für Allgemeinchirurgie, Universität Ulm

Zielsetzung

Schleimhautveränderungen nach intestinaler Ischämie und Reperfusion sind von wesentlicher klinischer Bedeutung. Es konnte in den letzten Jahren gezeigt werden, daß der Großteil dieser Schäden nicht in der Ischämie- sondern erst in der Reperfusionsphase entstehen. Verantwortlich hierfür sind freie Sauerstoffradikale (OR): Hypoxanthin (HX) akkumuliert während der Ischämiephase im Gewebe. Nach der Reperfusion wird Hypoxanthin zu Harnsäure (HS) verstoffwechselt. Hierbei fallen vermehrt OR an und überfordern die natürlichen Schutzmechanismen der Zelle. Katalysiert wird dieser Abbau über die Xanthinoxidase (XO). Es konnte gezeigt werden, daß nur ein geringerer Teil der Schleimhautschäden durch OR direkt verursacht wird, während der Großteil der Veränderungen auf aktivierte PMN-Leukozyten zurückzuführen sind. Durch Blockierung der XO mit Allopurinol (ALP) lassen sich die Reperfusionsschäden nahezu vollständig verhindern [1]. Ungeklärt ist bislang, ob PMN-Leukozyten durch OR im Blut direkt, oder über Gewebemediatoren aktiviert werden. Ziel dieser Untersuchung wasr es, in vitro festzustellen, ob OR PMN-Leukozyten *direkt* erregen können. Als Maß der Aktivierung der Leukozyten wurden deren Granulaveränderungen gewertet.

Methodik

Von 10 gesunden Probanden wurde heparinisiertes Vollblut entnommen. Hieraus wurden zum einen alle Leukozyten isoliert und zum anderen PMN-Leukozyten selektiv abgetrennt. Die Kulturen wurden bei 37°C in DMEM-Medium und 25% Humanserum bebrütet. Nach einer zweistündigen Stabilisierungsphase wurden sowohl den Gesamtleukozyten als auch den isolierten PMN-Leukozyten folgende Medien zugesetzt: 1. HX (5 mmol/l), 2. HS (5 mmol/l), 3. ALP (5 mmol/l)/HX (5 mmol/l)/XO (0,05 U/ml), 4. HX (5 mmol/l)/XO (0,05 U/ml). 0', 15', 30', 60' und 120' später wurden Proben entnommen. Es wurde die Leukozytenzahl, bezogen auf das Ausgangsvolumen, bestimmt. Bei Proben aus 5 Kulturen wurden Ausstrichpräparate angefertigt und modif. nach Giemsa gefärbt. Diese wurden im Mikroskop begutachtet und entsprechend der Anzahl großer Granula eingeteilt: 1. normal: mehr als 50 große Granula/Leukozyt,

Chirurgisches Forum 1993
f. experim. u. klinische Forschung
Becker/Beger/Hartel (Hrsg.)

2. vermindert: weniger als 51 und mehr als 5 große Granula/Leukozyt, 3. entgranuliert: weniger als 6 große Granula/Leukozyt. Der Granulationsgrad der übrigen 5 Versuchstiere wurde im Cell-Sorter semiquantitativ bestimmt. Statistische Signifikanzen der Verteilungen wurden nach dem t-Test errechnet.

Ergebnisse

1. Isolierte PMN-Leukozyten (Abb. 1a, 2)

Im Cell-Sorter läßt sich ein Reinheitsgrad von mehr als 99% an Granulozyten in diesen Kulturen dokumentieren (Abb. 2). 93% ± 2% dieser PMN-Leukozyten haben vor Versuchsbeginn normale Granula. Eine Inkubation über 120' mit HX oder HS führt zu keiner Änderung des Granulationsmusters. Dahingegen zeigt sich in der HX/XO- und in der ALP/HX/XO-Gruppe ein kontinuierlicher, langsamer Rückgang der Granulation. Nach 120' ist dieser in der HX/XO/ALP-Gruppe (84% ± 5%) gegenüber der HX/XO-Gruppe (79% ± 3%) deutlich weniger augenfällig.

2. Gesamtleukozytenkultur (Abb. 1b, 2)

Diese Kulturen enthalten sämtliche Zellen des weißen Blutbildes (Granulozyten, Monozyten, Lymphozyten, etc.) in nicht pathologischer Verteilung. 89% ± 3% der PMN-Leukozyten sind vor Versuchsbeginn normal granuliert und unterscheiden sich diesbezüglich nicht von den reinen PMN-Leukozytenkulturen. Auch in dieser Versuchsreihe bewirkt die Inkubation mit HX oder HS keine Veränderung im Grad der Granulation.

In der HX/XO-Gruppe zeigt sich bereits nach 30' ein Rückgang der normal granulierten PMN-Leukozyten auf 68% ± 5%. Diese Degranulation setzt sich weiter fort. Nach 120' findet sich nur noch bei 49% ± 3% der Neutrophilen eine normale Granulation. Die HX/XO/ALP-Gruppe läßt in den ersten 60' (87% ± 4% mit normaler Granulation) keine Änderungen erkennen. Erst der 120' Wert zeigt einen Rückgang normal granulierter PMN-Leukozyten auf 73% ± 4%.

Sowohl in den reinen PMN-Leukozyten- als auch in den Leukozytenkulturen bleibt die Gesamtzahl der Leukozyten bei allen Versuchen konstant.

Diskussion

Zu Beginn des Versuches unterscheiden sich die Kulturen der Gesamtleukozyten nicht von denen der isolierten Granulozyten. In beiden Versuchsreihen bewirken nach 120' weder HX noch HS eine Änderung des Granulationsgrades. In Anwesenheit von HX und XO kommt es in beiden Gruppen zu einem Abfall der Granulation. Diese fällt in der Gesamtleukozytenpopulation signifikant stärker ab. ALP bewirkt eine starke Protektion der PMN-Leukozyten nach 120'. Während der ersten 60' kann ALP die Degranulation sogar verhindern. Auf Grund dieser Ergebnisse ist davon auszugehen, daß OR PMN-Leukozyten im Blut direkt und ohne Gewebekontakt aktivieren können.

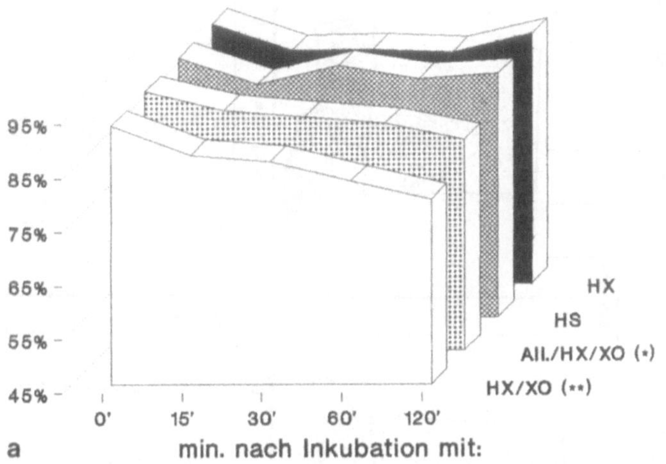

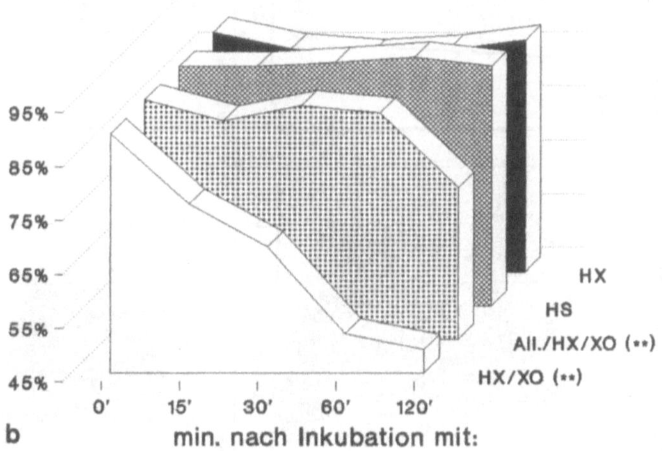

Abb. 1 a,b. Die Abbildung zeigt den Anteil normal granulierter Zellen nach Inkubation von PMN-Leukozyten und Gesamtleukozyten mit Hypoxanthin (HX), Harnsäure (HS), Xanthinoxidase (XO)/HX, bzw. Allopurinol (ALP)/XO/HX in Abhängigkeit von der Inkubationszeit. Signifikante Unterschiede gegenüber den Ausgangswerten: (*) $p < 0,01$, (**) $p < 0,001$

Diese Aktivierung wird vermutlich jedoch indirekt über Monozyten oder Lymphozyten kaskadenartig vermittelt. Eine leichte, wenn auch signifikante Degranulation nach OR-Exposition in den Granulozytenkulturen könnte über noch verbliebene Lymphozyten bzw. Monozyten vermittelt werden. Die Degranulation der PMN-Leukozyten nach Kontakt mit OR ist erstmals ein Hinweis auf eine weitere direkte Wirkung von OR auf PMN-Leukozyten ohne Endothelkontakt.

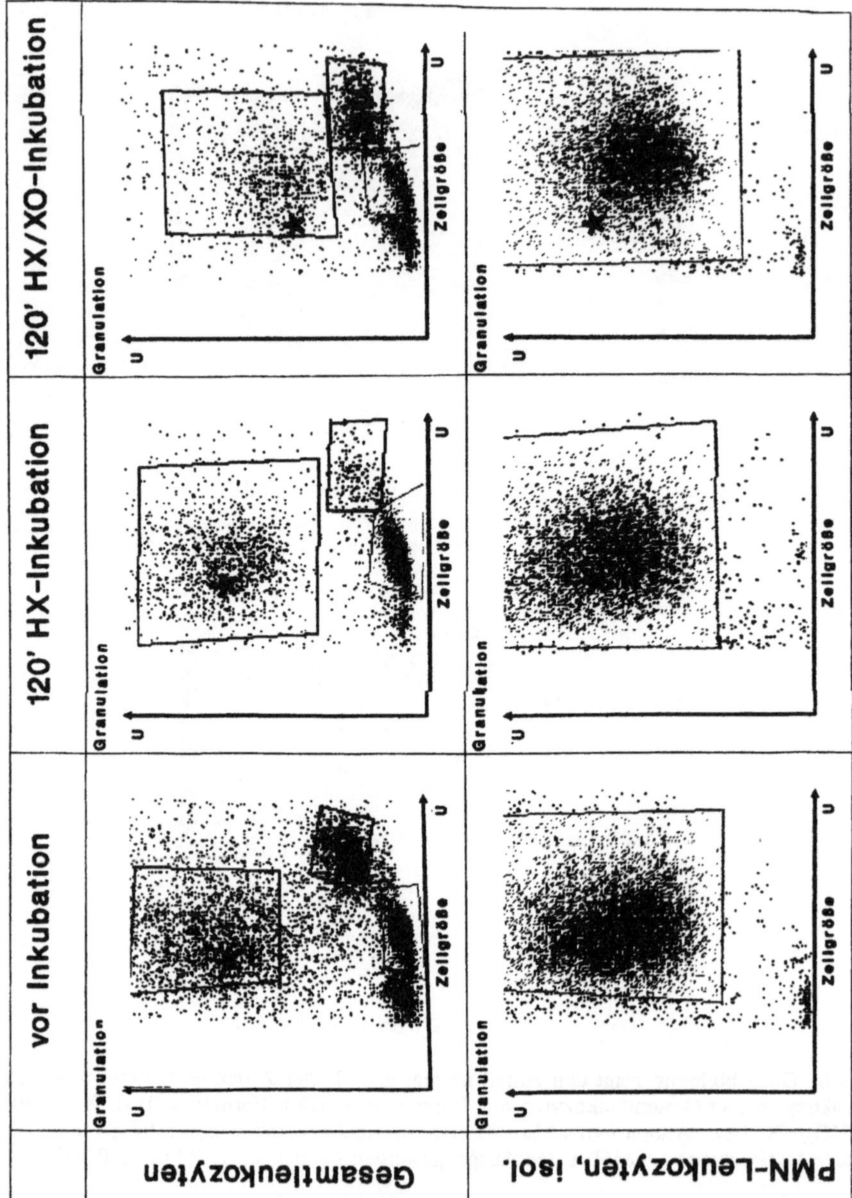

Abb. 2. Die Abbildung zeigt den Plot des Cell-Sorters. Jede untersuchte Zelle wird durch Granulationsgrad (y-Achse) und Zellgröße (x-Achse) definiert). Es sind isolierte PMN-Leukozyten und Gesamtleukozyten vor und nach 120' Inkubation mit HX bzw. HX/XO dargestellt. Das jeweilige Fenster der PMN-Leukozyten ist mit (*) markiert

Summary

After intestinal ischemia, oxygen radicals (OR) induce severe mucosal lesions, especially in the phase of reperfusion. They are generated by the xanthine oxidase (XO)/hypoxanthine (HX) system. Moderate lesions are generated by OR directly. Severe lesions, however, are induced by activated polymorphonuclear (PMN) leukocytes. We investigated whether OR are able to stimulate PMN leukocytes directly, without endothelial contact. From ten blood samples leukocytes and PMN leukocytes only were isolated and cultured. OR were generated by HX/XO. Every sample was divided into four samples and the following substances were added: a) HX, b) HX/uric acid, c) HX/allopurinol (ALP), and d) HX/XO. After 2 hours the probes were stained. The other part was examined by a cell sorter. These procedures were used to estimate the degree of degranulation. Samples containig *all leukocytes* and HX/XO in the medium showed a severe and significant degranulation of PMN leukocytes. ALP attenuated degranulation in all samples. Neither uric acid nor HX alone induced this reaction. In *isolated PMN leukocytes* cultures, HX/XO effected only a slight degranulation. OR seem to be able to activate PMN leukocytes without endothelial contact, probably mediated by lymphocytes or monocytes.

Literatur

1. Schoenberg MH, Poch B, Younes M, Schwarz A, Baczako K, Lundberg C, Haglund U, Beger HG (1991) Involvement of neutrophils in postischemic damage to the small intestine. GUT 32:905–912

Dr. B. Poch, Abteilung für Allgemeinchirurgie, Universität Ulm, Steinhövelstraße 9, W-7900 Ulm

Hepatozelluläre Stickoxidproduktion in der Sepsis: In vitro und in vivo Nachweis im Rattenmodell*

Hepatocellular Nitric Oxide Production in Sepsis: In Vitro and In Vivo Evidence in a Rat Model

J. Stadler[1], C.-D. Heidecke[1], T.R. Billiar[2] und J.R. Lancaster[2]

[1]Chirurgische Klinik und Poliklinik der TU München (Direktor: Prof. Dr. J.R. Siewert)
[2]Department of Surgery, University of Pittsburgh, Pittsburg, USA
(Direktor: Prof. Dr. R.L. Simmons)

Einleitung

Jüngste Forschungsergebnisse lassen vermuten, daß der Biosynthese von Stickoxid eine wesentliche Rolle in der Pathophysiologie der Sepsis zukommt. Als sog. "endothelium derived relaxing factor" (EDRF) reguliert Stickoxid sowohl den Gefäßwiderstand als auch die Thrombozytenaggregation und -adhäsion an den Gefäßwänden [1]. Die unter inflammatorischer Stimulation kontinuierlich erfolgende Produktion dieses hochreaktiven Radikals trägt daher entscheidend zur Entwicklung der typischen Kreislaufreaktion und Blutungsneigung septischer Patienten bei [2]. Außerdem führt Stickoxid zu einer Suppression zellulärer Stoffwechselprozesse wie z.B. der DNA-Replikation, des Energiehaushaltes oder der Proteinsynthese [3, 4]. Daraus resultiert zum einen eine Hemmung der Proliferation pathologischer Mikroorganismen [5], zum anderen aber auch eine Schädigung der Stickoxid produzierenden Zellen selbst, die zur Entwicklung von Organinsuffizienzen in der Sepsis beitragen dürfte. Unter diesem Aspekt konnte bereits gezeigt werden, daß Hepatozyten große Mengen an Endprodukten des Stickoxidmetabolismus produzieren [3, 4]. In den folgenden Studien sollte untersucht werden, ob Stickoxid in den Leberzellen tatsächlich in der Form des freien Radikals auftritt und mit welchen subzellulären Bestandteilen es reagiert.

Methodik

Isolation der Hepatozyten: Leberzellen wurden von Sprague-Dawley-Ratten durch Hepatektomie in Barbituratnarkose mit Hilfe einer *ex situ* Kollagenase Perfusionstechnik gewonnen. Die Parenchymzellen wurden von den nicht parenchymatösen Zellen durch mehrfache Zentrifugation bei 50 g getrennt.

* Mit Unterstützung der Deutschen Forschungsgemeinschaft: Sta 311/1-1.

Chirurgisches Forum 1993
f. experim. u. klinische Forschung
Becker/Beger/Hartel (Hrsg.)

Stimulation der Stickoxidbiosynthese: Zur *in vitro* Induktion der Stickoxidsynthese wurden frisch gewonnene Hepatozyten mit einer Kombination aus verschiedenen Zytokinen (500 U/ml MrTNFα, 5 U/ml hrIL -1, 100 U/ml rrIFN-gamma) und Endotoxin (10 μg/ml LPS, *E. coli* 0111:B_4) für 24 h inkubiert [3]. Die *in vivo* Stimulation der Stickoxidbiosynthese erfolgte durch Injektion einer Suspension von abgetötetem *Corynebacterium parvum* (28 mg/kg KG) intravenös, woraus eine chronische Entzündungsreaktion der Leber resultiert [4]. 7 Tage nach der Injektion wurden die Hepatozyten wie oben geschildert gewonnen und ebenfalls für 24 h inkubiert.

Nachweis der Stickoxidproduktion: Zur quantitativen Erfassung der Stickoxidsynthese wurden die stabilen Endprodukte Nitrit (NO_2) und Nitrat (NO_3) in den Kulturüberständen und im Serum der Tiere bestimmt. Dazu wurden in einer HPLC-Anordnung NO_3 über eine Cadmiumsäule zu NO_2 reduziert und dann durch einen calorimetrischen Assay gemessen. Der direkte Nachweis der Produktion und Bindung des Stickoxidradikals in den Hepatozyten wurde mit Hilfe der "electron paramagnetic resonance" (EPR) geführt. Dazu wurden ein Bruker 300 und ein Varian E-109 Spektrometer verwendet. Die Untersuchung des Zellextraktes wurde bei 77 Grad Kelvin mit einer Modulationsamplitude von 8 Gauss und einer Modulationsfrequenz von 100 kHz vorgenommen. Der untersuchte Frequenzbereich betrug 9,03–9,08 GHz und die Mikrowellenleistung wurde auf 1 mW eingestellt. Mit dieser Anordnung können Radikale wie das Stickoxid anhand der freien Elektronen nachgewiesen werden. Aus der Bindung an bestimmte, molekulare Strukturen, wie z.B. prosthetische Eisengruppen, ergeben sich spezifische Spektren.

Ergebnisse und Diskussion

Im Vergleich zu unbehandelten Hepatozyten, die in 24 h $17,7 \pm 5,8$ nmol NO_2/NO_3 pro 10^6 Zellen produzierten, stieg die NO_2/NO_3 Konzentration unter *in vitro* Stimulation mit Zytokinen und Endotoxin im selben Zeitraum auf $236,0 \pm 60,0$ nmol NO_2/NO_3 pro 10^6 Zellen an. Nach *in vivo* Induktion der Stickoxidsynthese durch Behandlung mit *Corynebacterium parvum* produzierten die Hepatozyten sogar $323,0 \pm 75,1$ nmol NO_2/NO_3 pro 10^6 Zellen in 24 h. Durch Zugabe des L-Argininderivates N^G-Monomethyl-L-Arginin (NMA) konnte in beiden Fällen die Stickoxidproduktion nahezu vollständig supprimiert werden. Nach Injektion von *Corynebacterium parvum* stiegen die Nitrit/Nitrat Spiegel im Serum auf 1759 ± 170 μmol/l gegenüber Werten von $17,4 \pm 0,4$ μmol/l bei unbehandelten Tieren an. Sowohl unter *in vitro* als auch unter *in vivo* Stimulation konnte in den Hepatozyten ein spezifisches EPR Signal bei g = 2,039 festgestellt werden, das bei unbehandelten Zellen und nach Hemmung der Stickoxidsynthese durch Zugabe von NMA nicht mehr nachzuweisen war (Abb. 1). Ein identisches Signal konnte in Hepatozyten gefunden werden, die mit Stickoxidlösungen oder mit Substanzen behandelt worden waren, die Stickoxid freisetzen. Der Vergleich mit dem Spektrum des Stickoxid-Ferredoxinkomplexes legt nahe, daß das Signal in den Hepatozyten durch Binden des Stickoxids an Eisengruppen der nicht Häm-Spezies hervorgerufen wird. Nach Ultrazentrifugation fand sich das Signal sowohl im Überstand, als auch in der zytosolischen Fraktion. Auf-

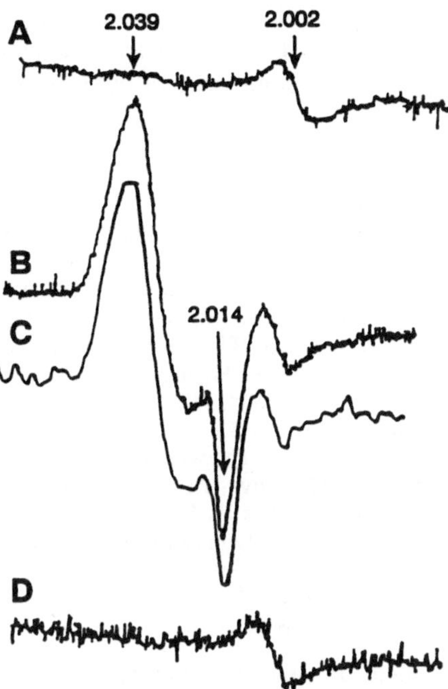

Abb. 1. EPR Signale von unbehandelten (*A*), mit Zytokinen und LPS stimulierten (*B*), mit Stickoxidlösung behandelten (*C*) und mit Zytokinen, LPS und NMA inkubierten Hepatozyten (*D*). Die Inkubationszeit betrug 24 h, die Expositionszeit mit Stickoxidlösungen 5 min

grund der zahlreichen Enzyme und anderer Proteine des Zytosols, die Eisengruppen in ihren aktiven Zentren aufweisen, kann man davon ausgehen, daß einige metabolische Alterationen des hepatozellulären Stoffwechsels in der Sepsis auf die Wirkung des Stickoxids zurückzuführen sind. Zukünftige Untersuchungen müssen aber erst klären, ob die Stickoxidbiosynthese tatsächlich auch zur Entwicklung der Leberzellinsuffizienz beiträgt.

Zusammenfassung

Nach Stimulation von Hepatozyten mit typischen Mediatoren der Sepsis konnten die stabilen Endprodukte des Stickoxidmetabolismus sowohl *in vitro* als auch *in vivo* nachgewiesen werden. Außerdem fand sich ein EPR Signal, das dem des Stickstoff-Ferredoxinkomplexes entspricht. Diese Ergebnisse belegen, daß Hepatozyten der Ratte in der Sepsis Stickoxid als freies Radikal produzieren, welches dann an prosthetische Eisengruppen von Zytoplasmaproteinen gebunden wird.

Summary

Following exposure of hepatocytes to septic stimuli, the stable endproducts of nitric oxide metabolism could be detected under *in vitro* as well as *in vivo* conditions. Furthermore, an electron paramagnetic resonance (EPR) signal was identified that closely resembles that of the nitric oxide ferredoxin complex. These results demonstrate that rat hepatocytes produce nitric oxide as a free radical in sepsis, which then binds to prosthetic iron complexes of cytoplasmic proteins.

Literatur

1. Ignarro LJ (1989) Endothelium-derived nitric oxide: actions and properties. FASEB J 3:31–36
2. Petros A, Bennet D, Vallance P (1991) Effect of nitric oxide synthase inhibitors on hypotension in patients with septic shock. Lancet 338:1557–1558
3. Stadler J, Billiar TR, Curran RD, Stuehr DJ, Ochoa JB, Simmons RL (1991) Effect of exogenous and endogenous nitric oxide on mitochondrial respiration of rat hepatocytes. Am J Physiol 260:C910–C916
4. Stadler J, Curran RD, Ochoa JB, Harbrecht BG, Hofman RA, Simmons RL, Billiar TR (1991) Effect of endogenous nitric oxide on mitochondrial respiration of rat hepatocytes in vitro and in vivo. Arch Surg 126:186–191
5. Nathan CF, Hibbs JB Jr (1991) Role of nitric oxide synthesis in macrophage antimicrobial activity. Current Opinion in Immunology 3:65–70

Dr. med. J. Stadler, Chirurgische Klinik und Poliklinik, Technische Universität München, Ismaninger Straße 22, W-8000 München 80

Hat die Hemmung der Lipoxigenase einen protektiven Effekt in der Frühphase der Sepsis?

Does Lipoxygenase Inhibition Have Any Protective Effect During the Early Septic State?

D. Moch[1], M. Schoenberg[2], S. Birk[1] und U.B. Brückner[1]

[1] Sektion Chirurgische Forschung, Chirurgische Universitätsklinik, Ulm
[2] Abteilung für Allgemeine Chirurgie, Chirurgische Universitätsklinik, Ulm

Endotoxin induziert über eine Stimulierung der Freisetzung von Arachidonsäure die Bildung von Lipoxi- und Zyklooxigenaseprodukten. Metabolite des Lipoxigenaseweges, wie Leukotriene (LT) und Hydroxyeicosatetraensäuren (HETE) wirken chemotaktisch auf PMN Leukozyten (insbes. LTB_4), erhöhen die Gefäßpermeabilität (LTC_4, D_4, E_4) und beeinträchtigen die Mikrozirkulation. Die Produktion von Leukotrienen im Endotoxinschock konnte nachgewiesen werden [1].

Stimulierte PMN-Leukozyten wiederum setzen toxische O_2-Radikale frei (sog. respiratory burst), welche durch Peroxidation von Membranlipiden direkt zellschädigend wirken und zu typischen Veränderungen der intrazellulären Schutzmechanismen, wie dem Glutathion-(GSH/GSSG)-System, führen.

Ziel der Arbeit war es daher zu untersuchen, inwieweit die Hemmung der 5- und 15-Lipoxigenase (LOX) in der Frühphase der Sepsis zu einer Minderung der durch O_2-Radikale induzierten Lipidperoxidation bzw. zur Verbesserung der Mikrozirkulation beiträgt.

Material und Methoden

Die Untersuchungen wurden randomisiert an insgesamt 70 männlichen Sprague-Dawley-Ratten mit einem mittleren Körpergewicht von 360 ± 60 g durchgeführt. Nach initialer Einleitung mit Äther wurde die Allgemeinnarkose mit Halothan (0,6–1 vol%) fortgeführt. Entsprechend der Randomisierung bekamen die Tiere danach entweder 50 mg/kg des 5- und 15-LOX-Hemmers mit sehr geringer Toxizität [2] FLM 5011 (Fahlberg-List Pharma, Magdeburg) oder gleiche Volumina des als Lösungsmittel fungierenden Olivenöls über eine Magensonde appliziert. Die Vena jugularis und Arteria carotis wurden zur Blutentnahme und Infusion bzw. zur Messung (Statham Db 23P) des Blutdruckes (MAP) kanüliert.

Nach medianer Laparotomie (Schnittlänge 3 cm) wurde die Durchblutung der Darmwand mittels Laser-Doppler-Flowmetrie (LDF) an der antimesenterialen Seite des Jejunums, 6 cm aboral der Einmündung des Ductus choledochus, gemessen (ALF 21, Advance Co., Ltd., Tokyo, Japan).

Chirurgisches Forum 1993
f. experim. u. klinische Forschung
Becker/Beger/Hartel (Hrsg.)

Die Sepsis wurde durch die Coecum-Ligatur-Punktions(CLP)-Technik induziert [3]. Vor sowie 30, 60 und 120 min nach Induktion der Sepsis wurden bei jeweils 10 Tieren MAP und LDF gemessen sowie 2 ml Blut zur Bestimmung von Endotoxin [Limulus-Test] und Prostanoiden ($PGF_{2\alpha}$, 6-keto $PGF_{1\alpha}$, TXB_2 mittels RIA]) entnommen. Mit einer in flüssigem N_2 vorgekühlten Wallenberg-Klemme wurde zu den entsprechenden Endzeitpunkten intravital 1 g Lebergewebe entnommen und darin anschließend folgende metabolische Parameter bestimmt: reduziertes (GSH) und oxidiertes (GSSG) Glutathion sowie die Myeloperoxidase (MPO) der Granulozyten [jeweils enzymatische Farbtests], die Lipidperoxidationsprodukte Malondialdehyd (MDA) [Fluoreszenzphotometrie] und konjugierte Diene [Spectralphotometrie] sowie die Purinmetabolite ATP, ADP und AMP [HPLC].

Da es sich um ein verbundenes bzw. unverbundenes Mehrstichprobenproblem handelt, wurden die parameterfreien Tests nach Friedman bzw. nach Kruskal-Wallis angewandt. Bei wiederholter Testung der gleichen Hypothese wurde der α-Fehler nach Bonferroni-Holm korrigiert.

Ergebnisse und Schlußfolgerungen

Die wichtigsten Ergebnisse sind in Tabelle 1 zusammengefaßt. Die Konzentration von Endotoxin im Blut stieg bereits 30 min nach Sepsisbeginn von 0,02 EU/ml auf $>$ 1,86 EU/ml und blieb während des gesamten Versuchszeitraumes sowohl bei den Kontroll- als auch bei den FLM-Tieren auf diesem erhöhten Niveau. Die ausgeprägte Endotoxinämie bereits nach 30 min beweist eindeutig die Effektivität der CLP-Technik als Sepsismodell.

Die Gewebskonzentrationen der MPO waren ab der 60. min in der FLM-gruppe im Vergleich zu den Kontrollen erniedrigt. Gleichzeitig lagen die Werte dieser Gruppe für GSH bzw. GSSG teilweise signifikant ($p < 0,05$) über bzw. unter den entsprechenden Werten der unbehandelten Ratten. Den gleichen Trend wiesen die Gewebekonzentrationen der konjugierten Diene bzw. von MDA auf. Der arterielle Druck sowie die Durchblutung der Dünndarmwand lagen zu allen Untersuchungszeitpunkten über dem der Kontrolltiere. FLM 5011 beeinflußt nicht die Produktion von Zyklooxigenaseprodukten, sondern hemmt lediglich die 5- und 15-LOX. Diese Inhibition bewirkt eine verbesserte Durchblutung des Dünndarms und weist somit indirekt auf eine Beteiligung von Lipoxigenasemetaboliten bei der Regulierung der Mikrozirkulation unter septischen Bedingungen hin.

Weder die Konzentrationen der einzelnen Prostanoide noch die der verschiedenen Purinmetabolite waren zwischen den Gruppen deutlich unterschiedlich.

LTB_4 besitzt eine starke chemotaktische Wirkung auf PMN-Leukozyten; bereits geringe Mengen induzieren eine Adhäsion von Leukozyten an das Endothel postkapillärer Venolen. Dies kann zu einer kurzzeitigen Stase führen und von einer (frühen) Diapedese und Migration der Leukozyten in den extravasalen Raum gefolgt sein [4]. Unter Behandlung mit FLM 5011 kommt es in der Leber im Vergleich zur Kontrolle zu einer Verminderung ($p < 0,05$) der MPO, welche als Marker der Stimulation von Leukozyten gilt. Diese Abnahme ist wahrscheinlich auf eine weniger ausgeprägte Bildung von LTB_4 zurückzuführen.

Tabelle 1. Änderungen von metabolischen und hämodynamischen Parametern vor (0-Wert) sowie 30, 60 und 120 min nach Induktion einer Sepsis

	0-Wert	30 min		60 min		120 min	
		KON	FLM	KON	FLM	KON	FLM
GSH [μmol/g Protein]	86 ± 4	60 ± 4	75[a] ± 3	48 ± 3	68[a] ± 3	46 ± 5	52 ± 5
GSSG [μmol/g Protein]	1,6 ± 0,2	2,2 ± 0,6	1,4[a] ± 0,2	2,9 ± 0,7	1,2[a] ± 0,2	2,4 ± 0,5	1,2[a] ± 0,2
MPO [μg/g Protein]	10,1 ± 1,5	18,2 ± 3,2	14,1 ± 1,1	19,1 ± 1,9	10,9[a] ± 1,4	13,7 ± 1,2	7,5[a] ± 0,9
KD [μmol/g Protein]	16,9 ± 4,1	12,6 ± 1,6	12,3 ± 0,8	12,5 ± 2,2	11,8 ± 0,4	11,6 ± 3,8	10,5 ± 1,2
MDA [μmol/g Protein]	411 ± 10	632 ± 10	557 ± 5	805 ± 15	739 ± 6	694 ± 4	538 ± 2
MAP [mm Hg]	102 ± 3,5	96 ± 2,7	113[a] ± 1,8	94 ± 2,5	106[a] ± 1,9	94 ± 3,4	103 ± 3,1
LDF [%]	100	45 ± 4,3	65[a] ± 3,1	40 ± 4,4	75[a] ± 3,2	57 ± 4,7	75 ± 4,1

GSH = reduziertes, GSSG = oxidiertes Glutathion; MPO = Myeloperoxidase der aktivierten Granulozyten; KD = konjugierte Diene; MDA = Malondialdehyd; MAP = Blutdruck; LDF = Durchblutung der Dünndarmwand; KON = Kontrolltiere; FLM = mit dem LOX-Hemmstoff vorbehandelte Ratten.

[a] $p < 0{,}05$ KON vs. FLM

Chemotaktisch akkumulierte Leukozyten wiederum setzen im Rahmen des "respiratory burst" über einen aktivierten Hexosemonophosphat-Shunt und das membranassoziierte NADPH-Oxidasesystem toxische O_2-Radikale frei. Diese besitzen eine hohe Affinität zu den Doppelbindungen von Membranlipiden und bewirken einerseits Membranschäden und andererseits wird die Freisetzung von Arachidonsäure aus der Phospholipidmembran stimuliert. Auf diese Weise wird der circulus vitiosus weiter unterhalten, woraus schlußendlich der Verlust der Zellintegrität resultiert. Metabolite und damit indirekte Parameter dieser Peroxidation von Membranlipiden sind die konjugierten Diene und das MDA. Nach Behandlung mit FLM 5011 ist in unserem Sepsismodell die Lipidperoxidation geringer ausgeprägt als bei den Kontrolltieren. Beweisend dafür ist auch das Verhalten des körpereigenen GSH/GSSG-Redoxsystems, welches als wirksamer Radikalenfänger fungiert. Bei den Kontrollratten kommt es bereits ab der 30. min zu einer Verminderung des reduzierten Glutathions, während das oxidierte GSSG ansteigt. Dies weist auf verstärkt abgelaufene oxidative Prozesse hin. Bei den FLM-Tieren sind diese Änderungen weit weniger stark ausgeprägt. Daraus kann auf einen abgeschwächten oxidativen Streß geschlossen werden.

Zusammenfassend kann man feststellen, daß die Hemmung der 5- und 15-Lipoxigenase zu einer Verbesserung der Mikrozirkulation und zu einer mäßiger ausgeprägten Generierung von O_2-Radikalen führt. Somit besitzt FLM 5011 in der Frühphase einer Sepsis (maximal 2 h nach Induktion) einen (indirekten) membranprotektiven Effekt.

Zusammenfassung

Am CLP-Sepsis-Modell der Ratte führt die Vorbehandlung mit einem 5- und 15-Lipoxigenase-(LOX)-Hemmer (FLM 5011) zu einer verminderten Aktivierung und somit Akkumulation von PMN-Leukozyten in der Leber während der Frühphase. Gleichzeitig fällt die Konzentration der reduzierten Form des Glutathions (GSH) im intrazellulären Redoxsystem deutlich geringer ab und ist nicht an einen simultanen Anstieg der oxidierten Form (GSSG) gekoppelt. Daraus sowie aus der (indirekt) nachgewiesenen geringeren Peroxidation der Membranlipide und aus den weniger stark ausgeprägten Mikrozirkulationsstörungen wird geschlossen, daß die Hemmung der 5- und 15-LOX eine mäßigere Generierung von O_2-Radikalen bedingt. FLM 5011 besitzt somit eine (indirekte) membranprotektive Wirksamkeit in der Frühphase der Sepsis.

Summary

The cecal ligation puncture (CLP) technique provides a feasible anomal model of sepsis for metabolic studies in rats. The aim of the study was to elucidate whether the pretreatment with the 5- and 15-lipoxygenase (LOX) inhibitor FLM 5011 attenuates the sequelae of the lipoxygenase pathway as well as the stimulation of polymorphonuclear (PMN) leukocytes and the generation of toxic oxygen radicals which occur during the early, compensatory phase of sepsis.

FLM pretreatment significantly reduced both the activation and accumulation of PMNs and hence the release of toxic oxygen species in liver tissue. The concomitant decrease in radical scavenger reduced glutathion (GSH) is, however, not accompanied by simultaneous increase in the oxidized metabolite (GSSG).

On the basis of these results as well as the lower lipid peroxidation of cell membranes – (indirectly) shown by the conjugated dienes ad malone dialdehyde – and the less pronounced deterioration of the microcirculation, respectively, we conclude that the inhibition of the 5- and 15-LOX leads to a moderate generation of O_2 radicals and hence mitigated tissue damage. Therefore, FLM 5011 seems suitable to protect (indirectly) the cell membranes during the early phase of sepsis.

Literatur

1. Hagmann W, Denzlinger C, Keppler D (1985) Production of peptide leukotrienes in endotoxin shock. FEBS Letters 180:309–313
2. Schewe T, Kühn H, Loose S, Lücke L (1991) Pharmacological profile, pharmacokinetics and biotransformation of the 5-lipoxygenase inhibitor FLM 5011. In: Bailey JM (ed) Prostaglandins, leukotrienes, lipoxins, and PAF. Plenum Press, New York, pp 383–397
3. Yelich MR (1990) Glucoregulatory, hormonal, and metabolic responses to endotoxicosis or cecal ligation and puncture sepsis in the rat. Circ Shock 31:351–363
4. Lindbom L, Hedqvist P, Dahlén SE, Lindgren JA, Arfors K-E (1982) Leukotriene B_4 induces extravasation and migration of polymorphnuclear leukocytes in vivo. Acta Physiol Scand 116:105–108

Dr. med. D. Moch, Sektion Chirurgische Forschung, Chirurgische Universitätsklinik Ulm, Oberer Eselsberg M25, W-7900 Ulm

Verlauf der Serumspiegel von TNF-α, IL-6 und CRP bei der postoperativen septischen Komplikation

Tumor Necrosis Factor (TNF) α, Interleukin (IL) 6, and C-Reactive Protein (CRP) in the Serum of Patients with Postoperative Septic Complications

W. Barthlen[1], N. Lehn[2], H. Bartels[1], M. Krönke[2], H. Wagner[2] und J.R. Siewert[1]

[1]Chirurgische Klinik und Poliklinik, Technische Universität München
[2]Institut für Medizinische Mikrobiologie und Hygiene, Technische Universität München

Einleitung

Postoperative septische Komplikationen, wie Peritonitis und Pneumonie, stellen die häufigste Ursache für die Letalität in der Abdominalchirurgie dar. Auch in der Unfallchirurgie sind es bei ständig verbesserten Therapiemöglichkeiten des initial hämorrhagisch-hypovolämischen Schocks heute hauptsächlich septische Spätkomplikationen, ausgehend von Weichteilen und Knochen oder vom Respirationstrakt, die für einen letalen Ausgang verantwortlich zu machen sind. Bei protrahiertem Verlauf oder nicht ausreichender chirurgischer Sanierung des septischen Fokus kommt es zu den bekannten Folgen der Sepsis wie akuter renaler Tubulusnekrose, mesenterialer Ischämie oder ARDS mit konsekutivem Multiorganversagen.

Die relativ stereotype Reaktion unterschiedlicher Organsysteme und Gewebeverbände legt als Ursache einen oder mehrere gemeinsame, humoral vermittelte Faktoren nahe. Tumornekrosefaktor α (TNF-α), ein 17-kD Polypeptid, scheint einer der wichtigsten proximalen Mediatoren in der gemeinsamen Endstrecke der Sepsis zu sein [1, 2, 3]. Es wird von Makrophagen und Kupfferzellen bei Aktivierung durch das Endotoxin gramnegativer Bakterien produziert [1, 4], spielt aber auch, wie in klinischen Studien vermutet [3] und tierexperimentell bereits nachgewiesen wurde, beim T-Zell vermittelten septischen Schock durch Endotoxine grampositiver Erreger eine entscheidende Rolle. Die zentrale Bedeutung von TNF-α bei Sepsis wird dadurch verdeutlicht, daß C3H/HeJ Mäuse mit einem genetischen Defekt der TNF-Synthese resistent gegen Endotoxin sind [2], und daß in mehreren tierexperimentellen Studien durch i.v. Gabe von monoklonalen TNF-Antikörpern ein vollständiger Schutz vor den Folgen einer LD100 Endotoxin- oder E. coli-Infusion erreicht werden konnte [1, 2]. Hohe Serumspiegel von zirkulierendem TNF-α wurden bei Freiwilligen nach i.v. Endotoxingabe [2] und bei Patienten im septischen Schock gefunden und korrelierten mit dem klinischen Verlauf und der Letalität [1, 3].

Ein weiteres wichtiges Mediator-Polypeptid ist das Interleukin-6 (IL-6), ebenfalls ein Produkt von Makrophagen, Kupffer- und Endothelzellen nach Aktivierung durch Endotoxin und TNF [1, 5]. IL-6 induziert die Produktion der Akutphasenproteine

Chirurgisches Forum 1993
f. experim. u. klinische Forschung
Becker/Beger/Hartel (Hrsg.)

durch Hepatozyten [4]. Bei chirurgischen Patienten wurden hohe Serumspiegel von IL-6 intra- und postoperativ gemessen, die mit der Dauer und dem Ausmaß des operativen Traumas korrelierten [5]. Das C-reaktive Protein (CRP) ist das bekannteste der Akutphasenproteine und findet weithin Verwendung als diagnostischer Parameter für akute und chronische Entzündungen.

Ziel der Studie war es, bei chirurgischen Patienten mit postoperativen septischen Komplikationen nach einer Korrelation der Serumspiegel von TNF-α, IL-6 und CRP mit dem Schweregrad von Sepsis und Multiorganversagen zu suchen.

Patienten und Methodik

13 Pat. mit postoperativer Peritonitis und 4 Pat. mit respiratorpflichtiger postoperativer Pneumonie wurden untersucht. Als Kontrollen dienten 20 Pat. nach großen viszeralchirurgischen Eingriffen und unkompliziertem Verlauf. Vollblut zur Bestimmung der Serumspiegel von TNF-α, IL-6 und CRP wurde über einen Zeitraum von 14 Tagen nach Beginn der Sepsis bzw. bei den Kontrollpatienten während der ersten 3 postoperativen Tage täglich um 9 Uhr abgenommen. Das Serum wurde bis zu einer Woche bei −30°C gelagert. TNF-α und IL-6 wurden mit Enzym-Immunoassays in Mikrotiterplatten mit 96 Vertiefungen bestimmt (Fa. Medgenix, Ratingen, BRD). Beide Tests basieren auf einem oligoklonalen System, bei dem verschiedene monoklonale Antikörper eingesetzt werden, die gegen unterschiedliche Epitope auf dem TNF-α bzw. IL-6 Molekül gerichtet sind. Als Marker-Enzym wird Meerrettich-Peroxidase verwendet. Die Nachweisgrenzen liegen bei 5 pg/ml und 3 pg/ml. Nach Herstellerangaben bestehen keine Kreuzreaktionen von TNF-α mit TNF-β oder von IL-6 mit TNF-α und TNF-β. CRP wurde im Serum mit partikelverstärkter Nephelometrie gemessen (Fa. Behring, Marburg, BRD). Die Obergrenze des Referenzbereichs für CRP im Serum gesunder Erwachsener liegt bei 5 mg/l und die Nachweisgrenze bei 2,5 mg/l.

Das Ausmaß von Sepsis und Organversagen wurde anhand etablierter Scores (APACHE II, Elebute-Stoner, Sepsis Severity Score) quantifiziert. Die statistischen Analysen wurden unter Benutzung von Pearson's Korrelationskoeffizient (SPSS, Chicago, Illinois, USA) durchgeführt.

Ergebnisse

Bei starken Schwankungen sowohl individuell als auch innerhalb der einzelnen Gruppen waren zum Krankheitsbeginn die Serumspiegel von TNF-α und IL-6 sowohl bei Patienten mit Peritonitis (38 ± 13 pg/ml / 1191 ± 253 pg/ml) als auch bei Pneumonie (26 ± 21 pg/ml / 1059 ± 588 pg/ml) deutlich gegenüber den Werten der Kontrollpatienten am 1. postop. Tag (11 ± 1 pg/ml / 435 ± 82 pg/ml) erhöht. Während des Verlaufs kam es bei den Patienten mit Peritonitis in der 2. Behandlungswoche noch zu einem Anstieg der TNF-α Werte (Abb. 1A), wohingegen die TNF-Spiegel in der Pneumonie-Gruppe konstant nur mäßig erhöht blieben (Abb. 1B). IL-6 war bei Patienten mit persistierender abdominaler Sepsis deutlich mit Spitzenwerten $>$ 2000 pg/ml erhöht (Abb. 1C), und fiel nach einem initialen Peak sowohl bei den Kontrollpati-

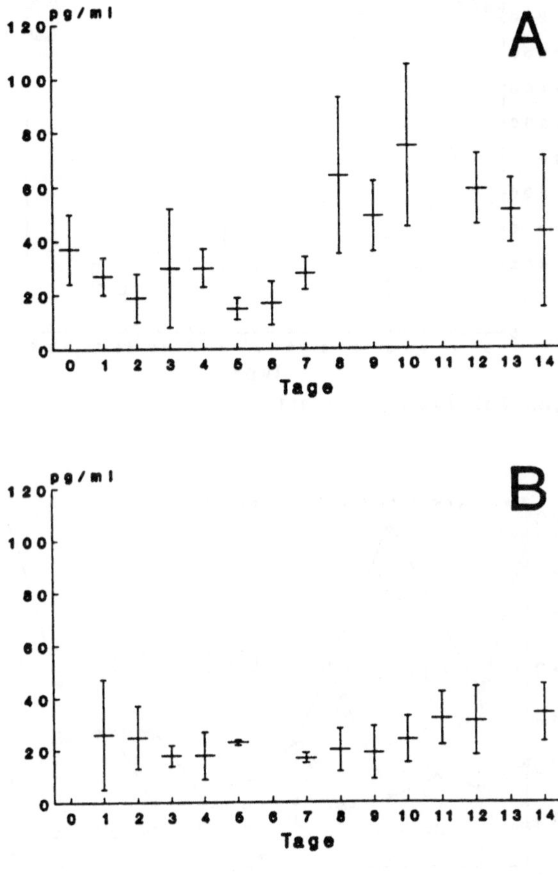

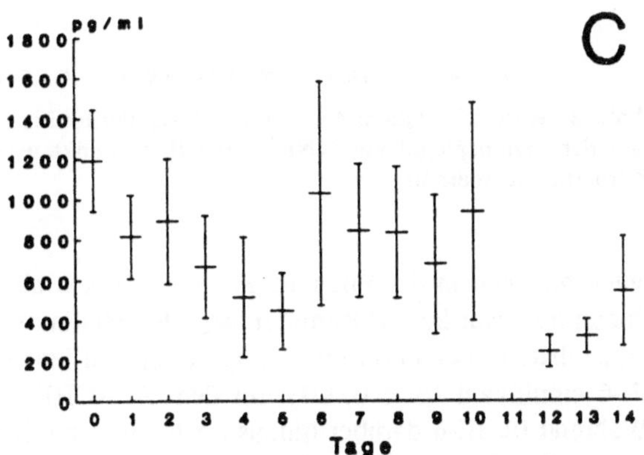

Abb. 1 A–D. Verlauf der Serumspiegel (Mittelwerte ± SEM) für TNF-α bei **A** Peritonitis (n = 13) und **B** Pneumonie (n = 4) und für Il-6 bei **C** Peritonitis (n = 13) und **D** Pneumonie (n = 4)

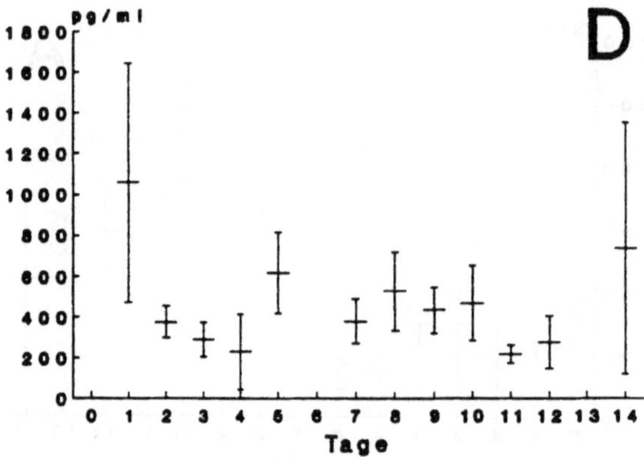

Abb. 1 D. Legende s. S. 411

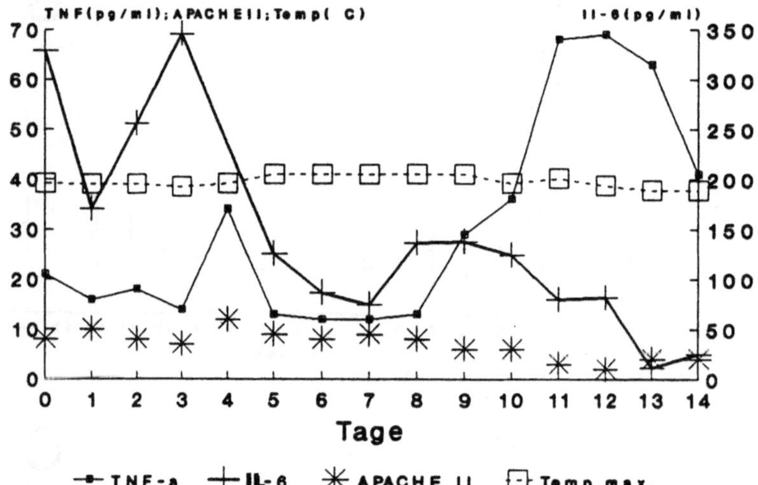

Abb. 2. Kasuistik Patient 45 J. mit diffuser Peritonitis aufgrund einer Duodenalleckage: Verlauf der Serumspiegel von TNF-α und IL-6, Punktewerte APACHE II Score und maximale Körperkerntemperatur

enten als auch in der Pneumonie-Gruppe rasch ab (Abb. 1D). Bei den Patienten mit Pneumonie war kein Zusammenhang der Mediatorspiegel mit dem klinischen Verlauf erkennbar. In der Peritonitisgruppe hingegen korrelierten die Werte von TNF-α und IL-6 signifikant ($p < 0{,}001$) mit dem APACHE II und dem Sepsis Severity Score. Während für IL-6 darüber hinaus noch eine signifikante Korrelation mit dem Elebute-Stoner Sepsisscore, Körperkerntemperatur und Organversagen nachgewiesen wurde, war dies für TNF-α nicht der Fall: Erhöhte Werte wurden sowohl präfinal (259 pg/ml), als auch bei klinischer Verbesserung des Patienten (98 pg/ml) mit sogar noch steigender Tendenz während der Erholungsphase vom Multiorganversagen gemessen (Abb. 2).

Das CRP lag während des gesamten Beobachtungszeitraums unspezifisch bei allen Patienten zwischen 100 und 300 mg/l und ließ bei den Studienpatienten zu keinem Zeitpunkt einen Zusammenhang mit dem postoperativen Verlauf erkennen. In der Kontrollgruppe war am 1. postop. Tag ein kurzfristiger Peak von IL-6 und am 2. postop. Tag von CRP zu beobachten.

Diskussion

Wir fanden bei chirurgischen Patienten mit postoperativen septischen Komplikationen erhöhte Serumspiegel von TNF-α gegenüber Kontrollpatienten mit unkompliziertem Verlauf. In der Peritonitisgruppe war im Mittel in der 2. Behandlungswoche noch ein Anstieg zu verzeichnen. Diese Daten müssen mit Vorsicht interpretiert werden, da bei TNF-α der Zeitpunkt der Blutabnahme im Sepsisverlauf von größter Bedeutung ist [2]. Ein septisches Geschehen bei Patienten entspricht mit wenigen Ausnahmen (z.B. fulminante Meningokokkensepsis) nicht der experimentellen Situation mit zeitlich und mengenmäßig definierter Toxingabe [3]. Viele Anhaltspunkte sprechen dafür, daß TNF-α während einer Endotoxinämie zum größten Teil initial ausgeschüttet wird [2], so daß bei der extrem kurzen Halbwertszeit von ca. 15 min hohe TNF-α Spiegel im Serum septischer Patienten nur ein transientes Ereignis sind [1, 2]. Hinzu kommt, daß der Anteil des biologisch inaktiven, an Rezeptoren, Proteine, Inhibitoren gebundenen TNF-α noch weitgehend unbekannt ist [3]. In der Pneumoniegruppe sprechen mäßig erhöhte, aber konstante Serumspiegel von TNF-α für einen "steady state" in der Konzentration der TNF-α Induktoren. Anders bei den Peritonitis-Patienten: Hier führen die Überschwemmung des Organismus mit Krankheitserregern bei nicht saniertem septischen Fokus sowie die Manipulationen des Intestinums während der chirurgischen Therapie wahrscheinlich zur multiplen Freisetzung von Endo- und Exotoxinen mit resultierender Mediatorausschüttung [3].

Das Fehlen einer Korrelation zwischen hohen Serumspiegeln von TNF-α und der Letalität bei septischen Patienten in dieser und anderen Studien [3] ist einerseits mit dem erwähnten Problem des Abnahmezeitpunkts der Serumproben erklärbar [2]. Zum anderen sprechen hohe TNF-α Serumspiegel während der Erholungsphase vom Organversagen für die Existenz nicht nur von deletären, sondern auch günstigen Effekten von TNF-α auf die Immunantwort des Patienten [1]. Hier sind noch viele Fragen offen, und die Rolle von TNF-α in der klinischen Situation des septischen Patienten, ob schädlich oder nützlich, ist weiterhin umstritten. Neben den Serumspiegeln von TNF-α wird in Zukunft auch die lokale TNF-α Konzentration, z.B. im RES oder ZNS, Beachtung finden müssen [1, 2].

Serumspiegel von IL-6 korrelierten in dieser und anderen Studien [3, 4, 5] bei Patienten mit postoperativen septischen Komplikationen signifikant mit der klinischen Schwere von Sepsis und Organversagen. IL-6 ist ein sensibler Maßstab für ein Gewebetrauma [5]. Eine mögliche Rolle als diagnostische Hilfe bei Therapieentscheidungen bedarf noch der weiteren Klärung.

Die Bestimmung von CRP bietet in der postoperativen Phase keine differentialdiagnostische Information. Die zeitliche Verzögerung des CRP-Peaks um 1 Tag im

Vergleich zu IL-6 in der Kontrollgruppe bestätigt die Induktion von CRP durch IL-6 [5].

Zusammenfassung

Ziel der Studie war es, nach einer Korrelation der Serumspiegel von TNF-α, IL-6 und CRP mit dem Schweregrad von Sepsis und Multiorganversagen während des Krankheitsverlaufs von 13 Pat. mit postoperativer Peritonitis und 4 Pat. mit respiratorpflichtiger postoperativer Pneumonie zu suchen. Bei starken Schwankungen sowohl individuell als auch innerhalb der einzelnen Gruppen waren zum Krankheitsbeginn die Serumspiegel von TNF-α / IL-6 sowohl bei Pat. mit Peritonitis (38 ± 13 pg/ml / 1191 ± 253 pg/ml) als auch bei Pneumonie (26 ± 21 pg/ml / 1059 ± 588 pg/ml) gegenüber den Werten von 20 Kontrollpatienten am 1. postoperativen Tag (11 ± 1 pg/ml / 435 ± 82 pg/ml) erhöht (Mittelwerte ± SEM). Das CRP lag unspezifisch bei allen Patienten zwischen 100 und 300 mg/l. Nach einem initialen Peak fiel IL-6 in der Pneumonie- und Kontrollgruppe rasch ab, blieb aber bei Pat. mit Peritonitis deutlich mit Einzelwerten > 2000 pg/ml während des Beobachtungszeitraums (14 Tage) erhöht. In der Pneumoniegruppe war keine Korrelation zwischen Mediatorspiegel und klinischem Verlauf feststellbar. Dagegen bestand in der Peritonitisgruppe eine signifikante Korrelation ($p < 0{,}001$, Perason's Korrelationskoeffizient) zwischen den Serumwerten von TNF-α und IL-6 mit dem APACHE II- und dem Sepsis Severity Score, jedoch nicht mit der Letalität. Hohe TNF-α Werte wurden sowohl präfinal (259 pg/ml), als auch bei klinischer Verbesserung des Patienten (98 pg/ml) mit sogar noch steigender Tendenz während der Erholungsphase vom Multiorganversagen gemessen.

Summary

The aim of the study was to look for a correlation of tumor necrosis factor α (TNF-α), interleukin 6 (IL-6), and C-reactive protein (CRP) serum levels with the severity of sepsis and multiple organ failure in 13 patients with postoperative peritonitis and 4 patients with postoperative pneumonia requiring ventilation. Values varied considerably. At the beginning, serum levels of TNF-α and IL-6 were increased in the peritonitis group (38 ± 13 pg/ml and 1191 ± 253 pg/ml, respectively) as well as in the patients with pneumonia (26 ± 21 pg/ml and 1059 ± 588 pg/ml) compared to controls (11 ± 1 pg/ml and 435 ± 82 pg/ml, respectively; mean ± SEM). CRP levels varied between 100 and 300 mg/l in all patients. After an initial peak, levels of IL-6 decreased quickly in the patients with pneumonia and controls, but remained high (> 2000 pg/ml) in patients with peritonitis. No correlation of the cytokine levels with the clinical course was found in the pneumonia group. In patients with peritonitis, however, a significant correlation ($p < 0{,}001$, Pearson's correlation coefficient) was found between serum levels of both TNF-α and IL-6 with the acute physiology and chronic health evaluation (APACHE) II and sepsis severity score. As far as survival was concerned, no correlation could be found in any group. High values of TNF-α

were observed in both moribund patients (259 pg/ml) and in patients recovering from multiple organ failure (98 pg/ml).

Literatur

1. Marano MA, Fong Y, Moldawer LL, Wei H, Calvano SE, Tracey KJ, Barie PS, Manogue K, Cerami A, Shires GT, Lowry SF (1990) Serum cachectin/tumor necrosis factor in critically ill patients with burns correlates with infection and mortality. Surg Gynecol Obstet 170:32–38
2. Michie HR, Manogue KR, Spriggs DR, Revhaug A, O'Dwyer S, Dinarello CA, Cerami A, Wolff SM, Wilmore DW (1988) Detection of circulating tumor necrosis factor after endotoxin administration. New Engl J Med 318:1481–1486
3. Calandra T, Baumgartner JD, Grau GE, Wu MM, Lambert PH, Schellekens J, Verhoef J, Glauser MP, and the Swiss-Dutch J5 Immunoglobulin Study Group (1990) Prognostic values of tumor necrosis factor/cachectin, interleukin-1, interferon-a, and interferon-y in the serum of patients with septic shock. J Infect Dis 161:982–987
4. Waage A, Brandtzaeg P, Halstensen A, Kierulf P, Espevik T (1989) The complex pattern of cytokines in serum from patients with meningococcal septic shock. J Exp Med 169:333–338
5. Cruickshank AM, Fraser WD, Burns HJG, Van Damme J, Shenkin A (1990) Response of serum interleukin-6 in patients undergoing elective surgery of varying severity. Clin Sci 79:161–165

Dr. W. Barthlen, Chirurgische Klinik und Poliklinik der Technischen Universität, Klinikum rechts der Isar, Ismaninger Straße 22, W-8000 München 80

Einfluß von AICA Ribosid auf die Reperfusionsschäden nach intestinaler Ischämie*

The Involvement of 5-Amino-4-Imidazolecarboxamide (AICA) Ribonucleotide on Reperfusion Damage After Intestinal Ischemia

M.H. Schoenberg[1], B. Poch[1], D. Moch[2] und H.G. Beger[1]

[1]Abteilung für Allgemeine Chirurgie, Chirurgische Universitätsklinik, Ulm (Direktor: Prof. Dr. H.G. Beger)
[2]Sektion Chirurgische Forschung, Chirurgische Universitätsklinik, Ulm (Leiter: Prof. Dr. U.B. Brückner)

Einleitung

Hämorrhagische Schleimhautschäden des Dünndarms werden häufig bei Patienten beobachtet, die nur kurzzeitig einen hämorrhagischen oder kardiogenen Schock überlebten und an einem akuten Verschluß der Mesenterialgefäße litten. Anhand tierexperimenteller Studien der zeitlich begrenzten und partiellen Ischämie konnte gezeigt werden, daß ein erheblicher Teil dieser Mukosaschäden nicht nur durch die vorangegangene Ischämie bedingt ist, sondern auch nach Wiederdurchblutung des Dünndarms entsteht. Nach Reoxygenierung des Darms entstehen sogenannte Sauerstoffradikale, die durch Lipidperoxidation die Zellmembran schädigen. Gleichzeitig induzieren Sauerstoffradikale die Akkumulation, Adhäsion und Aktivierung von PMN-Leukozyten im Darmgewebe. Einstrom und Aktivierung der PMN-Leukozyten sind in der späteren Reperfusionsphase hauptverantwortlich für die zu beobachtenden Mukosaschäden [1]. Verschiedene Pathomechanismen, die die gesteigerte Adhärenz der PMN-Leukozyten steuern, werden derzeit diskutiert. Nach ersten Untersuchungen scheinen jedoch der Adenosinstoffwechsel sowie die Adenosinrezeptoren der PMN-Leukozyten eine zentrale Rolle zu spielen. In in vitro-Versuchen wurde festgestellt, daß Adenosin die Adhärenz von PMN-Leukozyten und die weitere Freisetzung von Sauerstoffradikalen verhindert. Gleichzeitig jedoch steigert Adenosin paradoxerweise die Chemotaxis der PMN-Leukozyten [2]. Ungeklärt ist, welchen Einfluß Adenosin letztlich auf die postischämischen Schäden der Darmmukosa in vivo hat. 5-Amino-4-Imidazolcarboxamidribosid (AICAR) kann durch Hemmung der Adenosindeaminase den Abbau von Adenosin zu Inosin verhindern und damit die Adenosinkonzentration im Blut wie im Gewebe erhöhen. Ziel der vorliegenden Arbeit war es festzustellen, inwieweit durch die Behandlung mit AICAR der Purinstoffwechsel nach intestinaler Ischämie und Reperfusion verändert werden kann und welchen Einfluß

* Diese Studie wurde durch die Deutsche Forschungsgemeinschaft (Projekt Scho 309/1-4) gefördert.

Chirurgisches Forum 1993
f. experim. u. klinische Forschung
Becker/Beger/Hartel (Hrsg.)

eine Erhöhung der Adenosinkonzentration im Darmgewebe auf die Akkumulation der PMN-Leukozyten und damit auf die Mukosaschäden nach Reperfusion hat.

Methodik

Bei 12 Katzen wurde ein von der Arteria mesenterica superior perfundiertes Dünndarmsegment isoliert. Durch Stenosierung der Arteria mesenterica superior wurde der Blutfluß für 2 h auf 10% des Ausgangswertes vermindert. Anschließend wurde die Stenose entfernt und die Tiere eine weitere Stunde nachbeobachtet. 30 min vor Ischämie bis 30 min nach Reperfusionsbeginn wurden 6 Tiere mit AICAR (2,5 mg/min × kg KG) als kontinuierliche intravenöse Infusion behandelt. Vor und 2 h nach intestinaler Ischämie sowie 10 und 60 min nach Reperfusion wurden Gewebeproben entnommen. Im Gewebe wurden die Metabolite des Purinstoffwechsels ATP, ADP, AMP, Adenosin, Inosin, Hypoxanthin, Xanthin und Harnsäure mittels HPLC bestimmt [3]. Ebenso wurde als Maß der Leukozytenakkumulation die Myeloperoxidase (MPO) gemessen. Die Schleimhautschäden wurden konsekutiv nach Chiu et al. histologisch beurteilt [4].

Ergebnisse

Während der intestinalen Ischämie kommt es bei den *unbehandelten* Tieren zu einem deutlichen Abfall der energiereichen Phosphate und zu einem Anstieg der Adenosin- wie Hypoxanthinkonzentrationen. Nach Reperfusion steigen die energiereichen Phosphate deutlich an, ohne jedoch die Kontrollwerte zu erreichen. Die Adenosinkonzentrationen im Darmgewebe fallen innerhalb einer Stunde nach Reperfusion auf das Kontrollniveau ab (s. Abb. 1). Die MPO-Konzentrationen aller Tiere zeigen während der intestinalen Ischämie keinen wesentlichen Anstieg. Nach Reperfusion kommt es bei den *unbehandelten* Tieren jedoch zu einem vierfachen Anstieg der MPO-Konzentrationen als Zeichen einer erheblichen PMN-Leukozytenakkumulation im Gewebe (Abb. 2). In gleicher Weise entwickeln sich die histologischen Veränderungen. Nach intestinaler Ischämie zeigt die Mukosa nur geringfügige Schäden im Bereich der Zottenspitzen. Parallel zur Erhöhung der MPO jedoch lassen sich bereits 10 min nach Reperfusionsbeginn deutliche bis schwere Schleimhautschäden erkennen, die in der späten Reperfusionsphase (nach einer Stunde) deutlich zunehmen (s. Abb. 3).

Die Behandlung mit *AICAR* hat nur geringgradigen Einfluß auf ATP, ADP und AMP während Ischämie und Reperfusion. Die Adenosinkonzentrationen jedoch bleiben auch nach Reperfusion deutlich erhöht ($p < 0,05$) und fallen erst *nach* Beendigung der AICAR-Infusion deutlich ab (s. Abb. 1). Gleichzeitig verhindert AICAR über erhöhte Adenosinkonzentrationen im Gewebe die Akkumulation von PMN-Leukozyten in der Reperfusionsphase. Nach Beendigung der AICAR-Infusion jedoch steigen die MPO-Konzentrationen deutlich an ($p < 0,02$) (s. Abb. 2). Konsequenterweise verbessert AICAR durch Verhinderung der Akkumulation und Aktivierung der PMN-Leukozyten die schweren Schleimhautschäden wie sie bei den unbehandelten Tieren in der späten Reperfusionsphase beobachtet wurden. Bis zum Ende des Versuchszeit-

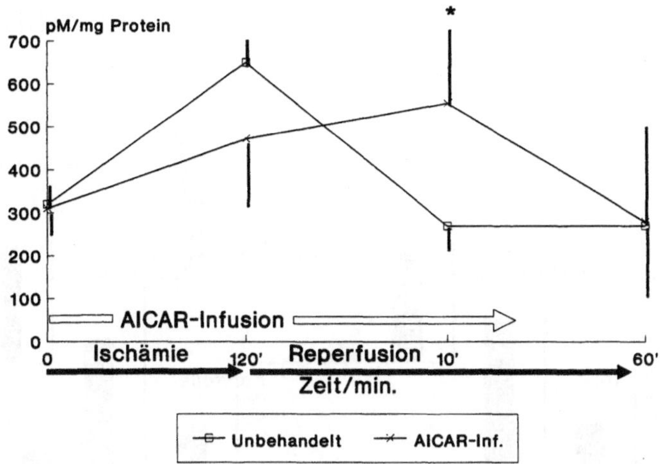

Abb. 1. Die Veränderungen der Adenosinkonzentration bei unbehandelten und AICAR-behandelten Tieren während intestinaler Ischämie und nach Reperfusion

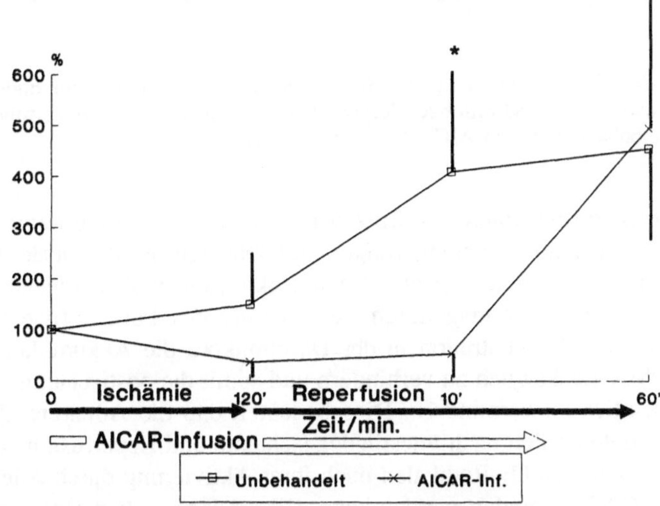

Abb. 2. Die Veränderungen der Myeloperoxidase als Maß der Akkumulation von PMN-Leukozyten bei unbehandelten und AICAR-behandelten Tieren während intestinaler Ischämie und nach Reperfusion in Prozent (Kontrolle ≙ 100%)

raumes überwiegen bei den AICAR-behandelten Katzen nur leichte Veränderungen der Darmmukosa (s. Abb. 3).

Diskussion

Nach intestinaler Ischämie kommt es zu einem Abfall energiereicher Phosphate und Anstieg des Adenosins. Die Schleimhautschäden sind eher gering ausgeprägt. Nach

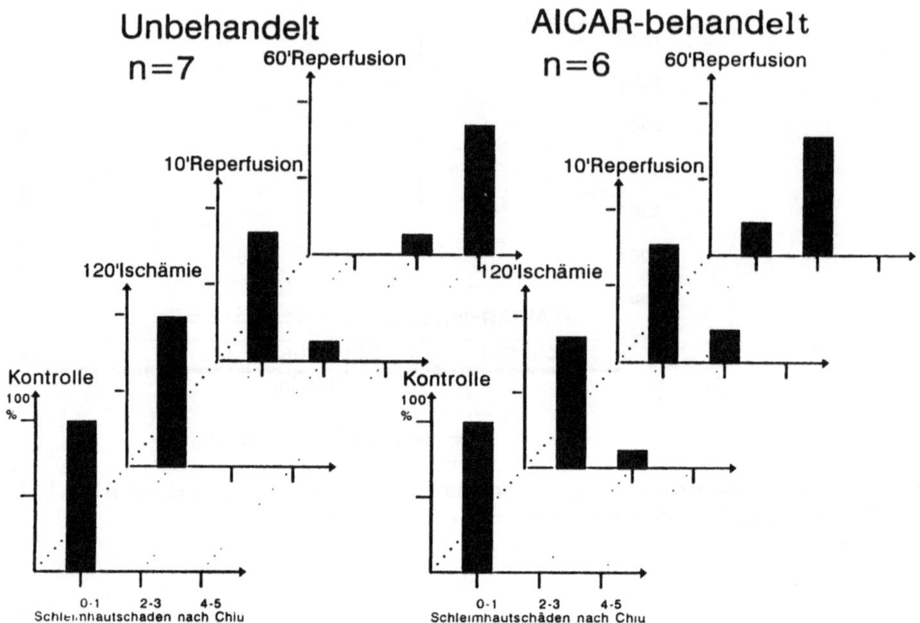

Abb. 3. Die Einteilung der Schleimhautschäden vor und am Ende der intestinalen Ischämie sowie 10 und 60 min nach Reperfusion nach dem Graduierungsschema von Chiu et al. [4] bei unbehandelten und AICAR-behandelten Tieren

Reperfusion kommt es trotz Wiederherstellung des Energiestoffwechsels zu schweren Schleimhautveränderungen des Dünndarms, die ursächlich mit der Akkumulation und Aktivierung der PMN-Leukozyten in Zusammenhang stehen [1]. AICAR-Behandlung vermag durch Veränderung des Purinstoffwechsels und Erhöhung der Adenosinkonzentration in der Darmmukosa die Akkumulation und Aktivierung von PMN-Leukozyten zu verhindern und somit die postischämischen Schleimhautschäden deutlich zu vermindern. Dies bedeutet, daß die Adhärenz der PMN-Leukozyten an Endothelzellen nach intestinaler Ischämie und Reperfusion sowie die vermehrte Freisetzung von O_2-Radikalen nach ihrer Aktivierung durch Adenosin bzw. Analoga wie AICAR verhindert werden kann. Eine Adenosin-bedingte Steigerung der Chemotaxis konnte anhand unserer Versuche nicht bestätigt werden.

Zusammenfassung

In einem Modell der intestinalen Ischämie und Reperfusion bei Katzen untersuchten wir die Wertigkeit des Adenosinstoffwechsels auf die postischämische Akkumulation und Aktivierung von PMN-Leukozyten. An 12 Katzen wurde eine intestinale Ischämie durch Stenosierung der Arteria mesenterica superior für zwei Stunden induziert, anschließend wurde die Stenose eröffnet und die Tiere eine Stunde nachbeobachtet. Sechs Katzen erhielten 30 min vor Ischämie bzw. 30 min nach Reperfusionsbeginn 5-Amino-4-Imidazolcarboxamidribosid (AICAR) in der Dosierung von 2,5 mg/min/kg

KG i.v. als kontinuierliche Infusion verabreicht. Im Gewebe wurden die Metabolite des Purinstoffwechsels und die Myeloperoxidase gemessen sowie die Schleimhautschäden histologisch beurteilt. AICAR führte durch Hemmung der Adenosindeaminase zu einer hohen Gewebskonzentration von Adenosin nicht nur während intestinaler Ischämie, sondern auch nach Reperfusion. Diese hohe Gewebskonzentration von Adenosin verhindert in dieser Phase die normalerweise zu beobachtende Akkumulation von PMN-Leukozyten. Folglich kam es zu keiner Zunahme der Schleimhautschäden in der Reperfusionsphase. Das heißt, die Schleimhautschäden waren wesentlich geringer als in der unbehandelten Gruppe. Die Modulation der Leukozytenadhärenz durch Adenosin scheint somit eine entscheidende Bedeutung für die Ausbildung der radikalisch bedingten Mukosaschäden zu haben.

Summary

We used a model of intestinal ischemia and reperfusion in 12 cats which were subjected to intestinal ischemia für 2 hours and 1 hour of reperfusion, respectively. Six cats were treated with 5-amino-4-imidazolecarboxamide ribonucleotide (AICAR) (dosage: 2.5 mg/min kg^{-1} body weight) as an continuous intravenous infusion. Treatment was started 30 min before ischemia lasting until 30 min after reperfusion. Before and 2 hours after ischemia as well as 10 and 60 min after reperfusion, tissue samples were excised for measurement of the purine metabolites and myeloperoxidase. Moreover, the tissue samples were examined histologically. AICAR treatment led to an increase of adenosine concentrations within the intestinal tissue, not only during ischemia but also during reperfusion. Consequently, these high adenosine concentrations inhibited the accumulation of polymorphonuclear (PMN) leukocytes as shown by low levels of myeloperoxidase. Concomitantly, histological examination revealed significant protection against postischemic damages after AICAR therapy. We conclude that high adenosine concentrations induced by AICAR treatment prevent PMN leukocyte accumulation and activation within the intestinal ischemia during the postischemic phase, thus preventing the aggravation of mucosal lesions normally observed in untreated cats.

Literatur

1. Schoenberg MH, Poch B, Younes M, Schwarz A, Baczako K, Lundberg C, Haglund U, Beger HG (1991) Involvement of neutrophils in postischemic damage to the small intestine. Gut 32:905–912
2. Cronstein BN, Daguma L, Nichols D, Hutchison AJ, Williams M (1990) The adenosine/neutrophil paradox resolved: human neutrophils possess both A1 and A2 receptors that promote chemotaxis and inhibit O_2-generation, respectively. J Clin Invest 85:1150–1157
3. Fredholm BB, Solevi A (1981) The release of adenosine/inosine from subcutaneous adiposed tissue by nerve stimulation and noradrenalin. J Physiol 313:351–367

4. Chiu CJ, McArdle AH, Brown R, Scott HJ, Fraser NG (1970) Intestinal mucosal lesions in low flow states. Arch Surg 101:478–483

PD Dr. med. M.H. Schoenberg, Abteilung für Allgemeine Chirurgie, Chirurgische Universitätsklinik Ulm, Steinhövelstraße 9, W-7900 Ulm

Serosa-Kalium-Aktivität, Elektromyographie und Schockmediator-Profile bei der experimentellen arteriellen und kombiniert arterio-venösen Dünndarmischämie

Serosa Potassium, Electromyography and Mediator Profiles in Arterial and Combined Arteriovenous Small-Bowel Ischemia

Ch. Töns[1], B. Klosterhalfen[1], M. Anurov[2], B.S. Titkova[2], A. Öttinger[2] und V. Schumpelick[1]

[1]Chirurgische Klinik, RWTH Aachen
[2]I. Medical Institute, Dept. Physiology of Digestion, Moskau, Rußland

Einleitung

Intestinale Ischämie und Mikrozirkulationsstörungen sind insbesondere hinsichtlich der als wesentlich diskutierten Rolle des Gastrointestinaltraktes im Geschehen der Sepsis und dem Übergang in ein Multiorganversagen von Bedeutung. Eine meßtechnisch gestützte qualitative Beurteilung der zellulären Integrität scheint mittels Elektromyographie und neuerdings auch mit dem nichtinvasiven Monitoring der Kalium-Aktivität auf der Serosa [1] möglich. In einem standardisierten Modell sollte mit diesen Meßverfahren und analogen Schockmediatorprofilen eine selektiv arterielle sowie eine kombiniert arteriovenöse Dünndarmischämie differenziert untersucht werden, um weiterreichende Erkenntnisse über die Bedeutung des Darmes in der Sepsis zu erhalten.

Methodik

Nach Erteilung der Tierversuchsgenehmigung durch den hiesigen Regierungspräsidenten und das Gesundheitsministerium in Rußland wurde die experimentelle Untersuchung an 12 Bastardhunden in Intubationsnarkose mit Thiopental und Fentanyl-Analgesie durchgeführt. Nach Laparotomie, Splenektomie und Katheterplazierung (V. femoralis, V. porta, A. femoralis) erfolgte die Präparation der Mesenterialwurzel und anschließende Isolierung je eines 150 cm langen Dünndarmsegmentes mit Skelettierung des Mesos sowie Querdurchtrennung des Darmes zur Vermeidung einer Kollateralperfusion. In der Mitte des ausgeschalteten Segmentes wurde eine 5 cm lange antimesenteriale Enterotomie für vergleichende Mukosamessungen durchgeführt. Die EMG-Bipolarelektrode wurde 10 cm oral der Enterotomiestelle mit 2 Serosanähten fixiert. Nach Klarspülung des ausgeschalteten Segmentes mit NaCl-Lösung wurde zur Normalisierung der traumatisch erhöhten Mediatoren eine manipulationsfreie 2stündige steady-state Phase eingehalten.

Chirurgisches Forum 1993
f. experim. u. klinische Forschung
Becker/Beger/Hartel (Hrsg.)

Die 12 Versuchstiere waren in 3 Gruppen eingeteilt: in der Gruppe A erfolgte die Auslösung einer selektiv arteriellen Ischämie der das isolierte Segment versorgenden Arterie, in der Gruppe B wurde entsprechend eine kombiniert arterio-venöse Ischämie erzeugt. Die Gruppe C war die Kontrollgruppe, bei der keine Gefäßokklusion durchgeführt wurde. Als Beobachtungsdauer waren 6 h nach Ablauf der steady-state Phase in allen Gruppen vorgesehen.

Die EMG-Ableitung erfolgte mit einem Mingograf-Gerät (Fa. Siemens) mit einer Eingangsempfindlichkeit < 1 mV. Die ionenselektive Messung der Kalium-Aktivität (a K^+) erfolgte mit dem OMS-Gerät der Fa. Medimon durch Aufsetzen des Sensors vergleichend auf die Serosa 5 cm aboral der EMG-Elektrode und auf die Mukosa im Bereich der Enterotomiestelle. Der Anpreßdruck des Sensors war durch sein Eigengewicht standardisiert.

Nach definiertem engmaschigen Profil erfolgten EMG und a K^+_{s+m}-Messungen. Zum Beginn sowie nach 2, 4 und 6 h der Ischämiedauer wurde ein Laborstatus (u.a. Mediatoren TNF, IL-1, IL-6, IL-8 und $PGF_{1\alpha}$ – in der Verarbeitungs- und Bestimmungstechnik wie in [2] dargestellt) durchgeführt. Zu den gleichen Zeitpunkten erfolgten Blutgasanalysen aus der A. femoralis, der V. porta und der betroffenen mesenterialen Segmentvene sowie Gewebsprobenentnahmen für die elektronenmikroskopische und histologische Aufarbeitung. Zur statistischen Analyse wurde der t-Test eingesetzt.

Ergebnisse

Das Versuchskonzept konnte bei 11 der 12 Hunde eingehalten werden, lediglich ein Tier der Gruppe B (kombinierte Ischämie) verstarb während der Versuchsdauer nach 180 min Ischämiedauer.

EMG Amplitude und Frequenz wie auch dic a K^+ auf Serosa und Mukosa zeigten bei der Gruppe A deutlich blandere Ischämiereaktionen als bei der Gruppe B.

Werte der a K^+ in mmol/l nach 60 min: Serosa Gr. A: 22,7 (SD 7,3), Gr. B: 31,6 (SD 3,9) [p = 0,038]; Mukosa Gr. A: 40,1 (SD 11,9), Gr. B: 56,1 (SD 14,7) [p = 0,07]. Im weiteren Verlauf zeigten die a K^+-Werte in beiden Gruppen einen Ausgleich des initialen Mukosa/Serosa-Gradienten, der entsprechend der erheblich drastischeren Gesamtreaktion in der Gr. B deutlich eher [bei 180 min] erfolgte als in der Gr. A [bei 230 min] (Abb. 1).

Auch die EMG-Auswertung belegte die blandere Reaktion der selektiv arteriellen Ischämie. Nach 60 min EMG-Frequenz Gr. A: 7,6 (SD 2,8), Gr. B: 1,3 (SD 1,7) [p = 0,004]. EMG-Amplitude Gr. A: 0,38 (SD 0,35), Gr. B: 0,04 (SD 0,08) [p = 0,08] (Abb. 2).

Auffällige Befunde zeigten sich beim mesenterialvenösen pO_2, der sich bei der selektiv arterielen Ischämie hochsignifikant erhöht fand: nach 120 min Gr. A: 34,1 (SD 1,96), Gr. B: 13,4 (SD 2,9) [p = 0,0001].

Bei der Analyse der humoralen Parameter zeigte IL-1 bei keiner der Ischämieformen eine signifikante Veränderung, IL-6 und IL-8 konnten wegen der fehlenden Kreuzreaktivität der humanen Antikörper beim Hund nicht ausgewertet werden. Bei allen weiteren Analysen fanden sich in allen drei Gruppen stets signifikant höhere Plasma-

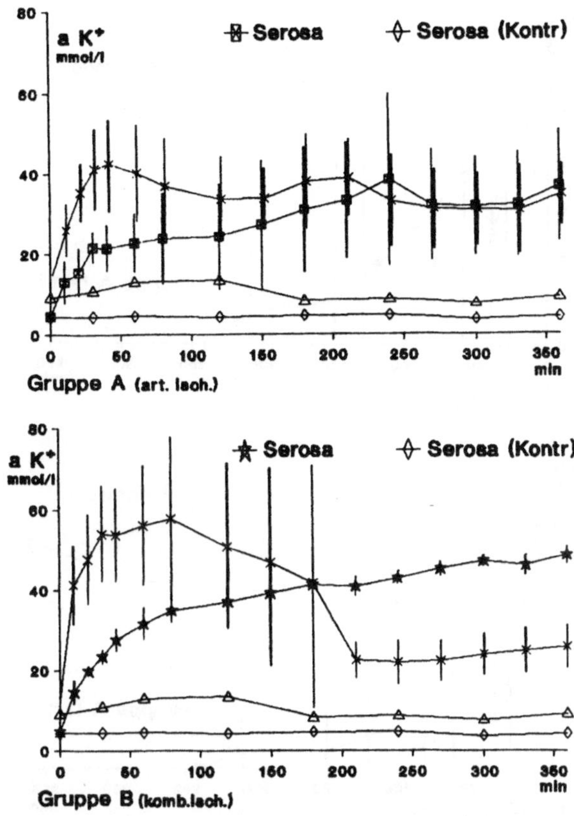

Abb. 1. Meßwerte der Kalium-Aktivität auf Serosa und Mukosa vergleichend zwischen arterieller und kombiniert arterio-venöser Ischämie

werte im Pfortaderblut gegenüber dem Cavablut. Die arterielle und kombiniert arteriovenöse Dünndarmischämie führt zu einer maximalen Dünndarmendothelaktivierung mit nachfolgender Endothelschädigung bis hin zur Endothelnekrose (Verlauf des endothelspezifischen 6-keto-$PGF_{1\alpha}$ als stabiler Metabolit des PGI_2). TNF_α korreliert als unspezifischer Marker der Gewebsschädigung durch seinen linear ansteigenden Verlauf mit der zunehmenden Darmwandschädigung. Sowohl die Endothelaktivierung bzw. -nekrose als auch die Darmwandschädigung ist orientiert an den Mediatorprofilen in der Gruppe B signifikant größer als in der Gruppe A (Abb. 3). Die Mediatorprofile korrelieren somit gut mit den elektromyographischen und a K^+-Ergebnissen. Die These, daß zum Zeitpunkt des Mukosa-Serosa a K^+-Gradientenausgleiches die Mukosabarriere aufgehoben ist und die Translokation begonnen hat [2], wird zwar anhand der Mediatorprofile gestützt, bedarf aber noch der Bestätigung durch die noch ausstehenden Endotoxinanalysen.

Als Erklärung für die signifikant blandere Reaktion der selektiv arteriellen Ischämie ist eine mögliche portal- bzw. mesenterialvenöse Stromumkehr als Ursache für die

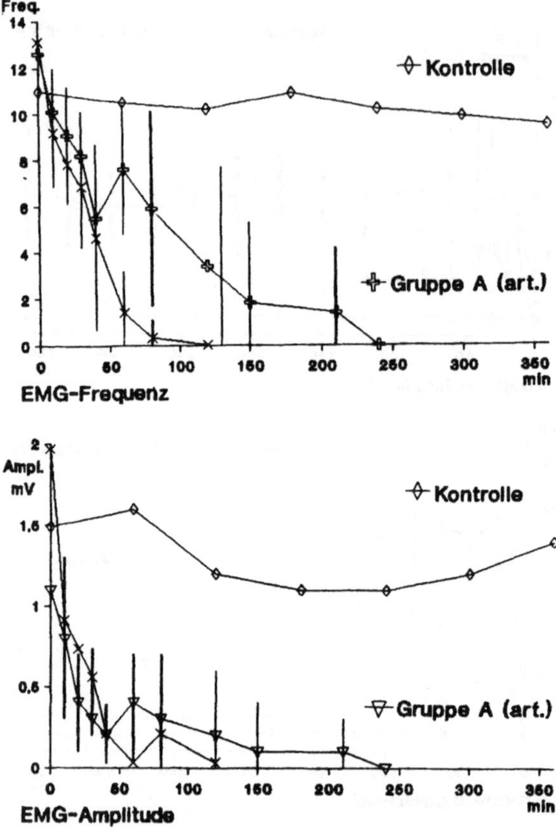

Abb. 2. Elektromyographische Ergebnisse vergleichend Frequenz und Amplitude jeweils mit Werten arterieller und kombiniert arterio-venöser Ischämie

hochsignifikant höheren pO_2-Werte der mesenterialen Segmentvene bei der selektiv arteriellen gegenüber der kombiniert arterio-venösen Ischämie zu diskutieren.

Zusammenfassung

In einem standardisierten Hundemodell wurden eine selektiv arterielle sowie eine kombiniert arterio-venöse Dünndarmischämie jeweils über 6 h vergleichend mit intestinaler Elektromyographie, Serosa- und Mukosa-Kalium-Oberflächenaktivität und Mediatorprofilen (PGF 1α, TNF, IL-1, -6 und -8) differenziert untersucht. EMG-Amplitude und Frequenz zeigten hochsignifikante ischämieabhängige Änderungen gegenüber der Kontrollgruppe sowie eine erheblich länger nachweisbare Aktivität bei der arteriellen gegenüber der kombinierten Ischämie. Bei der K^+-Aktivitätsmessung ergaben sich ebenfalls signifikante ischämieabhängige Befundänderungen, wobei bei beiden Ischämiearten ein Ausgleich des initialen Mukosa/Serosa-Gradienten erfolgte, der entsprechend der insgesamt heftigeren Reaktion bei der kombinierten Ischämie

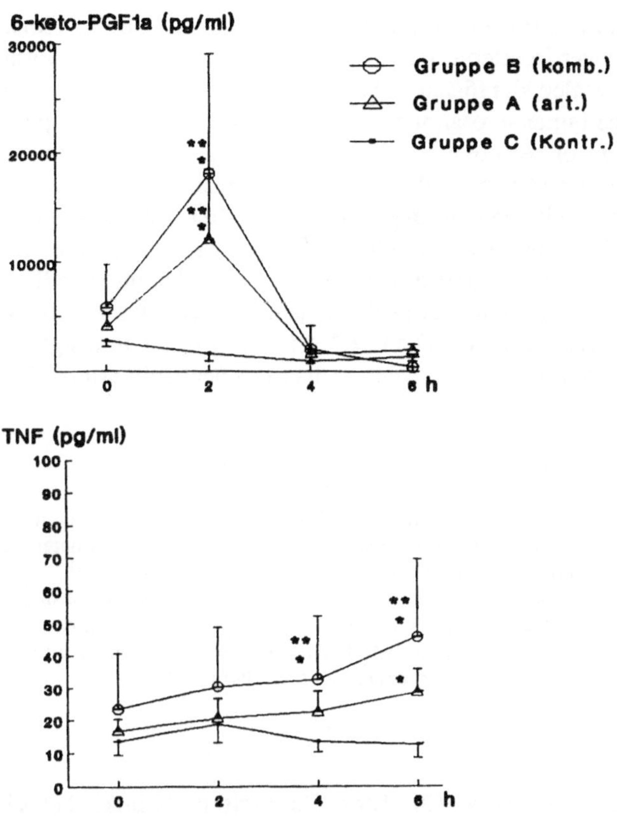

Abb. 3. Mediatorprofile von $PGF_{1\alpha}$ und TNF; * $p < 0{,}05$ A/B vs. C; ** $p < 0{,}05$ B vs. A

deutlich eher (nach 180 min) als bei der selektiv arteriellen Ischämie (nach 230 min) erfolgt. Die nach EMG- und K^+-Aktivitätswerten nach 180 bzw. 230 min zu erwartende Schockmediatoraktivierung läßt sich mit frühen $PGF_{1\alpha}$-Peaks als Ausdruck der primären Endothelaktivierung und nachfolgender Endothelschädigung bis zur Endothelnekrose (mit abfallenden $PGF_{1\alpha}$-Werten) nachvollziehen. TNF_α korreliert als Marker des Gewebeschadens mit den EMG- und Serosa-K^+-Aktivitätswerten und reagiert wie EMG- und K^+-Aktivitäten signifikant heftiger bei kombiniert arterio-venöser als bei der selektiv arteriellen Ischämie.

Summary

In a standardized dog model, both a 6-h selective arterial and a combined arteriovenous small-bowel ischemia were investigated comparatively by electromyography and by monitoring serosal and mucosal potassium surface activity. In addition, the profiles of various mediators – prostaglandin F (PGF)1α, tumor necrosis factor (TNF), and interleukin (IL)1,6, and 8 – were analyzed. The electromyogram (EMG) amplitude and frequency showed highly significant ischemia-dependent changes as compared to the control group. Furthermore, electrical activity remained detectable considerably longer in arterial than in combined ischemia. The measurement of K^+ activities also revealed significant ischemia-dependent changes. However, in both types of ischemia the initial serosa/mucosa K^+ gradient eventually disappeared. This occurred after 230 min of selective arterial ischemia and after 180 min of combined ischemia, which produced a generally more vigorous reaction. EMG results and K^+ activities suggested the activation of shock mediators after 180 min and 230 min, respectively. Early $PGF_{1\alpha}$ peaks as an indication of primary endothelial activation as well as subsequent endothelial damage and necrosis (with declining $PGF_{1\alpha}$ values) testify to that fact. TNF-α as a marker of tissue damage correlates well with EMG results and serosal K^+ activity. Like EMG and K^+ activity, it reacts in a significantly more vigorous fashion to combined arteriovenous than to selectively arterial ischemia.

Literatur

1. Töns C, Fenzlein PG, Winkeltau G, Büsser T, Schumpelick V (1991) Ionenselektives on-line Monitoring der Kalium-Aktivität als Parameter für die Dünndarmischämie. Langenbecks Arch Chir [Suppl] Chir Forum, S 271–275
2. Töns C, Klosterhalfen B, Klinge U, Kirkpatrick CJ, Mittermayer C, Schumpelick V (1993) Septischer Schock und multiples Organversagen in der chirurgischen Intensivmedizin. Ein tierexperimentelles Modell zur Analyse pulmonaler und intestinaler Dysfunktion. Langenbecks Arch Chir, eingereicht zur Publikation

Dr. med. H.W. Ch. Töns, Chirurgische Klinik, RWTH Aachen, Pauwelsstraße 30, W-5100 Aachen

Serosa- und Mucosa-Kaliumaktivität unter zeitlich begrenzter intestinaler Ischämie

Potassium Activity of Intestinal Serosa and Mucosa Due to Ischemia of Limited Duration

K.-H. Dietl[1], K. Redmann[2], B. Marschall[2], W. Pircher[1], B. Buchholz[1] und H. Bünte[1]

[1]Chirurgische Klinik und Poliklinik der Universität Münster
[2]Klinik und Poliklinik für Herz-Thorax-Gefäßchirurgie, Universität Münster

Einleitung

Die Vitalitätsdiagnostik des Intestinums bereitet bei verschiedenen Krankheitsbildern logistische Probleme:

1. Nach Literaturangaben treten bei vier Promille der Patienten, die herzchirurgischen Operationen unterzogen wurden, intestinale Probleme auf. In der Regel sind diese Patienten über längere Zeit herzinsuffizient und bedürfen hoher Katecholamindosen. Klinisch imponiert bei dieser Patientengruppe ein Darmversagen mit geblähtem Abdomen und Meteorismus bis zum Vollbild des akuten Abdomens mit beginnendem septischen Syndrom.

Bei der Laparotomie finden sich unterschiedlich starke Schädigungsgrade in unterschiedlichen Regionen des Darmes. Häufig ist isoliert ein Teil des Colons, das rechte Hemikolon mit Zoekalpol, oder Teile des Dünndarms betroffen. Therapeutisch kommen die Resektion gangränöser Darmabschnitte sowie die Anlage einer entlastenden Kolo- oder Zökostomie in Betracht.

Es ergeben sich in dieser Patientengruppe zwei Hauptprobleme: Erstens wird die Indikation zur Laparotomie oder Re-Laparotomie allein klinisch gestellt. Hilfreich wäre hier die genaue Fragestellung des Schädigungsgrades des Darmes auf laparoskopischem oder endoskopischem Wege, um eine überflüssige Laparotomie oder Re-Laparotomie zu vermeiden und die notwendige Operation frühzeitig in die Wege zu leiten. Zweitens ergibt sich am offenen Abdomen die Schwierigkeit der Festlegung der Resektionsgrenzen. Makroskopisch können die Farbe des Darmes, die Durchblutungsverhältnisse, die Motilität nach Bekopfen und der Tastbefund nur eine semiquantitative Beurteilung des Schädigungsgrades geben. Wichtig wäre hier ebenfalls ein objektiver Parameter zur Festlegung des Schädigungsgrades.

2. Eine zweite Patientengruppe ohne vorausgegangene Darmoperation mit akuten abdominellen Beschwerden, die im typischen Fall bei Darmischämie ein schmerzfreies Intervall aufweisen und deswegen die Indikation zur Laparotomie verzögert sein kann, wenn erst bei wieder erneut auftretender Bauchsymptomatik laparotomiert wird. Diese Patienten mit arteriellem oder venösem Mesenterialinfarkt oder chroni-

Chirurgisches Forum 1993
f. experim. u. klinische Forschung
Becker/Beger/Hartel (Hrsg.)

scher Darmischämie profitieren ebenfalls von einer frühzeitigen Vitalitätsdiagnostik des Darmes.

Methodik

Flowmessungen der A. mesenterica superior

Um die Auswirkungen hoher Katecholamindosen bei niedrigen arteriellen Drücken zu messen, wurden bei drei Schweinen elektromagnetische Flow-Meßköpfe an die A. hepatica communis, an die A. mesenterica sup., die A. carotis und an die A. iliaca communis gelegt. Das Herz-Zeit-Volumen wurde über einen Pulmonalis-Katheter und der arterielle Druck über einen Katheter in der kontralateralen A. carotis communis gemessen. Eine durch Entbluten ausgelöste Hypotonie mit systolischen Druckwerten um 50 mmHg und arteriellen Mitteldruckwerten um 35 mmHg wurde 30 bis 60 min beibehalten. Die Flowrate wurde nach Kalibration gegen Null und Korrelation mit einer dopplersonographischen Methode semiquantitativ bestimmt.

Erzeugung eines septischen Syndroms

Ein weiteres Tiermodell diente zur Klärung der Frage, ob allein durch eine extreme und anhaltende Minderperfusion des Darmes die Erzeugung eines septischen Syndroms induziert werden kann. Dazu wurde an sechs Versuchstieren (Schweinen) eine arterielle Hypotonie mit Werten von 50 mmHg über 90 min durch Ausbluten erzeugt. Nach Re-Transfusion des Eigenblutes wurden die Tiere im Steady-state in flacher Narkose geführt.

Die an verschiedenen Stellen eingelegten Temperatursonden maßen die Körpertemperatur an verschiedenen (acht) Stellen im Körper

1. A. pulmonalis
2. thorakaler Anteil des Oesophagus
3. im Leberhilus
4. und 5. an zwei Stellen des Dickdarm-Mesenteriums
6. und 7. an zwei Stellen des Dünndarm-Mesenteriums
8. an der V. porta ca. 15 cm vor dem Leberhilus

Gleichzeitig wurden über Katheter in die Vv. mesenterica inferior et superior Blutkulturen angelegt, um die Phasen der Bakteriämie nachzuweisen.

Messung des Sauerstoff-Partialdruckes und der Kalium-Aktivität in umschriebenen ischämischen Darmanteilen

Pathogenetisch fällt zunächst der Sauerstoff-Partialdruck im nicht mehr durchbluteten Darm auf Null. Danach beginnt die anaerobe Glykolyse mit der Folge der Entstehung saurer Stoffwechselprodukte, insbesondere Lactat. Nach Aufbrauchen der letzten ATP-Reserven kann die Natrium-Kalium-Pumpe das Ionenkonzentrationsgefälle an der Zellmembran nicht mehr aufrecht erhalten und es kommt zum Ausstrom des intrazellulären Kaliums in das Interstitium. Mit geeigneten Verfahren kann diese Phase der Zellschädigung durch Messung der Kalium-Aktivität im Interstitium erfaßt werden.

Sauerstoffmessungen am ischämischen Darm

Die O_2-Sonde wurde nach Kallibrierung auf die Serosa eines Darmanteiles aufgesetzt und unter stabilen Blutdruck- und Oxygenierungsverhältnissen der O_2-Partialdruck in diesem Darmanteil gemessen. Eine kontinuierliche Messung nach komplettem Ausklemmen des Darmes zeigt den Abfall des Sauerstoff-Partialdruckes im Gewebe nach kompletter Ischämie.

Messung der interstitiellen Kalium-Aktivität

Nach der Phase des Sauerstoffabfalls wird mit einer ionenselektiven Membran die Kalium-Aktivität im Interstitium der jeweiligen Darmanteile gemessen. Die ionenselektive Membran mißt dabei über eine Referenzelektrode das Potential der freien Kaliumionen. Die erhaltenen Meßwerte wurden flammenphotometrisch korreliert.

Durch Aufsetzen der ionenselektiven Membran auf eventerierte und unterschiedlich lange komplett ausgeklemmte Darmanteile im Intervall von 7 bis 10 min wurden die interstitiellen Kaliumwerte auf der Serosa und der Mucosa des Dünndarms, des Dickdarms und des Magens ermittelt. Gemessen wurde 1/2 h vor, während und 2 h nach der Ischämie des Darmes. Der Darm wurde in unterschiedlichen Intervallen ausgeklemmt; sie betrugen 40, 60, 80, 105, 120, 140, 180 min. Die Darmabschnitte wurden 5 h nach Re-Perfusion entnommen und histologisch aufgearbeitet, anschließend erfolgte die Korrelation der Ischämiezeit mit dem Kaliumwert und der histologisch nachgewiesenen Gewebeschädigung.

Ergebnisse

Flowmessungen der A. mesenterica superior

Die Flowmessung in den viszeralen und zentralen Arterien unter Hypotonie und hochdosierten Katecholamingaben zeigte, daß der zentrale arterielle Druck durch Katecholamine erhöht wird, der Flow in den Mesenterialarterien jedoch im Mittel um 30% vermindert wird.

Erzeugung eines septischen Syndroms

Die Erzeugung eines septischen Syndroms durch Hypotonie in den Mesenterialgefäßen und Resorption von Endo- und Exotoxinen aus dem Darm war bei einem normal ernährten Schwein im Mittel 8 h nach der anhaltenden Hypotonie zu beobachten. War der Darm der Versuchstiere entweder entleert oder dekontaminiert, so stieg das freie Intervall bis zum Einsetzen des Fiebers und des septischen Syndroms auf 16 bis 24 h.

Sauerstoff- und interstitielle Kaliummessungen am ischämischen Darm

Messungen des Sauerstoffpartialdruckes

Die Messung des Sauerstoffpartialdruckes bei Tieren mit einem stabilen Blutdruck und arteriellen Sauerstoffdruckwerten von 105 bis 120 mmHg ergaben im Mittel 70 mmHg. Bei kompletter Ischämie des Darmes fiel der Sauerstoffpartialdruck im Mittel innerhalb von 7 min auf Null ab. Die Kurve wird bei nur partieller Verlegung des Stromgebietes entsprechend verlängert.

Messungen der Kaliumaktivität

Die Kaliumwerte auf der Serosa und Mucosa des Magens, des Dünndarms und Dickdarms stiegen innerhalb von 15 bis 30 min auf Werte von 20 bis 30 mmol/l an. Nach Re-Perfusion der ischämischen Darmanteile stellte sich ein stabiles Kalium unter 5 mmol Aktivität innerhalb von maximal 30 min wieder ein.

Eine interstitielle Kaliumaktivität von über 15 mmol/l korrelierte histologisch eindeutig mit einer irreversiblen Mucosaschädigung. Eine Zerstörung der Darm-Blut-Schranke ermöglicht die Resorption von Ekto- und Endotoxinen aus dem Darm und bahnt somit die Entstehung eines septischen Syndroms.

Die Konsequenz bei Kaliumwerten über 15 mmol ist demnach zur Ausschaltung der Ursache des septischen Syndroms die Resektion der entsprechenden Darmanteile.

Die Zeitintervalle von 40 und 60 min zeigten keine Kaliumwerte über 15 mmol. Bei Ischämien über 105 min war in allen Fällen eine massiv erhöhte Kaliumaktivität zu messen und damit histologisch eine Mucosaschädigung nachzuweisen.

Diskussion

Die zur Zeit zur Verfügung stehenden ionenselektiven Membranen zur Messung der interstitiellen Kaliumaktivität können nur am offenen Abdomen eingesetzt werden. In Entwicklung befinden sich laparoskopisch und endoskopisch (koloskopisch und duodenoskopisch) anwendbare Sonden. Denkbar ist die beliebig wiederholbare Messung der Kaliumaktivität koloskopisch und duodenoskopisch bei besonderen Indikationen, die auch laparoskopisch auf der Serosa gemessene Kaliumaktivitätsbestimmung bei Patienten mit Verdacht auf ein ischämisches Darmsyndrom oder einen Mesenterialinfarkt.

Die kritische Grenze der Kaliumaktivität beträgt beim Schwein 15 mmol. Darüber ist in allen Fällen mit einer irreversiblen Schädigung der Mucosa zu rechnen. Entsprechende Werte für den menschlichen Darm müssen noch erarbeitet werden. Wegen der bekannten artspezifischen Unterschiede lassen sich die Meßwerte vom Versuchstier Schwein nicht direkt auf die klinische Anwendung übertragen.

Bei Verfeinerung der Meßsonden und Vereinfachung der Technik ist eine Routineanwendung zur Vitalitätsbeurteilung des menschlichen Darmes, zum Beispiel unter intensivmedizinischen Bedingungen oder bei Verdacht auf einen Mesenterialinfarkt denkbar.

Zusammenfassung

Mit der Messung der Kalium-Aktivität über eine ionenselektive Membran wurde eine direkte Korrelation zwischen der Dauer der Ischämie und dem Grad der histologischen Schädigung am Schweinedarm hergestellt. Bei einer Kaliumaktivität von mehr als dem Zwei- bis Dreifachen der Norm (> 15 mmol/l) entstehen irreversible Schädigungen der Schleimhaut.

Summary

The potassium activity of mucosa and serosa of the porcine intestines, measured by an ion-selective membrane, showed direct correlation to the duration of ischemia and the degree of histological cell damage. An increase in potassium activity higher than 15 mmol causes irreversible cell damage of the intestinal mucosal membrane.

Literatur

1. Bailey RW, Bulkley G, Hamilton S, Morris J, Haglund H (1987) Mesenteric ischemic injury due to cardiogenic shock. Am J Surg 153:108–116
2. Töns Ch, Fenzlein PG, Winkeltau G, Büsser Th, Schumpelick V (1991) Ionenselektives Online-Monitoring der Kaliumaktivität als Parameter für die Dünndarmischämie. Langenbecks Arch Chir [Suppl] Chir Forum, S 271–275

Dr. K.-H. Dietl, Chirurgische Klinik und Poliklinik, Universität Münster, Jungeblodtplatz 1, D-4400 Münster

Allopurinol verbessert die postischämische Muskelfunktion

Allopurinol Improves Postischemic Skeletal Muscle Function

A. Marx[1], L. Gürke[1], P.-M. Sutter[1], P. Erhard[2], J. Landmann[1] und M. Heberer[1]

[1]Departement für Chirurgie, Kantonsspital, Universität Basel (Vorsteher: Prof. Dr. F. Harder)
[2]Abteilung Biophysikalische Chemie, Biozentrum, Universität Basel (Leiter: Prof. Dr. J. Seelig)

Einleitung

Bei traumatologischen und orthopädischen Eingriffen gehört die Blutsperre zur täglichen Routine. Obwohl die obere Zeitgrenze der Tourniquet-Ischämie von 2 h rein empirisch festgelegt ist, wird diese in der Regel akzeptiert. Gerade aber bei komplexeren Eingriffen wäre es wünschenswert, diese Zeitspanne verlängern zu können. Es ist daher erstaunlich, daß die pharmakologische Beeinflußbarkeit des ischämie- und reperfusionsbedingten Schadens am Skelettmuskel bis jetzt wenig untersucht worden ist.

Allopurinol (AP) als kompetitiver Hemmer der Xanthinoxidase (XO) vermag die Ischämietoleranz vieler Organe zu verbessern. Für den Skelettmuskel ist dies jedoch nicht unbestritten.

Ziel dieser experimentellen Studie war es, den Effekt von Allopurinol auf die postischämische Muskelfunktion und den Energiemetabolismus zu untersuchen.

Methode

Für die Untersuchungen wurden männliche Wistar-Ratten (250–300 g, genehmigt durch das kantonale Veterinäramt) verwendet. Die Tiere wurden in zwei Gruppen eingeteilt: Gruppe A (n = 12) erhielt während 3 Tagen sowie 1 h vor Ischämie 40 mg/kg KG Allopurinol intraperitoneal. Tiere der Gruppe K (n = 12) wurden nicht medikamentös behandelt und erhielten die gleiche Menge Flüssigkeit als 0,9% NaCl-Lösung intraperitoneal. Nach Anästhesie (Pentothal i.p.), Analgesie (Fentanyl i.p.) und Tracheotomie wurde an den Hinterläufen der Tiere mittels eines pneumatischen Tourniquets (300 mmHg) eine 3-stündige Ischämie erzeugt, gefolgt von einer 2-stündigen Reperfusionsperiode. Die intramuskulären Temperaturen der Hinterläufe wurden während der Ischämie konstant bei 30°C ($\pm 0,2$) gehalten. Die Reperfusion bei Zimmertemperatur führte innert 10 min zu einem Anstieg der i.m. Temperatur auf $34,8$°C ($\pm 0,4$). Dieser gleichmäßige Temperaturanstieg auf präischemische Werte darf als Ausdruck einer homogenen Reperfusion gewertet werden. Nach Ischämie und Reperfusion wurden zwei in ihrer Faserzusammensetzung vergleichbare Muskeln [1]entnommen: Zur Funktionsmessung wurden die Mm. peronei bei 37° im Organbad gemäß dem Burke-Protokoll elektrisch stimuliert [2]. Als Parameter dienten

Chirurgisches Forum 1993
f. experim. u. klinische Forschung
Becker/Beger/Hartel (Hrsg.)

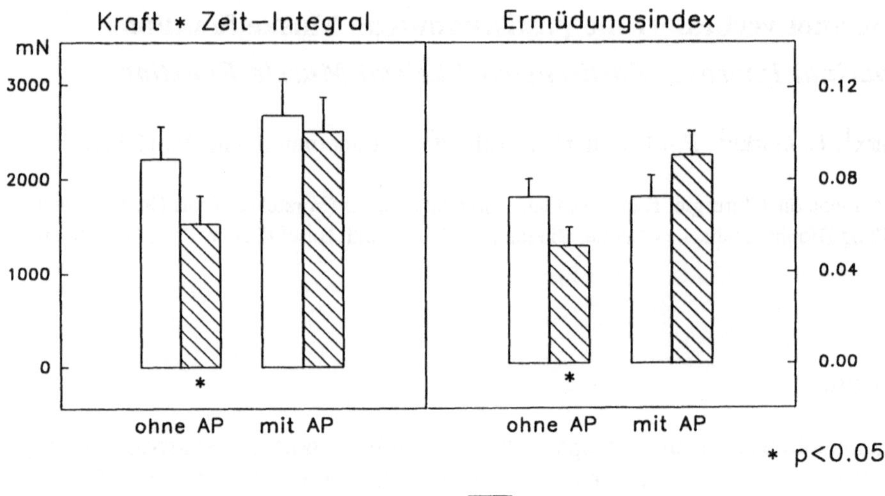

Abb. 1. Muskelfunktionsmessungen (Mm. peronei) nach 3 h Ischämie und 2 h Reperfusion

das Integral aus Kraft × Zeit (mN × sec), welches bei der isometrischen Kontraktion mit der Leistung korreliert [3] und der Ermüdungsindex nach Burke (Amplitude nach 1-minütiger Stimulation/maximale initiale Amplitude) [2]. Die Mm. gastrocnemii wurden zur Bestimmung von ATP, Phosphocreatin (PCr) und Creatin (Cr) bei der Entnahme mit flüssigem Stickstoff gefroren. Nach Perchlorsäureextraktion der Proben erfolgte die ^{31}P- und ^{1}H-MR-Spektroskopie (Bruker MEL 400, 9,8 Tesla). Als Maß des Energiestatus werden die Quotienten von β-ATP und Phosphocreatin zum Gesamtcreatin (PCr + Cr) angegeben.

Die kontralaterale nicht ischämische Seite diente sowohl bei den Funktionsuntersuchungen wie auch bei der MR-Spektroskopie in beiden Gruppen als Kontrolle. Die statistische Auswertung erfolgte mittels Varianzanalyse und anschließendem Diskriminationstest nach Scheffé. Als signifikant wurde ein $p < 0,05$ akzeptiert.

Ergebnisse

Durch Allopurinol konnte die postischämische Muskelfunktion signifikant verbessert werden. Während der ischämiegeschädigte Muskel der Kontrolltiere (Gruppe K) sich durch schlechtere Leistung und erhöhte Ermüdbarkeit signifikant von der kontralateralen Seite unterschied, konnten diese Unterschiede in der mit AP behandelten Gruppe A nicht gefunden werden. Die Resultate der Muskelfunktionsmessungen sind für beide Gruppen in Abb. 1 dargestellt. Die energiereichen Phosphate hingegen wurden durch die Gabe von Allopurinol nicht beeinflußt. Sowohl der Quotient von β-ATP/(PCr + Cr) wie auch PCr/(PCr + Cr) blieben unverändert (Abb. 2).

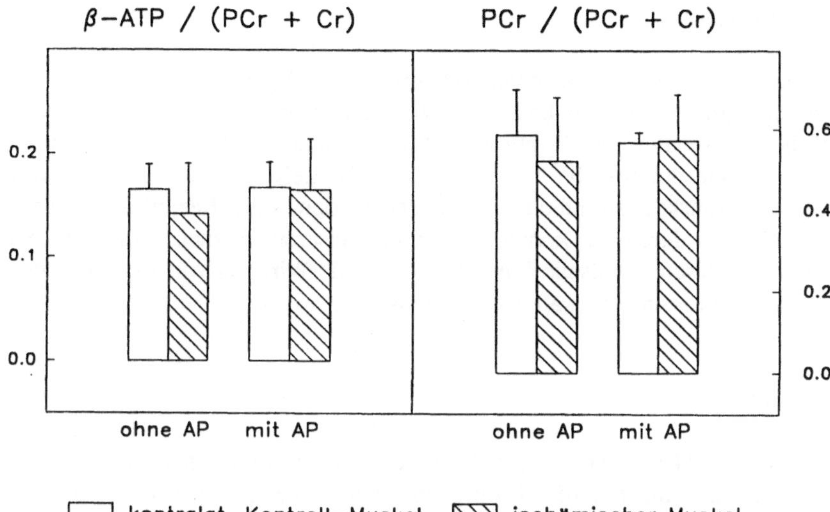

Abb. 2. Postischämischer Energiegehalt (Mm. gastrocnemii); ^{31}P- und ^{1}H-MR-Spektroskopie nach 3 h Ischämie und 2 h Reperfusion

Diskussion

Einer Verbesserung der Ischämietoleranz des Skelettmuskels durch Allopurinol wurde bis jetzt meist nur durch indirekte Parameter (Verbesserung der Mikrozirkulation, Reduktion von Muskellogen-Druck etc.) nachgewiesen. Die wenigen Arbeiten, welche direkt den Einfluß von AP auf die postischämische Funktion des Muskels untersuchen, kommen zu unterschiedlichen Resultaten [4, 5]. In unserem Tierexperiment konnte Allopurinol nach 3-stündiger temperaturkontrollierter Ischämie und 2-stündiger Reperfusion sowohl die Muskelleistung als auch die Ermüdbarkeit signifikant verbessern. Eine Beeinflussung des Energiemetabolismus durch AP konnten wir nicht nachweisen. Der in unserem Experiment gesetzte Schaden hat bei den Kontrolltieren (Gruppe K) zwar zu einer signifikanten Funktionseinbuße, nicht aber zu einer deutlichen Reduktion von β-ATP und PCr geführt. AP führte also unter diesen Bedingungen zu einer Funktionsverbesserung, ohne den Energiestoffwechsel beeinflussen zu können. Dies spricht dafür, daß Allopurinol die postischämische Funktionsverbesserung nicht über den salvage pathway (Blockierung der XO mit entsprechender Kumulation von wieder zu ATP synthetisierbarem Hypoxanthin im Gewebe), sondern eher über andere Mechanismen beeinflußt.

Die Verbesserung der postischämischen Leistung und der Ermüdbarkeit durch AP darf natürlich nicht direkt auf die klinische Situation übertragen werden. Da Allopurinol aber ein bekanntes Medikament mit großer therapeutischer Breite ist, drängen sich entsprechende Untersuchungen bei traumatologischen oder orthopädischen Operationen in Blutsperre auf.

Zusammenfassung

Allopurinol vermag die Ischämietoleranz vieler Organe zu verbessern. Dies ist für den Skelettmuskel nicht unbestritten. Nur wenige Arbeiten haben den Einfluß von AP auf die postischämische Funktion des Muskels untersucht. In unserer experimentellen Studie konnte durch Gabe von AP sowohl die Leistung wie auch die Ermüdbarkeit des Skelettmuskels signifikant verbessert werden. Eine Beeinflussung des Energiemetabolismus durch AP konnten wir unter unseren Versuchsbedingungen hingegen nicht nachweisen. Klinische Studien, welche die Wirkung von AP bei Operationen in Blutsperre untersuchen, wären wünschenswert.

Summary

Allopurinol (AP) is known to reduce postischemic organ damage. Few papers have addressed the influence of AP on postischemic skeletal muscle function. Our experimental study discovered a significant improvement of postischemic muscle performance and fatigue. β-ATP and phosphocreatine levels, however, remained unchanged after the administration of AP. Studies of allopurinol administration during clinical surgery with tourniquet-induced ischemia are necessary.

Literatur

1. Armstrong RB, Phelps RO (1984) Muscle fibre type composition of the rat hindlimb. Am J Anat 171:259–272
2. Burke RE (1961) Motor unit types of cat triceps surae muscle. J Physiol 193:141–160
3. Burke RE, Rudomin P, Zajac III FE (1976) The effect of activation history on tension production by individual muscle units. Brain Res 109:515–529
4. Feller AM, Roth AC, Russell RC (1990) Tissue protection by elimination of oxygen free radicals in the post-ischemic reperfusion phase. Handchir Mikrochir Plast Chir 22:4–13
5. McCutchan HJ, Schwappach JR, Enquist EG, Walden DL, Terada LS, Reiss PK, Leff JA, Repine JE (1990) Xanthine oxidase-derived H_2O_2 contributed to reperfusion injury of ischemic skeletal muscle. Am J Physiol 258:H1415–H1419

Dr. A. Marx, Oberarzt, Departement Chirurgie, Kantonsspital der Universität, CH-4031 Basel, Schweiz

Renovaskuläre Hypertonie – Ist eine präoperative Evaluierung des Therapieerfolges möglich?

Renovascular Hypertension – Can the Response to Therapy Be Predicted?

T. Hupp[1], J.H. Clorius[2], C. Kartak[1] und J.R. Allenberg[1]

[1]Sektion Gefäßchirurgie (Leiter: Prof. Dr. J.R. Allenberg), Chirurgische Universitätsklinik Heidelberg (Dir.: Prof. Dr. Ch. Herfarth)
[2]Forschungsschwerpunkt Radiologische Diagnostik und Therapie (Dir.: Prof. Dr. G. van Kaick), Deutsches Krebsforschungszentrum, Heidelberg

Einleitung

Die kritische Analyse der chirurgischen oder endovaskulären Ergebnisse bei der Therapie der renovaskulären Hypertonie zeigt, daß bei allen Therapieformen eine nicht unerhebliche Prozentzahl an Therapieversagern zu verzeichnen ist. Eine Hypertonieheilung ist nur bei 50–80% der Patienten zu erreichen. Nimmt man die Normalisierung des Blutdrucks als Wertmaßstab des chirurgischen oder endovaskulären Erfolges, stellt speziell bei der renovaskulären Hypertonie ein Untersuchungsverfahren zur Prädiktion des Therapieerfolges eine vielfach geforderte Notwendigkeit dar [1, 2].

Studienziel

Mit Hilfe der Belastungs-Szintigraphie sollte an Patienten mit einer renovaskulären Hypertonie eine Prädiktion des Therapieerfolges vor chirurgischer oder interventioneller Therapie vorgenommen werden. Es sollte die Hypothese überprüft werden, ob Patienten mit einer renovaskulären Hypertonie und einer belastungsabhängigen bilateralen Hippurattransportstörung einen "renal fixierten" Hypertonus haben, der weder durch eine chirurgische Revaskularisation oder durch eine Dilatationsbehandlung der Nierenarterienstenose heilbar sei. Die Szintigramme unter fahrradergometrischer Belastung wurden benutzt, um den Einfluß einer sympathomimetischen "Streß"-Situation auf den Hippurattransport zu dokumentieren. Die gewonnenen Daten der Belastungsszintigraphie sollten mit dem klinischen Verlauf des Blutdruckes (prä-, postoperativ und im follow-up) verglichen werden. Die Sensitivität, Spezifität und die Bedeutung

Chirurgisches Forum 1993
f. experim. u. klinische Forschung
Becker/Beger/Hartel (Hrsg.)

des positiven sowie negativen Vorhersagewertes dieser Untersuchungsmethode sollte an Hand des sog. "Gold-Standard" Renin diskutiert werden.

Methode

Präoperative Szintigraphie (6 μCi (I 123)-Jod-Hippurat/kg KG) im Liegen und unter Streßprovokation (fahrradergometrische Belastung, 40/60 Watt) zur Erfassung von bilateralen Hippurattransportstörungen. Prä- und postoperative Dokumentation des Blutdruckes (Klassifikation nach Maxwell 1972 [3]), der antihypertensiven Medikation und von Kreatinin und Harnstoff. Der Nachuntersuchungszeitraum erstreckte sich von 3 Monaten bis zu 24 Monaten, im Mittel war er 14,2 Monate.

Patienten

Aus dem Gesamtkrankengut aller Patienten mit Nierenarterienrekonstruktionen an der Chirurgischen Universitätsklinik Heidelberg im Zeitraum 1/80–12/91 konnten 84 der 196 Patienten in eine prospektive Studie zur Evaluierung der Prädiktion des Therapieerfolges (Hypertonieheilung) mittels einer prätherapeutischen Belastungsszintigraphie eingebracht werden. Für die endgültige Analyse verblieben 58 Patienten in der Studie.

Ergebnisse

36 von 58 Patienten (62%) entwickelten unter fahrradergometrischer Belastung eine passagere, bilateral pathologische Hippurattransportstörung (= pathologisches Belastungs-Szintigramm). 22 von 58 Patienten (38%) zeigten während der fahrradergometrischen Belastung keine verzögerte bilaterale Hippurattransportstörung in den Nieren (= normales Belastungs-Szintigramm). Bei 8 freiwilligen, normotensiven männlichen Kontroll-Probanden konnte kein pathologisches Belastungs-Szintigramm aufgezeichnet werden.

Bei den Patienten mit einem pathologischen Belastungs-Szintigramm resultierte die Hippurattransportstörung in einer verzögerten Exkretion des radioaktiv markierten Hippurates aus beiden Nieren in die Blase (verzögerte Blasenerscheinungszeit der Aktivität). Die mittlere Tracer-Erscheinungszeit in der Blase veränderte sich von 3,5 min (SD 1,1/SEM 0,2 min) während der Ruheszintigraphie in einen deutlichen pathologischen Bereich unter fahrradergometrischer Belastung von 9,1 min (SD 5,6/SEM 1,0 min) (Abb. 1).

Zwischen den zwei Patientenkollektiven (pathologisches und normales Belastungs-Szintigramm) waren deutliche Unterschiede im posttherapeutischen Blutdruckverlauf und in der Notwendigkeit einer fortzusetzenden medikamentösen Therapie zu verzeichnen. Die Patienten mit einem normalen Belastungsszintigramm hatten posttherapeutisch einen mittleren Blutdruck von 132/79 mmHg. Im Vergleich dazu war der mittlere Blutdruck bei den Patienten mit einem pathologischen Belastungsszintigramm 151/85 mmHg (P systolisch $< 0{,}001$/P diastolisch $= 0{,}01$). Der Bedarf an antihyperten-

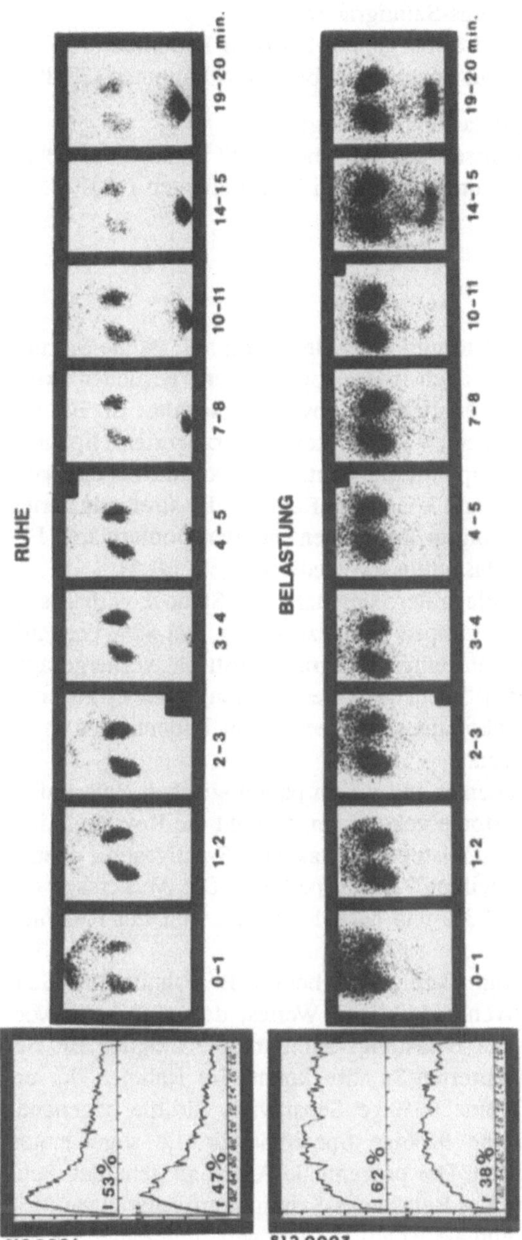

Abb. 1. Pathologisches Belastungs-Szintigramm. Die Kurven zeigen eine deutlich verzögerte bilaterale Aktivitätsauswaschung unter Belastung (*untere Bildreihe links*). Unter Ruhebedingungen erscheint die Aktivität regelrecht nach 3–4 Minuten in der Blase (*obere Bildreihe: viertes Bild von rechts*), unter Belastungsbedingungen jedoch deutlich verzögert erst nach 10–11 Minuten (*untere Bildreihe: siebentes Bild von links*). Klinische Daten: 54jähriger Patient, Nierenarterienstenose rechts (Arteriosklerose), renovaskuläre Hypertonie, Kreatinin 1,1 mg/dl

siver Medikation nach Revaskularisation war in beiden Patientengruppen signifikant unterschiedlich: 0,3 im Vergleich zu 1,5 Substanzgruppen an Antihypertensiva pro Tag (Patienten mit normalem versus pathologischem Belastungsszintigramm; $P < 0{,}001$).

Hypertonieverlauf (Pat. mit path. Belastungs-Szintigramm):
Die Hypertonie war nach der Revaskularisation geheilt bei 6/36 Patienten (16,7%), verbessert bei 20/36 Patienten (55,5%) und unverändert bei 10/36 Patienten (27,8%).

Hypertonieverlauf (Pat. mit normalem Belastungs-Szintigramm):
Die Hypertonie war durch die Revaskularisation geheilt bei 17/22 Patienten (77,3%), verbessert bei 2/22 Patienten (9,1%) und unverändert bei 3/22 Patienten (13,6%).

Diskussion

Tritt das Phänomen der Hippurattransportstörung unter Belastung auf, ist die Störung immer bilateral zu verzeichnen, das heißt auch in der sogenannten "gesunden" kontralateralen Niere, der prärenal keine Nierenarterienstenose vorgeschaltet ist. Bei der Ruhe(Basis)-Szintigraphie zeigen die Patienten jedoch keinen verzögerten Hippurattransport. Das Phänomen der bilateralen Hippurattransportstörung könnte als eine kortikale Perfusionsstörung gedeutet werden und könnte im Rahmen der streßinduzierten Sympathikusstimulation eine Dysregulation im Zusammenspiel der glomerulären Filtrationsrate und des effektiven renalen Plasmaflusses wiederspiegeln [4, 5].

Bei der Wertung von Patienten mit unilateraler Nierenarterien-Stenose verhält sich die Heilung der Hypertonie in den zwei Gruppen geradezu invers. Bei 82% der Patienten mit einem präoperativ normalen Belastungsszintigramm tritt die vorhergesagte Heilung der Hypertonie ein. Bei 3 der 4 "nicht geheilten" Patienten ist es zu einer deutlichen Besserung der Hypertonie gekommen. Nur bei einem Patienten ist es zu keiner Heilung der Hypertonie gekommen.

Umgekehrt ist es nur bei 6 der 36 Patienten mit einem pathologischen Belastungs-Szintigramm zu einer Heilung der Hypertonie gekommen, obwohl die Revaskularisationsergebnisse alle regelrecht waren. Also leistet die Belastungs-Szintigraphie ebenso eine Vorhersage bezüglich einer "Nichtheilung" der Hypertonie. Die Vorhersage der "Nichtheilung" traf im Frühergebnis bei 83% und nach 1 Jahr bei 94% der Patienten zu.

Für das Zielkriterium "Hypertonieheilung" zeigt sich bei der Berechnung der Sensitivität und des positiven oder negativen prädiktiven Wertes, daß eine hohe Vorhersagekraft des Therapieerfolges mit der Belastungs-Szintigraphie möglich ist. Bei Patienten mit einer unilateralen Nierenarterien-Stenose konnte im Rahmen der ersten Nachuntersuchung (Follow-up I) eine 93%ige Sensitivität für die sogenannten Hypertonie-"Nonresponder" und eine 92%ige Spezifität für die sogenannten Hypertonie-"Responder" errechnet werden. Der prozentuale Anteil an geheilten Patienten von allen, die präoperativ ein normales Belastungs-Szintigramm hatten, war 86% (= negativer Vorhersagewert). Der prozentuale Anteil an nicht geheilten Patienten von allen, die präoperativ ein pathologisches Belastungs-Szintigramm hatten, war 96% (= positiver Vorhersagewert). Aus der Anzahl der "richtig positiven" und "richtig negativen" Patienten konnte in dem Patientenkollekiv mit unilateraler Nierenarterienstenose (40 Patienten) eine Treffsicherheit für die Vorhersagekraft der Untersuchungsmethode (Hypertonieheilung) von 92,5% errechnet werden.

Wollenweber [6] wies als Erster im Rahmen von diagnostischen Bemühungen um die renovaskuläre Hypertonie auf den Bedarf einer Untersuchungsmethode hin, mit der man eine Trennung zwischen Hypertonie-"Responder" und Hypertonie-"Nonresponder" vornehmen kann. In regelmäßigen Abständen wird seitdem auf die Notwendigkeit einer solchen Untersuchungsmethode hingewiesen. Nach Peters [2] stellt die größte Herausforderung bei der Diagnostik der renovaskulären Hypertonie ein Nachweisverfahren dar, mit dem die funktionelle Bedeutung einer Nierenarterienstenose verifiziert werden kann. Unterschiedlichste Reninbestimmungsmethoden haben wegen ihrer hohen Fehlerquote im Routinediagnostikablauf und wegen zu hoher falsch positiver und falsch negativer Ergebnisse enttäuscht. Je nach Literaturangabe schwanken die Angaben über falsch negative Renin-Befunde zwischen 16 und 44% und über falsch positive Renin-Befunde zwischen 7 und 39%. Die Renindaten unserer Patienten erbrachten für die Prädiktion des Therapieerfolges eine Spezifität von 71% und eine Sensitivität von nur 38%.

Das Phänomen der bilateralen Hippurattransportstörung, ein anfängliches Epiphänomen bei szintigraphischen Untersuchungen von Senknieren [4], stellte sich als ein passageres Phänomen dar, das anfänglich unter Orthostasebedingungen und später gezielt unter genormter fahrradergometrischer Belastung beobachtet wurde. Die Besonderheit dabei war, daß die Hippurattransportstörung dann immer bilateral zu beobachten war, also auch in der sog. "gesunden" unauffälligen Niere. Bei Normotonikern (Kontroll-Probanden) war solch eine bilaterale Hippurattransportstörung nicht zu beobachten. Das Phänomen der Hippurattransportstörung trat in unserem Krankengut bei 62% der untersuchten Hypertoniker auf und zeigte auch in früheren Untersuchungen eine fast konstante prozentuale Verteilung von 60 zu 40% auf (pathologischer Hippurattransport zu normalem Hippurattransport) [4, 5]. Eine szintigraphische Hypertonieform war entdeckt. Sie war jedoch weder der Goldblatt-Hypertonie noch der essentiellen Hypertonie in irgend einer Form zuzuordnen. Erst durch die Unterscheidung in die zwei Untergruppen (pathologisches oder normales Belastungs-Szintigramm) und durch die klinische Beobachtung des unterschiedlichen Blutdruckverhaltens nach einer revaskularisierenden Therapie war eine Deutung der Szintigraphiebefunde möglich. Dadurch war jetzt mit Hilfe der Belastungs-Szintigraphie eine präoperative Selektionierung der Patienten in sogenannte Therapie-"Responder" und "Non-Responder" möglich geworden.

Zusammenfassung

Durch die Behandlung einer Nierenarterien(NA)-Stenose kommt es nur bei 50 bis 80% aller Patienten zu einer Heilung der renovaskulären Hypertonie. Bei 20 bis 50% der Patienten liegt demzufolge eine andere Hypertonieursache als der "Goldblatt"-Mechanismus vor. In einer prospektiven Studie wurde untersucht, ob mit einer szintigraphischen Spezialuntersuchung der Effekt einer Nierenarterien-Rekonstruktion in Bezug auf den postoperativen Hypertonieverlauf vorhergesagt werden kann. Bei 58 von 196 Patienten mit einer NA-Revaskularisation und Hypertonie (1/80 bis 12/91) wurde eine prätherapeutische Belastungs-Szintigraphie (BS) zur Evaluierung des postoperativen Therapieerfolges durchgeführt. Nach der Nierenarterien-Revaskularisation (49× chirurgisch und 9× endovaskulär); (Follow-up mean 14,2 Monate [3–24 Mon.]) wurde der präoperative szintigraphische Befund mit dem postoperativen Blutdruckverhalten korreliert. 36/58 Patienten (62%) entwickelten eine Belastungsinduzierte passagere, bilaterale Hippurat-Transportstörung (= pathologisches BS). Nur 2 dieser 36 Patienten wurden nach erfolgreicher NA-Rekonstruktion normotensiv ohne antihypertensive Medikation (mittlerer Blutdruck präop. 183/103 mmHg, postop. 151/85 mmHg, mittlere antihypertensive Medikation/Tag präop. 2,9, postop. 1,5 Substanzgruppen/Tag). 22/58 Patienten (38%) zeigten einen unauffälligen Hippurat-Transport bei der präop. szintigraphischen Untersuchung (= normales BS). 17 dieser 22 Patienten wurden nach der NA-Rekonstruktion normotensiv ohne antihypertensive Medikation (mittlerer Blutdruck präop. 169/97 mmHg, postop. 132/79 mmHg, antihypertensive Medikation präop. 1,3 , postop. 0,3 Substanzgruppen/Tag). Die belastungsinduzierte bilaterale Hippurat-Transportstörung deckt einen intrarenalen Befund auf, der klinisch einem renal fixierten, nicht heilbaren Hypertonus gleichzusetzen ist. Bei einer unilateralen NA-Stenose kann mit der Belastungs-Szintigraphie der Therapieerfolg mit einer Sensitivität von 93% und einer Spezifität von 92% vorhergesagt werden (96%iger positiver Vorhersagewert, 86%iger negativer Vorhersagewert).

Summary

Renal artery stenosis with resultant renovascular hypertension has attracted clinical attention because the disease is potentially curable and because numerous diagnostic and therapeutic modalities compete for clinical acceptance. Despite all available presurgical diagnostic methods, the therapeutic result of renovascular reconstruction is not predictable as far as the postoperative course of hypertension is concerned. In order to make a preoperative prediction of the final course of renovascular hypertension, we carried out a prospective study to verify the predictive value of a new scintigraphic method, exercise hippurate scintigraphy. Fifty eight patients with hypertension and angiographically documented uni- or bilateral renovascular stenosis were referred to rest and exercise hippurate scintigrams before operation. The results of the examination at rest served as standard and were compared with the exercise scintigrams. Out of 58 patients, 36 (62%) developed an exercise-induced bilateral hippurate transport disturbance, whereas 22 (38%) patients failed to respond to exercise with altered hippurate kinetics. After renal artery reconstruction (surgical in 49 cases and endovascular [PTA] in nine), 17 of 22 (77%) patients who had normal exercise renograms were cured of hypertension. In comparison, blood pressure values were little influenced by therapy in patients with abnormal exercise scintigrams. Out of 36 patients, 34 (94%) continued to have hypertensive disease after therapy. The study shows that exercise scintigraphy helps to identify patients with crurable and noncrurable renovascular hypertension (sensitivity 93%, specifity 92%, positive predictive value 96%, and negative predictive value 86%).

Literatur

1. Bardram L, Helgstrand U, Bentzen MH, Hansen HJB, Engell HC (1985) Late results after surgical treatment of renovascular hypertension. A follow-up study of 122 patients 2–18 years after surgery. Ann Surg 201:219–224
2. Peters AM (1990) Renal artery stenosis, reno-vascular hypertension and predicting the blood pressure response to renal revascularization. Nucl Med Com 11:1–5
3. Maxwell MH, Bleifer KH, Franklin SS, Varady PD (1972) Cooperative study of renovascular hypertension. Demographic analysis of the study. JAMA 220:1195–1204
4. Clorius JH, Allenberg JR, Hupp T, Strauss LG, Schmidlin P, Irngartinger G, Wagner R, Mukhopadhyay C (1987) Predictive value of exercise renography for presurgical evaluation of nephrogenic hypertension. Hypertension 10:280–286
5. Hupp T, Corius JH, Allenberg JR (1991) Renovascular hypertension: predicting surgical cure with exercise renography. J Vasc Surg 14:200–207
6. Wollenweber J, Sheps SG, Davis GD (1968) Clinical course of atherosclerotic renovascular disease. Am J Cardiol 21:60–71

Dr. med. Th. Hupp, Sektion Gefäßchirurgie, Chirurgische Universitätsklinik Heidelberg, Kirschnerstraße 1, W-6900 Heidelberg

Behandlung medikamentenrefraktärer ventrikulärer Tachykardien durch Defibrillatorimplantation, Rhythmuschirurgie oder Herztransplantation

Treatment of Drug-Resistant Ventricular Tachycardia by Implantation of Automatic ,Defibrillators, Antiarrhythmia-Surgery or Heart-Transplantation

E. Kreuzer[1], R. Haberl[2], B. Meiser[1], B. Kemkes[1], G. Steinbeck[2] und B. Reichart[1]

[1]Herzchirurgische Klinik, Klinikum Großhadern, Universität München
[2]Medizinische Klinik I, Klinikum Großhadern, Universität München

Einleitung

Herzrhythmusstörungen als Symptom und als Komplikation zahlreicher Erkrankungen enden häufig letal. Kardiale Arrhythmien dauerhaft zu beherrschen, setzt sorgfältige differentialdiagnostische Überlegungen voraus, wobei unabdingbar dafür das Verstehen pathogenetischer Mechanismen ist, das sich aus den elektrophysiologischen Eigenschaften des pathologisch veränderten Myokards durch das Experiment ableiten läßt. Das Spektrum des heute therapeutisch Möglichen reicht von physikalischen Maßnahmen über eine vielfältige und gut fundierte medikamentöse Behandlung, über Elektrotherapie bis hin zu chirurgischen Eingriffen am Myokard selbst. Die Herzchirurgie bietet zur Behandlung medikamentenrefraktärer ventrikulärer Tachykardien die Implantation des automatischen Defibrillators, den rhythmuschirurgischen Eingriff oder auch die Herztransplantation an. Wir werten nach dem aktuellen Stand der Dinge alle rhythmuschirurgischen Eingriffe am offenen Herzen vorsichtig als eine mehr oder minder fundierte, alternative Therapieform, die nur einem relativ schmalen Bereich bekannter Rhythmusstörungen als Hilfe sich anbietet.

Unsere Studie vergleicht die Ergebnisse dieser verschiedenartigen Möglichkeiten in Bezug auf das Überleben und die Lebensqualität der betroffenen Patienten.

Patienten und Methode

Die Gruppen wurden je nach Allgemeinzustand und Indikationen in 3 verschiedene Unterteilungen geordnet:

Patientengruppe I (n = 84), mit einem mittleren Alter von 64 Jahren, wiesen als Erkrankung eine ischämische oder dilatative Kardiomyopathie auf. Die Ejektionsfraktion lag im Durchschnitt bei 20%. Die polymorphen und polytropen Extrasystolen wurden in 37 Fällen epikardial und 52 Fällen transvenös/subcutan mit automatischen Defibrillatoren versorgt. Die Implantationszeit lag zwischen 1987 und 1992.

Chirurgisches Forum 1993
f. experim. u. klinische Forschung
Becker/Beger/Hartel (Hrsg.)

Die Patienten der Gruppe II (n = 32), mit einem mittleren Alter von 62 Jahren, ausschließlich ätiologisch mit einer ischämischen Kardiomyopathie behaftet, erbrachten eine durchschnittliche Auswurfleistung von 25%. Ihre Rhythmusstörungen wurden im Elektrokardiogramm lediglich mit monomorph und monotop charakterisiert. Sie wurden deshalb konservativ chirurgisch behandelt. Dabei schlossen die angewandten operativen Techniken die partielle Endokardresektion, das partielle Encircling sowie die Ablation mittels Kryosonde ein. Wegen eines vorhandenen Vorderwandaneurysmas wurde bei 7 Patienten die sog. DOR-Plastik durchgeführt.

Die Patienten mit einem mittleren Alter von 35 Jahren, welche die Gruppe III darstellten, litten sowohl an einer ischämischen bzw. dilatativen Kardiomyopathie. Ihre durchschnittliche Auswurfleistung betrug 19%. Das klinische Erscheinungsbild bestand im Auftreten polymorpher und polytoper Extrasystolen. Diese Patienten, die mehrfach präoperativ defibrilliert werden mußten, wurden orthotop herztransplantiert.

Ergebnisse

Drei Monate post operationem lebten in Gruppe I 95%, in Gruppe II 78% und in Gruppe III 70% der Patienten.

Ein Jahr post operationem registrierten wir eine Überlebensrate für Gruppe I mit 91%, während die konservativ-rhythmuschirurgisch versorgten Patienten zu 75% überlebten. Die orthotop herztransplantierten Patienten der Gruppe III erreichten eine Überlebensrate von 60%.

Zwei Jahre post operationem hatte sich die Überlebensrate der mit einem Defibrillator versorgten Patienten nicht geändert. Das gleiche galt für die konservativ-rhythmuschirurgisch versorgten Patienten. Lediglich die orthotop herztransplantierten Patienten der Gruppe III (n = 10) zeigten keine Veränderung der Überlebensrate im Vergleich zum 1. postoperativen Jahr.

Zum Vergleich der 3 genannten Gruppen wurde ein Kontingent von 32 Patienten erfaßt, das lediglich medikamentös behandelt wurde. Hier überlebten die ersten 3 Monate 80%. 58% waren nach einem Jahr als Überlebensrate registriert worden. Diese Rate entsprach auch dem erhobenen Wert nach 2 Jahren. Während die Patienten in Gruppe I unter Beibehaltung der medikamentösen Therapie zum Teil mehrfach täglich wegen ventrikulärer Tachykardien automatisch defibrilliert werden, bieten alle übrigen Patienten der Gruppe II und III keinerlei ventrikuläre Rhythmusstörungen. Somit sind auch keine antiarrhythmischen Medikamente notwendig. Die Lebensqualität dieser beiden Gruppen ist als "gut" zu bezeichnen.

Diskussion

Alle 3 genannten operativen Methoden herzchirurgischer Therapie bieten bei ventrikulären Tachykardien eine echte Alternative zur rein medikamentösen Behandlung. Die Defibrillationsimplantation ergibt die höchste Überlebensrate zumindest nach 2 Jahren, hat jedoch im Gegensatz zu anderen Methoden den Nachteil, daß die Herzleistung nicht verbessert und der Patient durch häufige tägliche Defibrillationen belastet ist. Die Lebensqualität ist somit als eingeschränkt zu bezeichnen. Die Rhythmuschirurgie stellt deshalb sicherlich die überlegenere Alternative dar. Sie ist allerdings nur bei lokalisierbaren monomorphen und monotopen Extrasystolen möglich. Bedenkt man weiterhin, daß bei ischämischen Kardiomyopathien mit ausgebildeten Aneurysmen durch Resektion dieser Aneurysmen bzw. durch Anlegen der sog. DOR-Plastiken auch die ventrikuläre Leistung des Restmyokards deutlich verbessert wird, scheint die konservativ-rhythmuschirurgische Therapieform in unseren Augen der optimalste Eingriff. Die Herztransplantation sollte als letzte Möglichkeit jeglicher chirurgischen Intervention offen bleiben. Die Kontraindikation sowie die post transplantationem auftretenden Komplikationen beeinflussen deutlich die Lebensqualität.

Entscheidend ist eine individuelle Indikationsstellung aufgrund der Morphologie der Rhythmusstörung, der Mono- oder Polytopie, dem Allgemeinzustand des Patienten, seinem Alter sowie der noch vorhandenen regionalen Kontraktilität des Myokards.

Summary

The implantation of automatic defibrillators, antiarrhythmia surgery or heart-transplantation (HTx) serve as therapeutic options for treatment of drug resistant ventricular tachycardia (VT). This study compares the results of the different methods with regard to survival rate and quality of life.

According to their general condition and indication, the patients were subdivided into three different groups. In group I (n = 84, mean age 64 years) patients suffered from ischemic or dilative cardiomyopathy (CMP), with a cardiac ejection-fraction of 20% on average and polymorph and polytopic extrasystolies (ES); in 32 cases automatic defibrillators were implanted using epicardial leads and in 52 cases using transvenous/subcutaneous leads. Patients in group II (n = 32, mean age 62 years) with ischemic CMP, and with an EF of 25% on average and exclusively monomorph and monotopic ES received antiarrhythmic surgery. Patients in group III (n = 10, mean age 35 years) suffered from ischemic or dilative CMP with an EF of 19% on average and polymorph and polytopic ES. These patients underwent cardiac transplantation.

Survival rate after 3 months was 95% in group I, 78% in group II and 70% in group III; the corresponding 1 year survival rates were 93%, 74% and 70%. Patients in group I continued to receive antiarrhythmic drugs and were defibrillated several times per day in certain cases. Patients in group II and III were completely free of ventricular arrhythmias not necessitating any antiarrhythmic drugs.

All three cardiac surgical methods for treatment of VT serve as an alternative treatment when compared to conservative therapy. The best survival rates were achieved after implantation of automatic defibrillators, but, in contrast to the other methods, cardiac function was not improved and quality of life reached a lower level when compared to the other groups. Antiarrhythmia surgery obtains excellent results but is, however, indicated only in case of localized monomorph and monotopic ES. Cardiac transplantation remains as last option of surgical intervention. The indication for the different surgical procedures is based on morphology of VT, general condition of the patients and cardiac function.

Prof. Dr. E. Kreuzer, Herzchirurgische Klinik, Klinikum Großhadern, Marchioninistraße 15, W-8000 München 70

Entwicklung und Test des Laser-Speckle-Verfahrens zur Quantifizierung der Hautdurchblutung

Development and Test of the Laser-Speckle Method for the Quantification of the Skin Blood Flow

D. Abendroth[1], J. Schmand[2], B. Ruth[2] und L. Sunder-Plassmann[1]

[1]Abteilung für Gefäß-, Thorax- und Herzchirurgie, Klinikum der Universität Ulm
[2]GSF-Forschungszentrum für Umwelt + Gesundheit, Neuherberg

Einleitung

Die Mikrozirkulation in Hautniveau bei arterieller Verschlußerkrankung ist von besonderer Bedeutung, denn sie entscheidet u.a. über den Erhalt der Gliedmaße. Als optimal werden diejenigen Meßmethoden angesehen, welche bereits im Frühstadium, d.h. vor dem Auftreten morphologischer Veränderungen, funktionelle Störungen erfassen. Die Laser-Speckle-Methode (L.S.) stellt einen neuen, einfachen und nichtinvasiven Ansatz dar, Mikrozirkulationsstörungen in Hautniveau zu messen. Die Besonderheit des Laser-Speckle-Verfahrens liegt in der Berührungslosigkeit sowie in der erstmalig realisierten Ausschaltung von Störfaktoren der unbewußten Hautbewegung. Gerät und Meßmethode wurden bereits an anderer Stelle ausführlich beschrieben [1, 2].

Patienten und Methoden

Ziel der Untersuchung war ein Methodenvergleich dieses neuen Prototyps eines Laser-Speckle-Gerätes (LS) für die berührungsfreie Messung der Hautdurchblutung mit der bekannten transkutanen Sauerstoffdruckmessung (tcpO_2) [3, 4] (44°C). Die Messungen erfolgten in komfortabler liegenden Position in einem klimatisierten Raum (21°C ± 0,7) in Ruhe nach einer 20minütigen Akklimatisationszeit sowie nach 3 min einer suprasystolischen Blutzufuhrunterbrechung oberhalb des Meßortes (Fußdorsum) Mittels einer Blutdruckmanschettte zur Erfassung der postokklusiven und posthypoxischen Reoxygenierungskapazität.

Untersucht wurden vier Gruppen:

1. gesunde Kontrollpersonen (Gruppe I Nichtraucher = 26, 53 Untersuchungen, mittleres Alter 29,4 Jahre [25–52 Jahre]).
2. gesunde Raucher ohne klinische Anzeichen einer peripheren arteriellen Verschlußerkrankung (Gruppe II = 9, 17 Messungen, durchschnittliches Alter 27,8 Jahre [23–31 Jahre]).
3. Patienten mit arterieller Verschlußerkrankung im Stadium IIb nach Fontaine (Gruppe III = 15, 29 Messungen, durchschnittliches Alter 69,6 Jahre [54–84 Jahre]) sowie

Chirurgisches Forum 1993
f. experim. u. klinische Forschung
Becker/Beger/Hartel (Hrsg.)

4. Patienten nach simultaner Pankreas- und Nierentransplantation als Vertreter der Gruppe des Typ I-Diabetes mit 20 Patienten und 40 Messungen im durchschnittlichen Alter von 37 Jahren [im Bereich 25–53 Jahre].

Statistik

Die Ergebnisse werden als Mittelwert mit Standardabweichung angegeben. Die Unterschiede wurden nach dem student-t-Test sowie Mann-Whitney-rank-sum-Test bestimmt. Das Signifikanzniveau wurde bei 5% bei beiden Tests angenommen.

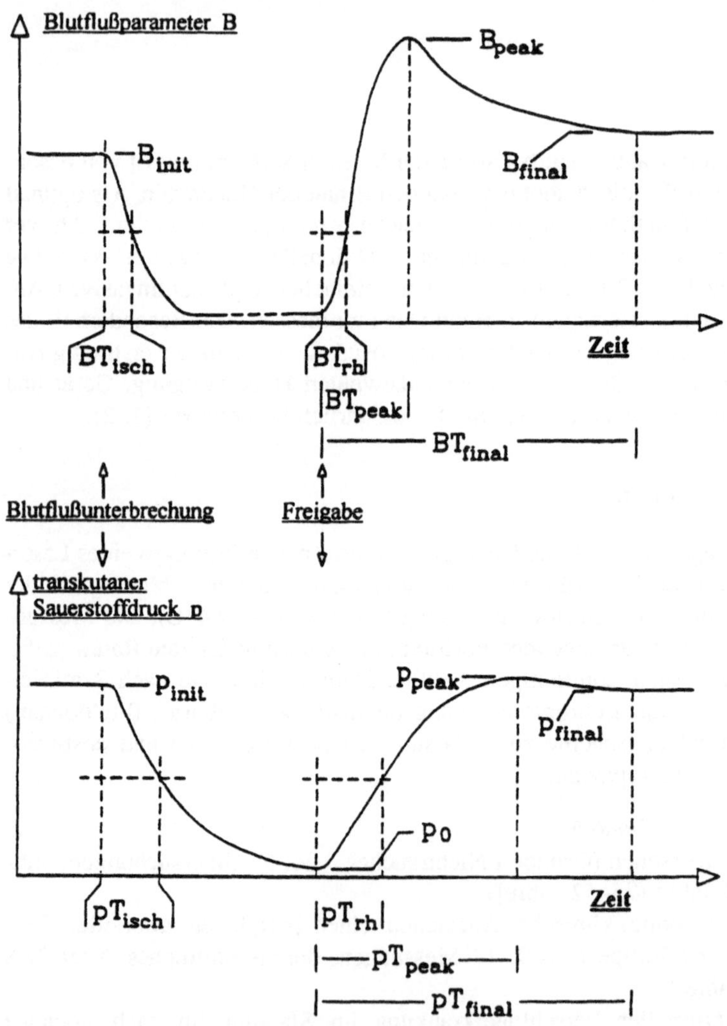

Abb. 1. Beispiele für die Blutflußparameter B und den Sauerstoffdruckparameter p während Ischämie und nach suprasystolischer Blutzufuhrunterbrechung mit reaktiver Hyperämie. Darstellung der absoluten und zeitabhängigen Meßparameter

Ergebnisse

Die Reproduzierbarkeit des LS-Verfahrens zeigte sich gut genug, um die erwarteten Änderungen der Durchblutungsqualität zu erfassen. Die parallel zur $tcpO_2$-Messung durchgeführte L.S.-Messung zeigte mit dem B_{init}-Wert des Blutflußparameters B den sog. "steady state" Blutfluß an.

Die Definition einer steady state Situation war gegeben, wenn die Variation des $TcpO_2$-Wertes kleiner ± 2 mmHg für mindestens 3 min betrug. Zunächst wurden der Blutflußparameter B sowie der $tcpO_2$-Wert p nach Akklimatisation in Ruhe vor und nach Okklusion und nachfolgender reaktiver postokklusiver Hyperämie gemessen. Beide Methoden zeigten einen charakteristischen Verlauf ihrer Signale während der gesamten Untersuchung und werden in der Abb. 1 mit folgenden charakteristischen Werten beschreiben: Bestimmung des Absolutwertes B und p bei der initialen "steady state" Situation (B_{init} für den Blutflußparameter und p_{init} für die $tcpO_2$-Werte) sowie die Kontrollwerte während der totalen Blutzufuhrunterbrechung, anschließend

Tabelle 1. Mittelwerte, Standardabweichungen und Signifikanz-Niveau der Meßwerte des Blutflußparameters B [relative Einheiten, Sekunden]. Die Signifikant-Niveaus beziehen sich auf die Hypothese, daß kein Unterschied zur Kontrolle vorhanden ist

Meßparameter	Gruppe I Kontrolle	Gruppe II Raucher	Gruppe III AVK	Gruppe IV Diabetiker
B_{init}	5,95 ± 2,55	5,29 ± 2,64 n.s.	4,07 ± 1,69 0,027	3,81 ± 1,51 0,0005
B_{peak}	8,90 ± 2,91	8,52 ± 2,81 n.s.	10,64 ± 5,71 n.s.	5,71 ± 2,68 < 0,0001
B_{final}	6,10 ± 3,23	4,76 ± 2,14 n.s.	5,26 ± 2,51 n.s.	3,27 ± 1,82 0,0002
BT_{isch}	4,87 ± 2,38	18,4 ± 15,2 < 0,0001	21,2 ± 33,1 0,006	3,79 ± 1,52 0,0002
BT_{rh}	4,10 ± 2,06	14,5 ± 15,4 < 0,0001	17,6 ± 32,7 0,004	5,31 ± 3,55 0,043
BT_{peak}	17,9 ± 8,0	76,6 ± 62,3 < 0,0001	68,6 ± 51,6 < 0,0001	25,4 ± 21,7 n.s.
BT_{final}	50,6 ± 38,7	234 ± 144 < 0,0001	126 ± 75 < 0,0001	46,5 ± 33,0 n.s.

die Spitzenwerte der hyperämischen Antwort (B_{peak} und p_{peak}) sowie die Endwerte in erneuten steady state (B_{final} und p_{final}). Der zeitliche Verlauf kann wie folgt beschrieben werden: 1. die Halbwertzeiten des Blutflußparameters B und $tcpO_2$-Messung p fallend vom initialen Wert zu dem Kontrollwert während der Blutzufuhrunterbrechung als BT_{isch} und pT_{isch} sowie der Anstieg dieser Werte von der Okklusion BT_{rh} sowie pT_{rh}. 2. Die absoluten Zeiten von L.S. und $tcpO_2$-Messung vom Anstieg des Kontrollwertes zu dem Spitzenwert der Hyperämie nach Blutzufuhrunterbrechung als BT_{peak} und pT_{peak} sowie beim Erreichen des "steady states" nach Blutzufuhrunterbrechung als BT_{final} und pT_{final}.

Die Gesamtzeit einer Einzelmessung betrug ca. 20 min bei gesunden Normalpersonen und 30–35 min bei Patienten mit fortgeschrittener arterieller Verschlußerkrankung.

Der Wert B_{init} fiel signifikant von $5,95 \pm 2,55$ für die Kontrollgruppe über $4,07 \pm 1,60$ für die Gruppe der peripheren arteriellen Verschlußerkrankung auf $3,81 \pm 1,51$ für die Gruppe der Diabetiker ab. Die Halbwertzeit BT_{rh} im Anstieg

Tabelle 2. Mittelwerte, Standardabweichungen und Signifikanz-Niveau der Meßwerte des Sauerstoffdruckmessung pI [Torr, Sekunden] (s. Tabelle 1)

Meßparameter	Gruppe I Kontrolle	Gruppe II Raucher	Gruppe III AVK	Gruppe IV Diabetiker
p_{init}	62,1 ± 7,2	64,2 ± 7,6 n.s.	29,7 ± 18,7 0,0001	54,3 ± 13,4 0,0032
p0	5,8 ± 7,1	3,8 ± 2,0 n.s.	7,1 ± 10,0 n.s.	20,0 ± 18,2 < 0,0001
p_{peak}	64,3 ± 7,8	67,3 ± 7,1 n.s.	37,2 ± 17,8 < 0,0001	57,2 ± 13,2 < 0,0051
p_{final}	63,6 ± 7,8	66,0 ± 7,0 n.s.	33,4 ± 17,3 < 0,0001	56,6 ± 13,4 0,0076
pT_{isch}	82,3 ± 21,5	79,8 ± 11,1 n.s.	60,1 ± 40,1 0,018	99,3 ± 95,8 n.s.
pT_{rh}	72,0 ± 18,4	79,3 ± 17,9 n.s.	184 ± 84 0,0006	63,3 ± 28,6 n.s.
pT_{peak}	319 ± 85	357 ± 93 n.s.	389 ± 206 n.s.	263 ± 104 0,0054
pT_{final}	341 ± 92	381 ± 105 n.s.	425 ± 226 n.s.	282 ± 121 0,0096

des Blutflußparameters B im Rahmen der reaktiven Hyperämie war signifkant erhöht von $4,10 \pm 2,06$ auf $14,5 \pm 15,4$ sek für die Raucher sowie auf $17,6 \pm 32,7$ sek für die Werte der peripheren arteriellen Verschlußerkrankung. Die Diabetiker zeigten hier einen Wert von $5,31 \pm 3,55$ sek. Die anderen charakteristischen Parameter wie B_{peak} und BT_{peak} während der reaktiven Hyperämie sowie die Werte B_{final} und BT_{final} zeigten ähnliche Effekte (Tabelle 1 und 2). Der Korrelationskoeffizient zwischen den verschiedenen charakteristischen Werten der Laser-Speckle-Methode zeigte in seinem Verhalten im Rahmen der Absolutwerte von B sowie der charakteristischen Zeiten während der dynamischen Untersuchung ein unterschiedliches Variationsverhalten und scheint somit eine zusätzliche Information zur transkutanen Sauerstoffdruckmessung darzustellen.

Zusammenfassung

Die Bestimmung der Mikrozirkulation im Hautbereich bei arterieller Verschlußerkrankung ist von großer Bedeutung. Die Laser-Speckle-Methode stellt hier einen neuen, einfachen und berührungsfreien Ansatz dar, Mikrozirkulationsstörungen in Hautniveau zu erfassen. Ziel dieser Untersuchung war ein Methodenvergleich eines Prototypen des Laser-Speckle-Gerätes mit der bekannten transkutanen Sauerstoffdruckmessung. Messungen an Gesunden, asymptomatischen Rauchern, AVK-Patienten (Stad. IIb) und Typ I-Diabetikern mit diabetischen Spätsymptomen zeigten, daß sowohl die Absolutwerte als auch die Zeitwerte nach suprasystolischer Blutflußunterbrechung sich im Vergleich zu gesunden Testpersonen unterschiedlich änderten. Diese unterschiedliche Beobachtung der Variation und Dynamik während Ischämie und reaktiver Hyperämie erlaubt eine zusätzliche Information im Vergleich zu anderen klinisch etablierten Methoden.

Summary

Measurement of microcirculation of the skin is of great importance in arterial occlusive disease. The Laser-Speckle device is a new, simple approach to measure microcirculatory disorders of the skin without any contact. Aim of this study was a methodological comparison of a prototype of the Laser-Speckle device with the established transcutaneous oxygen pressure measurement. Measurements on healthy controls, asymptomatic smokers, patients with peripheral arterial occlusive disease and on type I diabetic patients with late diabetic complications showed that the absolute values as well as the time-related values after suprasystolic blood flow occlusion were affected differently when compared to measurements on healthy controls. This different observation of different variation and dynamics during ischemia and reactive hyperemia provides an additional information for comparison with other clinical methods employed.

Literatur

1. Ruth B (1990) Blood flow determination by the laser speckle method. Int J Microcirc Clin Exp 9:21–45
2. Kvernebo K, Slagsvold E, Straden E, Kroese A, Larsen S (1988) Laser Doppler flowmetry in evaluation of lower limb resting skin circulation. A study in healthy controls and atherosclerotic patients. Scand J Clin Lab Invest 48:621–626
3. Karanfilian RG, Lynch TG, Zirul VT, Padberg FT, Jamil Z, Hobson RW (1986) The value of laser Doppler velocimetry and transcutaneous oxygen tension determination in predicting healing of ischemic forefoot ulcerations and amputations in diabetic and nondiabetic patients. J Vasc Surg 4:511–516
4. Allen PIM, Goldman M (1987) Skin blood flow: a comparison of cutaneous oxymetry and laser Doppler flowmetry. Eur J Vasc Surg 1:315–318

Priv.-Doz. Dr. D. Abendroth, Abteilung für Gefäß-, Thorax- und Herzchirurgie, Klinikum der Universität Ulm, Steinhövelstraße 9, W-7900 Ulm

Screening potentiell anti-arteriosklerotisch wirksamer Substanzen anhand der Migrationsaktivität humaner Gefäßwandmyozyten im Zellkulturmodell

Screening Substances with Potentially Antiarteriosclerotic Effects by Investigating the Migratory Activity of Human Vessel Wall Myocytes in a Cell Culture Model

R. Brandl[1], B. Höfling[2], J. Heimerl[2] und G. Bauriedel[2]

[1]Chirurgische Klinik und Poliklinik, Universität Regensburg
[2]Medizinische Klinik I, Universität München, Klinikum Großhadern

Einleitung

Die Einwanderung glatter Muskelzellen (SMC) aus der Media in den subendothelialen Raum wird im Rahmen der Plaqueformierung als wesentlicher, der Proliferation dieser Zellen vorgeschalteter pathogenetischer Prozeß angesehen. Die Analyse des zellulären Motilitätsverhaltens in vitro könnte für das Verständnis zugrundeliegender Pathomechanismen und damit für die Entwicklung kausaler Therapiekonzepte von Bedeutung sein.

Material und Methoden

Zellkultur-Technik

Aus intraoperativ und perkutan mittels Simpson-Atherektomiekatheter abgetragenen Plaques (Primärstenosen aus 5 Koronarien, 7 Femoralarterien, 2 Aorten von 14 symptomatischen Patienten) wurden Zellkulturen glatter Muskelzellen (SMC) mittels enzymatischer Disaggregierung (Kollagenase/Elastase) angelegt. Bezüglich des detaillierten methodischen Vorgehens siehe [1–4].

Immunfluoreszenzmikroskopie

Die Typisierung der Zellen erfolgte immunfluoreszenzmikroskopisch nach Markierung mit monoklonalen Primärantikörpern gegen glattmuskuläres α-Aktin und von Willebrand-Faktor sowie mit FITC-konjugierten Zweit-Antikörpern (goat anti mouse IgG) [1–4].

Motilitätsanalyse

Die spontane zelluläre Motilität wurde an SMC-Primärkulturen bei einer Zelldichte von 2000–5000 Zellen/cm^2 untersucht. Die Kulturen wurden während des gesam-

Chirurgisches Forum 1993
f. experim. u. klinische Forschung
Becker/Beger/Hartel (Hrsg.)

ten Meßvorgangs bei 37°C in Standard-Zellkulturmedium inkubiert. Die Analyse der Zellbewegungen erfolgte anhand eines computergestützten Video-Analysesystems (vergleiche [2, 3]).

Ergebnisse

Lichtmikroskopisch zeigten die kultivierten Zellen ungeachtet der ursprünglichen Plaqueabtragungsstelle eine polygonale bis spindelförmige Gestalt. Der immunfluoreszenzmikroskopische Nachweis von glattmuskulärem α-Aktin und die negative Reaktion mit Antikörpern gegen von Willebrand-Faktor charakterisierte 80–90% und damit die Mehrzahl der Zellen als glatte Muskelzellen.

Die Spontanmotilität der kultivierten SMC folgte einem zufälligen Verteilungsmuster. Richtungsänderungen der Zellbewegungen lagen zwischen 0° und 180°. Eine Synchronisation der Einzelzellbewegung mit der benachbarter Zellen war nicht erkennbar.

Die mittlere Geschwindigkeit der SMC-Migration (v), definiert als Zentroidverlagerung pro Zeiteinheit, lag für unbehandelte Zellen bei $21,7 \pm 2,1$ μm/h (Kontrolle als Bezugsgröße = 100%). Nach Zugabe von Israpidin, einem Calcium-Antagonisten der Dihydropyridingruppe, war bei einer Wirkstoffkonzentration von 10^{-7} M eine signifikante Abnahme der mittleren Migrationsgeschwindigkeit auf 67% zu verzeichnen. Das Antitubulin Colchizin bewirkte in gleicher Wirkstoffkonzentration eine Minderung auf 34% ($p < 0,05$).

Diskussion

Unsere Ergebnisse zeigen, daß die Migrationsaktivität kultivierter SMC aus menschlichem Plaquegewebe anhand eines computergestützten Videodokumentationssystems quantifizierbar charakterisiert werden kann. Die ursprüngliche Lokalisation der Plaqueabtragungsstelle hatte keinen Einfluß auf die Meßwerte. Die immunfluoreszenzmikroskopische Typisierung bestätigt in Übereinstimmung mit früheren Untersuchungen [1, 4] die hohe Homogenität der Zellkulturen mit einem SMC-Anteil von 80 bis 90%. Eine signifikante Abhängigkeit von der Serumkonzentration des Zellkulturmediums, wie sie für die Proliferation dieser Zellen besteht [1, 4], ist in den in unserem Experiment angewandten Konzentrationsbereichen (FCS 15%) nicht zu beobachten gewesen. Dies spricht dafür, daß es sich bei dem Parameter SMC-Migrationsaktivität um eine Meßgröße handelt, die unabhängig ist von der streng Serum-abhängigen SMC-Proliferationsaktivität [2, 3]. Wiederholte Motilitätsstudien an ein und derselben Kultur zeigten über einen Zeitraum von 5 Tagen keine Unterschiede in den gemessenen Migrationsgeschwindigkeiten von statistischer Signifikanz. In ihrer Gesamtheit sprechen die vorgenannten Bedingungen dafür, daß von einer hinreichenden Konstanz der Motilitätsanalysen in unserem in-vitro-Modell ausgegangen werden darf.

Somit sind die Voraussetzungen gegeben, um den Einfluß verschiedener Pharmaka auf den Aktivitätsparameter Migrationsgeschwindigkeitsverhalten glatter Muskelzellen in vitro zu quantifizieren. Sicherlich ist das beschriebene SMC-Zellkulturmodell nicht in der Lage, die komplexe in vivo-Situation der arteriosklerotischen Läsion zu repräsentieren. Trotzdem finden sich Zusammenhänge zwischen quantifizierbaren in-vitro-Parametern und spezifischem Ausgangsmaterial, die für beteiligte pathophysiologische Mechanismen sprechen: Hier liegen tierexperimentelle Befunde [5] vor sowie Beobachtungen am Zellkulturmodell humaner SMC aus Arterioskleroseläsionen symptomatischer Patienten [1–4]. Wie die Untersuchungen von Bauriedel u. Mitarb. [3] zeigten, sind Zellen aus humanen Restenoseläsionen durch eine signifikant erhöhte Migrationsaktivität gegenüber Zellen aus Primärstenosegewebe charakterisiert. Die Möglichkeit einer wirksamen Hemmung dieser zellulären Aktivität könnte somit nicht nur neue Perspektiven für die sekundäre Prävention nach revaskularisierenden Eingriffen, sondern auch für die Primärprophylaxe eröffnen.

Zusammenfassung

Neben der Proliferation wird die Migration glatter Muskelzellen (SMC) als wesentlicher zellulärer Mechanismus bei der Plaqueformierung angesehen. Kulturen humaner SMCs wurden von koronaren (n = 5), femoralen (n = 7) und aortalen (n = 2) arteriosklerotischen Läsionen angelegt. Durch ein computergestütztes standardisiertes Video-Analysesystem wurde die spontane SMC-Migrationsaktivität mit 21,7 ± 2,1 μm/h (n = 14; x ± SD) gemessen. Zugabe des Calcium-Antagonisten Israpidin (10^{-7} M) oder Colchizin (10^{-7} M) hatte jeweils eine signifikante Abnahme der SMC-Migrationsgeschwindigkeit zur Folge.

Die Ergebnisse zeigen, daß die SMC-Migrationsgeschwindigkeit als Parameter für das Screening potentiell antiarteriosklerotisch wirksamer Substanzen von Bedeutung sein könnte.

Summary

In addition to proliferation, migration of smooth muscle cells (SMC) is considered to be an essential cellular mechanism involved in human plaque formation. SMC's were cultured from 14 coronary (n = 5), femoral (n = 7), and aortic (n = 2) arteries of symptomatic patients. Using a semiautomatic standardized video analysis system, SMC migratory activity was quantified to 21.7 ± 2.1 μm/h (n = 14; $x \pm$SD). Addition of different drugs such as isradipine ($10^{-7} M$) or colchicine ($10^{-7} M$) resulted in a significant reduction of SMC migratory velocity. These results indicate that SMC migratory velocity may be a parameter to screen-selected substances for potential antiarteriosclerotic effects.

Literatur

1. Bauriedel G, Beyer RW, Überfuhr P, Brandl R, Heimerl J, Heidemann P, Becker HM, Höfling B (1991) Zellkultivierung aus operativ angetragenem Plaquegewebe. Angio Archiv 21:29–35

2. Bauriedel G, Windstetter U, Brandl R, Plas E, Kandolf R, Höfling B (1991) Erhöhte In-vitro-Motilität humaner Gefäßwandmyozyten aus Restenose-Läsionen peripherer und koronarer Gefäße. Z Kardiol 80:494–499
3. Bauriedel G, Windstetter U, DeMaio SJ, Kandolf R, Häfling B (1992) Migratory activity of human smooth muscle cells cultivated from coronary and peripheral primary and restenotic lesions removed from percutaneous atherectomy. Circulation 85:554–564
4. Dartsch PC, Voisard R, Bauriedel G, Höfling B, Betz E (1990) Growth characteristics and cytoskeletal organization of cultured smooth muscle cells from human primary stenosing and restenosing lesions. Arteriosclerosis 10:62–75
5. Grünwald J, Haudenschild CC (1984) Intimal injury in vivo activates vascular smooth muscle cell migration and explant outgrowth in vitro. Arteriosclerosis 4:183–188

Dr. R. Brandl, Oberarzt, Klinik und Poliklinik für Chirurgie, Universität Regensburg, Franz Josef Strauß Allee 11, W-8400 Regensburg

Intraoperative Qualitätssicherung nach gefäßchirurgischer Intervention an den Mesenterialgefäßen durch Serosa-Monitoring der Kalium-Aktivität

Potassium Monitoring on Serosa Surface as Indicator for Small-Bowel Viability in Vascular Surgery

Th. Büsser, Ch. Töns, G. Winkeltau und V. Schumpelick

Chirurgische Klinik, RWTH Aachen (Direktor: Univ.-Prof. Dr. med. V. Schumpelick)

Einleitung

Akute intestinale Ischämien zwingen bei gefäßchirurgischen Interventionen zu bisher lediglich klinisch begründeten Entscheidungen bezüglich primärer Resektion oder rekonstruktiven Maßnahmen. Farbstoffanflutungstests, Dopplersonographie o.ä. haben sich als objektive Entscheidungshilfe nicht durchsetzen können. Zwar ist die wiederhergestellte Perfusion darstellbar, eine Objektivierung der zellulären Integrität zur Vermeidung fibrotischer Spätstenosen ist bisher nicht möglich.

Ziel der Untersuchung war zum einen eine Validitätsprüfung der klinischen Beurteilung, zum anderen sollte das ionenselektive Kalium-Oberflächenmonitoring [1] in seiner Wertigkeit zur Reperfusionsbeurteilung überprüft werden.

Methodik

In Äther/Hypnomidate-Narkose wurde bei 50 Sprague Dawley Ratten eine Dünndarmischämie durch Abklemmen der Arteria und Vena mesenterica superior erzeugt. Eine mittlere Dünndarmschlinge wurde für postoperative radiologische Spätkontrollen mit einem röntgendichten Faden markiert. Während der Ischämie- und späteren Reperfusionsphase wurde in 2 und 5minütigen Abständen die Kalium-Serosa-Aktivität (a K^+) mit einem ionenselektiven Meßgerät (Fa. Siegert GmbH) durch nichtinvasives Aufsetzen des Sensors auf die Serosa des zuvor ausgewählten Dünndarmsegmentes gemessen. Durch Applikation einer Wärmelampe und Befeuchten des Darmes mit angewärmter Kochsalzlösung wurden konstante Außenbedingungen sichergestellt. Der Anpreßdruck des Sensors wurde jeweils durch sein Eigengewicht standardisiert.

Nach 40, 60 und 80 min erfolgte die klinische Beurteilung der intraoperativen Ischämiesituation durch zwei erfahrene Chirurgen in Unkenntnis der zuvor ermittelten Meßwerte. War nach 80 min noch keine adäquate Ischämiesituation festgestellt, wurde beurteilungsunabhängig bei diesen Tieren nach 120 min reperfundiert. Bei den übrigen Ratten wurde die Reperfusion eingeleitet, wenn von den Beurteilern zu einem der Untersuchungszeitpunkte eine eindeutige aber noch nicht resektionspflichtige

Chirurgisches Forum 1993
f. experim. u. klinische Forschung
Becker/Beger/Hartel (Hrsg.)

Ischämiesituation konstatiert wurde. Die Reperfusionsphase wurde einheitlich über 30 min klinisch und mittels a K^+ Messung überwacht. Nach Beurteilung des Erholungsverhaltens über 30 min erfolgte eine erneute Stellungnahme der klinischen Beobachter bezüglich der endgültig einzuschätzenden Viabilität des Darmes.

Bei der aus 5 weiteren Ratten bestehenden Kontrollgruppe wurden ohne Anlage einer Ischämie die Meßdaten wie oben angegeben über 120 min erhoben.

Bei den langzeitüberlebenden Ratten erfolgte am 8. postoperativen Tag eine radiologische Passagedarstellung nach Gabe von bariumhaltigem Futter. Nach Mikroangiographie des markierten Darmsegmentes sowie Euthanasie der Tiere wurde abschließend eine histologische Klassifizierung nach Chiu [2] durchgeführt.

Ergebnisse und Diskussion

Operationstechnisch bedingt verstarben 4 Tiere der Untersuchungsgruppe, so daß die Ischämie- und Reperfusionsuntersuchung bei 46 Ratten ausgewertet werden konnte.

Die Kontrollgruppe zeigte sowohl nach klinischer Beurteilung als auch bei der Messung der Kalium-Aktivität (a K^+) auf der Dünndarmserosa ein völlig stabiles Bild mit einer mittleren a K^+ über 120 min von 8,2 mmol/l SD-max $\pm$ 1,2 mmol/l. In der Ischämiegruppe fand sich ein hochsignifikanter Zusammenhang zwischen Ischämiedauer und Anstieg der a K^+ ($p < 0{,}001$). Der Anstieg der K^+-Aktivitätswerte während der ersten 60 min war linear. Nach 20 min (n = 46) bis auf $22,3 \pm 7,7$ mmol/l, nach 40 min (n = 46) $44,1 \pm 7,6$ mmol/l, nach 60 min (n = 34) $64,9 \pm 10,8$ mmol/l, nach 80 min (n = 22) $78,6 \pm 10,5$ mmol/l, nach 100 min (n = 7) $84,1 \pm 12,8$ mmol/l, nach 120 min (n = 7) $93,2 \pm 14,0$ mmol/l a K^+.

Nach kritischer Beurteilung lag eine eindeutige Ischämiewirkung ohne Resektionspflichtigkeit und damit die Indikation zur Reperfusion bei 26,1% (n = 12) nach 40minütiger Ischämiezeit vor, bei 26,1% (n = 12) nach 60 min, und bei 32,6% (n = 15) nach 80 min. Die restlichen 7 Tiere zeigten auch nach 80 min keine eindeutige Ischämiewirkung, so daß bei diesen 15,3% nach 120 min reperfundiert wurde.

Vermeintlich korrelierend zum klinischen Eindruck zeigten auch die Mittelwerte der a K^+ unter Reperfusion einen steilen Abfall: nach 10 min $47,5 \pm 22,6$ mmol/l, nach 20 min $35,7 \pm 20,9$ mmol/l und nach 30 min $34,4 \pm 21,7$ mmol/l.

Bei der abschließenden klinischen Beurteilung der Ischämie und des Reperfusionsverhaltens legten sich die Gutachter bei 28 Ratten auf eine gesicherte Darmviabilität fest. Bei den übrigen 18 Tieren läge ein zweifelhafter Befund und damit doch eine Resektionspflichtigkeit vor.

Innerhalb der ersten 24 h nach Beendigung des Ischämieversuches kamen spontan 29 Ratten (63%) ad exitum, darunter alle 22 der nach 80 und 120 min reperfundierten sowie 7 der 12 nach 60 min reperfundierten Tiere. Bei der Sektion fanden sich überwiegend vollständige Darmnekrosen mit Spontanperforationen sowie histologisch ausschließlich Grad 4 und 5 nach Chiu.

Gemäß klinischem Eindruck überlebten leidensfrei 17 Versuchstiere (37%) 8 postoperative Tage. Bei der Sekundärdiagnostik (MDP, Mikroangiographie und Histologie) fand sich bei 5 Tieren allerdings eine Defektheilung mit fibrotischer Stenosierung und vorliegendem Subileus. Bei diesen Tieren zeigte sich mikroangiographisch eine

Rarefizierung der segmentalen Gefäße sowie histologisch Ischämiegrade 3 und 4 nach Chiu [2].

Die Fehlerhaftigkeit der klinischen Beurteilung der Darmviabilität ist evident. Zum Zeitpunkt der Reperfusion sollten 100% der beurteilten Darmischämien voll rückbildungsfähig sein – tatsächlich überlebten aber nur 37% der Tiere diese klinisch als voll rückbildungsfähig eingeschätzte Ischämiesituation. Auch die Beurteilungskorrektur nach Beobachtung des Erholungsverhaltens geht noch von 28 Tieren mit einer zu erwartenden restitutio ad integrum aus. Zu diesem Zeitpunkt beträgt beim Beurteilungskriterium "Überleben" der klinisch falsch positive Fehler 37,9% und orientiert an der restitutio ad integrum sogar 47,1%.

Prüft man die Wertigkeit der a K^+-Messung auf der Dünndarmserosa an dem Ergebnis des Überlebens und der Sekundärdiagnostik, findet sich entsprechend eine Zuordnung in drei Gruppen (Abb. 1): alle Tiere haben eine restitutio ad integrum erreicht, deren maximaler a K^+-Ischämiewert (a K^+_{is}) $< 42,3 \pm 6,1$ mmol/l und der 10 min Reperfusionswert (a K^+_{rp10}) $< 16,6 \pm 3,3$ mmol/l betrug (n = 12).

Eine überlebte radiologisch und histologisch belegte Defektheilung bestand bei a K^+-Konstellationen von a K^+_{is} $54,7 \pm 8,5$ mmol/l und a K^+_{rp10} $24,6 \pm 4,0$ mmol/l (n = 5).

Hochzuverlässig bestand eine durch exitus letalis, Sektion und Histologie dokumentierte Darmnekrose bei a K^+_{is} $78,2 \pm 14,8$ mmol/l und a K^+_{rp10} $36,7 \pm 13,6$ mmol/l (n = 29).

Das nichtinvasive ionenselektive Monitoring der Kalium-Aktivität auf reperfundiertem Dünndarm zeigt sich der rein klinischen Beurteilung deutlich überlegen. Falsch positive klinische Beurteilungen von 38 bzw. 47% belegen die Notwendigkeit zu einem objektivierenden metrischen Verfahren [3]. Gegenüber bisher zu diesem Zweck erprobten Verfahren scheint das Monitoring der a K^+ auch die zelluläre Integrität

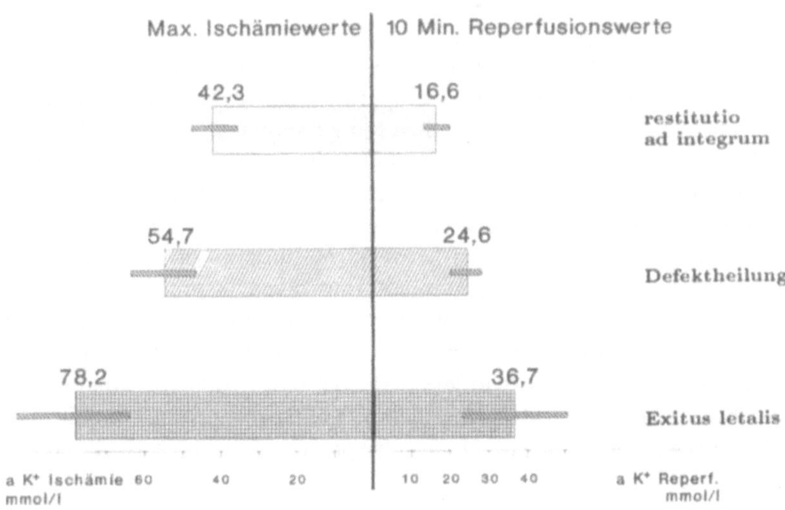

Abb. 1. Serosa a K^+-Werte der maximalen Ischämie und nach 10 min Reperfusion, differenziert nach Spätergebnissen

erfassen zu können. Nur Darmgewebe, das bei erneuter Perfusion auch damit ATP-Zufuhr über die reaktivierte Na^+/K^+-Pumpe bei der Reperfusion die a K^+-Werte nach 10 min unter 20 mmol/l senken kann, scheint der fibrotischen Spätstenose oder gar Darmnekrose zu entgehen.

Basierend auf den experimentellen Ergebnissen hat das ionenselektive Serosa-Monitoring der a K^+ bei abdominellen gefäßchirurgischen Eingriffen als intraoperatives metrisches Kontrollverfahren Eingang in die Klinik gefunden.

Zusammenfassung

Die intraoperative Entscheidung, passager ischämisch geschädigten Darm zu resezieren oder belassen zu dürfen, basiert auch heute noch allein auf chirurgischer Empirie. In einem Dünndarmischämiemodell an 55 Sprague Dawley Ratten wurde die Validität klinischer Beurteilung sowie ein ionenselektives Kalium-Monitoring der Dünndarmserosa zur intraoperativen Ischämiebeurteilung erprobt. Die klinische Beurteilung erweist sich mit 47% falsch positiver Beurteilung als unzuverlässig. Neben einem hochsignifikanten ($p < 0,001$) linearem Zusammenhang zwischen Ischämiedauer und Anstieg der K^+-Aktivität lassen sich durch ionenselektives K^+-Monitoring relevante Reperfusionsprofile darstellen. Gesicherte Darmviabilität (klinisch, histologisch und röntgenologisch) zeigt sich bei maximalen Ischämiewerten < 45 mmol/l K^+-Akt. und unmittelbarem Rückgang der K^+-Akt. nach 10 min Reperfusion auf Werte < 20 mmol/l. Basierend auf den experimentellen Daten findet das ionenselektive K^+-Oberflächenmonitoring als intraoperatives metrisches Kontrollverfahren bei intestinalen gefäßchirurgischen Eingriffen derzeit Eingang in die Klinik.

Summary

The intraoperative decision whether or not to resect bowel segments compromised by transient ischemia is still based on purely empirical surgical judgement. A model of reversible small-bowel ischemia involving 55 Sprague Dawley rats was used to test the validity of both clinical judgement and of ion-selective, serosal potassium monitoring with respect to the intraoperative assessment of ischemic damage. Clinical evaluation proved to be unreliable, with 47% false positive results. Apart from a highly significant ($p < 0.001$) linear correlation between the duration of ischemia and the rise in K^+ activity, the ion selective K^+ monitoring revealed prognostically relevant patterns of reperfusion. Verified gut viability (clinically, histologically, and radiologically) is indicated by maximum K^+ activities less than 45 mmol/l under ischemic conditions and a decline in K^+ values to less than 20 mmol/l within 10 min of reperfusion. Based on these experimental data, the method of ion-selective K^+ monitoring is now being clinically applied in intestinal vascular procedures to objectively predict gut viability.

Literatur

1. Töns Ch, Fenzlein PG, Winkeltau G, Büsser Th, Schumpelick V (1991) Ionenselektives on-line Monitoring der Kalium-Aktivität als Parameter für die Dünndarmischämie. Langenbecks Arch Chir [Suppl] Chir Forum, S 271–275
2. Chiu C-J, McArdle AH, Brown R, Scott HJ, Gurd FN (1970) Intestinal mucosal lesion in low-flow states. Arch Surg 101:478–483
3. Bulkley GB, Zuidema GD, Hamilton SR, O'Mara C, Klacsmann PG, Horn SD (1981) Intraoperative determination of small intestinal viability following ischemic injury. Arch Surg 193:628–635

Dr. med. H.W.Ch. Töns, Chirurgische Klinik, RWTH Aachen, Pauwelsstraße 30, W-5100 Aachen

Transplantation von humanen Endothelzellen auf biologische Herzklappenprothesen

Transplantation of Human Endothelial Cells onto Cardiac Valve Bioprostheses

T. Fischlein, G. Lehner, W. Lante und B. Reichart

Herzchirurgische Klinik, Ludwig-Maximilians-Universität, München

Einleitung

Biologische Herzklappenprothesen weisen im Gegensatz zu normalen Herzklappen kein vitales Endothel auf. Auch lange nach Implantation dieser gewöhnlich mit Glutaraldehyd oder Formaldehyd fixierten Xenografts konnte eine Endothelialisierung bisher nicht beobachtet werden. Gerade das Fehlen dieser natürlichen Schutzbarriere wird neben der zytotoxischen Aldehyd-Konservierung für die frühe Degeneration und die dadurch bedingten schlechten Langzeitergebnisse dieser Bioimplantate verantwortlich gemacht. Trotz der bekannten Vorteile gegenüber den mechanischen Klappenmodellen scheint deshalb die Verwendung dieser Prothesen in erster Linie nur mehr beim alten Patienten gerechtfertigt zu sein. Nun könnte eine Endothelialisierung der biologischen Herzklappenprothesen durch Transplantation von autologen Endothelzellen (EC), wie es bereits an Kunststoffprothesen in der peripheren Gefäßchirurgie klinisch erfolgreich praktiziert wurde [1, 2], die rasche Klappen-Degeneration verhindern. Ein funktionstüchtiges, intaktes Endothel könnte nicht nur die Oberflächenthrombogenität und die Ablagerung von Thrombusformationen verhindern, sondern vor allem den vermehrten Plasmaprotein-Einstrom in die Klappensegel und die dadurch bedingte rasche Kalzifizierung des Klappenapparates unterbinden [3]. Inwieweit eine EC-Beschichtung von mit Glutaraldehyd fixierten Bioklappen möglich ist, soll in dieser experimentellen Studie gezeigt werden.

Material und Methoden

Als biologisches Material zur Endothelialisierung wurden kommerziell erwerbbare Schweineklappenprothesen (n = 6) und nach dem gleichen Verfahren fixiertes bovines Pericard (n = 20) verwendet. Als Zellquelle dienten humane Vena saphena EC, welche von Venenresten nach koronaren Bypassoperationen gewonnen wurden.

Präparation des biologischen Materials

Beide Materialien waren in 0,25% Glutaraldehyd (GA) konserviert. Zur Verminderung der Zytotoxizität freier Aldehyd-Gruppen mußten alle Präparate vor der Zellbeschich-

Chirurgisches Forum 1993
f. experim. u. klinische Forschung
Becker/Beger/Hartel (Hrsg.)

tung nach einem speziellen Verfahren gespült werden. Dabei wurden diese in kalter, gepufferter saliner Flüssigkeit (PBS) mehrfach gewaschen und in L-Glutaminsäure bei niederem pH-Wert für 48 h und Raumtemperatur gelagert. Nach einem zusätzlichen Waschvorgang in PBS wurden die Präparatstücke in 24-Lochplatten gelegt und unter Teflonringen (1,1 cm Durchmesser) fixiert. Anschließend wurden die Klappensegel und die Serosaoberflächen der Perikardstücke mit einer Heparin-Fibronectin Lösung vorbeschichtet. Alle Präparate wurden mit einem Wachstumsfaktor behandelt; ein Teil der Perikardstücke mit "Endothelial Cell Growth Supplement" (ECGS, 30 000 ng/ml, Seromed), der Rest mit "basic Fibroblast Growthfactor" (nFGF, 7 ng/ml).

Endothelialisierung

Die humanen EC wurden nach einem bewährten und bereits früher beschriebenen Verfahren aus den Venenstücken isoliert und anschließend im Brutschrank kultiviert [4]. Nach Erreichen einer geeignet hohen Zellzahl wurden die EC auf die vorbereiteten Präparate, bei einer Zelldichte von 50 000 EC/cm^2 ausgesät. Zur Heranreifung des Zytoskeletts sowie des Zellgefüges wurden die endothelialisierten Paäparate für 7 Tage bei 37°C und 5% CO_2 in Medium M-199 mit 20% humanem Serum nachkultiviert. Drei kommerziell erwerbbare Bioprothesen wurden in toto an beiden Seiten auf die gleiche Weise endothelialisiert. Dem Zellmedium wurde entweder ECGS oder bFGF Wachstumsfaktor zugesetzt.

EC Proliferation, Morphologie und Metabolismus

Die Zellproliferation wurde im beta-Counter, nach Inkorporation von ^{3}H-Thymidin in die Zellen, mittels angegebener "Counts" bestimmt. Als Stoffwechsel-Parameter diente das von den EC produzierte Prostacyklin (PGI_2), welches im Medium als 6-keto-prostaglandin F1alpha mit Hilfe von RIA (DuPont) nachgewiesen wurde. Morphologische Untersuchungen wurden mit dem Rasterelektronenmikroskop (REM) und dem Lichtmikroskop durchgeführt.

Ergebnisse

Proliferationsstudien haben gezeigt, daß die beste Wachstumsstimulation mit bFGF (die optimale Konzentration betrug 7 ng/ml) – im Vergleich mit ECGS – zu erreichen war. So konnten am 3. Tag 14102 $\pm$ 628 Counts mit bFGF vs. 1177 $\pm$ 98 Counts mit ECGS im beta-Counter bestimmt werden. Am 7. Tag betrug der Unterschied 288727 $\pm$ 39668 nach bFGF vs. 91924 $\pm$ 1123 Counts nach ECGS Stimulation ($p < 0{,}001$).

Die beibehaltene Stoffwechselfunktion der transplantierten EC konnte durch die nachgewiesene PGI_2 Produktion bestätigt werden. Die mit bFGF aktivierten transplantierten EC produzierten am 7. Tag durchschnittlich 3750 pg $PGI_2/10^6$ EC, welches als der sogenannte Basis-Level angesehen werden kann. Die Stimulation mit 25

μM Na-Arachidonsäure ergab durchschnittlich 8750 pg/10^6 EC, die Hemmung mit 10 mMol Acetylsalicylsäure 1500 pg/10^6 EC, jeweils nach 2 h gemessen.

Die REM Auswertungen zeigten, daß eine Endothelialisierung auf unbehandelten GA fixierten Präparaten nicht möglich erscheint. Auf diesen Oberflächen konnten nur tote, nicht adhärente EC gefunden werden. Die speziell vorbehandelten Perikard- oder Klappenpräparate zeigten am 7. Tag nach bFGF Stimulation einen durchwegs konfluenten EC-Rasen, während die mit ECGS stimulierten Zellkulturen als präkonfluent erschienen. Auch auf den in toto endothelialisierten Bioprothesen fand sich eine schöne und konfluente Zellschichte, darunter ein intaktes und unauffälliges Kollagen-Maschenwerk.

Zusammenfassung

In dieser Arbeit konnte demonstriert werden, daß eine in-vitro Endothelialisierung von speziell vorbereiteten Glutaraldehyd fixierten Herzklappenprothesen möglich ist. Die Proliferation der ausgesäten Endothelzellen wird dabei durch den Zusatz von bFGF optimal verstärkt. Eine Reduzierung der Toxizität von freien Aldehyd-Gruppen durch Aminosäuren-Behandlung scheint damit bewiesen worden zu sein. Als besonders wichtig in diesem Zusammenhang erscheint die Feststellung, daß die Endothelzellen auch nach Transplantation ihre Stoffwechselfunktionen aufrechterhalten können. Inwieweit jedoch diese transplantierten Zellen den einwirkenden Scherkräften der turbulenten Blutströmung im Klappenbereich standhalten können, bleibt weiteren Versuchen auf diesem Gebiet vorbehalten. Anzunehmen ist, daß die erfolgreiche autologe Endothelialisierung, zusammen mit einer Neutralisierung des toxischen Glutaraldehyds, die rasche Degeneration von biologischen Klappenprothesen verhindern kann. Die Möglichkeit der biologischen Beschichtung könnte zu einer Neuentwicklung dieser Implantate beitragen und die Zukunft der Klappenchirurgie entscheidend beeinflussen.

Summary

The main focus of this study was to investigate the possibility of endothelialization of biological artificial cardiac valves. As confirmed by scanning electron microscopy, our final results show that in vitro endothelialization of specially prepared biological valves fixed with glutaraldehyde by human endothelial cells is possible. In order to reduce the toxicity of free aldehydes, valve specimens were treated with L-glutamic acid. Subsequently, the growth factor bFGF was utilized to ensure optimal proliferation of transplanted endothelial cells. In this context, our findings of prostacyclin (PGI_2) production showed that even after transplantation these cells were able to maintain their metabolic activity. However, future experiments have to evaluate the shear stress resistance of the newly created host endothelium. The possibility of biological coating via a vital and autologous endothelium could improve the clinical outcome of these implants and significantly contribute to progress in cardiac surgery.

Literatur

1. Örtenwall P, Wadenvik H, Kutti J, Risberg B (1990) Endothelial cell seeding reduces thrombogenicity of Dacron grafts in humans. J Vasc Surg 11:403–10
2. Fischlein T, Zilla P, Eberl T, Puschmann R, et al. (1992) Initial clinical data on human in vitro endothelialization of vascular prostheses. In: Zilla P et al. (eds) Applied cardiovascular biology, 1990–91, pp 131–138
3. Frater RWM, Gong G, Hoffman D, Liao K (1992) Endothelial covering of biological artificial heart valves. Ann Thorac Surg 53:371–2
4. Zilla P, Fasol R, Dudeck U, Fischlein T, Reichart B et al. (1990) In situ cannulation, micregrid follow-up and low-density plating provide first passage endothelial cell masscultures for in vitro lining. J Vasc Surg 12:180–189

Dr. T. Fischlein, Herzchirurgische Klinik, LMU München, Klinikum Großhadern, Marchioninistraße 15, W-8000 München 70

Funktionsstörungen neutrophiler Granulozyten in bestrahlten Haut- vs. Haut-Muskel-Lappen

Neutrophil Function in Irridated Skin Flaps and Skin-Muscle-Flaps

C.J. Gabka[1], P. Benhaim[2], K. Fu[3], H. Scheuenstuhl[2] und S.J. Mathes[2]

[1]Chirurgische Klinik und Poliklinik, Klinikum Großhadern (Dir.: Prof. Dr. F.W. Schildberg), Ludwig-Maximilians-Universität München
[2]Division of Plastic and Reconstructive Surgery (Head: Prof. Dr. S.J. Mathes), University of California, San Francisco, USA
[3]Department of Radiation Oncology, University of California, San Francisco, USA

Einleitung

Die natürliche Resistenz von chirurgischen oder traumatischen Wunden gegenüber pathogenen Keimen ist primär abhängig von dem unspezifischen Immunsystem, also der ungestörten Funktion phagozytierender Zellen [1]. Dieses Prinzip gilt auch für Eingriffe in bestrahltem Gewebe, die durch eine auffällig hohe postoperative Komplikationsrate belastet sind.

Tatsächlich konnte in Vorversuchen an einem Kaninchenmodell eine Minderfunktion neutrophiler Granulozyten mit verminderter Phagozytoseaktivität und eingeschränktem maximalen "oxidative burst" nachgewiesen werden [2].

Ziel der vorliegenden Untersuchungen war die Evaluierung dieser Ergebnisse an einem anatomisch dem Menschen mehr entsprechenden Modell, sowie die Suche nach den maßgeblichen Faktoren für die verminderte Neutrophilenfunktion in bestrahltem Gewebe. Da in der Literatur als wesentliches verantwortliches Kriterium eine strahleninduzierte Minderperfusion mit konsekutivem pO_2-Abfall angegeben wird, sollte die Abhängigkeit der Neutrophilenfunktion von der jeweiligen Sauerstoffversorgung des Gewebes (pO_2) untersucht werden. Die Versuchsanordnung mit Bildung muskulokutaner Lappen (= gute Durchblutung, hoher pO_2)) sowie "random pattern" Hautlappen (= mäßige Durchblutung, niedriger pO_2) bot gleichzeitig den Vorteil, einen direkten Vergleich der beiden in der Plastischen Chirurgie am häufigsten zur Defektdeckung eingesetzten Lappenarten durchführen zu können.

Chirurgisches Forum 1993
f. experim. u. klinische Forschung
Becker/Beger/Hartel (Hrsg.)

Material und Methoden

Es wurden Yucatan Mini Schweine verwendet, da der anatomische Aufbau der Haut dieses Tieres dem des Menschen entspricht.

Bei insgesamt 12 Tieren wurden rechtsseitig am Rücken 2 Felder von je 10 × 15 cm Größe bestrahlt: ein kraniales Feld über dem M. latissimus dorsi und ein kaudales Feld an der Flanke. 6, 12 und 16 Wochen nach Radiatio wurden in den Strahlen- und den entsprechenden Kontrollfeldern kontralateral muskulo-kutane (M. latissimus dorsi) und "random pattern" Haut-Lappen (Flanke) gehoben. Die Bestrahlung erfolgte als nicht-fraktionierte Einzeitbestrahlung mit einer Leistung von 6 Millionen-Elektronen-Volt (MeV) und einer Dosis von 20 Gy.

Gleichzeitig mit der Lappenhebung wurden zur Ansammlung von Wundflüssigkeit metallene Zylinder (4 × 1,5 cm) unter die Lappen implantiert. Die Aspiration der Wundflüssigkeit erfolgte perkutan am 3. und 5. postoperativen Tag. Nach Quantifizierung der Leukozyten wurden folgende Funktionen mittels Durchflußzytometrie (FACScan, Fa. Becton-Dickinson) untersucht:

- Die *Phagozytose-Aktivität* der PMN wurde gemessen nach Inkubation der Zellen mit fluoreszierenden Latex Microspheres.
- Der *"respiratory burst"* wurde durch die Messung der Produktion von Wasserstoffperoxid (H_2O_2) mit dem Dichlorofluorescein (DCF) Assay ermittelt. Messungen erfolgten an nicht-stimulierten und an mit 100 mm PMA (Phorbol-Myristat-Azetat) stimulierten Zellen.

Der *partielle Sauerstoffpartialdruck* (pO_2) wurde unterhalb des jeweiligen Lappens gemessen, indem eine sogenannte "Optode" (Fa. InnerSpace; Irvine, Kalifornien, USA) perkutan in die unter den Lappen implantierten Wundzylinder eingebracht wurde. Messungen erfolgten am 3. postoperativen Tag unter standardisierten Bedingungen.

Ergebnisse

Die *Phygozytoseleistung* der Neutrophilen aus bestrahlten RP- und MC-Lappen war in allen Versuchen quantitativ und mit Zunahme der Beobachtungszeit auch statistisch signifikant niedriger als die der Kontrollzellen. Darüberhinaus gab es einen deutlichen Unterschied zwischen den betrahlten RP- und MC-Lappen: Während sich die Phagozytoseaktivität in den MC-Lappen nur marginal von 90 auf 77% im Vergleich zur Kontrolle verminderte, fiel diese in den bestrahlten RT-Lappen von 66% nach 6 Wochen auf nur noch 30% der entsprechenden Kontrollen nach 16 Wochen post Radiatio.

Die Analyse des relativen Anstiegs der *Wasserstoffperoxid-Produktion* von nicht-stimulierten zu PMA-stimulierten Zellen zeigte, daß die maximale H_2O_2-Produktion von Neutrophilen aus bestrahlten Lappen signifikant geringer ($p < 0,001$) war als in den entsprechenden Kontrollzellen aus nicht-bestrahlten Feldern. Darüberhinaus fiel auf, daß die H_2O_2-Produktion in den bestrahlten RP-Lappen mit Zunahme der Zeit abnahm, während sie in den bestrahlten MC-Lappen über den Beobachtungszeitraum konstant blieb (RP-Lappen: 47%, 37%, 32% der Kontrolle nach 6, 12, 16 Wochen; MC-Lappen: 50%, 51%, 49%).

Die subkutanen bzw. submuskulären *pO_2-Messungen* ergaben quantitativ und größtenteils statistisch signifikant niedrigere pO_2-Werte unter den bestrahlten Lappen im Vergleich zu den nicht-bestrahlten Lappen. Darüberhinaus lagen die pO_2-Werte in den RP Lappen unter denen der MC Lappen. Mit Zunahme der Beobachtungszeit nach Bestrahlung kam es zu einer immer schlechter werdenden Sauerstoffversorgung unter den bestrahlten RP-Lappen (65%, 60%, 42% der Kontrolle nach 6, 12, 16 Wochen), während dies in bestrahlten MC-Lappen nicht zu beobachten war (80%, 78%, 76%). Diese Unterschiede zwischen den bestrahlten RP- und MC-Lappen waren statistisch signifikant für die 12- und 16-Wochen-Gruppen (student t-Test: $p < 0{,}05$).

Diskussion

Die ungestörte Migration von neutrophilen Granulozyten und Makrophagen aus der Blutbahn zum Ort der Infektion mit nachfolgender Phagozytose und Vernichtung pathogener Organismen durch Bildung von Lysosomen und Produktion toxischer Sauerstoffmetabolite ist Voraussetzung für die primäre Infektionsresistenz chirurgischer Wunden [1].

In der vorliegenden Untersuchung wird nachgewiesen, daß es in bestrahltem Gewebe zu Funktionsstörungen der neutrophilen Granulozyten kommt. Offensichtlich sind die Neutrophilen bei der Migration durch das bestrahlte Gewebe supprimierenden Einflüssen ausgesetzt, die in verminderter Phagozytoseleistung und erniedrigter maximaler H_2O_2-Produktion resultieren. Damit wurden die in einem Kaninchenmodell gewonnenen Erkenntnisse bestätigt [2] und der Nachweis erbracht, daß diese Ergebnisse auch auf den Menschen übertragbar sind, da das hier verwendete Modell vom anatomischen Aufbau her dem des Menschen gleicht.

Die Messungen des Sauerstoffpartialdruckes direkt im Wundbereich zeigten einen kontinuierlichen Abfall des pO_2 unter den bestrahlten Lappenplastiken. Dieser war besonders deutlich im Falle der Hautlappen, während der gefäßreiche Muskelstiel des M. latissimus dorsi trotz Bestrahlung ein relativ hohes pO_2 Niveau gewährleistet. 16 Wochen nach Bestrahlung betrug der pO_2 unter den bestrahlten RP-Lappen nur noch 40% des nicht-bestrahlten Hautlappens, der entsprechende Wert unter dem bestrahlten Haut-Muskel-Lappen betrug fast 80%. Diese Ergebnisse weisen darauf hin, daß in bestrahltem Gewebe durch die Anwendung von muskulo-kutanen Lappenplastiken trotz eingetretener Strahlenfolgen noch eine gute Durchblutung des Wundbereiches zu erwarten ist. Die plastische Verschiebung von reinen Hautlappen in bestrahltem Gewebe ist dagegen nicht zu empfehlen.

Der partiell mit dem Absinken des pO_2 einhergehende Abfall von Phagozytose und "respiratory burst" der PMN aus den bestrahlten Feldern weist auf eine Abhängigkeit dieser Funktionen von einer adäquaten inter- und intrazellulären Sauerstoffversorgung hin. Besonders auffällig ist diese Beziehung bei Analyse der maximalen H_2O_2-Produktion in PMN von bestrahlten Hautlappen: Im Vergleich zur Kontrolle fielen im Beobachtungszeitraum sowohl die H_2O_2-Produktion als auch der pO_2 um mehr als 20%. Tatsächlich ist der "oxidative burst" der Neutrophilen abhängig von einer ausreichenden intrazellulären Sauerstoffspannung [3]. Zumindest zum Teil ist daher die eingeschränkte maximale H_2O_2-Produktion darauf zurückzuführen.

Allerdings war auch der "respiratory burst" der PMN aus bestrahlten Haut-Muskel-Lappen auf fast 50% der Kontrolle erniedrigt, obwohl der pO_2 Wert auf nur ca. 80% der Kontrolle absank. Die hierbei gemessenen Werte von ca. 20–30 mmHg pO_2 können nicht für eine derartig hohe Einschränkung verantwortlich sein [4]. Von daher sind weitere die Granulozytenfunktion beeinträchtigende Faktoren zu postulieren. In erster Linie kommen dabei im bestrahlten Gewebe freigesetzte Zytokine in Betracht. Die modulierende Wirkung dieser Stoffklasse von Glykoproteinen auf die Granulozyten ist bekannt [5], wobei bisher jedoch mehr stimulierende als supprimierende Effekte beschrieben wurden. Die Identifizierung dieser Faktoren ist Ziel weiterer Forschungen.

Zusammenfassung

Untersuchungen über die Funktion neutrophiler Granulozyten in bestrahlten Haut- und Haut-Muskel-Lappenplastiken zeigten eine verminderte Phagozytosekapazität und eingeschränkte maximale Stimulierbarkeit des "respiratory burst" dieser für die Wundresistenz wichtigen Zellen. Als ein wesentliches Kriterium hierfür muß die in bestrahltem Gewebe erniedrigte partielle Sauerstoffspannung gelten, die in der vorliegenden Arbeit besonders bei den bestrahlten Hautlappenplastiken erniedrigt war, während bestrahlte Haut-Muskel-Lappenplastiken – wahrscheinlich aufgrund des gefäßreichen Muskelanteils – trotz Bestrahlung ausreichende pO_2-Werte im Vergleich zur Kontrolle aufwiesen.

Summary

Investigations on neutrophil function in irradiated random pattern and myocutaneous flaps in Yucatan mini pigs demonstrated decreased phagocytosis and impaired maximal respiratory burst of polymorphonuclear neutrophils (PMN) when compared to nonirradiated controls. Certainly, lower tissue oxygen levels in the irradiated areas contributed to this finding, being clearly decreased in the irradiated random pattern flaps, whereas irradiated myocutaneous flaps – probably due to their muscle predicle – maintained a fairly high pO_2 level (80%) compared to nonirradiated controls. However, other factors, most likely cytokines, must be considered for these findings as well.

Literatur

1. Benhaim P, Hunt TK (1993) Natural resistance to infection: leukocyte functions. J Burn Care Rehabil, in press (April 1993)
2. Gabka CJ, Benhaim P, Chan AS, Scheuenstuhl H, Mathes SJ (1992) Evaluation of neutrophil function in irradiated tissue. In: Mason SK, Oliver KC (eds) Surgical Forum XLIII. American College of Surgeons, New Orleans, pp 656–659

3. Curnutte JT, Kurver R, Babior BM (1987) Activation of the respiratory burst oxidase in a fully soluble system from human neutrophils. J Biol Chem 262:6450–6452
4. La Van FB, Hunt TK (1990) Oxygen and wound healing. Clinics Plast Surg 17:463–468
5. Kapp A, Zeck-Kapp G (1990) Activation of oxidative metabolism in human polymorphnuclear neutrophilic granulocytes: the role of immuno-modulating cytokines. J Invest Dermatol 95 [Suppl]:94–99

Dr. C.J. Gabka, Chirurgische Klinik und Poliklinik, Klinikum Großhadern, Ludwig-Maximilians-Universität, Marchioninistraße 15, W-8000 München 70

Gewebeprotektion bei akuter Ischämie durch transdermale Wirkstoffapplikation über Liposomen

Tissue Protection After Acute Ischemia by Transdermal Drug Administration with Liposomes

F. Rösken[1], E. Uhl[1], M.D. Menger[1], S.B. Curri[2] und K. Meßmer[1]

[1]Institut für Chirurgische Forschung, LMU München
[2]Centro di Biologica Molecolare, Milano, Italy

Einleitung

Die Nekrose von transplantiertem Hautgewebe stellt in der plastischen Chirurgie eine folgenschwere Komplikation dar. Unzureichende mikrovaskuläre Perfusion und Gewebehypoxie sind die entscheidenen Ursachen für die Ausbildung einer Hautlappennekrose. Durch vasoaktive Substanzen kann eine Verbesserung der Perfusion ischämiegefährdeten Gewebes erreicht werden [1]. Die orale oder parenterale Gabe solcher Substanzen ist jedoch oft von systemischen Nebenwirkungen begleitet. Lokale Applikation durch Koppelung des Wirkstoffes an einen Liposomen-Carrier [2] eröffnet die Möglichkeit einer streng lokalen Behandlung bei gleichzeitig verlängerter Wirkdauer unter Vermeidung systemischer Nebenwirkungen. Ziel der vorliegenden Studie war es deshalb, den Einfluß der transdermalen Applikation der vasoaktiven Substanz Buflomedil, gekoppelt an Liposomen, auf die Mikrozirkulation und die Entstehung von Hautlappennekrosen zu untersuchen. In früheren experimentellen Studien war nachgewiesen worden, daß durch intravenöse Applikation von Buflomedil das Ausmaß der Hautlappennekrose signifikant reduziert werden kann [3].

Methodik

Als Modell verwendeten wir das Ohr der homozygoten haarlosen Maus (hr/hr, 8–10 Wochen alt, Gewicht 25–30 g). Das Ohr wird von 3 großen, an der Basis eintretenden Gefäßnervenbündeln versorgt. Zur Stimulation eines gestielten Hautlappens wurden 4/5 des Ohres nahe der Basis unter Schonung eines schmalen Gewebestreifens und des darin verlaufenden anterioren Gefäßnervenbündels durchtrennt [4]. Hierdurch entwickelt sich über einen Zeitraum von 5 Tagen eine Nekrose von 35–45% der Gesamtfläche des Hautlappens.

Zur Behandlung verwendeten wir an Liposomen-gekoppeltes Buflomedil-Hydrochlorid [5]. In dieser Applikationsform wird Buflomedil von sphärischen Lipidvesikeln, bestehend aus einer Doppelmembran amphiphiler Moleküle (Phosphatidylcholin 33,33 mg/ml) mit einem Durchmesser von 6–10 μm, umschlossen. Die Therapie er-

Chirurgisches Forum 1993
f. experim. u. klinische Forschung
Becker/Beger/Hartel (Hrsg.)

folgte täglich durch standardisierte lokale Applikation des Liposomenkomplexes über einen Zeitraum von 30 min. Die Behandlung begann direkt nach Hautlappenanhebung und erstreckte sich über einen Zeitraum von 5 Tagen (Gruppe 1, n = 8). In einer zweiten Gruppe (n = 7) wurden die Hautlappen zusätzlich 5 Tage präoperativ behandelt. Als Kontrolle diente in beiden Gruppen das kontralaterale Ohr, welches mit einer Liposomenlösung ohne Buflomedil behandelt wurde.

Zur Beurteilung der Mikrozirkulation des Ohres wurden die Tiere in einer Plexiglasplattform immobilisiert und das Ohr über einem Objektträger flach ausgespannt. Die mikrovaskuläre Perfusion wurde im proximalen, zentralen und distalen Teil des Hautlappens mittels Laser Doppler Flowmeter (MBF3D; Moor Instruments LTD., Axminster, England) einen Tag vor Hautlappenhebung und anschließend täglich bis zum fünften postoperativen Tag gemessen. Das Ausmaß der nichtperfundierten Fläche/Hautlappennekrose wurde durch intravitale Kapillaroskopie nach i.v. Injektion des Fluoreszenzmarkers FITC-Dextran (MW: 150 000) erfaßt und per Videorecorder aufgezeichnet. Auf diese Weise konnte die Grenze zwischen perfundierten und nichtperfundierten Kapillaren exakt definiert werden. Die nichtperfundierte Fläche wurde planimetrisch unter Zuhilfenahme eines computergestützten Mikrozirkulationsanalysesystems (CAMAS) offline bestimmt. Für den statistischen Vergleich zwischen Kontroll- und behandelten Tieren kam der Wilcoxon Test zur Anwendung. Als Signifikanzniveau wurde $p < 0,05$ festgelegt.

Ergebnisse

Makroskopisch ließ sich in den beiden mit Buflomedil behandelten Gruppen gegenüber der Kontrolle ein geringergradiges Gewebeödem erkennen. Bei fünftägiger

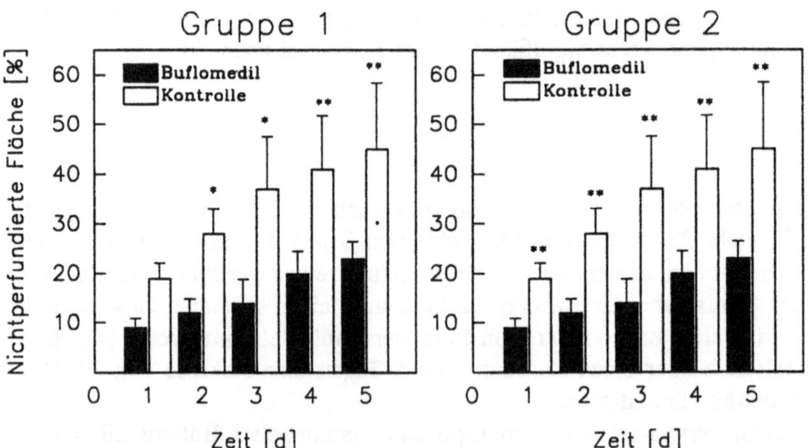

Abb. 1. Wirkung transdermal applizierter Buflomedil-Liposomen auf den Anteil der nichtperfundierten/nekrotischen Fläche in Prozent der Fläche des Hautlappens. Gruppe 1 (postoperative Behandlung, Gruppe 2 (prä- und postoperative Behandlung), Mittelwert ± SD, Wilcoxon Test mit Bonferroni-Holm Korrektur; * $p < 0,05$, ** $p < 0,01$ vs. Kontrolle

Behandlung mit Buflomedil postoperativ (Gruppe 1) zeigte sich im Vergleich zur Kontrolle schon am ersten Tag nach Hautlappenhebung eine signifikante Verbesserung der mikrovaskulären Perfusion von bis zu 81%. Die Hautlappennekrose war 5 Tage nach Lappenhebung von 45% auf 22% reduziert (Abb. 1). Die fünftägige Vorbehandlung mit Liposomen-gebundenem Buflomedil erbrachte keinen zusätzlichen therapeutischen Effekt (Abb. 1).

Zusammenfassung

Die transdermale Applikation von Buflomedil in liposomaler Form verbessert die mikrovaskuläre Perfusion von gestielten Hautlappen. Im Vergleich zu unbehandelten Hautlappen konnte die Nekrosefläche um mehr als die Hälfte reduziert werden. Eine fünftägige Vorbehandlung mit Liposomen-Buflomedillösung erbrachte keinen weiteren Therapieerfolg. Die transdermale Therapie war damit in ihrer Wirkung vergleichbar dem Effekt der intravenösen Gabe von Buflomedil [3].

Der gewebeprotektive Effekt des Liposomenpräparates beruht wahrscheinlich auf den für Buflomedil bekannten Eigenschaften Vasodilatation, Verbesserung der Erythrozyten-Verformbarkeit, Hemmung der Plättchenaggregation und Anstieg der intrazellulären cyclo-AMP Konzentration, welche eine geringere Exprimierung von Adhäsionsrezeptoren und somit eine Hemmung der Leukozytenadhärenz bewirkt [5]. Die transdermale Behandlung über Liposomen bietet somit einen neuen wirkungsvollen Weg zur Protektion ischämie-gefährdeten Hautgewebes unter Vermeidung systemischer Nebenwirkungen.

Summary

The effect of the vasoactive drug buflomedil contained in liposomes on microcirculation and skin flap necrosis was studied in the hairless mouse ear skin flap model. The animals were allocated to a 5-day pretreatment (group 2) and a non-pretreated group (group 1). The contralateral ear was used as a control. Tissue perfusion was measured 1 day prior to and daily following flap creation over a 5-day period by laser-Doppler flowmetry. Skin flap necrosis was evaluated by intravital fluorescence capillaroscopy. Local administration of buflomedil-liposomes (daily) markedly increased microvascular perfusion in single-pedicle flaps and reduced skin flap necrosis from 45% to 22% (group 1). Additional 5-day pretreatment (group 2) before flap creation did not further enhance the protective effect of liposome-bound buflomedil. We conclude that transdermal treatment by vasoactive substances docked to liposomes could represent a new approach to prevent skin flap necrosis.

Literatur

1. Sunder-Plassmann L, v. Hesler FW, Abendroth D, Bohmert H (1989) Protective effect of Buflomedil in TRAM flap procedures. In: Messmer K (ed) Ischemic diseases and the microcirculation – New Results. Zuckschwerdt, München, pp 123–125

2. Mezei M (1988) Liposomes in the topical application of drugs: a review. In: Gregoriadis G (ed) Liposomes as drug carriers. Wiley, Chichester, pp 663–678
3. Galla TJ, Barker JH, Saetzler RK, Hammersen F, Messmer K (1991) Increase in skin flap survival by the vasoactive drug Buflomedil. Plast Reconstruct Surg 87:130–136
4. Barker JH, Hammersen F, Bondar I, Galla TJ, Menger MD, Gross W, Messmer K (1989) Direct monitoring of nutritive blood flow in a failing skin flap: The hairless mouse ear skin flap model. Plast Reconstruct Surg 84:303–313
5. Clissold SP, Lynch S, Sorkin EM (1987) Buflomedil: A review of its pharmacodynamic and pharmacokinetic properties, and therapeutic efficacy in peripheral and cerebral vascular diseases. Drugs 33:430–460

F. Rösken, Institut für Chirurgische Forschung, Ludwig-Maximilians-Universität, Marchioninistraße 15, W-8000 München 70

Welchen Einfluß haben Änderungen der Plasmaviskosität durch Volumenersatzmittel auf Gewebsoxygenierung und Organperfusion?

Does Elevated Plasma Viscosity Alter Tissue Oxygenation and Organ Blood Flow?

H. Krieter[1], F. Kefalianakis[1], U.B. Brückner[2] und K. Meßmer[3]

[1]Abteilung für Experimentelle Chirurgie, Chirurgische Kliniken, Universität Heidelberg
[2]Sektion Chirurgische Forschung, Chirurgische Universitätsklinik I, Universität Ulm
[3]Institut für Chirurgische Forschung, Klinikum Großhadern, Universität München

Einleitung

Kolloidale Volumenersatzmittel werden in großem Umfang sowohl zur Substitution akuter Blutverluste als auch im Rahmen einer isovolämischen Hämodilution eingesetzt. Der dilutionsbedingt geringere arterielle O_2-Gehalt wird dabei in einem weiten Hämatokritbereich durch ein gesteigertes Herzzeitvolumen kompensiert [1]. Neben einer konsequent aufrechterhaltenen Isovolämie ist die verbesserte Fluidität des Blutes und der dadurch erhöhte venöse Rückstrom zum Herzen für die Funktion dieses Regelmechanismus unabdingbar [1].

In-vitro Messungen ergaben, daß die Infusion größerer Mengen eines Kolloids die Plasmaviskosität zu steigern vermag. Hieraus wurde teilweise auf eine kritische Verminderung der nutritiven Organperfusion geschlossen, welche weiterhin (insbesondere bei den längerkettigen Dextranmolekülen) die O_2-Versorgung des Gewebes negativ beeinflussen würde [2, 3].

Ziel der hier vorgestellten Untersuchung war daher zu prüfen, ob und in welchem Maße eine Steigerung der Plasmaviskosität die Organdurchblutung *in vivo* beeinträchtigt. Hierzu wurde in einem Tiermodell die Plasmaviskosität artifiziell durch Infusion extrem hochmolekularen Dextrans auf das Doppelte bzw. Dreifache der Norm angehoben.

Methodik

Nach Genehmigung des Versuchsprotokolls durch die zuständige Behörde wurden 7 splenektomierte Beagle-Hunde ($13,4 \pm 1,3$ kg) prämediziert (20 mg/kg Propionyl-Promazin i.m.), narkotisiert (15 mg/kg Pentobarbital + 7,5 mg Piritramid i.v.; anschließend kontinuierlich 0,45 μg/kg/min Piritramid), intubiert und kontrolliert beatmet (FiO_2: 0,3; Frequenz: 12/min; Atemzeitvolumen: 150 ml/kg/min bzw. $paCO_2$ = 38–40 mmHg).

Chirurgisches Forum 1993
f. experim. u. klinische Forschung
Becker/Beger/Hartel (Hrsg.)

Chirurgische Präparation: Zur Bestimmung von hämodynamischen und blutchemischen Parametern wurden folgende Katheter unter Röntgenkontrolle plaziert: ein PVC-Katheter (Ø 1,8 mm) über einen Ast der rechten V. jugularis externa in die V. cava superior in Höhe des rechten Vorhofes (Druck; venöse Blutproben); je ein PE-Katheter (Ø 2,0 mm) in die Arteria (Druck; Blutproben) und Vena femoralis (Infusion der Dextran-Lösung); ein 7-5F-Swan-Ganz-Katheter über einen Ast der rechten V. jugularis in die A. pulmonalis (Druck; gemischtvenöse Blutproben; Körpertemperatur; Herzzeitvolumen = HZV). Zur Injektion der radioaktiv markierten Mikrosphären (s.u.) diente ein Angiographiekatheter (Cordis Corp, Miami/USA), der über die linke A. carotis in den linken Vorhof vorgeschoben worden war.

Hämodynamik: Alle Drucke wurden über Statham P23ID-Wandler (Gould Inc, Oxnard/USA) zusammen mit dem über drei Stichelektroden abgeleiteten EKG auf einem 8-Kanalschreiber (Brush Mk-481, Gould Inc, Oxnard/USA) kontinuierlich aufgezeichnet. Zu jedem Meßzeitpunkt wurde der pulmonalkapilläre Verschlußdruck bestimmt. Das HZV wurde jeweils 3-fach in der endexspiratorischen Phase gemessen (9310 Lung Water Computer, Edwards Lab, Santa Anna/USA) und gemittelt.

Blutchemie: Arterielle und gemischtvenöse Blutproben wurden mit einem Blutgasanalysator (ABL 3, Radiometer, Kopenhagen/DK) analysiert. Des weiteren wurden folgende Parameter mit herkömmlichen Labormethoden bestimmt: Hämatokrit (Hk), Hämoglobingehalt (Hb) sowie die Konzentrationen im Plasma von Laktat, Natrium, Kalium, Gesamteiweiß und Albumin.

Viskosimetrie: Zur Messung der Plasmaviskosität wurde arterielles Blut in EDTA-Röhrchen gesammelt und sofort bei Raumtemperatur für 5 min mit 4 500 U/min zentrifugiert. Die Viskosität des Plasmaüberstandes wurde mit einem Kapillar-Viskosimeter (Ø 0,38 mm; Viscometer, Coulter Electronics, Luton/GB) jeweils 3-fach bei 37°C gemessen und arithmetisch gemittelt.

Messungen des Gewebs-pO_2: Die Leber wurde durch eine mediane Laparotomie (Schnittlänge 10 cm) dargestellt und die Verteilung des Gewebs-pO_2 auf der Oberfläche mit einer Platin-Mehrdraht-Oberflächen-Elektrode (MDO) nach Kessler und Lübbers gemessen [4]. Pro Meßzeitpunkt wurden 300–400 Einzelmessungen zu Histogrammen zusammengefaßt.

Regionale und globale Organperfusion: Die nutritive Organdurchblutung wurde mit der Mikrosphärentechnik bestimmt [5]. Etwa $3–4 \cdot 10^6$ Mikrosphären (Ø15μm) wurden in den linken Vorhof injiziert. Gleichzeitig wurden arterielle (Aorta abdominalis) und gemischtvenöse (A. pulmonalis) Referenzproben mit einer Harvardpumpe entzogen. Die Injektionsfolge der Nuklide (^{141}Ce, ^{114m}In, ^{85}Sr, ^{95}Nb) war randomisiert. Die regionale Durchblutung wurde in 280 Gewebsproben aus 18 Organen bestimmt.

Versuchsprotokoll: Nach Abschluß der chirurgischen Präparation wurden alls Tiere heparinisiert (250 U/kg) und mit 6% Dextran 60 (Schiwa, Glandorf/D) isovolämisch auf einen Hämatokrit von 30 vol% diluiert. Nach einer 30minütigen Stabilisierungsphase wurden die Ausgangswerte aller Parameter gemessen (Zeitpunkt: VISK 1). Durch Infusion von nur 4% des gemessenen Blutvolumens in Form einer 50%igen hochmolekularen Dextran 500-Lösung (MW: 500 000 d, Pharmacia, Uppsala/Schweden) wurde die Plasmaviskosität schrittweise auf Werte von 2 bzw. 3 mPas eingestellt. Nach jeweils 30 min Ausgleichsphase wurden erneut alle Parameter gemessen (Zeitpunkte: VISK 2 und VISK 3).

Statistik: Nach Prüfung auf Normverteilung wurden die Daten einer Varianzanalyse für wiederholte Messungen (Zeitreihenanalyse) unterzogen. Signifikante Unterschiede wurden mit dem gepaarten t-Test lokalisiert. Bei wiederholter Testung gleicher Hypothesen wurde das α-Niveau nach Bonferroni-Holm sequentiell korrigiert.

Ergebnisse

Die wichtigsten Ergebnisse sind in Tabelle 1 zusammengefaßt. Sowohl das HZV als auch die nutritive Durchblutung von Herz, Gehirn und Leber nahmen mit Steigerung der Plasmaviskosität auf 2 bzw. 3 mPas deutlich zu ($p < 0,01$, VISK 3 vs. VISK 1), während die Herzfrequenz unverändert blieb. Gleichzeitig sank der Hämatokrit auf 24 bzw. 20 vol%, und die Summenhistogramme auf der Leberoberfläche wurden nach rechts zu höheren Werten verschoben. Zum Zeitpunkt VISK 2 erreichte der mittlere Gewebs-pO_2-Wert ein Maximum und sank bei VISK 3 wieder auf den Ausgangswert ab; zu diesem Zeitpunkt fanden sich erstmals hypoxische pO_2-Werte unterhalb von 5 mmHg.

Tabelle 1. Änderungen (MW ± SD) von Plasmaviskosität (PVisk), Herzzeitvolumen (HZV), mittlerem arteriellen Druck (MAP), Herzfrequenz (HF), Hämatokrit (Hk) sowie der Durchblutunf von Herz (Q_{Herz}), Gehirn (Q_{Gehirn}) und Leber (Q_{Leber}). Aus den mehr als 1200 Meßwerten der MDO sind der mittlere pO_2 der Histogramme (MDO-pO_2-MW) sowie der prozentuale Anteil von Meßwerten mit einem $pO_2 < 5$ mmHg (MDO-$pO_2 < 5$) angegeben

Parameter	VISK 1	VISK 2	VISK 3
PVisk [mPas]	1,10 ± 0,05	2,05 ± 0,11	3,00 ± 0,21
HZV [ml/kg/min]	156 ± 26	182 ± 44	249 ± 64
MAP [mmHg]	113 ± 7	116 ± 12	116 ± 16
HF [S/min]	124 ± 18	128 ± 28	129 ± 30
Hk [vol%]	30,3 ± 0,7	24,0 ± 0,5	19,8 ± 1,9
Q_{Herz} [ml/min/100g]	102 ± 18	191 ± 32	213 ± 48
Q_{Gehirn} [ml/min/100g]	34 ± 9	45 ± 11	57 ± 15
Q_{Leber} [ml/min/100g]	17 ± 5	29 ± 9	45 ± 12
MDO-pO_2-MW [mmHg]	20,8 ± 2,1	30,1 ± 3,5	22,1 ± 4,1
MDO-$pO_2 < 5$ [%]	0	0	4

Diskussion

Durch Infusion kleiner Volumina hochmolekularen Dextrans (4% des Blutvolumens) konnte jeweils die gewünschte Hyperviskosität des Plasmas erzielt werden. Trotz der extrem gesteigerten Plasmaviskosität nahmen bei konstanter Herzfrequenz sowohl das HZV als auch die nutritive Organdurchblutung zu. Die pO_2-Werte auf der Leberoberfläche waren homogener verteilt, und der Mittelwert war deutlich erhöht. Bei der weiteren Steigerung der Plasmaviskosität auf 3 mPas fiel der mittlere Gewebs-pO_2 wieder auf Basiswerte ab. Zu diesem Zeitpunkt fanden sich erstmals hypoxische Werte < 5 mmHg. Dies weist darauf hin, daß möglicherweise bei einer Plasmaviskosität um 3 mPas eine kritische Grenze der Kompensation erreicht ist. Solche Extremwerte werden jedoch bei klinischer Anwendung von Kolloidlösungen sowohl zum Blutersatz als auch bei der Hämodilution niemals erzielt.

Diese Ergebnisse untermauern einmal mehr die zentrale Rolle des Hämatokrits als Determinante der rheologischen Eigenschaften des Vollblutes; ungeachtet der massiven Änderungen der Plasmaviskosität steigt die Durchblutung der vitalen Organe bei gleichzeitig abnehmendem Hämatokrit weit über Ausgangswerte an und stellt somit trotz des verminderten arteriellen O_2-Gehaltes eine ausreichende Sauerstoffversorgung sicher.

Schlußfolgerungen

Selbst bei extremer Steigerung der Plasmaviskosität auf 3 mPas bleibt der Hämatokrit die bestimmende Größe der Blutfluidität. Da bei klinischer Anwendung von Dextranlösungen zum einen nur wesentlich geringere Erhöhungen der Plasmaviskosität (< 0,5 mPas) beobachtet werden und zudem der Einsatz von Volumenersatzmitteln immer mit einer Reduktion des Hämatokrits einhergeht, sind tatsächlich keine negativen Auswirkungen auf die nutritive Organdurchblutung und die O_2-Versorgung des Gewebes zu erwarten.

Zusammenfassung

Die Infusion von Volumenersatzmitteln kann zu einer geringfügigen Steigerung der Plasmaviskosität um bis zu 0,5 mPas führen. Um den Einfluß dieses Effektes auf Organdurchblutung und O_2-Versorgung des Gewebes zu prüfen, wurde bei 7 Beagle-Hunden die Plasmaviskosität mittels eines hochmolekularen Dextrans (MW: 500 000 d) schrittweise auf das Doppelte bzw. Dreifache der Norm eingestellt. Die Organdurchblutung wurde mit radioaktiv markierten Mikrosphären (Ø15μm), die Gewebsoxygenierung der Leber mit einer Mehrdraht-Platin-Oberflächen-Elektrode (MDO) gemessen.

Ungeachtet der erheblich gesteigerten Plasmaviskosität (2 bzw. 3 mPas) nahmen sowohl das HZV als auch die nutritive Durchblutung von Herz, Gehirn und Leber kontinuierlich zu. Die Mittelwerte der mit der MDO gemessenen pO_2-Histogramme erreichten bei einer Plasmaviskosität von 2 mPas bei homogener Verteilung ein Maximum, das über den Ausgangswerten ($p < 0{,}01$) lag. Eine weitere Steigerung der Plasmaviskosität auf 3 mPas ließ die pO_2-Werte wieder in den Bereich der Norm absinken. Gleichzeitig nahm der Hämatokrit auf 24 bzw. 20 vol% ab. Diese Ergebnisse belegen, daß der Hämatokrit auch bei extrem hoher Plasmaviskosität für die rheologischen Eigenschaften des Vollblutes entscheidend ist. In der klinischen Anwendung von Volumenersatzmitteln ist somit – zumindest bei gefäßgesunden Patienten – keinesfalls mit einer Verschlechterung der Organdurchblutung oder -oxygenierung zu rechnen.

Summary

The administration of colloids (e.g., dextran) for blood replacement was found to induce hyperviscosity of the plasma. To evaluate the clinical relevance of this phenomenon, the effects of artificially elevated plasma viscosity on organ blood flow and tissue oxygenation were investigated in a canine model. Plasma viscosity was raised to 2 and 3 mPas, i.e., two and three times the normal value, by infusion of 4% of the blood volume of a high molecular weight dextran (500 000 Da). Organ blood flow was measured by the microsphere ($\emptyset 15 \mu m$) technique, while the distribution of the pO_2 values on the surface of the liver was determined by a multiwire platinum electrode (MDO). Despite the tremendous increase in plasma viscosity, both the cardiac output and the organ blood flow were highest at a viscosity of 3 mPas. Simultaneously, the hematocrit dropped to 24 and 20 vol%, respectively. The mean pO_2 value on the liver surface peaked at a viscosity of 2 mPas and returned to baseline when the plasma viscosity reached 3 mPa. Hence it follows that the reduction in hematocrit not only compensates the higher plasma viscosity, but governs the blood rheology. Thus, the slight changes in plasma viscosity observed during the administration of colloids in the clinical setting will never induce negative effects on organ blood flow or tissue oxygenation.

Literatur

1. Messmer K (1989) Acute preoperative hemodilution: Physiological basis and clinical application. In: Tuma RF, White JV, Messmer K (eds) The role of hemodilution in optimal patient care. Zuckschwerdt, München, pp 54–74
2. Jung F, Roggenkamp HG, Kiesewetter H (1984) Das Kapillarschlauch-Viskosimeter: Methodik und Qualitätskontrolle. In: Kiesewetter H, Ehrly AM, Jung F (Hrsg) Hämorheologische Meßmethoden. Münchner Wissenschaftliche Publikationen, München, pp 134–139
3. Landgraf H, Ehrly AM (1984) Möglichkeiten und Bedeutung der Quantifizierung der Plasmaviskosität. In: Kiesewetter H, Ehrly AM, Jung F (Hrsg) Hämorheologische Meßmethoden. Münchner Wissenschaftliche Publikationen, München, pp 35–41
4. Kessler M, Härrison DK, Höper J (1986) Tissue oxygen measurement techniques. In: Baker CH, Nastuk WL (eds) Microcirculatory technology. Academic Press, Orlando, pp 391–425
5. Gross W, Schosser R, Messmer K (1990) MIC-III: An integrated software package to support experiments using the radioactive microsphere technique. Comput Meth Progr Biomed 33:65–85

Dr. med. H. Krieter, Abteilung für Experimentelle Chirurgie, Chirurgische Kliniken, Universität Heidelberg, Im Neuenheimer Feld 347, W-6900 Heidelberg

Einflußfaktoren perioperativer Histaminfreisetzung in der Posteinleitungsphase: Maligne Grunderkrankung als Risiko

Factors Influencing Perioperative Histamine Release Throughout the Postinduction Period: Malignant Disease as a Risk Factor

B. Stinner[1], H. Menke[2], H. Sitter[3], D. Duda[4], W. Lorenz[3] und W. Dick[4]

[1]Klinik für Allgemeinchirurgie, Universität Marburg
[2]Klinik für Allgemeinchirurgie, Universität Mainz
[3]Institut für Theoretische Chirurgie, Universität Marburg
[4]Klinik für Anästhesiologie, Universität Mainz

Einleitung

Die erste Auswertung der Mainz-Marburg Studie zeigte einen extrem hohe Inzidenz (72%) von Histaminfreisetzungsereignissen in der Narkoseeinleitung und Operationsvorbereitung bei 240 allgemeinchirurgischen Patienten [2]. Der naheliegende Schluß, daß es sich hierbei um streßinduzierte Schwankungen der Plasmahistaminspiegel handelte, wurde aber durch mehrere Begleitstudien an Patienten auf einer Normalstation bzw. vor und während der gastrointestinalen Endoskopie widerlegt [2]. Besonders fiel aber auf, daß in der Posteinleitungsphase (hämodynamische Stabilisierung nach Einleitung der Narkose mit gleichzeitiger Infusion eines Plasmasubstitutes) die Häufigkeit von Histaminfreisetzung mit 30% etwa doppelt so hoch lag wie in allen anderen präoperativen Phasen. Dieser überraschende Befund stand in völligem Widerspruch zu einer früheren kontrollierten klinischen Studie an 450 orthopädischen Patienten, bei denen keine einzige klinisch relevante Histaminfreisetzung durch genau dieses Plasmasubstitut (Haemaccel-35) aufgetreten war [3]. Vor allem drei Ursachen kommen hierfür in Frage: eine Herstellungsänderung des Plasmasubstituts über den Zeitraum von 10 Jahren, veränderte Applikationsbedingungen (*vor* gegen *nach* Narkoseeinleitung) oder Unterschiede in der Patientenpopulation (orthopädische gegen allgemeinchirurgisches Krankengut). Der erste Grund scheidet nach unlängst erfolgter erneuter Überprüfung von Haemaccel-35 an Hunden, Probanden und 600 Patienten aus, die beiden anderen Gründe sind aber nicht von der Hand zu weisen. Eine Risikoanalyse der Patientengruppen, vor allem von Tumorpatienten, sollte deshalb den dritten Faktor evaluieren.

Patienten und Methoden

Eine prospektive randomisierte Doppelblindstudie wurde 1988–1991 an 240 allgemeinchirurgischen Patienten in Mainz durchgeführt (Alter: 18–83 Jahre, 116 männlich, 124 weiblich, ASA I–III, 70 Patienten mit maligner Grunderkrankung, 9 drop outs).

Chirurgisches Forum 1993
f. experim. u. klinische Forschung
Becker/Beger/Hartel (Hrsg.)

Nach Prämedikation mit Flunitrazepam per os und Legen zweier peripherer venöser Zugänge wurden die Ausgangswerte für Herzfrequenz, Blutdruck und Plasmahistamin gewonnen. Danach erfolgten nach einem exakten Zeitschema [2] weitere Messungen und Blutabnahmen nach doppelblind verabreichten H1- und H2-Rezeptorantagonisten (Dimetinden-Maleat plus Cimetidin (H1 und H2) oder Placebo). Die Narkoseeinleitung erfolgte mit Fentanyl und Thiopental sowie Succinylcholin zur Intubation. Danach wurde die Narkose mit N20/02 und Enfluran weitergeführt, es wurde mit Alcuronium vollrelaxiert und in der Posteinleitungsphase wurden 500 ml eines Plasmasubstitutes (Haemaccel oder Ringer) randomisiert in 20 min verabreicht. Blutdruck, Herzfrequenz, klinische und EKG-Zeichen sowie alle Eingriffe des verantwortlichen Anästhesisten wurden von einem unabhängigen Fachkollegen als Beobachter im Studienbogen dokumentiert. Histaminbestimmung, Klassifikation der Reaktionsarten und Risikoanalyse erfolgten entsprechend dem vorher publizierten Studienprotokoll (Details in [2]).

Die Risikoanalyse erfolgte mit den allgemeinen Parametern Alter, Geschlecht und ASA-Klasse, die als binäre Variable (ja/nein) behandelt wurden (z.B. Alter über 65-jährige gegen Jüngere, ASA-Klasse III gegen I + II). Danach wurden spezielle Parameter als binäre Variable einbezogen, wie die Vorerkrankungen an Herz, Lunge, Gefäßsystem, Stoffwechsel, Leber sowie Niereninsuffizienz, Blutpathologie und Überempfindlichkeitsreaktionen. Schließlich wurde das Fehlen der Antihistaminikaprophylaxe und das Vorliegen maligner Grunderkrankungen als binäre Variable einbezogen. Jede dieser Variablen wurde als potentieller Risikofaktor zuerst für sich allein mit dem χ^2-Test hinsichtlich Histaminfreisetzung überprüft, dann folgte die weitere Analyse mit einem schrittweisen, vorwärtsgerichteten logistischen Regressionsmodell, in dem die Wahrscheinlichkeit für das Auftreten einer Histaminfreisetzung unter der Bedingung berechnet wurde, daß gewisse Risikoparameter vorliegen.

Ergebnisse

In der Posteinleitungsphase kam es bei 231 Patienten (9 drop outs) zu 73 Histaminfreisetzungsereignissen (HFE) und 31 Histaminfreisetzungsreaktionen (HR) mit klinischer Symptomatik, aber in der Regel *ohne Hautreaktion*. Bei der Einzelfaktoranalyse der Risikofaktoren erwies sich allein das Fehlen der Antihistaminikaprophylaxe mit dem 2%-Niveau als signifikant. Die Grundkrankheit Karzinom (p = 0,12) und die Niereninsuffizienz (p = 0,2) zeigen aber Trends. Diese wurden bei der stufenweisen Variablenselektion im logistischen Regressionsmodell verstärkt, so daß neben dem Fehlen einer Antihistaminikaprophylaxe die Grundkrankheit maligne Erkrankung und die Niereninsuffizienz als Risikofaktor identifiziert werden konnten.

Das relative Risiko für Karzinompatienten im Vergleich zu Nicht-Karzinompatienten betrug für Histaminfreisetzungsereignisse 137, für Histaminfreisetzungsreaktionen (mit klinischen Symptomen) 1,66 (Tabelle 1). Bei der quantitativen Auswertung der Histaminfreisetzungsereignisse zeigte sich aber, daß für Karzinompatienten das Risiko mit hohen Plasmahistaminspiegeln deutlich zunahm (Tabelle 1). Alle histaminassoziierten Schwerstreaktionen (1 intraoperativer letaler Ausgang, 2 Zwischenfälle mit ungeplanter Intensivtherapie) fielen auf Karzinompatienten. Keiner dieser Patienten hatte eine H1- + H2-Antihistaminikaprophylaxe erhalten. Insgesamt traten in der Antihistaminika-Prophylaxegruppe überhaupt keine klinisch relevanten Histaminfreisetzungsreaktionen mehr auf, d.h. in keinem Fall war der Routineanästhesist (blind hinsichtlich Prophylaxe und Blutersatzmittel) gezwungen, medikamentös oder durch physikalische Maßnahmen (Lagerung) zu intervenieren ($p < 0{,}004$ im χ^2-Test).

Tabelle 1. Relatives Risiko für Histaminfreisetzungsereignisse (HFE), Histaminfreisetzungsreaktionen mit klinischer Symptomatik (HR), histaminassoziierte Schwerstreaktionen (SR) und für Histaminfreisetzungsereignisse oberhalb kritischer Plasmahistaminspiegel (HIS) in der Posteinleitungsphase für Patienten mit maligner Grunderkrankung

	Inzidenz der Histaminfreisetzungsereignisse (n)		
Freisetzungsklasse	Patienten *mit* maligner Grunderkrankung	Patienten *ohne* maligne Grunderkrankung	relatives Risiko
HFE	24 / 70	46 / 161	1,37
HR	13 / 70	18 / 161	1,66
HIS > 1 ng/ml	16 / 70	21 / 161	1,75
HIS > 2 ng/ml	10 / 70	6 / 161	3,83
HIS > 5 ng/ml	5 / 70	1 / 161	11,50
HIS > 10 ng/ml	4 / 70	1 / 161	9,20
SR	3 / 70	0 / 161	n.d.

Diskussion

In letzter Zeit häufen sich Berichte, daß speziell hinsichtlich Histaminfreisetzung als harmlos angesehene Medikamente der operativen Vorbereitung des Patienten durch vorherige Gabe von Arzneimitteln der Narkoseeinleitung "scharfgemacht" werden. Dies wurde für Etomidate nach Lormetazepam [4] und Midazolam, aber auch nach Pancuronium und Alcuronium [4] gezeigt, wobei letzteres in dieser Studie angewandt wurde. Noch drastischer fiel diese pharmakologische Sensibilisierung für Thiopental-Suxamethonium nach vorheriger Gabe des Optoids Nalbuphin auf [5]. Vieles spricht deshalb dafür, daß dies auch im vorliegenden Fall für Haemaccel-35 gilt. Die extrem hohe Inzidenz der pseudoallergischen Reaktionen paßt nicht zur guten Verträglichkeit in *gleichzeitig* durchgeführten Versuchen an Hunden, Probanden und 600 Patienten in 3 Zentren (Ulm, Heidelberg und Hamburg), bei denen nur 35 Hautreaktionen und eine systemische Reaktion ohne lebensbedrohliches Ausmaß auftraten. Es paßt auch nicht zu verschiedenen kontrollierten Studien vor 10 Jahren [3].

In der hier vorliegenden Risikoanalyse wurde auch Ringer-Lösung mit einbezogen, die mit einer Inzidenz von 5/59 Patienten behandlungsbedürftige Herzkreislaufreaktionen mit Histaminfreisetzung eine unglaublich hohe "Nebenwirkungsrate" aufweist. Diese Rate wird durch eine Anthistaminikaprophylaxe drastisch reduziert (1/59 Patienten) [2].

Das Modell der "pharmakologischen Sensibilisierung" des chirurgischen Patienten für mediatorbedingte kardiovaskuläre Reaktionen und Zwischenfälle paßt auch zum Tumorkranken. Veränderte Spiegel an Cytokinen, vor allem Tumornekrosefaktor α und Interleukinen, erleichtern die Freisetzung von Mediatoren aus Mastzellen (histamine releasing factors [1]). Dies könnte die Häufing von klinisch relevanten Histaminfreisetzungsreaktionen in der vorliegenden Studie als zweite Ursache neben der medikamentösen Sensibilisierung erklären.

Zusammenfassung

In einer prospektiven, randomisierten Studie an 240 allgemeinchirurgischen Patienten zur Überprüfung der Wirksamkeit einer perioperativen H1/H2-Antihistaminikaprophylaxe konnte nachgewiesen werden, daß in der Posteinleitungsphase (nach Narkoseeinleitung, bei Infusion Plasmasubstitut, vor Hautschnitt) eine deutlich erhöhte Inzidenz von Histaminfreisetzungsereignissen und -reaktionen vorliegt (30%). Durch multivariate Datenanalyse konnte hierfür das Fehlen einer H1/H2-Prophylaxe und eine maligne Grunderkrankung als wesentliches Risikomerkmal identifiziert werden. Seine Erklärung findet dieses Phänomen in einer pharmakologischen Sensibilisierung durch die Medikamente der Narkoseeinleitung und durch eine erhöhte Histaminfreisetzungsneigung als Folge veränderter Cytokinmuster beim Tumorpatienten ("histamine releasing factors").

Summary

In a prospective, controlled, randomized trial in 240 patients undergoing general surgery, a significantly high incidence of histamine release events and reactions could be shown after induction of anesthesia and before skin incision throughout the infusion of a plasma substitute. By multivariate data analysis, lack of H1/H2 prophylaxis and malignant disease could be identified as relevant risk factors for these reactions. "Pharmacological sensitizing" of the patient by the anesthetic drugs together with an altered cytokine environment ("histamine releasing factors") in tumor patients is suggested as a possible explanation for the increased tendency to release histamine.

Literatur

1. Kaplan AP, Reddigari S, Baeza M, Kuna P (1991) Histamine releasing factors and cytokine-dependent activation of basophils and mast cells. Adv Immunol 50:237–260
2. Duda D, Lorenz W, Menke H, Stinner B, Hasse Ch, Nies Ch, Schäfer U, Sitter H, Junginger T, Rothmund M, Doenicke A, Dick W (1993) Perioperative non-specific histamine release: A new classification by aetiological mechanisms and evaluation of their clinical relevance by demonstrating clinical pictures without skin reactions. Ann Fr Anaest Reanim (in press)
3. Lorenz W, Doenicke A, Schöning B, Karges H, Schmal A (1980) Incidence and mechanism of adverse reactions to polypeptides in man and dog. Joint WHO/IABS Symposium on the standardization of albumin, plasma substitutes and plasmapheresis. Develop Biol Standard 48:207–234

4. Lorenz W, Doenicke A (1978) Anaphylactoid reactions and histamine release by intravenous drugs used in surgery and anaesthesia. In: Watkins Jm Ward AM (eds) Adverse response to intravenous drugs. Academic Press, London, pp 83–112
5. Dick W, Lorenz W, Heintz D, Sitter H, Doenicke A (1992) Histaminfreisetzung bei der Einleitung von Kombinationsnarkosen mit Nalbuphin oder Fentanyl. Anaesthesist 41:239–247

Dr. med. B. Stinner, Klinik für Allgemeinchirurgie, Philipps-Universität Marburg, Baldingerstraße, W-3550 Marburg

4. Lorenz W, Doenicke A (1978) Anaphylactoid reactions and histamine release by intravenous drugs used in surgery and anaesthesia. In: Watkins J, Ward AM (eds) Adverse response to intravenous drugs. Academic Press, London, pp 83–112
5. Dick W, Lorenz W, Heinz D, [illegible], Doenicke A (1979) Histaminfreisetzung bei der Einleitung von [illegible] mit [illegible]. Anaesthesist [illegible]
247

[illegible], Philipps-Universität Marburg, Baldingerstraße, W-3550 Marburg

Initialtherapie mit hypertonen-hyperonkotischen Infusionslösungen nach hämorrhagischem Schock zur Verbesserung der Lebermikrozirkulation

Influence of Hypertonic-Hyperoncotic Fluid Resuscitation for Initial Treatment After Hemorrhagic Shock for Attenuation of the Hepatic Microcirculation

V. Bühren[1], I. Marzi[1], G. Seeck[1] und M. Bauer[2]

[1]Abteilung Unfallchirurgie, Chirurgische Universitätsklinik, Homburg/Saar
[2]Klinik für Anästhesiologie und Intensivmedizin, Universität des Saarlandes, Homburg/Saar

Einleitung

In neueren Untersuchungen konnte die Wirksamkeit geringer Volumina hypertoner-hyperonkotischer Infusionslösungen in der Initialtherapie nach hämorrhagisch/traumatischem Schock auch für den klinischen Einsatz nachgewiesen werden [3]. Relativ wenig untersucht wurden bisher organspezifische Auswirkungen dieses therapeutischen Ansatzes, insbesondere auch im Hinblick auf das zentrale Schockorgan Leber. So konnte für den bezüglich Kreislaufparametern suffizienten Volumenersatz mit Kristalloiden gezeigt werden, daß weder die Mikrozirkulation noch die hepatozelluläre Funktion auf die Ausgangswerte zurückgeführt werden [5]. In eigenen Untersuchungen wurde darüberhinaus gefunden, daß trotz konventioneller Schocktherapie eine langdauernde Engstellung der Sinusoide resultiert [1].

Ziel der vorliegenden Studie ist die Erfassung der Auswirkungen eines hypertonen-hyperonkotischen Volumenersatzes auf die Mikrozirkulation der Leber mit den Parametern Sinusoidweite und Leukozytenadhäsion. In einem druckgesteuerten hämorrhagischen Schockmodell an der Ratte kommen als Prüfsubstanzen 7,2% NaCl/10% Dextran 60 Lösung (HSDex; Hyperdex, Schiwa) und 7,2% NaCl/10% Hydroxyethylstärkelösung (HSHes; Hyperhes, Schiwa) zur Anwendung, als Vergleichsgruppe wird eine adäquate Therapie mit Ringerlaktat durchgeführt. Zur Erfassung der systemischen Therapieeffizienz werden arterieller Blutdruck, Hämatokrit und Basenüberschuß herangezogen. Die Beurteilung der hepatischen Parameter erfolgte in der von uns beschriebenen Methodik mittels direkter Visualisierung durch intravitale Videomikroskopie [2].

Material und Methodik

Weibliche Sprague-Dawley Ratten (Körpergewicht 190–240 g, n = 6 pro Gruppe) erhielten nach Pentobarbitalnarkose (50 mg/kg i.p.) eine Tracheostomie sowie Kanülie-

Chirurgisches Forum 1993
f. experim. u. klinische Forschung
Becker/Beger/Hartel (Hrsg.)

rungen (0,5×0,9, Braun, Melsungen, Deutschland) der linken A. carotis und der rechten V. jugularis. Nach medianer Laparotomie mit nachfolgendem Bauchdeckenverschluß wurde außer in der Sham-Gruppe der mittlere arterielle Blutdruck (MAP) mittels Entblutung für 45 min auf 40 mmHg abgesenkt. Die Volumensubstitution erfolgte anschließend mit Ringerlaktat (RL-Gruppe, 3facher Ersatz des Blutabzugvolumens über 30 min), HSDex (HSD-Gruppe, 4 ml/kg über 3 min) oder HSHes (HSH-Gruppe, 4 ml/kg über 3 min). Bei fortlaufender Kontrolle von MAP und Körpertemperatur wurden die Blutgase (STAT profile 5, Nova biomedicals, Rödermark) und der Hämatokrit (Mikrozentrifuge) als Ausgangswert sowie am Ende der Schockphase bzw. nach Volumenersatz bestimmt. Zur Intravitalmikroskopie wurde das Abdomen erneut eröffnet und der linke Leberlappen nach Mobilisation mit der Fascies abdominalis auf einer Plexiglasplattform plaziert. Nach Injektion von Acridine Orange (1 μmol/kg) erfolgte die Mikroskopie in Epifluoreszenztechnik (Nikon MM 11, Hg-Lasmpe, 545 nm Filter, Endvergrößerung 330×). Über eine CCD-Kamera (FK 6990, Pieper, Schwerte) wurden jeweils 5 Leberlobuli erfaßt und auf Videoband (SVHS, Panasonic FS1) unter paralleler Zeitcodierung (VTG 33, FOR-A company, Tokyo) aufgezeichnet. Die Auswertung der Leukozyten-Endothel-Interaktionen sowie die Messung der Sinusoide wurde verblindet über eine rechnergestützte frame-by-frame Analyse vorgenommen (Lobulus, Medvis, Saarlouis, Deutschland). Adhärente Leukozyten wurden in temporär (> 0,2 und < 20 sec) und permanent (> 20 sec) haftende differenziert. Die Größenordnung der Leukozyten-Endothel-Interaktionen wurde als Verhältnis der temporären Haftungen zur Gesamtzahl markierter Zellen definiert. Die Ergebnisse werden als mean ± SEM angegeben. Statistische Signifikanz wird mit einem $p \leq 0{,}05$ definiert.

Tabelle 1. Systemische Parameter zum Schockverlauf: Mittlerer arterieller Blutdruck [mmHg], Hämatokrit [%], Basenüberschuß [mmHg], Hämatokrit [%], Basenüberschuß [mmol/l] ($p \leq 0{,}05$: [a]vs. Sham-Gruppe, [b]vs. Schockphase)

	Ausgangswert	Schockphase	Volumenersatz
Mitt. art. Druck			
Sham	130,7 ± 5,2	126,2 ± 7,1	124,8 ± 6,0
RL	138,0 ± 8,1	40,8 ± 1,8[a]	93,4 ± 6,8[b]
HSDex	134,7 ± 6,4	40,5 ± 0,9[a]	98,3 ± 5,7[b]
HSHes	128,5 ± 5,0	38,5 ± 0,8[a]	109,7 ± 3,8[b]
Hämatokrit			
Sham	42,3 ± 1,8	41,0 ± 2,4	39,3 ± 2,9
RL	43,3 ± 0,9	32,7 ± 1,0[a]	18,0 ± 1,5[b,a]
HSDex	43,5 ± 0,6	31,7 ± 0,6[a]	20,6 ± 1,3[b,a]
HSHes	44,8 ± 1,7	32,5 ± 1,1[a]	22,6 ± 0,9[b,a]
Basenüberschuß			
Sham	–0,2 ± 0,8	–0,8 ± 1,2	–1,7 ± 1,0
RL	–0,5 ± 0,7	–7,1 ± 0,6[a]	–7,5 ± 1,8[a]
HSDex	–1,1 ± 0,8	–7,0 ± 0,5[a]	–5,6 ± 0,7[a]
HSHes	0,0 ± 0,9	–8,1 ± 1,1[a]	–3,1 ± 0,8[b]

Ergebnisse

Der MAP stieg unmittelbar nach Beginn der Therapie in allen Schockgruppen vergleichbar an (s. Tabelle 1). Für den Basenüberschuß ließ sich in der HSH-Gruppe eine verbesserte Erholungstendenz beobachten. Tendenziell bestätigte sich diese Beobachtung auch in den Hämatokritwerten, jedoch ohne statistische Signifikanz.

Für die Mikrozirkulationsparameter in der Leber fanden sich keine Unterschiede zwischen den Therapiegruppen mit gegenüber der Shamgruppe durchschnittlich um 30% reduzierten Durchmessern der Sinusoide (s. Abb. 1). Im Gegensatz dazu wurde die im Vergleich zu den Sham-Kontrollen massiv gesteigerte Leukozytenadhärenz in der RL- und HSH-Gruppe in der HSD-Gruppe signifikant auf Basiswerte reduziert.

Diskussion

Der Volumenersatz mit hypertonen-hyperonkotischen Lösungen (HHL) führt auch bei geringer Dosierung von lediglich 4 ml/kg Körpergewicht zur prompten Restauration der systemischen und regionalen Zirkulation. Als wesentlicher Mechanismus gilt neben positiv inotropen und vasomotorischen Effekten die Füllung des vaskulären Kompartments durch Einstrom intrazellulären Wassers. Diese Flüssigkeitsverschiebung soll über das Abschwellen der Endothelzellen auch mittelbar potentiell zu einer Verbesserung der Mikrozirkulation führen.

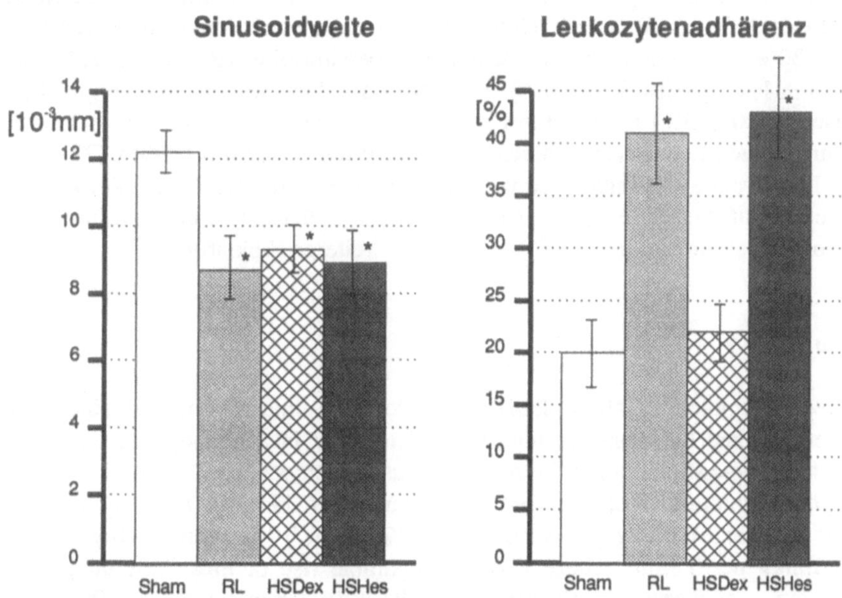

Abb. 1. Weite der Lebersinusoide [μm] und relative Leukozytenadhärenz (temporär haftende im Verhältnis zu allen markierten Leukozyten [%]) nach Volumenersatz ($p \leq 0{,}05$: * vs. Sham-Gruppe)

In den systemischen Parametern erwiesen sich in der vorliegenden Studie die HHL-Lösungen gegenüber der Substitution mit RL als vergleichbar, wobei in Übereinstimmung mit anderen Untersuchern für HSHes die günstigen Effekte im Hinblick auf den Basenüberschuß deutlicher nachweisbar waren. Demgegenüber konnte ein für Muskelkapillaren beschriebener dilatierender Mechanismus [4] überraschenderweise für hepatische Sinusoide nicht bestätigt werden. Mögliche Erklärungen waren ein auf Grund erhöhter Glukoneogenese fehlender osmotischer Gradient und/oder die speziellen morphologischen Verhältnisse im Leberstrombett mit Fensterung des Endothels.

Im Kontrast sowohl zu RL wie auch HSHes zeigte die HSDex-Gruppe eine deutliche Reduzierung der Leukozytenadhärenz. Bei identischer Engstellung des Strombetts in allen Gruppen muß ein spezifischer Effekt des Dextrans auf Adhäsionsmoleküle und hier insbesondere auf Selektine diskutiert werden.

Zusammenfassung

Lebermikrozirkulation, hepatische Leukozyten-Endothelzell-Interaktion und Sinusoiddurchmesser wurden unter Anwendung der Intravitalmikroskopie in einem nicht heparinisierten druckgesteuerten hämorrhagischen Schockmodell an der Ratte untersucht. Als Infusionslösungen zur Initialtherapie wurden Ringerlaktat (RL; dreifaches Entblutungsvolumen/30 min), 7,2% hypertone NaCl/10% Dextran 60 Lösung (HSDex; 4 ml/kg/3 min) oder 7,2%/10% Hydroxyethylstärkelösung (HSHes; 4 ml/kg/3 min) verwendet. Der mittlere arterielle Blutdruck stieg unmittelbar nach Volumentherapie in allen Schockgruppen vergleichbar an (RL 93 ± 16,8 mmHg, HSDex 99 ± 5,7, HSHes 110 ± 3,8). Keine Unterschiede ergaben sich hinsichtlich der generell um ca. 30% reduzierten Durchmesser der Lebersinusoide (RL 8,7 ± 1,6 μm, HSDex 9,3 ± 1,1, HSHes 8,9 ± 0,6). Im Gegensatz dazu war die im Vergleich zu Sham-Tieren (20 ± 3%) nach hämorrhagischem Schock bekannte massive Steigerung der kurzzeitigen Leukozytenadhärenz (< 20 sec) nur in der mit HSDex (22 ± 3%) behandelten Gruppe signifikant reduziert (RL 41 ± 5%, HSHes 43 ± 5%). Die Ergebnisse weisen auf die Rolle von Dextran bindenden Adhäsionsmolekülen hin und bedürfen hinsichtlich ihrer klinischen Relevanz der weiteren Abklärung.

Summary

Hepatic microcirculation, leukocyte-endothelial interaction, and sinusoidal widths were studied by means of intravital microscopy in a nonheparinized fixed pressure hemorrhagic shock model in the rat. Resuscitation was performed either with lactated Ringers solution (RL; threefold shed volume per 30 min), 7.2% saline/10% Dextran 60 (HSDex; 4 ml/kg per 3 min), or 7.2% saline/10% hydroxylethylstarch (HSHes; 4 ml/kg per 3 min). There was a comparable rise of mean arterial pressures after initiation of therapy in all groups (RL 93 ± 16.4 mmHg; HSDex 98 ± 5.7; HSHes 110 ± 3.8). No differences were observed between groups regarding a 30% narrowing of sinusoids compared to the sham group after induction of shock (RL 8.7 ± 1.6 μm; HSDex 9.3 ± 1.1; HSHes 8.9 ± 0.6). In contrast, temporary leukocyte adhesion

(< 20 s) compared to controls (20% ± 3%) was reduced only by HSDex (22 ± 3) to baseline (RL 41 ± 5, HSHes 43 ± 5). These results may indicate an involvement of dextran-binding adhesions molecules and need further evaluation regarding their clinical relevance.

Literatur

1. Marzi I, Bauer M, Secchi A, Hower R, Larsen R, Bühren V (1992) Time course and pattern of hepatic leukocyte-endothelial interaction after hemorrhagic shock in the rat. Circ Shock 37:15
2. Marzi I, Knee J, Bühren V, Menger M, Trentz O (1992) Reduction by superoxide dismutase of leukocyte-endothelial adherence after liver transplantation. Surgery 111:90–97
3. Mattox KL, Maningas PA, Moore EE, Mateer JR, Aprahamian C, Burch JM, Pepe PE (1991) Prehospital hypertonic saline/dextran infusion for post-traumatic hypotension – The USA multicenter trial. Ann Surg 213:482–491
4. Mazzoni MC, Borgström P, Intaglietta M, Arfors KE (1990) Capillary narrowing in hemorrhagic shock is rectified by hyperosmotic saline-dextran reinfusion. Circ Shock 31:407–418
5. Wang P, Ayala A, Dean RE, Hauptman JG, Zheng F, DeJong GK, Chaudry IH (1991) Adequate crystalloid resuscitation restores but fails to maintain the active hepatocellular function following hemorrhagic shock. J Trauma 31:601–607

Priv.Doz. Dr. med. V. Bühren, Abteilung Unfallchirurgie, Chirurgische Universitätsklinik, W-6650 Homburg/Saar

Die Cholesterinester-Konzentration im Serum als Parameter der Leberfunktion nach chirurgischen Operationen im Abdomen

Serum Cholesterol Ester Concentration as a Parameter of Liver Function After Abdominal Surgery

M. Sachs[1], U. Männl[2], C. Gurlitt[2], H. Förster[2] und A. Encke[1]

[1] Klinik für Allgemeinchirurgie, Klinikum der Johann Wolfgang Goethe-Universität, Frankfurt am Main
[2] Abteilung für Experimentelle Anaesthesiologie, Klinikum der Johann Wolfgang Goethe-Universität, Frankfurt am Main

Einleitung

Nach Lapatoromien ist eine Abnahme der Gesamt-Cholesterinkonzentration im Serum nachweisbar [3, 5], deren Pathogenese bisher nicht geklärt werden konnte. In Voruntersuchungen konnten wir nachweisen, daß vor allem die Cholesterinester von dieser Konzentrationsabnahme des Gesamt-Cholesterins betroffen sind. Für die Veresterung des freien Cholesterins im Blut an den alpha-Lipoproteinen ist das nur in der Leber synthetisierte und in das Blut sezernierte Enzym Lecithin:Cholesterin-Acyl-Transferase (LCAT) verantwortlich. Deshalb sollte ermittelt werden, ob die intra- und postoperative Verminderung der Cholesterinesterkonzentration im Serum Ausdruck einer gestörten Exkretionsfunktion der Leber ist und ob sie nach Operationen an der Leber und bei "postoperativer Leberinsuffizienz" [1] stärker ausgeprägt ist ("Estersturz" [2]).

Methodik

In die *prospektiv* durchgeführte Studie wurden 30 stoffwechselgesunde Patienten aufgenommen, die sich elektiven Laparotomien, meist wegen Tumoren der Leber, des Pankreas oder des Magens (jeweils n = 10), unterziehen lassen mußten. Die näheren klinischen Daten dieser Patienten sind in Tabelle 1 aufgeführt. Ferner wurden in einer retrospektiven Studie 5 Patienten mit klinisch manifester Leberinsuffizienz nach großen leberchirurgischen Eingriffen untersucht: erweiterte Hemihepatektomie wegen Lebertumor [n = 3], Blutstillung und Tamponade nach traumatischer Leberruptur [n = 1], orthotope homologe Lebertransplantation wegen hepatocellulären Carcinoms bei Lebercirrhose [n = 1]. Die Liegezeit dieser Patienten auf der Intensivstation betrug mindestens 20 Tage. Analysiert wurden neben den üblichen Routinelaborparametern die wichtigsten Parameter des Lipidstoffwechsels im Serum (Cholesterin[-ester], Triglyceride, Freie Fettsäuren, Phospholipide). Die Blutentnahmen erfolgten unmittelbar präoperativ, intraoperativ 30 min nach Beginn der Organpräparation, unmittelbar

Chirurgisches Forum 1993
f. experim. u. klinische Forschung
Becker/Beger/Hartel (Hrsg.)

Tabelle 1. Übersicht über die prospektiv erfaßten Patienten nach elektiven Eingriffen am Leber, Magen und Pankreas

Gruppe	Geschlechtsverteilung [m:w]	Alter (Jahre) [x̄]	Liegezeit Intensivstation [x̄]	Diagnosen		Operationsverfahren	
Magen	5 : 5	64,4	0,6 Tage	Magencarcinom	(n = 8)	Gastrektomie [Roux]	(n = 8)
				Magenausgangsstenose	(n = 2)	Billroth II	(n = 2)
Leber	5 : 5	51,9	2,2 Tage	HCC	(n = 3)	Segmentresektionen	(n = 5)
				FNH	(n = 1)	Hemihepatektomie (li.)	(n = 2)
				Haemangiom	(n = 1)	Hemihepatektomie (re.)	(n = 3)
				Filia [Colon]	(n = 5)		
Pankreas	5 : 5	59,8	1,8 Tage	Pankreas-Ca.	(n = 9)	Op. n. Whipple	(n = 6)
				Papillenpolyp	(n = 1)	Linksresektion	(n = 1)
						transduoden.Polypektomie	(n = 1)
						biliodigest. Anastom.	(n = 1)

Tabelle 2. Cholesterin-Esterquotient bei stoffwechselgesunden Patienten nach elektiven Eingriffen an Leber, Magen, Pankreas (jeweils n = 10) und bei Patienten mit postoperativer Leberinsuffizienz (n = 5) [$\bar{x}$, s, $p < 0{,}005$]

	präop.		postop.		1.		2.		3.		4.	
					postoperativer Tag							
Magen-Op	1,82	(0,30)	1,61	(0,46)	1,31	(0,26)	1,24	(0,29)	1,19	(0,16)	1,29	(0,18)
Leber-Op.	2,15	(0,92)	1,47	(0,33)	1,40	(0,36)	1,00	(0,40)	1,04	(0,37)	1,14	(0,36)
Pankreas-Op.	1,42	(0,57)	1,30	(0,43)	1,12	(0,41)	1,07	(0,31)	1,00	(0,32)	1,05	(0,30)
postop. LI.	1,95	(0,66)	1,73	(0,51)	1,17	(0,45)	0,64	(0,39)	0,45	(0,25)	0,29	(0,13)

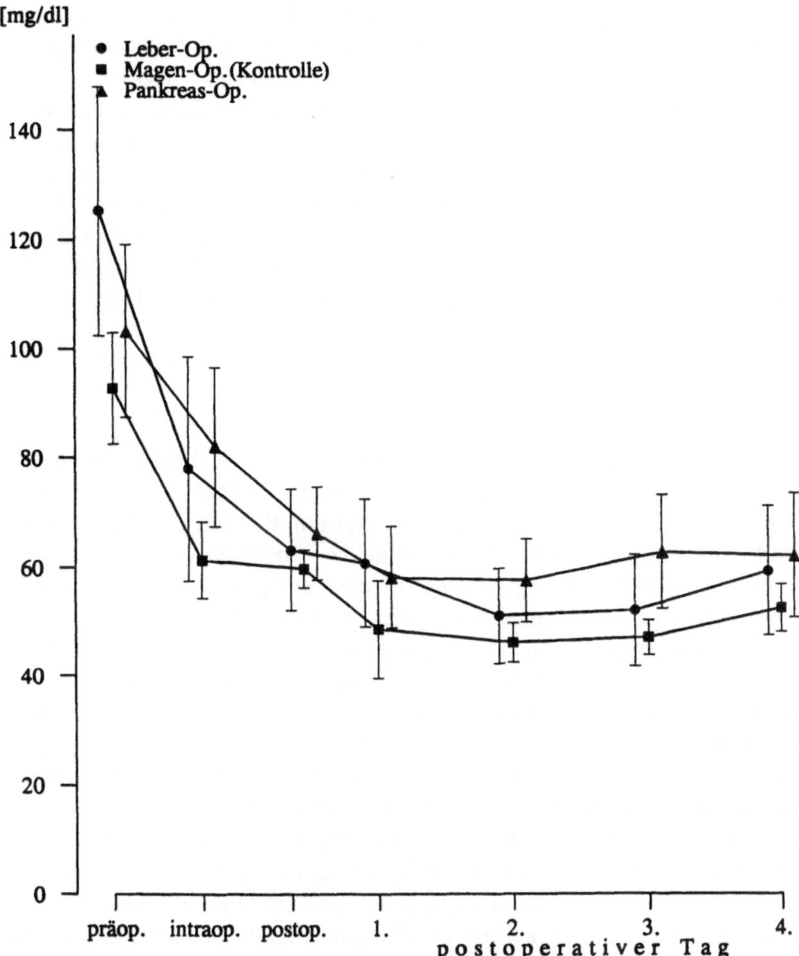

Abb. 1. Der Einfluß von elektiven Operationen an Leber, Pankreas oder Magen (Kontrolle) auf die Konzentration der Cholesterinester (mg/dl) im Serum bei stoffwechselgesunden Patienten [jeweils n = 10, Median, ± Standardfehler]

postoperativ (Hautnaht) und am Morgen des 1.–4. postoperativen Tages jeweils um 6.45 Uhr.

Außerdem wurde bei narkotisierten männlichen Wistar-Ratten (Körpergewicht 300–400 g) ein Leberschaden durch eine zentrale (hilusnahe) Gallengangsliteratur hervorgerufen. Das Ausbluten der narkotisierten Tiere (Pentobarbital 40 mg/kg KG s.c.) erfolgte 3, 6, 12, 24, 48 und 72 h nach Gallengangsliteratur (näheres zur Methodik bei [4]).

Analytik: Die Bestimmung der Konzentration des freien (unveresterten) Cholesterins im Serum erfolgte enzymatisch mittels Cholesterinoxidase und Peroxidase, während für die Gesamt-Cholesterinkonzentration zusätzlich noch Cholesterinesterase verwendet wurde. Die Konzentration der Cholesterinester im Serum wurde rechnerisch durch Subtraktion der Konzentration des freien Cholesterins von der Gesamt-Cholesterinkonzentration errechnet. Außerdem wurde der sog. Cholesterin-Esterquotient (Q_E) berechnet: Q_E = [Cholesterinester] : [freies Cholesterin]. Referenzbereiche dieser Methoden im Serum von stoffwechselgesunden Patienten: Gesamtcholesterin (bis 200 mg/dl), freies Cholesterin (40–70 mg/dl), Cholesterinester (80–130 mg/dl) und Esterquotient (1,5–2,5 [bei Ratten 2,8–3,8]).

Ergebnisse

Intra- und postoperativ ist nach allen Operationen unabhängig vom betroffenen Organsystem und unabhängig vom verwendeten Narkoseverfahren eine Abnahme der Serumkonzentrationen der Cholesterinester um 30–50% des präoperativen Ausgangswertes nachweisbar (Abb. 1), während das Absinken der Konzentration des freien (unveresterten) Cholesterins schwächer ausgeprägt ist. Signifikante Unterschiede zwischen den einzelnen Patientengruppen ergeben sich aber nur, wenn das Verhältnis der Cholesterinester zum freien Cholesterin (sog. Esterquotient Q_E) ermittelt wird (siehe Tabelle 2). Nach Eingriffen am Pankreas und an der Leber ist der Esterquotient postoperativ signifikant niedriger als nach Operationen am Magen (Kontrollgruppe). Bei Patienten mit Leberinsuffizienz (LI) nach ausgedehnten Leberoperationen (n = 5) läßt sich ein "Estersturz" (Tabelle 2) nachweisen, d.h. die Konzentration der Cholesterinester liegt deutlich unter der des freien Cholesterins ($Q_E < 0,5$). Bei diesen Patienten läßt sich eine positive Korrelation (r = 0,73) des Esterquotienten zur Aktivität der Cholinesterase (CHE) im Serum statistisch nachweisen (Abb. 2), aber keine Korrelation zu anderen Parametern der Leberfunktion (Bilirubin, Quick, AT III, Albumin, GLDH, Lactat). Auch nach Gallengangsligatur bei der Ratte ist nach etwa 12 h ein signifikantes Absinken des Cholesterin-Esterquotienten nachweisbar, parallel zum Ansteigen des Serumbilirubinspiegels (Tabelle 3).

Tabelle 3. Der Einfluß einer hilusnahen Gallengangsligatur bei der Wistar-Ratte auf das Verhältnis der Cholesterinester zum freien Cholesterin (Esterquotient) im Serum ($p < 0,01$)

Parameter	Einheit	Stat.	Kontr.	3 h	6 h	12 h	24 h	48 h	72 h
direktes Bilirubin	mg/dl	x	0,12	0,56	1,36	1,34	3,47	5,42	8,12
		s	0,04	0,14	0,53	0,64	0,82	1,23	1,30
Cholesterin-Esterquotient	–	x	3,3	3,7	2,1	1,6	0,9	1,4	1,2
		s	0,3	2,3	0,7	0,4	0,4	0,4	0,3

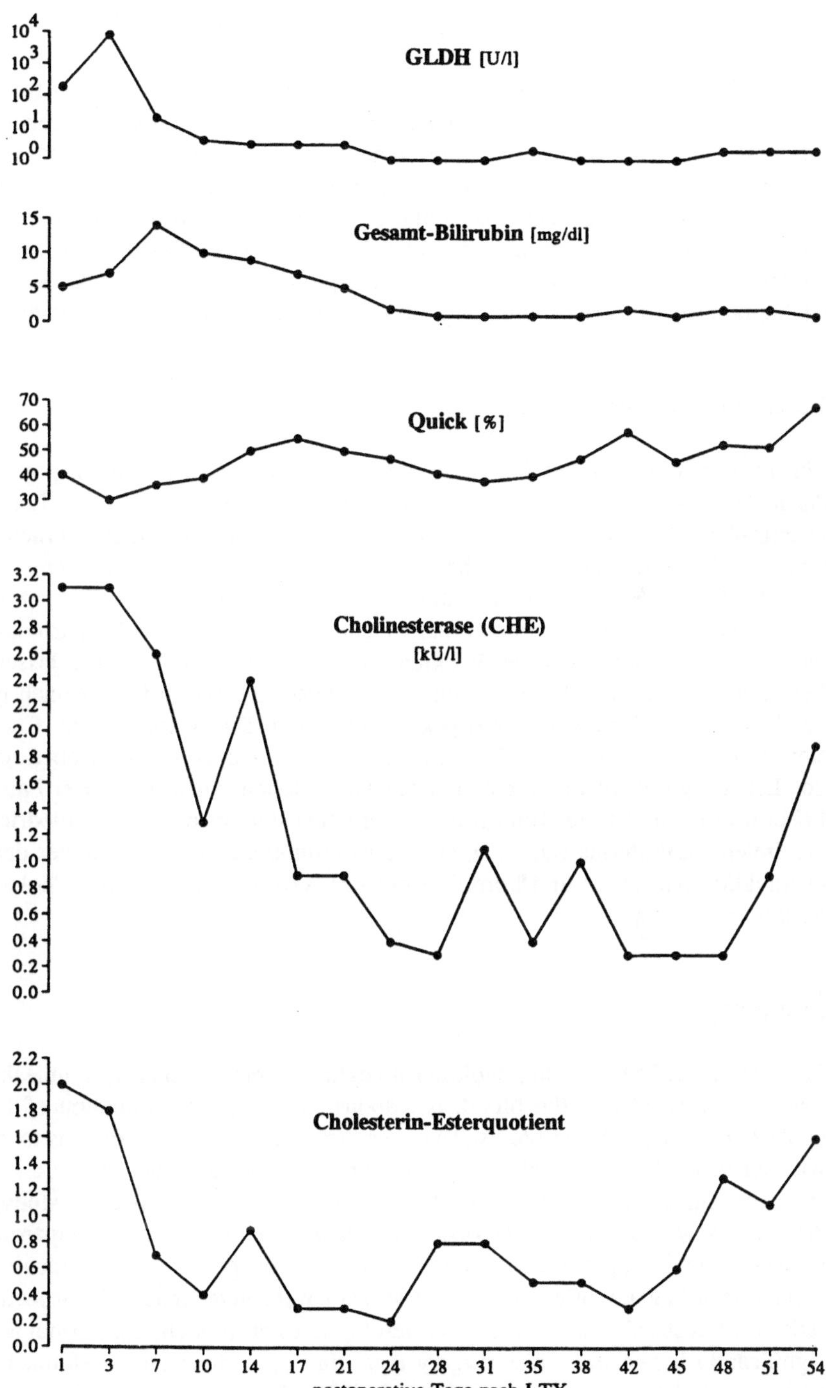

Abb. 2. Verlauf verschiedener Parameter der Leberfunktion bei einem 58jährigen Patienten nach orthotoper homologer Lebertransplantation: Korrelation zwischen dem Verlauf der Aktivität der Cholinesterase im Serum und dem Esterquotienten

Diskussion und Schlußfolgerungen

Das Verhältnis der Serumkonzentrationen der Cholesterinester und des freien Cholesterins (Esterquotient) ist *ein* Parameter der Exkretionsfunktion der Leber und korreliert mit der Aktivität der Cholinesterase im Serum. Da LCAT und CHE beide Sekretionsenzyme der Leber sind, erklärt sich das parallele Verhalten beider Parameter. Ein "Estersturz", d.h ein Absinken des Esterquotienten von normal ca. 2 auf Werte unter 0,5 ist als Symptom einer postoperativen Leberinsuffizienz zu werten. Weitere Untersuchungen müssen klären, ob der Esterquotient als Parameter der Leberfunktion auch eine prognostische Bedeutung bei Patienten mit Leberinsuffizienz hat.

Zusammenfassung

Für die Veresterung des freien Cholesterins im Serum an den alpha-Lipoproteinen ist das in der Leber synthetisierte und in das Blut sezernierte Enzym LCAT (Lecithin:Cholesterin-Acyl-Transferase) verantwortlich. Deshalb sollte ermittelt werden, ob nach Operationen an der Leber oder bei postoperativer Leberinsuffizienz eine Verminderung der Cholesterinesterkonzentration im Serum nachweisbar ist. Prospektiv wurden 30 stoffwechselgesunde Patienten untersucht, die sich elektiven Lasparotomien meist wegen Tumoren der Leber, des Pankreas oder des Magens unterziehen lassen mußten. Ferner wurden 5 Patienten mit klinisch manifester Leberinsuffizienz nach großen leberchirurgischen Eingriffen retrospektiv untersucht. Das Verhältnis der Cholesterinester zum freien Cholesterin (Esterquotient Q_E, normal 2–3) war nach Eingriffen an der Leber signifikant niedriger als nach Operationen am Magen. Bei Patienten mit Leberinsuffizienz ist die Konzentration der Cholesterinester deutlich niedriger als die des freien Cholesterins ($Q_E < 0,5$). Der Esterquotient ist ein Parameter der Exkretionsfunktion der Leber und korreliert mit der Aktivität des Enzyms Cholesterase im Serum.

Summary

The enzyme LCAT (lecithin:cholesterol acyltransferase), which is synthesized in the liver and secreted into the blood, is responsible for the esterification of free serum cholesterol in alpha-lipoproteins. Thus, the aim of the present study was to investigate whether reduced serum cholesterol ester concentrations are registered after surgery of the liver and in postoperative hepatic insufficiency. The prospective study admitted 30 patients with healthy metabolism who had to undergo elective laparotomies for tumors of the liver, pancreas, or stomach. Another five patients with clinically manifest hepatic insufficiency after major liver surgery were investigated retrospectively. The ratio of cholesterol ester to free cholesterol (i.e., ester quotient Q_E normal at 2–3) was significantly lower after liver surgery than after operations on the stomach. In those patients with hepatic insufficiency, the cholesterol ester concentration is substantially lower than that of free cholesterol ($Q_E < 0.5$). The ester quotient is a parameter for the secretory function of the liver and correlates with the activity of the enzyme cholinesterase in the serum.

Literatur

1. Brölsch ChE, Neuhaus P, Ringe B, Sturm J, Pichlmayr R (1985) Postoperative Leberinsuffizienz nach leberchirurgischen Eingriffen. In: Encke A et al. (Hrsg) Chirurgische Intensivmedizin. Urban & Schwarzenberg, München Wien Baltimore, pp 237–244
2. Brunner W (1935) Beitrag zur pankreatogenen Lipämie. Klin Wochenschr 14:1853–1855
3. Georgieff M, Kattermann R, Geiger K, Storz LW, Bethke U, Lutz H (1979) Unterschiede im postoperativen Stoffwechselverhalten bei prä- und postoperativem Beginn der totalen parenteralen Ernährung. Z Ernährungswiss 18:160–183
4. Sachs M, Gurlitt C, Förster H, Encke A (1992) Einfluß der extrahepatischen Cholestase auf den Aminosäurenstoffwechsel im Tierversuch. Z Gastroenterol [Suppl] 4:30
5. Wolfram G, Doenicke A, Zöllner N (1973/74) Die essentiellen Fettsäuren in den Cholesterinestern des Serums vor und in den Tagen nach einer Magenoperation. Infusionstherapie 1:537–540

Dr. med. M. Sachs, Klinik für Allgemeinchirurgie, Klinikum der Johann Wolfgang Goethe-Universität, Theodor-Stern-Kai 7, W-6000 Frankfurt am Main 70

for the secretory function of the liver and correlates with the activity of the enzyme cholinesterase in the serum.

Literatur

1. [illegible] (1981) [illegible] nach [illegible] Eingriffen. In: [illegible] A et al. (Hrsg) Chirurgische [illegible] Urban & Schwarzenberg, München Wien Baltimore, pp 237–244
2. Brunner W (1959) Beitrag zur pathologischen Lipämie. Klin Wochenschr 14: [illegible]
3. [illegible] W, [illegible] (1979) [illegible] bei prä- und postoperativ [illegible] der [illegible] Z [illegible] 78:160–[illegible]
4. [illegible] (1982) Einfluß der [illegible] auf den [illegible] im Tierversuch. Z Gastroenterol (Suppl) 4:50
5. [illegible] (1983) Die extrahepatische [illegible] und Cholesterin [illegible] Infusionstherapie [illegible]

Dr. med. H. [illegible], Klinik für Allgemeinchirurgie, Klinikum der Johann Wolfgang Goethe-Universität, Theodor-Stern-Kai 7, W-6000 Frankfurt am Main 70

Chirurgisches Forum 1994

München, 111. Kongreß, 13.–17. April 1994

Vortragsanmeldungen

Die Sitzungen des FORUMs für experimentelle und klinische Forschung sind ein fester Bestandteil im Gesamtkongreßprogramm. Sie bestehen aus 6-Minuten-Vorträgen mit ausreichender Diskussionszeit über Ergebnisse aus der experimentellen und klinischen Forschung. Zur Beteiligung sind bevorzugt der chirurgische Nachwuchs, aber auch junge Forscher aus anderen medizinischen Fachgebieten zur Pflege interdisziplinärer Kontakte aufgefordert. Verhandlungssprachen sind Deutsch und Englisch.

Als Leitthemen der einzelnen Sitzungen sind vorgesehen: Trauma; Schock; Herz, Lunge und Gefäßsysteme; Transplantation; Onkologie; Magen-Darm; endokrine Chirurgie; Leber-Galle-Pankreas; perioperative Pathophysiologie-Intensivmedizin; Organersatz-Biomechanische Unterstützung; laparoskopische Operationstechniken.

Die Auswahl der Sitzungstitel für das endgültige Programm richtet sich nach dem zahlenmäßigen Überwiegen der eingereichten Beiträge zu den verschiedenen Themenkreisen auf der Basis der Qualitätsbewertung.

Bedingungen für die Anmeldung

1. Für die Anmeldung ist eine Kurzfassung in **sechsfacher Ausfertigung** bis spätestens **30. September** des Vorjahres vor dem Kongreßjahr an den FORUM-Ausschuß der Deutschen Gesellschaft für Chirurgie einzusenden:

   Sekretariat „Chirurgisches FORUM“
   Chirurgische Universitätsklinik
   Steinhövelstraße 9

   D-W 7900 Ulm/Donau

   Bereits veröffentlichte Arbeiten dürfen nicht eingesandt werden!

2. Der Erstautor bestätigt durch seine Unterschrift, daß die gesetzlichen Bestimmungen des Tierschutzes bei tierexperimentellen Untersuchungen eingehalten worden sind.

3. Grundsätzlich ist die Anmeldung mehrerer verschiedener Beiträge möglich. Die Auswahl durch den wissenschaftlichen Beirat orientiert sich dahingehend, daß der Erstautor im endgültigen Programm nur einmal genannt werden kann.

4. Die Anmeldung eines Beitrags zum FORUM schließt die Anmeldung eines Vortrages mit dem gleichen Grundthema für eine andere Kongreßsitzung aus.

Kurzfassung

5. Die Kurzfassung soll in klarer Gliederung ausschließlich objektive Fakten über die Zahl der Untersuchungen oder Experimente, die angewandten Methoden und endgültigen Ergebnisse enthalten. Ausführliche Einleitungen, historische Daten und Literaturübersichten sind zu vermeiden. Nur Mitteilungen von wesentlichem Informationswert ermöglichen eine sachliche Beurteilung durch die Mitglieder des wissenschaftlichen Beirates.

6. Auf dem Formblatt (Beilage in den MITTEILUNGEN, ansonsten über die Deutsche Gesellschaft für Chirurgie oder Sekretariat „Chirurgisches FORUM") sind die Namen der Autoren, beginnend mit dem Vortragenden, mit akademischem Grad sowie Anschrift der Klinik oder Institut und der Arbeitstitel einzutragen.

7. Da sich die Deutsche Gesellschaft für Chirurgie einer „Empfehlung über die Begrenzung der Autorenzahl" angeschlossen hat (siehe MITTEILUNGEN Heft 4/1975, Seite 140), können einschließlich des Vortragenden nur 4 Autoren genannt werden. Lediglich bei interdisziplinären Arbeiten sind insgesamt 6 Autorennamen möglich.

8. Dem Text der Kurzfassung wird nur der Arbeitstitel ohne Autorennamen vorangestellt, damit eine anonyme Weiterbearbeitung gesichert ist (siehe 9). Der Umfang darf das angegebene Feld nicht überschreiten. Die Einsendung hat per Einschreiben zu erfolgen. Die eigene Klinik (Institut) darf im Text nicht erwähnt oder zitiert werden.

9. Jeder Beitrag soll von dem Autor durch einen Vermerk für eines der oben angegebenen Leitthemen vorgeschlagen werden.

Anonyme Bearbeitung

10. Vor der Sitzung des FORUM-Ausschusses werden die Beiträge anonym (ohne Nennung der Autoren und der Herkunft) zur Beurteilung an die Mitglieder des wissenschaftlichen Beirats versandt. (Bestimmungen für den FORUM-Ausschuß, siehe MITTEILUNGEN Heft 5/1990, Seite 24).

11. Die Autoren der angenommenen Beiträge werden bis Mitte November des Vorjahres vor dem Kongreß verständigt.

Manuskript

12. Das Manuskript ist in **doppelter Ausfertigung mit folgender Gliederung** (deutscher und englischer Titel, sämtliche Autoren, beteiligte Institutionen, Einleitung, Methodik, Ergebnisse, Zusammenfassung auf Deutsch und Englisch, Literaturangaben, vollständige Korrespondenzadresse des Autors) einzureichen.

    Es werden auch Disketten angenommen. Senden Sie bitte 5¼" Disketten mit reinem Textfile (ASCI) ohne Befehl. Ein identischer Ausdruck ist ebenfalls mitzusenden.

Wenn **keine Bilder oder Tabellen** eingereicht werden, darf das gesamte Manuskript **maximal 5 Schreibmaschinenseiten** (bei 4 cm Rand allseitig, maximal 35 Zeilen pro Seite bei 1½-zeiligem Abstand) umfassen.

Jede Schwarzweiß-Abbildung (schematische Strichabbildung) oder Tabelle verkürzt den zulässigen Schreibmaschinentext mindestens um ½ Textseite. Es werden Positivabzüge (tiefschwarz) in Endgröße erbeten. Abbildungen und Tabellen sind arabisch zu numerieren, die Abbildungen sind mit einer Überschrift zu versehen. Für jede Abbildung oder Tabelle ist eine prägnante Legende auf besonderem Blatt erforderlich, dabei müssen die Autoren darauf achten, daß sämtliche in den Abbildungen oder Tabellen vorkommenden Abkürzungen in der Legende erklärt werden. Halbtonbilder oder Röntgenbilder werden nicht angenommen. Strichabbildungen, die mit einem PC erstellt werden, müssen über Laserdrucker ausgegeben werden (kein Nadeldrucker).

Das Literaturverzeichnis darf 5 Zitate nicht überschreiten. Es sind 1. sämtliche Autorennamen mit den Initialen der Vornamen (grundsätzlich nachgestellt); 2. Jahreszahl in Klammern; 3. vollständiger Titel der zitierten Arbeit; abgekürzter Titel der Zeitschrift nach Index medicus; 5. Bandzahl (arabische Ziffer); 6. Anfang- und Endseitenzahl der Arbeit anzugeben; z. B.:

Sawasti P, Watanabe M, Weronawati T (1979) Gallensteine in Asien. Chirurg 50: 57 – 64.

Bei Büchern sollten 1. sämtliche Autorennamen mit den Initialen der Vornamen (grundsätzlich nachgestellt) und 2. Titel des Kapitels; 3. Erscheinungsjahr; 4. vollständiger nicht abgekürzter Buchtitel; 5. Namen der Herausgeber (Initialen des Vornamens nach den Herausgebernamen gestellt); 6. Verlag; 7. Verlagsort; 8. Anfangs- und Endseitenzahl des zitierten Kapitels; z. B.:

Enke A, Hanisch E (1990) Management inklusive intensivmedizinischer Überwachung und Therapie bei gastrointestinaler Blutung. In: Häring R (Hrsg) Gastrointestinale Blutung. Blackwell Überreuter, Berlin, S. 39 – 43.

13. Die redaktionellen Vorschriften sind sorgfältig zu beachten. Gelegentlich trotzdem erforderlich werdende redaktionelle Änderungen im Rahmen der gegebenen Vorschriften behält sich die Schriftleitung vor.

14. Das Manuskript wird in einem zitierfähigen FORUM-Band als Supplement von Langenbecks Archiv vor dem nächsten Kongreß gedruckt vorliegen.

Einsendeschluß

15. Manuskripte, die bis zum **31.12.1993** nicht eingegangen sind, können im FORUM-Band nicht berücksichtigt werden und **schließen eine Aufnahme in das endgültige Kongreßprogramm aus.**

16. Lieferung von Sonderdrucken nur bei sofortiger Bestellung nach Aufforderung durch den Verlag und gegen Berechnung.

Wissenschaftlicher Beirat im FORUM-Ausschuß der Deutschen Gesellschaft für Chirurgie

H.G. Beger, Ulm	M. Büchler, Ulm
Vorsitzender des Beirats	Für das FORUM-Sekretariat